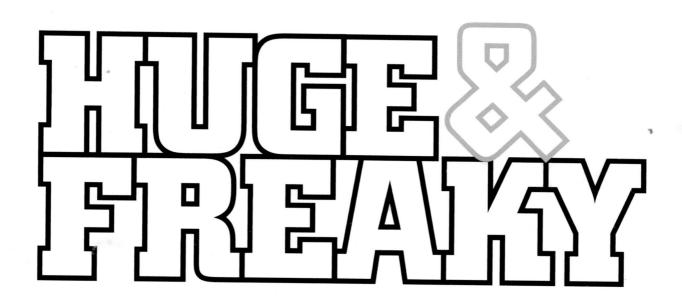

HUGE & FREAKY

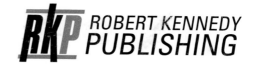

RKP ROBERT KENNEDY
PUBLISHING

Published by Robert Kennedy Publishing
400 Matheson Boulevard West
Mississauga, ON
L5R 3M1 Canada
Visit us at www.emusclemag.com or www.rkpubs.com

Art Directors: Jason Branidis and Darrell Leighton
Managing Senior Production Editor: Wendy Morley
Copy Editor: James De Medeiros
Cover Photos: Robert Reiff
Cover Model: Joel Stubbs

Library and Archives Canada Cataloguing in Publication

Weis, Dennis B., 1945-

Huge & freaky : muscle mass and strength secrets : build a body

fortress naturally / by Dennis B. Weis and Robert Kennedy.

Includes index.

ISBN 978-1-55210-083-7

1. Bodybuilding--Training. 2. Weight training. 3. Muscle strength.

I. Kennedy, Robert, 1938- II. Title. III. Title: Huge & freaky.

IV. Title: Musclemag presents Huge & freaky.

GV546.5.W484 2010   613.7'13   C2010-903402-3

10 9 8 7 6 5 4 3 2 1

Distributed in Canada by NBN (National Book Network)
67 Mowat Avenue, Suite 241
Toronto, ON
M6K 3E3

Distributed in USA by NBN (National Book Network)
15200 NBN Way
Blue Ridge Summit, PA
17214
Printed in Canada.

Build a Body Fortress Naturally

HUGE & FREAKY

MUSCLE MASS AND STRENGTH SECRETS

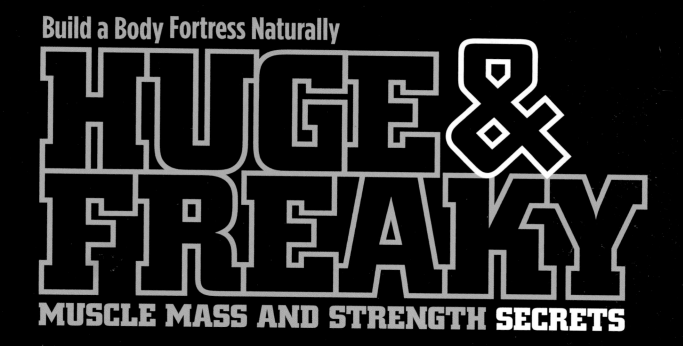

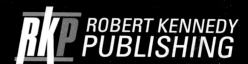

ROBERT KENNEDY
PUBLISHING

TABLE OF CONTENTS

TABLE OF CONTENTS

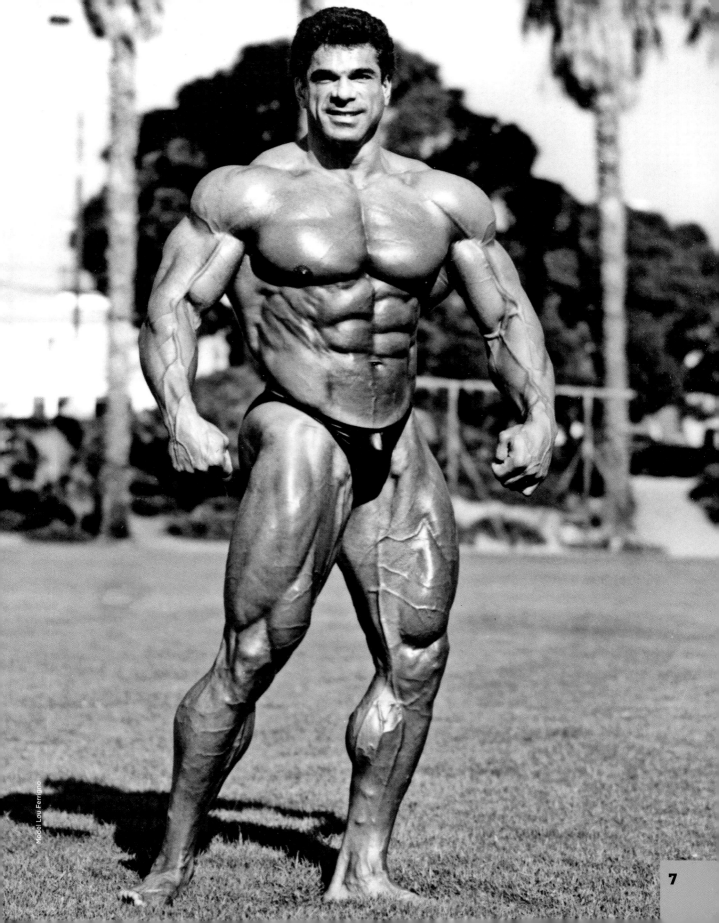

Model Lou Ferrigno

7

FOREWORD

Catch the bodybuilding wave for huge and freaky muscle mass and strength.

Try the "flick test" with this book. You know, flick the pages, check out the photos and get an instant sense of the enormous amount of standout strategies for bodybuilders within these pages. Don't read any more of this foreword. The next paragraphs won't run away; this section will be here when you return. Indulge, enjoy. Go ahead, flick the pages ...

See what we mean? This book is a gem. If you are one of the 36.2 million North Americans training with weights to improve your fitness, strength and physique, *Huge & Freaky Muscle Mass and Strength* is for you. Using the information in this resource, you'll be well on your way to maximizing your potential for building mass and strength.

If you adopt and incorporate our advice, your bodybuilding efforts will also take on extra meaning. You will reach a new level of development. You will enjoy better progress. You will have more productive workouts. You will grow muscle like never before.

For the advanced bodybuilder, *Huge & Freaky Muscle Mass and Strength* reveals priceless nuggets of behind-closed-doors information on every page. This isn't your unrealistic bodybuilding book filled with empty promises. By combining 100-percent muscle talk with a bounty of photos of the stars you've come to admire, we've created a manual that offers a veritable wealth of up-to-date, exciting, exclusive training secrets for stimulating untapped muscle-fiber development and strength.

This book starts where others have left off. We have a deep-rooted interested in getting to the very soul of bodybuilding knowledge. Be warned, however: *Huge & Freaky Muscle Mass and Strength* is an advanced book. It is not geared toward the beginner (zero to six months of actual training) and isn't even appropriate for lukewarm intermediates (seven months to one-and-a-half years of dedicated training). It is specifically designed for the advanced bodybuilder who has performed serious training for longer than a year and a half. We therefore assume that you are already familiar with the bodybuilding basics.

The late Vince Gironda once said, "There are more gyms, books, magazines and training courses about bodybuilding than ever before. Hardly a day goes by when we don't see a new 'progressive-resistance' apparatus being released on the market, yet people are still in the dark about this sport. They crave one element over everything else: Bodybuilding know-how in the form of good information."

Huge & Freaky Muscle Mass and Strength is founded on a wealth of credible, clear and concise advanced-level information for achieving unsurpassed gains in muscle mass and strength. Use this book to infuse your personal bodybuilding adventure with new-found enthusiasm. If you have the willpower to make improvements, we will show you the way! Now, at last, you are in a position to force-feed your muscles to titanic new dimensions.

We have put an incredible amount of time and effort into the production of *Huge & Freaky Muscle Mass and Strength*. This book is not based on mere theory – its contents have been arrived at through many years of empirical discovery, extensive research and data collection. Within the pages, we broach subjects such as super muscle and strength specialization, 28-red-line intensity-manipulation techniques for muscle building, and 100-plus cherry bomb exercise tips, topics that have hardly merited mention in other bodybuilding books. *Huge & Freaky Muscle Mass and Strength* has even focused an entire chapter on the master plan of phase training; we take you through every phase, step by step.

You'll also find a section expressly detailing the 12-week weight-gaining blitz cycle and a strategy for busting through training plateaus. A special exercise selection chart will help you choose exactly the right movements for your muscle-building needs, and the instruction doesn't end there, as we've also outlined a complete one-day upper-arm blitz program. We offer extensive advice on developing abdominals that really show, even when you're adding unsurpassed huge and freaky muscle mass.

As an advanced bodybuilder, you've already put some beef on your frame. Now let's take your progress even further – let's make your next workout a first step toward mastering total muscle success and confidence. Muscle building is a way of life; it's your life. We know it. You know it. Let this book be your go-to source for the most effective methods to increase muscle mass and strength. We are with you every step along your journey.

With the willpower to succeed, you can take your bodybuilding efforts to the next level of progress and muscular development.

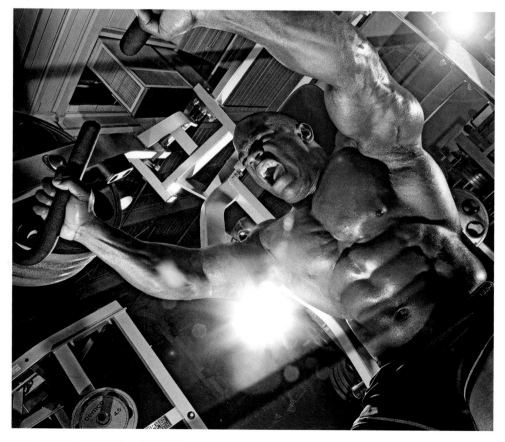

Photo by Paul Buceta
Model Johnnie Jackson

INTRODUCTION

Step into the world of huge and freaky muscle mass and strength!

Of all the letters and e-mails we have received during our 30-plus years of writing bodybuilding books, at least 75 percent are from people who want to add a large amount of quality muscle mass and considerably improve their strength levels.

Many individuals begin training because they are unsatisfied with their bodies and want to achieve the "ideal" physique. Our years of active involvement in the iron game have taught us that bodybuilders are perpetually searching for greater muscle size, regardless of their body type. Most bodybuilders also reach a point in their training when they feel their strength would increase substantially if they could just add a few pounds of muscular bodyweight.

A number of factors affect a person's ability to gain muscle mass, including genetics, nutrition and body type along with training frequency, approach and intensity. While the basic concepts are straightforward, packing on muscle has become a deep science complicated by sophisticated advertisements, research findings and articles about metabolic programming. The average bodybuilder who desperately wants to attain more solid mass and make remarkable strength increases shouldn't be afraid to face the challenges of muscle building. The "science of bodybuilding" may seem overwhelming, but gaining quality muscle weight doesn't have to be difficult – the process can still be simple, quick and effective.

We have designed an innovative but proven basic multi-phase program that will accelerate your muscular weight gains and dramatically increase your present strength level. Here's a very brief overview of the six main parts of the plan:

1. Three total-body primary and secondary muscle-gain workouts performed on non-consecutive days.
2. Basic core-growth exercises such as the barbell back squat, bench press, deadlift, bent-over row, upright row, parallel bar dip and barbell curl. This program does not include any isolation "shaping" exercises such as the dumbbell concentration curl, flye, lateral raise and kickback.
3. Three or four sets of six to eight reps (high reps are counterproductive, except when training abs and calves, for which you should do 15 to 40 reps) for each exercise in the primary workout and one set of varying rep schemes in the secondary workout.
4. Longer rest periods between sets (four to six minutes in some exercises) and on non-scheduled workout days.
5. Gradual consumption of 1,000 to 1,500 calories more than your daily basal metabolic and activity exertion requirements. This ex-

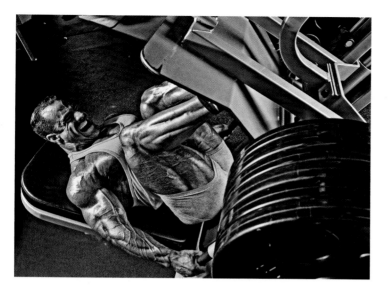

Challenging your body with specific exercises and techniques is a crucial part of strength and mass building.

Photo by Ralph DeHaan
Model Mark Dugdale

tra amount will be taken in through five or six calorie-dense whole-food meals or muscle-mass shakes over the course of a day, each spaced 2.5 to 3 hours apart.

6. Gains in muscle mass should be no less than 0.5 pounds and no more than 2 to 2.5 pounds a week.

The plan will stimulate muscle growth and strength developments without overtaxing your recovery ability; the program is challenging but not unrealistic. Before beginning our discussion of each phase, we have a few important points to note about the human body. A healthy individual maintains an average bodyweight by taking in a certain number of calories per day. If you continue consuming that same number of calories but reduce your daily physical activity level, you will gradually become heavier. If you increase your daily caloric intake but maintain your daily physical activities, you will also gain weight. The process seems basic enough, so why do certain bodybuilders fail to add the muscle mass and strength they desire as readily as others? Because though they are training hard, they are not eating enough or not getting the proper nutrients to promote growth.

Understanding the process of metabolism and knowing how your system functions are key components of successful muscle growth.

Some trainers have metabolic systems that interfere with the proper absorption and use of food (nutrients) to facilitate muscular gains. Other bodybuilders have body chemistries naturally more prone to developing specific deficiencies in vital muscle-building minerals, vitamins and/or enzymes.

Nutrition is another critical aspect when you are working to improve your physique. If you overlook the importance of your meal plans and do not consume the vitamins and natural elements needed to support growth, instead merely shoveling in "empty calories," you will never add healthy weight, no matter how hard you train. Digestive difficulties can also disrupt your efforts to build muscle, as certain conditions prevent food from being fully utilized before it gets passed from the body as waste. With a proper diagnosis, however, most individuals with digestive problems respond well to regular exercise with heavy weights, modified diets based on food tolerances and the use of natural supplements.

In designing this program, we have talked to, studied and observed many of the world's elite bodybuilders, powerlifters and strongmen to learn the techniques they use to achieve superior physiques. These champions agree that success in building Herculean muscle mass and strength is based on these six phases:

1. *Huge & Freaky Muscle Mass and Strength* Workout Plan
2. Powerful nutrition and supplementation tactics and strategies
3. Proper sleep and recovery
4. Genetic potential, motivation and realistic goal-setting
5. Mind-power doctrine of an iron warrior
6. Sufficient physical and mechanical restorative modalities

Bodybuilding has become a complex science that is continually growing with new research on training, physiology, nutrition, supplements and psychology. Though we realize the proposed six-phase muscle-gain and strength program may seem simplistic, this plan will work for you, if you stay highly motivated and 100-percent disciplined.

ABOUT THE AUTHORS

Dennis B. Weis is a Ketchikan, Alaska-based power bodybuilder. He is a hard-hitting, uncompromising professional freelance writer and investigative research consultant in the fields of bodybuilding, nutrition, physiology and powerlifting.

Dennis was first published over three decades ago (1976) in the pages of *Iron Man* magazine. Since that time, he has become known to the vast majority of those who read mainstream bodybuilding and physique magazines throughout the United States, Canada and Europe. His works have appeared in such magazines as *Bodybuilding Monthly* (U.K. publication), *Exercise For Men Only, Hardgainer* (Cyprus publication), *Iron Man, Muscle & Fitness, MuscleMag International, Natural Bodybuilding & Fitness* and *Reps!*

The credentials of this prolific writer extend beyond the scope of article writing – he is also the co-author of three critically acclaimed bestselling books: *Mass!* (1986), *Raw Muscle* (1989) and *Anabolic Muscle Mass: The Secrets of Anabolic Reinforcement Without Steroids* (1995). His most recent work, The Bodybuilding Brain Stack CD – 19 Master Data eReports, is fast becoming a bestseller on Internet bodybuilding sites.

In recognition of his writing accomplishments, he has received Meritorious Service Awards for published works as a magazine consultant and published book author. He has been a guest on numerous radio talk shows around the country, sharing his knowledge and experience.

During the past three decades, Dennis has established a small but dynamic one-man business servicing male and female bodybuilders and powerlifting enthusiasts of all types. Using his expertise, he offers very personal (one-to-one or

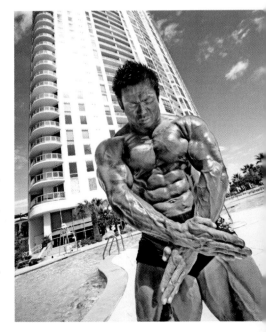

mail order) and highly professional instruction on all phases of physical excellence.

Dennis is modest about his own accomplishments in the iron game, but his lifetime lifts are noteworthy and inspirational.

DENNIS B. WEIS' PERSONAL FEATS OF STRENGTH

- Bench press: 325 pounds; conventional deadlift: 650 pounds; squat: 530 pounds;
- Barbell deadlift (behind-the-back): One rep – 595 pounds
- High-bar full squat: 75 consecutive reps – 300 pounds (at the time, this was an unofficial world record); 27 reps – 405 pounds; and, 15 reps – 450 pounds, all performed at a bodyweight of 207 pounds
- Barbell front squat: 15 reps – 355 pounds
- Quarter squat (in a power rack): 4–6 sets/20 reps – 1,000 pounds
- Vertical leg press: 4–6 sets/20 reps – 800 pounds
- Two-handed barbell straight-arm pullover: 20 consecutive reps – 140 pounds; one-rep – 190 pounds (a mere 20 pounds short of the listed world record at the time)
- Barbell overhead press: Three strict reps – 225 pounds
- Barbell overhead push press: One rep – 270 pounds
- Barbell clean from "hang:" 3–4 sets/10 reps – 225 pounds
- Vertical dip on parallel bars: 3–4 sets/6 reps – 150 pounds
- Strict two-handed barbell curl: Three reps – 185 pounds
- Cheat two-handed barbell curl: 10 consecutive reps – 250 pounds
- Preacher bench barbell curl: 40 reps – 125 pounds; one rep – 185 pounds
- Preacher bench reverse barbell curl: 100 consecutive reps – 100 pounds
- Bodyweight-only push-up: 150 reps
- Pull-ups: 10 sets/10 reps – 100 pounds
- Bodyweight-only pull-ups: 27 reps

Dennis achieved many of these feats of strength and muscular endurance at a bodyweight of 215 pounds and standing 6'1½", with a 48.5-inch chest (normal), 18.25-inch upper arms (contracted) and 17.5-inch calves.

These personal-best lifetime achievements of strength and impressive muscle group measurements didn't happen by chance; Dennis boasts more than 45 years of experience as a power bodybuilder.

Web site: www.dennisbweis.com
E-mail: yukonherc@kpunet.net

ROBERT KENNEDY

Robert Kennedy is the president of RK Publishing, a company with a strong focus on health, fitness, nutrition and lifestyle titles, the most successful of which is Tosca Reno's *Eat-Clean Diet* series. Robert is also well known in the realm of bodybuilding as the publisher of *MuscleMag International*, a monthly magazine for male and female bodybuilders that he established in 1974. He is also publisher of *Clean Eating, Reps!, Maximum Fitness, Oxygen* and *American Curves.*

Like co-author Dennis B. Weis, Robert has trained for many years and has successfully competed in both weightlifting and bodybuilding contests. He was born in Europe in 1938 and emigrated from the U.K. to Canada at the age of 30.

Robert has written dozens of books about bodybuilding, including bestsellers *Hardcore Bodybuilding* (1982), *Beef It!: Upping the Muscle Mass* (1983), *Pumping Up!* (1985) (co-authored with Ben Weider), *1,001 Musclebuilding Tips* (2007) and his most recent, *Encyclopedia of Bodybuilding: The Complete A–Z Guide on Muscle Building* (2008). Robert also pursued formal education and training as an artist, specializing in oil painting and stone carving, and to this day he keeps up with both. He has hosted art exhibitions in London, England; Salzburg, Austria; and, Toronto, Ontario. He uses his late father's name for his artwork – visit www.wolfgangkals.com for more information about his work in the art world.

His avid interest in and enthusiasm for bodybuilding, a sport he still practices, has made Robert one of the most knowledgeable and respected people in this field.

DISCLAIMER

The information contained in *Huge & Freaky Muscle Mass and Strength Secrets* is provided for the reader's use as a guide for achieving superior muscle mass and strength. No information herein should be construed as medical advice, and the exercises, high-intensity workouts, restorative modalities and nutritional systems of body care information covered in this book should not be taken as a substitute for professional medical advice. Not all of the workouts and practices in this report are suitable for everyone.

The reader should consult a licensed primary care physician before attempting the types of workouts and practices recommended herein. Weight training poses a significant risk of injury, and the reader should take due care to use proper equipment and exercise in a safe training environment.

All recommendations contained in this book are made without guarantee on the part of the author and/or publisher who, as a result, disclaim any and all liability in connection to use of this information.

ACKNOWLEDGMENTS

Dennis B. Weis would like to thank these wonderful people for their assistance with the book project.

TRANSCRIBERS:
Elizabeth "Eli" (Weis) Brown, Dennis' daughter; Tristan Weis, aka "Roo," Dennis' grandson

MUSCLE-TRAINING RESEARCH JOURNALISTS:
Dan Gallapoo
Nick Nilsson
Alan Palmieri
Greg Sushinsky
Denie Walter
Billy G. Weis (Tristan's Dad)

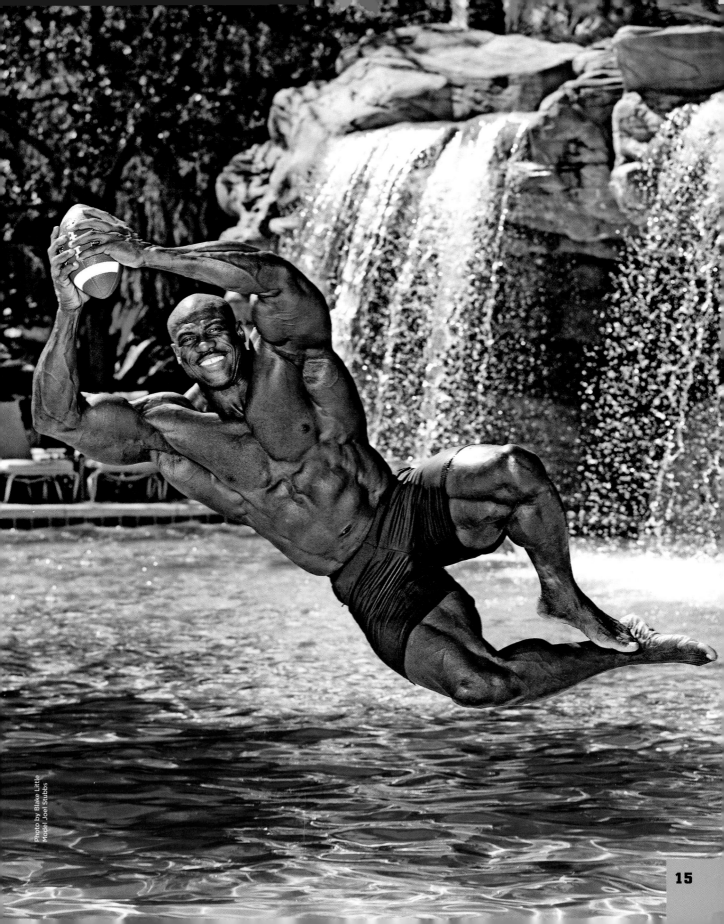

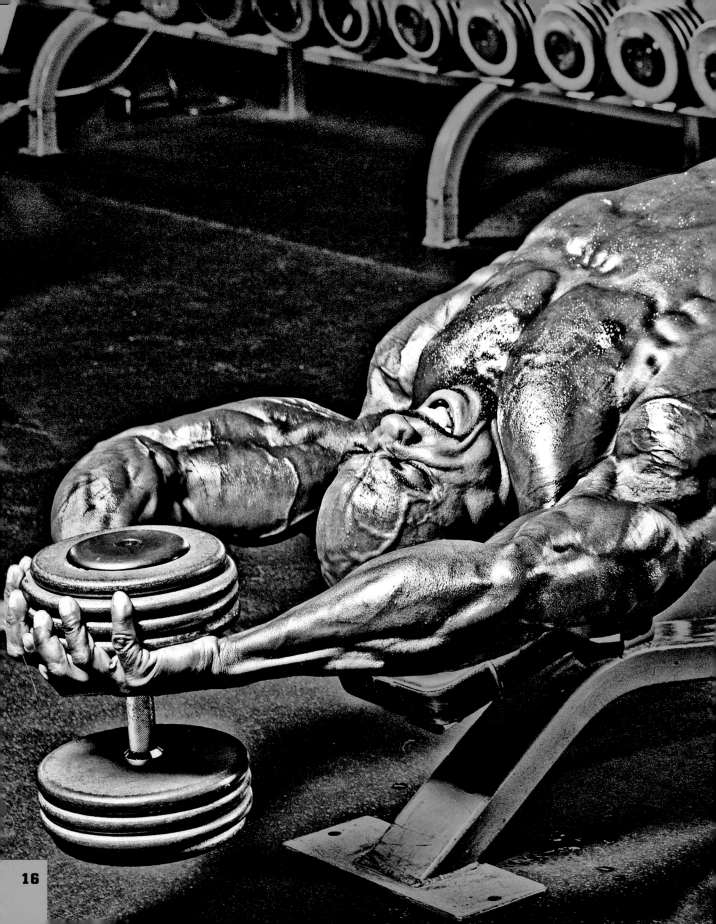

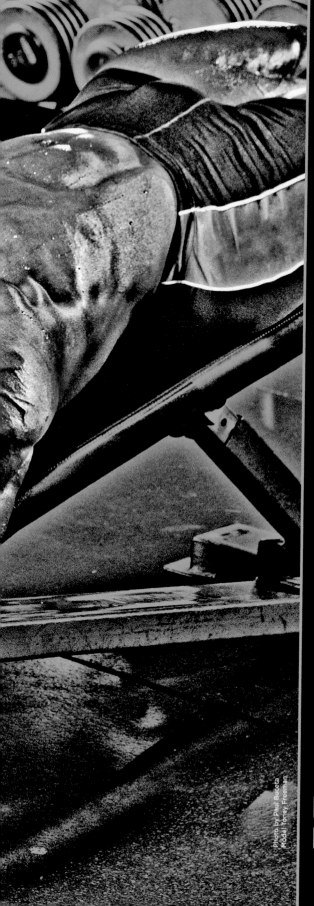

BOOK 01

Phase 1: Huge & Freaky Muscle Mass and Strength Program

CHAPTER 1

PHASE 1: HUGE & FREAKY MUSCLE MASS AND STRENGTH WORKOUT PLAN

You have the potential to add 40 to 50 pounds of muscle mass to your body and make increases in over-all strength by 400 percent.

Our research in gyms throughout the U.S. and abroad has shown that many individuals don't first build a solid foundation to prime their physiques for successful long-term muscle gains. Most bodybuilders just choose a particular routine, figure out a split that works for them and follow the program week after week. Then, when progress slows, they focus on trying to increase their muscle-gain factor by adding more sets and reps to their present regimen, and in some extreme cases, up their training frequency. A lot of guys never branch out from their basic concepts or approaches to training.

A few genetically fortunate individuals will achieve muscular gains with this type of strategy. More often, however, trainers hit a plateau with their workouts, fail to solve the problem, try something else, get frustrated and end up taking a layoff from the gym. But one of the simplest ways to jump-start muscle gains is by simply returning to the old-fashioned, basic programs – workouts that include a few exercises to work large groups of muscles rather than the detail moves to target smaller muscle groups.

Using a simplified training schedule two or three times a week, getting plenty of rest and recuperation along with following a proper nutrition and supplementation plan is often all that is necessary to overcome a sticking point. After six to twelve weeks using a fundamental program, the power bodybuilder usually kick-starts his or her progress and can return to regular training schedules with renewed success.

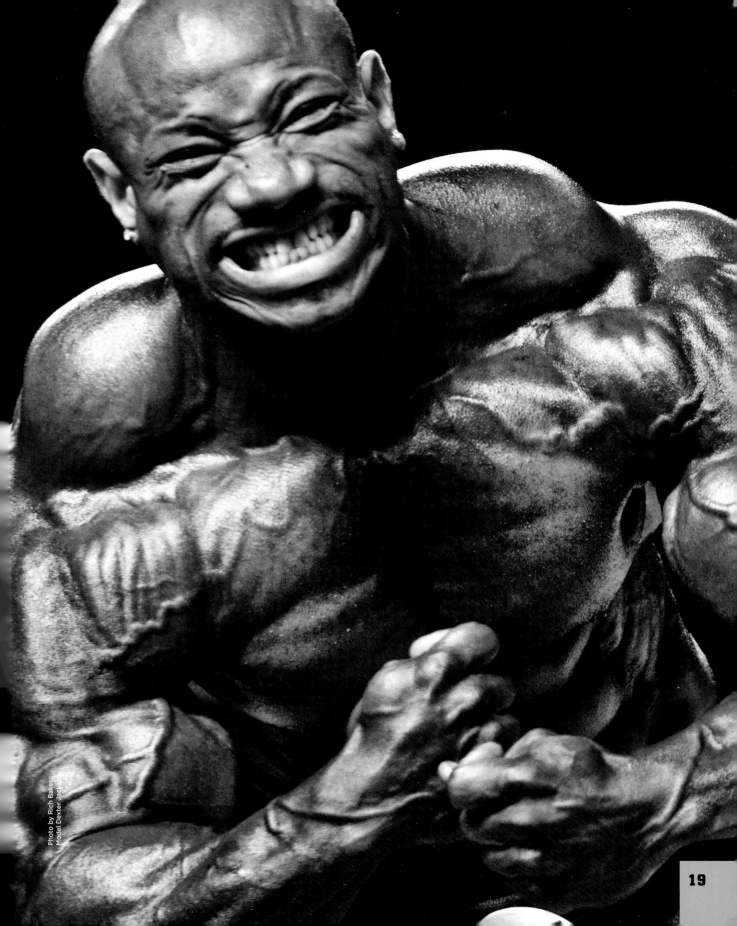

19

We recognize that bodybuilding is an important part of your life, but we also realize you likely have many responsibilities that may affect your ability or freedom to train as much as you'd like. Over the course of your training career, chances are you will at some point have to sacrifice some of your workout time to focus on other pursuits.

Getting off-track from your training schedule can happen for many reasons: Family obligations, long work hours, shift work, school commitments and responsibilities at home, just to name a few. When time is in short supply, many bodybuilders shorten their workouts, and this change can have a negative impact, depending on how they train. Less time for a gym session makes certain full-length muscle fiber-alerting routines (i.e., multiple exercises and sets per muscle group) impossible to complete. That being said, a lack of training time should never become an excuse for procrastinating or missing workouts completely.

While his training wasn't always orthodox, Arnold recognized the importance of time spent in the gym.

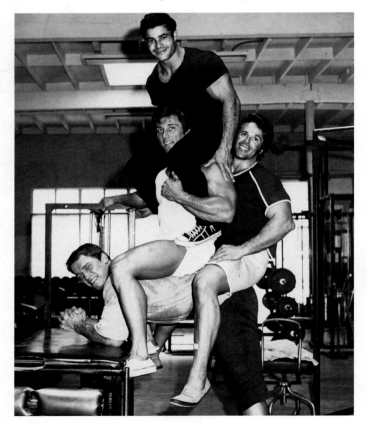

The best solution when you're strapped for time is to devise a 70-minute workout plan. During the first 20 minutes of an intense workout, natural resting blood testosterone and glucose levels rise dramatically. They peak at approximately 20 minutes and remain steady through the middle portion of the session. The levels then decrease from about the 55- to 70-minute marks. These amounts are still slightly elevated at the end of the workout, as the window for testosterone and glucose to return to their original resting levels is at least two hours post-workout. (See Appendix 1a for a detailed graph of testosterone levels over the course of an intense 70-minute session.)

By limiting your workout to approximately 70 minutes, you will maintain a positive nitrogen balance in your body. This bodily state encourages a high level muscle-tissue activation and strength-gain factor, even if you are a hardgainer or someone who has a tendency to overtrain and not allow enough time for recovery. One of the best ways to achieve the positive nitrogen balance is by employing the Total-Body Blast Workout.

THE TOTAL-BODY BLAST WORKOUT

The exercise plan is set up on a 45- to 90-day schedule in which you do an eight-point total-body blast (including thighs, calves, chest, back, deltoids, biceps, triceps and abdominals). You'll follow a one-day-on/one-day-off split (except for weekends, when you'll rest Saturday and Sunday) using a modified version of the popular push/pull system. The following chart reveals how this will be accomplished:

TOTAL-BODY BLAST TRAINING SPLIT	
Monday	Schedule A
Tuesday	Off
Wednesday	Schedule B
Thursday	Off
Friday	Schedule C
Saturday	Off
Sunday	Off
All workouts should last a total of 70 minutes.	

Models (top to bottom) Franco Columbu, Frank Zane, Peter Caputo and Arnold Schwarzenegger

HUGE & FREAKY MUSCLE MASS AND STRENGTH MODIFIED PUSH/PULL SYSTEM CHART

SCHEDULE A PRIMARY WORKOUT

BODYPARTS TRAINED	EXERCISES
Thighs	Barbell Back Squat
Calves	Standing Calf Raise
Abs	Crunch

ECONO-TIME SECONDARY WORKOUT

BODYPARTS TRAINED	EXERCISES
Back	Bodyweight-Only Pull-Up
Chest	Incline Barbell Bench Press
Delts	Barbell Upright Row
Triceps	Parallel Bar Dip
Biceps	Barbell Curl

SCHEDULE B PRIMARY WORKOUT

BODYPARTS TRAINED	EXERCISES
Chest	Flat Barbell Bench Press
Delts	Barbell Upright Row
Triceps	Parallel Bar Dip

ECONO-TIME SECONDARY WORKOUT

BODYPARTS TRAINED	EXERCISES
Thighs	Leg Press
Calves	Machine Calf Raise
Back	Hyperextension (prone)
Biceps	Dumbbell Curl (standing)
Abs	Reverse Ab Crunch

SCHEDULE C PRIMARY WORKOUT

BODYPARTS TRAINED	EXERCISES
Back	Deadlift Bent-Over Row
Biceps	Barbell Curl

ECONO-TIME SECONDARY WORKOUT

BODYPARTS TRAINED	EXERCISES
Thighs	Hack Squat
Calves	Donkey Calf Raise
Chest	Incline Dumbbell Press
Delts	Barbell Overhead Press
Triceps	EZ-Bar Triceps Extension (lying)
Abs	Seated Knee Pull-In

The plan includes nine primary "Core Growth" exercises, seven of which (1, 4–9) will stimulate enhanced neuromuscular activation to facilitate muscle gains and strength enhancements. These seven are also top movements for triggering an anabolic hormone response to help you add quality mass in a short amount of time.

CORE GROWTH EXERCISES

1. Barbell back squat
2. Standing calf raise
3. Crunch
4. Barbell bench press
5. Barbell upright row
6. Parallel bar dip
7. Deadlift
8. Bent-over row
9. Barbell curl

Once you turn on the anabolic switch with this program, giving your body adequate recovery time (for both the central nervous system and muscles at cellular level) becomes vital. The split is set up with a minimum of one rest day between select workouts and the exercises within each routine.

Primary workout exercises listed for calves and abs (standing calf raise and crunch) are structured into schedule "A," not to stimulate anabolic hormones, but to improve your muscular body mass proportions. For example, adding muscle mass to your pecs is worthless if your waist expands at the same rate because of a lack of ab training. Timely and proper ab training, combined with eating smaller meals and having a well-rounded nutrition plan will also keep your waistline in check. (For a detailed discussion, see Phase 2 – Powerful Nutrition and Supplement Tactics.)

The primary "Core Growth" exercises should be performed in the order listed within your split (A, B, C). The movements have been arranged in such a way that the muscle groups are worked in order of their relative size from largest to smallest. For example, in schedule "A" the thighs are targeted first with the barbell back squat followed by calf work with the machine calf raise. Regardless of what specific

training schedule you follow, there is a definite benefit to doing your calf exercises after thigh movements. Thigh training causes a huge influx of blood flowing in the legs that carries over to your calf work, giving those muscles a better contraction and pump than if they were done elsewhere in a workout.

Regular leg workouts are crucial to the overall success of your training because they help improve blood circulation through the body, and most leg moves indirectly call other muscle groups into play. (Some leg exercises can even contribute to muscle growth in your arms!) Because of these all-important functions, leg day is scheduled first in this particular training schedule.

LOW SETS, LOW-MEDIUM REPS, HEAVY POUNDAGE

Schedules A, B and C each include primary and secondary workouts. Here are the recommended sets and reps for the "Core Growth" exercises in the primary workouts:

PRIMARY WORKOUTS: (SIZE AND STRENGTH ENHANCEMENT)

EXERCISES	SETS	REPS
Back Squat*	4	6–8
Bench Press*	4	6–8
Deadlift*	4	6–8
Bent-Over Row*	4	6–8
Upright Row*	3	6–8
Curl*	3	6–8
Parallel Bar Dip (with weight, if possible)	3	6–8
Standing Calf Raise	3	15–20
Crunch	3	15–20
*Move should be performed with a barbell.		

Three or four sets of these exercises is the optimal range for developing muscle mass and strength (excluding warm-up sets). This approach, combined with proper nutrition and supplementation, will increase levels of key muscle-growth hormones such as HGH and improve enzyme chemical amounts so your body adapts to the workout stress. Stick to this recommended number of sets for the entire six to twelve weeks of using this program. At the end of that time period, if you aren't satisfied with your progress, you can vary the sets slightly to best suit your individual needs, physique goals and body type.

Performing only three or four mass- and strength-building sets is also one of the best ways to avoid overtaxing your muscles and creating an environment of catabolism rather than one of anabolism. As Lee Haney, eight-time IFBB Mr. Olympia, has advocated on many occasions, "Stimulate, don't annihilate!"

ECONO-TIME SECONDARY WORKOUTS

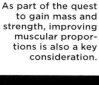

As part of the quest to gain mass and strength, improving muscular proportions is also a key consideration.

Each move in the Econo-Time Secondary Workouts should be completed using a Four-Component Set (i.e., Total-Intensity Set). Select a weight that allows you to complete eight reps to positive failure. Continue the set with two or three (partner assisted) forced reps. Perform your final rep with a static, or iso-tension, hold at peak contraction for 10 to 15 seconds. Finish the rep with a five- to eight-second negative. Each exercise listed under Econo-Time Secondary Workout is performed just once using the Four-Component Set (i.e., one set of eight normal reps, two or three forced reps, static hold at peak contraction on final rep, negative on final rep).

Note: If you train alone, doing forced reps with proper form won't be possible. If you don't have a spotter, use brief rests between reps to achieve the extra two or three reps beyond failure. Take a short rest (about 10 seconds) at the end of your eighth regular rep. Repeat two more times in the same manner.

Rep-Outs: For calf and ab exercises, complete one set of 15 to 40 reps. On bodyweight-only (no attached poundage) exercises such as parallel bar dips and pull-ups, perform one set to positive failure.

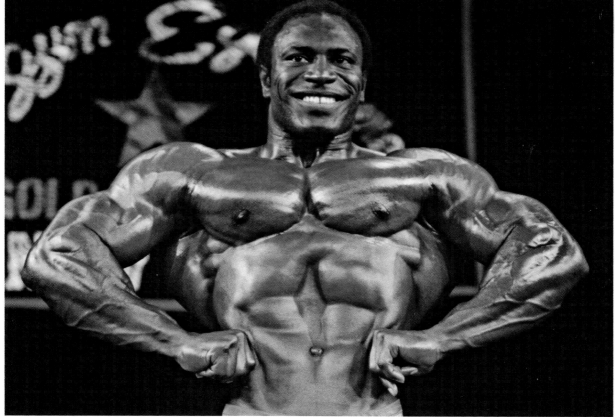

Model Lee Haney

CHAPTER 2

MUSCLE FIBERS: TYPE-SPECIFIC TRAINING

Determining optimal rep ranges for each bodypart, based on your body type and individual genetics, will maximize you potential for muscle shape and size.

Over the course of your power bodybuilding career, you will likely make quite a few changes to your regimen in the forms of equipment choice, exercise technique, training frequency, number of reps and sets, and rest periods. Specifically, the rep count you use for each bodypart is crucial when trying to achieve muscular gains. Incorporating a wide variety of rep ranges will benefit your effort to reach absolute potential in muscle size, shape and vascularity.

In 1980 Fred C. Hatfield, or "Dr. Squat," confirmed fast- and slow-twitch muscle fibers need to be trained differently in a feature interview in *Iron Man* magazine. He stated: "Bodybuilders, in order to achieve the tremendous musculature they possess, have to do slow movements (reps) and fast movements (speed reps), use light poundage, heavy poundage and every weight in between, to increase the mechanisms of the muscle structures."

The following chart lists the optimal rep range for each muscle group to stimulate strength gains and metabolic endurance in relation to the type of muscle fiber.

BODYPART	REP RANGE
Thighs	5–25
Lower Back, Lats, Traps	6–15
Chest, Delts, Triceps, Biceps	5–12
Calves, Abs	15–40

Research has demonstrated that rep ranges of five to eight will build the most amount of contractile (fast-twitch) muscle fiber (this type has more potential for growth than slow-twitch). For the purposes of the *Huge & Freaky Muscle Mass and Strength* program, we have chosen a rep range of six to eight per set for seven of the primary exercises listed. We developed this plan using a six- to eight-rep range based on physiological research on the general breakdown of muscle fibers within the human body.

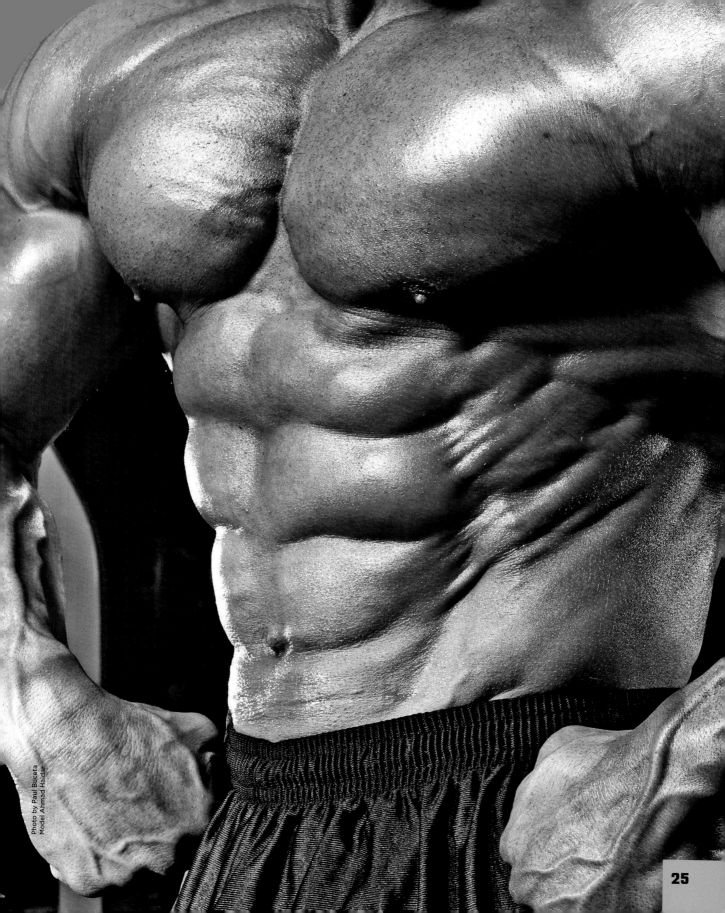

25

Have you ever wondered how much of each type of muscle fiber you have (fast- versus slow-twitch)? The average individual has an approximate 50:50 ratio, but the exact proportions differ depending on genetics. There is a general test that can be useful for determining whether a select muscle in your body is composed more of Type I (slow) or Type II (fast) muscle fibers.

MUSCLE FIBER TEST

Use a weight that is 80 percent of your unfatigued one-rep maximum for a particular exercise and do one set of as many reps as possible. The rep cadence should be two seconds in the positive phase and four seconds in the negative phase.

Evaluating your results is simple: If you can do seven reps (hitting failure at that point), the muscle has a 50:50 average makeup of fast- and slow-twitch fibers. If you achieve fewer than seven reps, the muscle contains more of the fast-twitch variety. Conversely, if you can perform more than seven reps, the muscle is composed of a greater proportion of slow-twitch fibers. In other words, the fewer reps you can do (below seven) the higher the muscle's fast-twitch percentage; the further you can go past seven, the greater the slow-twitch composition in the muscle.

Because the two types of fibers respond differently to various forms of training, it's important to understand how each functions in your body. Type I fibers have a high aerobic capacity for oxidation, they contract slowly and they are crucial for endurance activities – this type benefits from higher-rep training. Type II fibers assist with short, heavy lifting and quick bursts of power – they are engaged during brief, high-intensity workouts. If you train your body using only one scheme (either low-rep or high-rep), you are likely neglecting a large number of muscle fibers, therefore limiting your potential for growth. To target and build your muscles optimally, you have to vary your rep ranges in order to recruit the largest possible number of both Type I and Type II fibers. Training to activate both types can be achieved through an approach called Slow/Fast-Twitch Muscle Fiber Sets.

SLOW/FAST-TWITCH MUSCLE FIBER SETS

SLOW-TWITCH SETS	REPS
1. Lightest weight	15
2. Add weight	12
3. Add weight	10
4. Add weight	8
FAST-TWITCH SETS	REPS
5. Add weight	7
6. Add weight	6
7. Add weight	5
8. Add weight	4*
*Include 1 or 2 forced reps.	

Many bodybuilders have achieved remarkable results from using the above sets-and-reps formula for one compound exercise (e.g., barbell back squats, flat-bench presses, barbell curls) for only a select muscle group. You can also switch the order of the sets to add a bit of variety to your workouts and help ensure your muscles do not get accustomed to the exercise order. We have used eight total sets as the benchmark for this type of training, a number that was reached from research findings on optimum workout overload.

DETERMINING OPTIMUM WORKOUT OVERLOAD

About 15 years ago, Dr. Kevin A. Pezzi discovered two methods for figuring out an individual's optimal workout load (so trainers could customize their routines to maximize and accelerate muscle gains to new levels).

Method 1: This particular concept will help you determine whether you are overtraining. If, for example, you are a right-handed individual, you should experience marked strength improvements on the right side when the muscles are trained unilaterally (i.e., one limb at a time). If you don't notice a strength increase on the dominant side of your body when employing unilateral or asymmetric training (or that side actually gets weaker) after a predetermined period of time, you may be training your muscles too hard.

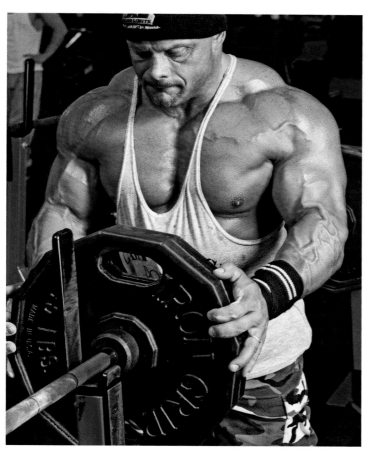

A skilled training partner can help on certain exercises by adding weight to the bar between sets.

Photo by Kevin Horton
Model Rodney Roller

Method 2: This concept allows a person to determine his or her optimal workout load and objectively evaluate variables such as number of sets, reps and frequency of exercise for their effects on muscular development. To use this method, select one move for evaluation (for the purpose of this example we'll use the standing barbell curl). If you have been performing a total of four heavy sets for this exercise but aren't sure if more would produce greater gains, try six total heavy sets for two or three weeks.

At the end of the predetermined time period, compare the results to what you achieved when using four sets (during an equal time frame). You should be keeping an accurate training log of exercises used, number of sets and reps, dates of workouts, along with miscellaneous factors such as lack of sleep, injuries and illnesses, as these are important considerations when you are trying to complete a fair assessment. If your progress has accelerated after the switch from four to six total heavy sets, then you were likely undertraining that particular muscle group. Increase the total number of heavy sets for that specific movement from six to eight (but never go beyond eight) and repeat the process as described. Because this method involves an element of trial and error using calculated testing periods, it may take a couple of months to determine your optimal workout loads for a particular muscle group.

If your strength level and/or muscle size decrease while you are evaluating optimal workout loads, this is a clear indication of overtraining. Should this occur, you need to immediately reduce your workload on the specific bodypart you are testing to previously accepted workout loads. Do not complete the entire predetermined period (i.e., two or three weeks) for that exercise.

Method 2 can also be tested using a unilateral approach to see how each limb responds to varying reps and sets (this is a good way to evaluate and correct any muscular imbalances). For example, substitute the standing barbell curl with the alternating dumbell curl, and perform a different number of sets and reps for each arm. Use a period of two or three weeks for this evaluation. On this exercise you might do six heavy sets of six reps for the right arm and eight sets of four reps for the left. At the end of the time frame, reverse the sets-and-reps protocol for each arm and repeat for an equal amount of time. Continue to monitor your response to the differing numbers of sets and reps until you find the optimal scheme for that muscle group.

The second method will work on any major or minor muscle group. Generally, when using this approach to test your muscles and training responses, the number of sets should not exceed eight total heavy sets per select muscle group.

Note: Use the Slow/Fast-Twitch Muscle Fiber Sets or Method 1 or 2 only when you return to your regular training schedules. Do not use any of these strategies during the Modified Push/Pull Workout System presented in this book.

CHAPTER 3

PROGRAM SPECIFICS: REPS, SETS & REST PERIODS

A successful workout is more than just a series of exercises – it's a calculated combination of reps–and–sets schemes, technique and rest time.

Your main priority when performing reps is to work as heavily as possible. And by that, we do not mean using cheating movements just for the sake of handling huge poundage. Perform each repetition over a full range of motion and use the concentration techniques (which will be discussed in a later chapter). You should aim to use as much weight as you can and constantly push for more. Work slowly, and pause to take a breath or two between each rep (i.e., the rest-pause principle).

Certain movements in this program require that you take precautions for safety. Having a training partner or spotter can be beneficial for many reasons during your workouts, but specifically, you should always use a competent and knowledgeable spotter when doing barbell bench presses and squats. The spotter should:

1. Be alert.
2. Check that the correct poundage is being used on the bar, plus make sure the collars are securely fastened on the bar.
3. Know how many reps are to be performed.
4. Help unrack the bar, assist as necessary (and only as necessary) during the lift and return the bar to the rack at the end of the set.
5. Encourage you and monitor your exercise form throughout.

Generally, the total time for one set of an exercise is a sum of the seconds it takes to move the weight through the positive and negative phases (over the full range of motion), multiplied by the number of repetitions in that set. Some bodybuilders take about three seconds to complete the positive phase and six seconds to finish the negative phase (doubling the time on the reverse portion of the rep is called slow negatives). This rep tempo is the ideal pace for the rep schemes in the secondary workout phase of the Modified Push/Pull System.

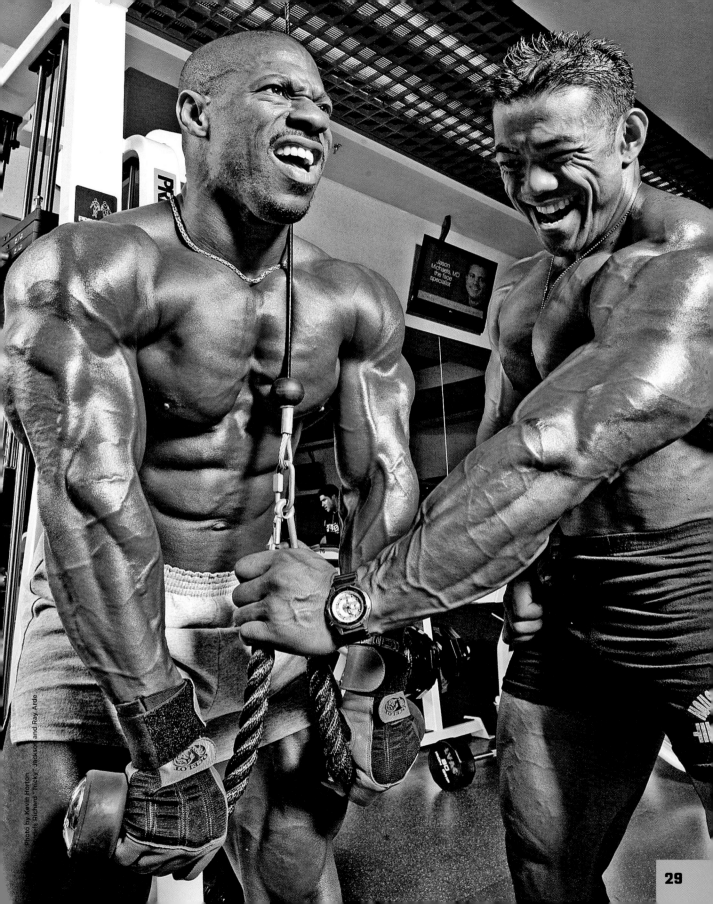

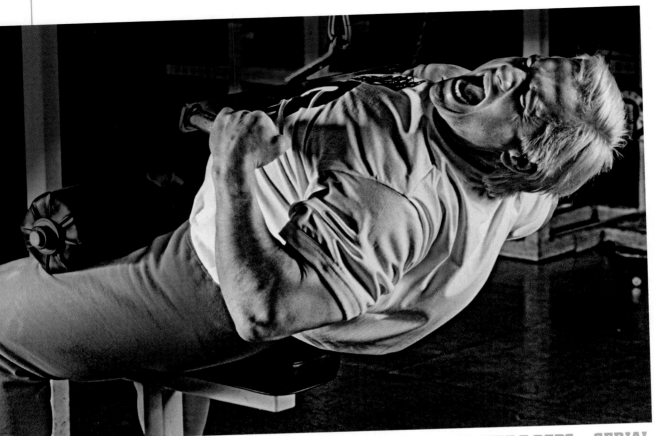

What may look like poor form and bad technique can sometimes be an intentional loosening of style to achieve mechanical advantage – a cheat rep.

Many of you, however, want to build incredible mass and make huge strength gains, so a slight modification to rep speed may be beneficial. For the exercises listed in the primary workout phase, accelerating the positive phase of the reps will help stimulate the target muscles.

HIGH-SPEED REPS

The positive phase of each rep should be completed as fast as possible (without compromising safety and proper form), taking less than two seconds to complete. Make sure you use limited ancillary muscle momentum and minimal leverage factors. The negative phase should be at least two times slower than the positive (around four or five seconds). The bar should travel along the same path and your form should be identical from the first to the final reps of a set. Remember, in order to make gains and improvements, you must control the weight – don't let it control you.

LOOSE-STYLE REPS – SERIAL DISTORTION TECHNIQUE

While precise form and proper technique are crucial to prevent injury and to make successful gains, there are certain instances when a move can and should be done with loose form. Cheat reps, or loose-style reps, refers to the momentary loss of precision biomechanical integrity of the structured exercise movement. This strategy can be used within the rep structure of the "Core Growth" exercises (see "Core Growth" Exercise Selection Chart). The definition may sound complex, but the motion itself is fairly easy to master.

For example, in almost all types of rowing and curling moves (and various laterals and or front raises), you can incorporate a bit of cheating technique in a rhythmic rocking motion. You first bend forward at the waist, then, with a controlled thrust of your body, you get the weight moving through the sticking point

Model Tom Platz

as you bend backward slightly. On a movement such as heavy standing barbell triceps extensions, you would reverse the order of waist motion (lean back, body thrust forward, lean forward). Another example where cheat reps can be helpful is when bench pressing; some power bodybuilders will quickly lower the bar to their abdominal regions. Then, by simultaneously arching their backs and giving a mighty thrust of abdominal power, they drive the barbell upward to lockout.

To those who aren't familiar with this approach, doing reps in loose or serial distortion style on the exercises noted above simply looks like exaggerated body movements. However, they serve a very important function by giving a micro-second of mechanical advantage helping you pass a sticking point of the lift while never compromising maximum tension within the muscle cell structure.

The late Chuck Sipes was an advocate for the value of both cheating and strict exercises in a training program. He believed, on certain exercises, that loose form helped to develop tendon and ligament power. On other moves, he rationalized that precise form was necessary for optimal development. For more infor-

mation on programs designed to use both techniques, check out the eBook *Echoes From the Power Storm that Was...Chuck Sipes!*

Chuck's take on cheating and strict movements is logical because the body is only as strong as its weakest link. If each and every rep of each and every set were done in strict form, you would have to continually use light poundage, therefore making ongoing progress impossible. For the best results, we recommend doing the first 70 percent of your reps in a set with strict form then finishing off the last 30 percent with controlled cheat reps.

It is interesting to note that many power bodybuilding champions over the years have been observed using what seems like horrendous forms of cheating in their precontest training exercises. But when they compete in, say, a powerlifting meet, when each lift has a title and a code of conduct for performance, their form is perfect and they do exceptionally well. Essentially what's happened is the cheating in their precontest workouts conditioned their muscles to deal with the heavier resistance in powerlifting events.

OPTIMAL REST PERIODS BETWEEN SETS

As you begin a multi-rep set, blood gets pumped into the muscle, causing it to congest. With each rep you force out within a particular set, you will experience an increasing burning sensation as the lactic acid starts to build up. Finally the muscle will begin to cramp or cease its contraction, and this is when the muscle reaches a state of momentary exhaustion. Muscle failure, as it's also called, is caused by lactic acid buildup and the absence of oxygen, an environment created by the retention or backup of the blood supply in the muscle being exercised.

Bob Gajda, former AAU Mr. USA, Mr. America and Mr. Universe winner, carried out some research about oxygen debt and lactic acid buildup in muscle tissue. He found when lactic acid accumulates in a muscle it must be neutralized by buffers (bicarbonates, cell phosphates, hemoglobin and plasma proteins) in the blood to prevent the chemical pH balance from being greatly altered. A normal pH bal-

For safety, an experienced and competent spotter should always be on hand for moves such as the barbell bench press.

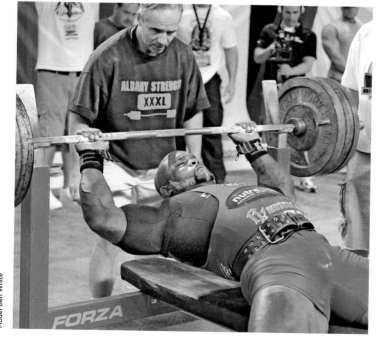

Photo by Garry Bartlett
Model Ben White

ance is 7.35; when the lactic acid is not neutralized, the balance is skewed ever so slightly, and you end up feeling fatigued and tired.

The only way the pH balance can remain steady and lactic acid can be neutralized is by having a continuous supply of fresh oxygenated blood, because oxygen is required to convert blood lactic acid to glycogen. This is the exact physiological process the rest-pause principle is founded upon. When you rest between reps for a period of 10 seconds or more, a fresh supply of oxygenated blood gets reintroduced into the contracting muscle. Therefore, the muscle isn't forced to work as long without oxygen and lactic acid accumulation levels are much lower than normal.

Extensive research on the theories of muscle fatigue indicates that when muscle-building repetitions are done in a continuous manner with one deep breath between reps (or only one breath per six reps, as nine-time world powerlifting champion Larry Pacifico occasionally preferred in the bench press), the decline in your starting strength can be anywhere from 20 to 42 percent.

Therefore, you need to consider what the optimal duration of rest should be between every set in your workouts. Take, for example, the 300-pound barbell bench press for four sets of six to eight mentioned earlier. At the completion of your first set (reps done to momentary failure), you may experience a starting strength loss of 20 to 42 percent. In other words, your first all-out set of six to eight reps will now be between 240 (300 – [300 x 0.2] = 240 pounds) and 174 pounds (300 – [300 x 0.42] = 174 pounds).

The human body houses an internal structure with an amazing capacity to recover at a fast rate. In the first 10 seconds of a rest period, 56 percent of the decreased starting strength is recouped; at the 35-second mark, 84 percent of that lost strength is regenerated. From that point onward, it takes another 35 seconds to regain another 12 percent. Therefore, at the 70-second rest period, the muscle has recuperated 96 percent of the initial decline. It generally takes an additional three minutes (studies have noted an exact time of two minutes and 50 seconds) to gain the final four percent to reach

100-percent recovery. (See Appendix 3a.) For the primary and secondary workout phases in this program, the rest-pause sequences between exercise sets are recommended as follows:

PRIMARY WORKOUTS (SCHEDULE A – B – C)

When you complete each size- and strength-enhancing set of a primary "Core Growth" exercise, your rest period should be three-and-a-half to six minutes. Make sure you rest at least the minimum amount, as any shorter will not allow the body to remove lactic acid and other byproducts of fatigue from the muscles – you don't want fatigue to be your enemy during these sets.

Conversely, the calves and abs can recover with minimal rest periods of one-and-a-half to two minutes. You can use this same time frame for your "Dress Rehearsal" warm-up sets, which we will be outlining in the next chapter.

SECONDARY WORKOUTS (SCHEDULE A – B – C)

When performing the secondary exercises, you should use rest periods that are one-and-a-half to two minutes from set to set, and do plenty of deep breathing. Also, in this workout phase, perform only one "Dress Rehearsal" warm-up set per exercise, if necessary.

Though your muscles have an incredible capacity to recuperate strength after rest periods within a workout, muscle groups vary in the length of time needed to fully recover between workouts. The following chart shows an approximate figure of adequate rest days needed for four major and minor muscle groups.

MUSCLE	DAYS TO RECOVER
Quads	4.5
Pecs	3.5
Biceps	3
Calves	1

Of course, a number of factors impact the specific recovery period of each muscle group. Use the following list to help you plan your training split to allow for ample rest days between workouts for the same muscles.

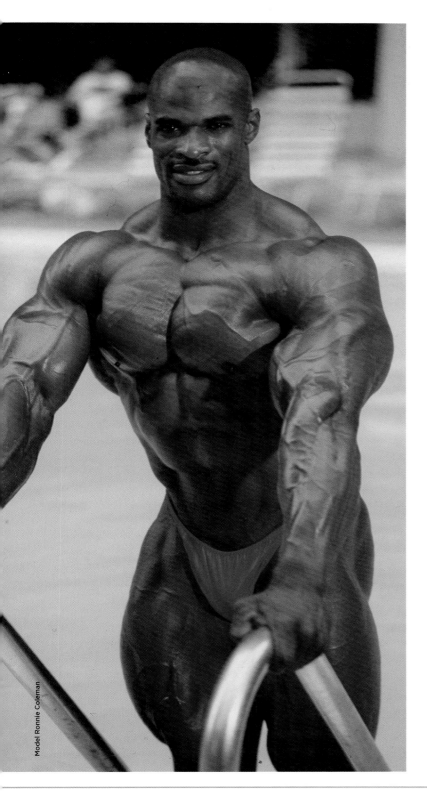

Model Ronnie Coleman

NINE VARIABLES AFFECTING RECOVERY TIME

1. Large muscles take longer to recover than smaller muscles.
2. Fast-twitch muscle fibers generally take longer to recover, as they are responsible for strength and power, whereas slow-twitch muscle fibers rejuvenate faster because they are suited to localized muscle endurance.
3. High-intensity exercise with poundage exceeding 80 percent of a one-rep maximum requires greater recuperation time than lifting with weights that are less than 80 percent of your one-rep maximum.
4. Exercises that use a full range of motion typically cause greater amounts of connective tissue damage, therefore necessitating greater recovery time than partial-movement exercises.
5. In general, as you get older you'll need to schedule longer recovery periods. If you are over 35, adjust your workouts accordingly to allow for more recuperation time.
6. Bigger bodybuilders (think Jay Cutler and Ronnie Coleman) will need more muscle recovery time than comparatively smaller guys (Mark Dugdale and David Henry).
7. Adhering to a proper nutrition plan and following a muscle-building supplement regimen can significantly shorten recuperation time, while poor dietary and supplementation practices can prolong it.
8. Anabolic steroids can reduce recovery time, but this is not a recommendation to take these drugs. And many recreational and prescriptive drugs can dramatically increase the time it takes for muscles to recover from a workout. Prolonged use of corticosteroid class drugs such as prednisone (used for treating asthma, emphysema, arthritis, lupus and other autoimmune diseases) can hinder recovery time.
9. States of overtraining, whether the cause is biological, physiological or psychological, negatively impact recovery time requirements. The same is true for undertraining. Don't be guilty of either.

CHAPTER 4

WARM-UP PROCEDURES, WORKOUT PROGRESSION & STRETCHING

Avoid injury, improve blood flow, help prevent muscle soreness and increase flexibility with three pre- and post-workout strategies: warm-up, stretching, cool-down.

Before beginning any workout within *Huge & Freaky Muscle Mass and Strength Secrets*, we strongly suggest you perform a carefully planned general warm-up to increase your body's core and skeletal muscle temperatures slightly (these muscles represent 35 to 40 percent of total body mass).

A basic warm-up will encourage maximum blood supply in the skeletal muscles and vascular system. Begin with five to ten minutes (enough to break a sweat) on a piece of equipment such as the stationary bike, stair climber, cross-country ski machine, stepper, treadmill or elliptical. Start with a slow cadence and work up to a relatively brisk pace for the last minute or so. To use different muscles, avoid injury and for interest's sake, use different equipment from workout to workout. For example, if you use the stair stepper in Schedule A, try the elliptical in Schedule B, etc.

AEROBIC THREE-MINUTE SYSTEM

When training for ultimate mass and strength, it is important that you avoid extended periods of intense aerobic activity (30 minutes or more). Long bouts of cardio will increase the likelihood that you'll burn up hard-earned muscle mass. When limited to an appropriate length and level of intensity, however, aerobics can serve an important function for developing the cardio respiratory system without compromising your gains.

We suggest the Aerobic Three-Minute System. Using a treadmill, stationary bike or other cardio machine, work at a sprint pace for 20 seconds (i.e., 80 to 90 percent of your target pulse). Then, without pause, coast for 10 seconds (i.e., about 60 to 65 percent of your target heart rate).

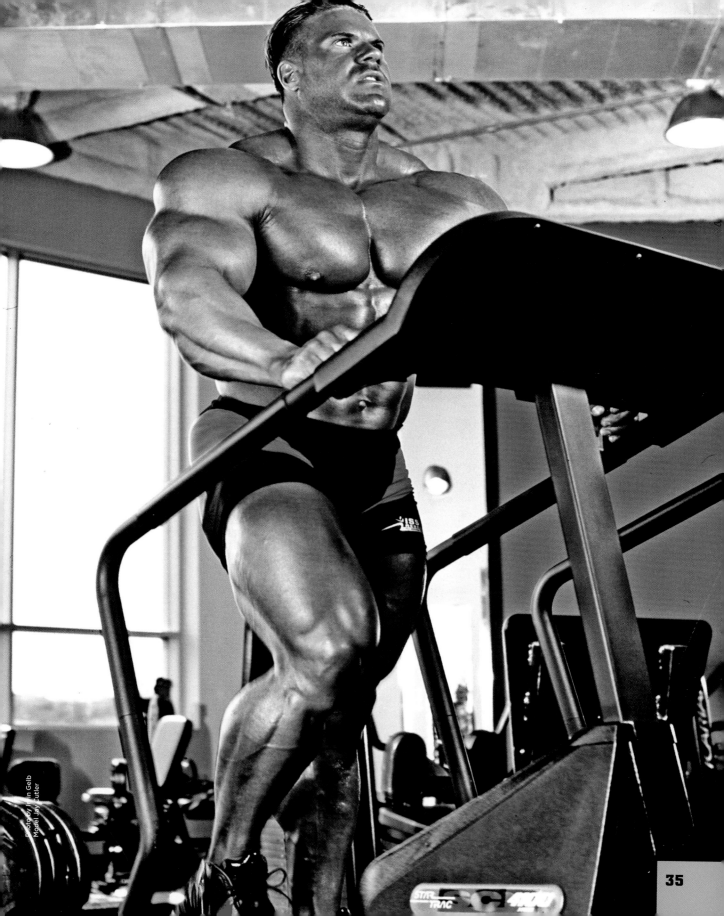

Repeat this fast-slow 20-10 sequence non-stop six times (for a total of three minutes). You should aim to use this sequence two nonconsecutive days a week. If you are over 40 years of age, lead a sedentary lifestyle or have not had an active cardiac stress test, do not use this high-low intensity method of aerobic conditioning, as your body may not be able to tolerate the rapid change in pace.

Keep in mind that every aerobic training session should always begin with a five- to ten-minute warm-up and conclude with a five- to ten-minute cool-down.

"DRESS REHEARSAL" WARM-UPS

Proper warm-ups specific to your muscles are an integral aspect of training, yet many bodybuilders overlook or neglect them. One of the worst errors a bodybuilder can make is to fatigue a muscle with too many warm-up sets prior to attacking the area with heavy poundage. Overworking the muscle and exacerbating lactic acid buildup and then exposing the muscle to working sets and reps will not help you build muscular size and strength.

In addition to a general warm-up, a non-fatiguing "dress rehearsal" (exercise specific) warm-up is necessary for seven of the nine "Core Growth" exercises (machine calf raises and ab crunches are excluded). This form of warm-up will force blood into the muscles and tendons and ensure the central nervous system is maximally stimulated (you can further activate the CNS by eating foods rich in tyrosine and sulfur such as meat and eggs). Warming up the specific muscles you're going to work will also create a highly alert contractile state in the skeletal muscle fibers.

This type of warm-up also preps the muscle by rehearsing the exercise range of motion and introducing progressively heavier poundage. You'll notice in the following example that the reps stay fairly low, counting down from five to one – higher-rep warm-ups would create a pH imbalance and lactic acid buildup. The end result would then be early fatigue at the chemical level, a state when the brain cannot recruit the high-threshold muscle fibers nec-

essary for completing the size- and strength-enhancing sets.

The correct process for "dress rehearsal" warm-ups sets is to use 30 to 90 percent of the poundage you will be using for your working sets of a particular exercise. For example, if you are performing the barbell bench press with 300 pounds for four sets of six to eight reps, the "dress rehearsal" warm-up sets will look like this:

WARM-UP SET	WEIGHT (IN POUNDS)	REPS
Rest 1.5–2 min.	90 (30% of 300)	5
Rest 1.5–2 min.	135 (45% of 300)	4
Rest 1.5–2 min.	180 (60% of 300)	3
Rest 1.5–2 min.	210–215 (70–75% of 300)	3
Rest 1.5–2 min.	270 (90% of 300)	1

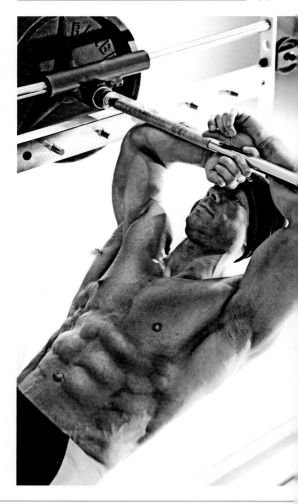

Photo by Paul Buceta
Model Adam Headland

A critical mistake bodybuilders can make is doing too many warm-up sets, essentially overworking the muscle before heavy working sets.

Upon completion, you will load the bar to 300 pounds for the first of four working sets of six to eight reps. Once you're properly warmed up, it is of utmost importance that you push your training intensity to the absolute limits of your pain threshold in order to maximize your mass and strength gains. Building progression into your workouts is a key factor to achieving optimal results. The following chart outlines how you can intensify your workout over a span of 14 weeks (we've used the barbell bench press as the exercise example).

Both options illustrate how the reps and poundage progressions are made, using a hypothetical weight of 300 pounds. On primary exercises for larger muscles such as the thighs, back and chest, you can increase the poundage by increments of 5 to 10 pounds; on exercises for smaller muscle groups such as the deltoids, triceps and biceps, weight increases can range from 2.5 to 5 pounds. The best amount of weight to add will vary from bodybuilder to bodybuilder and from muscle group to muscle group. You need to determine what works best for your body and level of training, but an increase anywhere in the range of 2 to 10 pounds is reasonable.

Follow the progression formulas as outlined until you are capable of performing four sets of eight reps (i.e., Option 1 – Workout 9) and/or four sets of eight reps with an additional 5 to 10 pounds than your base weight at the beginning of the program (i.e., Option 2 – Workout 9). When you reach that point, increase your poundage by 2.5 to 5 pounds, reduce your reps to six and begin a new progression sequence.

PNF STRETCHING

Many bodybuilders, from beginner to advanced level, completely avoid warming up and instead immediately begin a stretching routine as soon as they walk onto the gym floor. This all-too-common practice only invites injury or damage to muscles and tendons, as they haven't received an appreciable influx of blood flow via a general and "dress rehearsal" warm-up. Therefore, it's imperative you always perform both types of warm-ups before stretching prior to training.

INTENSITY-BOOSTING PROGRESSION CHARTS

WORKOUT	SETS/REPS	WEIGHT (IN POUNDS)
OPTION 1		
1	4/6	300
2	1/7	300
	3/6	300
3	2/7	300
	2/6	300
4	3/7	300
	1/6	300
5	4/7	300
	1/8	300
6	1/8	300
	3/7	300
7	2/8	300
	2/7	300
8	3/8	300
	1/7	300
9	4/8	300
10	4/6	305–310
11	4/7	305–310
	3/6	305–310
12	2/7	305–310
	2/6	305–310
13	3/7	305–310
	1/6	305–310
14	4/7	305–310
OPTION 2		
1	4/6	300
2	1/7	300
	3/6	300
3	1/8	300
	3/6	300
4	1/8	305–310
	1/7	300
	2/6	300
5	2/8	305–310
	2/6	300
6	2/8	305–310
	1/7	300
	1/6	300
7	3/8	305–310
	1/6	300
8	3/8	305–310
	1/7	300
9	4/8	305–310
10	4/6	310–315
11	1/8	310–315
	1/7	310–315
	2/6	310–315
12	2/8	310–315
	2/6	310–315
13	2/8	310–315
14	2/8	310–315
	1/7	310–315
	1/6	310–315

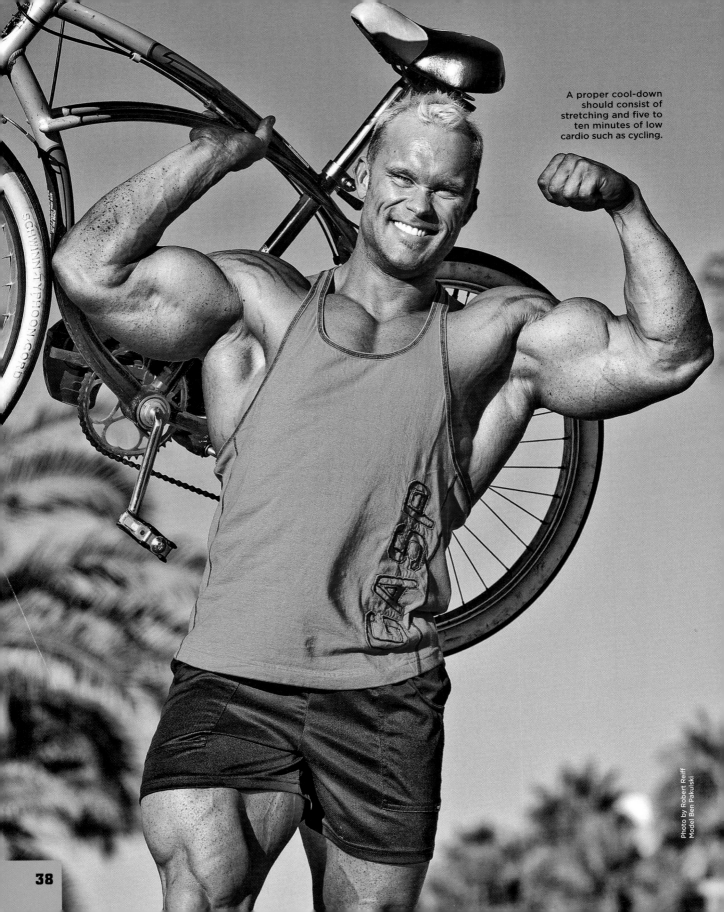

A proper cool-down should consist of stretching and five to ten minutes of low cardio such as cycling.

Of equal importance is completing a proper cool-down at the end of your sessions. Some experts actually argue that the cool-down is even more crucial than the warm-up because light movement and stretching immediately post-workout will help prevent muscle soreness and improve flexibility and range of motion. Your cool-down should include five to ten minutes with a mixture of very low-impact cardio (i.e., walking on the treadmill, cycling at a low speed and resistance on the stationary bike) and stretching elements. PNF (Proprioceptive Neuromuscular Facilitation) stretching with a partner is a technique you may want to incorporate at the conclusion of certain workouts. This approach is considered one of the most effective forms of flexibility training. Techniques under the PNF system can be ac-

tive (with voluntary muscle contraction) or passive (without any muscular contraction). And while there are many PNF stretching variations, one common feature is facilitating muscular inhibition.

If you have never routinely stretched your muscles post-workout, keep in mind that it can take upward of six weeks for a stretching program to become effective. If you do stretch but not consistently, the positive effects will be limited. If you get out of the habit, just three weeks without proper stretching will cause your previous improvements to diminish. For more information on stretching protocols, we suggest visiting the Web site www.dragondoor.com or searching for books and DVDs on Russian stretching secrets by our good friend, the world-renowned Pavel Tsatsouline.

Routine stretching can have a positive impact on flexibility and range of motion in as little as six weeks when done consistently.

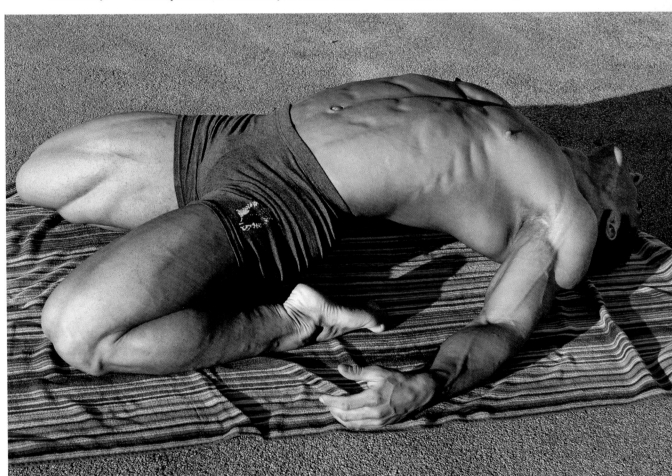

Photo by Irvin Gelb
Model Antoine Vaillant

CHAPTER 5

MODIFIED PUSH/PULL SYSTEM WORKOUT SCHEDULE

You'll target every major muscle group in this training schedule, activating your muscles in a new way to overcome stagnation and spark new growth.

SCHEDULE A PRIMARY WORKOUT — MONDAY

BODYPARTS TRAINED: Thighs, Calves, Abs

EXERCISE	SETS	REPS
Barbell Back Squat	4	6–8
Standing Calf Raise	3	15–20
Weighted Crunch	3	15–20

ECONO-TIME SECONDARY WORKOUT

BODYPARTS TRAINED: Chest, Delts, Triceps, Biceps

EXERCISE	SETS/REPS
Bodyweight Pull-Up	1 set to positive failure
Incline Barbell Bench Press	4-component set*
Upright Row	4-component set*
Parallel Bar Dip	1 set to positive failure
Barbell Curl	4-component set*

*The 4-component set should consist of 1 set of 8 reps to positive failure, 2 to 3 forced reps with a 10- to 20- second static hold on last forced rep and a 5- to 8-second negative.

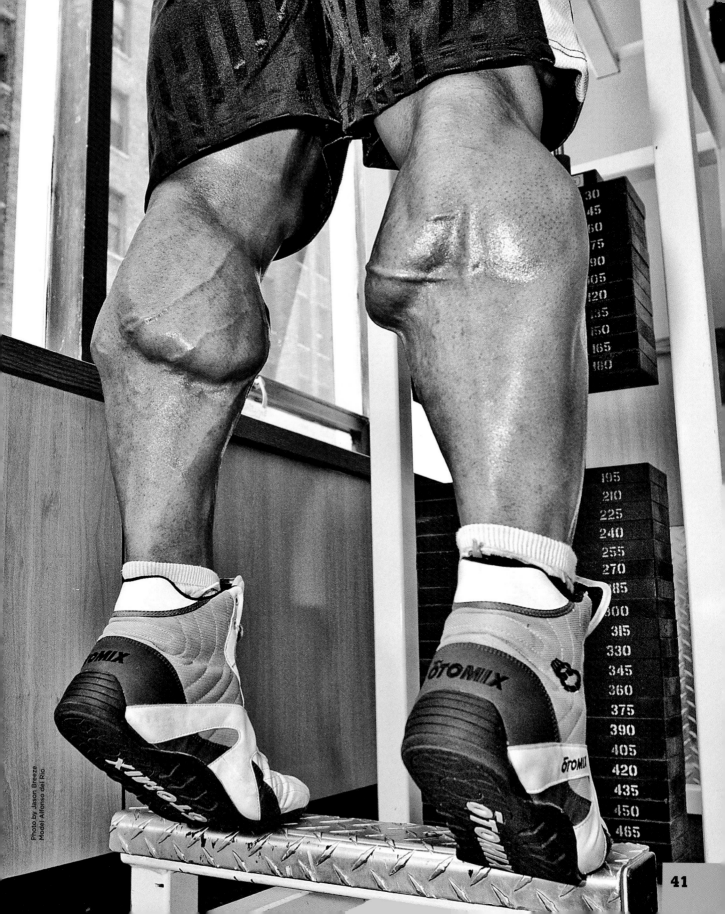

Photo by Jason Breeze
Model Alfonso del Rio

30
45
60
75
90
105
120
135
150
165
180

195
210
225
240
255
270
285
300
315
330
345
360
375
390
405
420
435
450
465

41

SCHEDULE B PRIMARY WORKOUT — WEDNESDAY

BODYPARTS TRAINED: Chest, Delts, Triceps

EXERCISE	SETS	REPS
Barbell Bench Press (flat)	4	6–8
Barbell Upright Row	3	6–8
Parallel Bar Dip (with weight, if possible)	3	6–8

ECONO-TIME SECONDARY WORKOUT

BODYPARTS TRAINED: Thighs, Calves, Back, Biceps, Abs

EXERCISE	SETS/REPS
Leg Press	4-component set*
Seated Calf Raise	1 set to positive failure
Hyperextension (prone)	1 set to positive failure
Dumbbell Curl	4-component set*
Reverse Ab Crunch	1 set to positive failure

*The 4-component set should consist of 1 set of 8 reps to positive failure, 2 to 3 forced reps with a 10- to 20-second static hold on last forced rep and a 5- to 8-second negative.

While the leg press isn't one of the seven core growth exercises, it's a great move to encourage leg development.

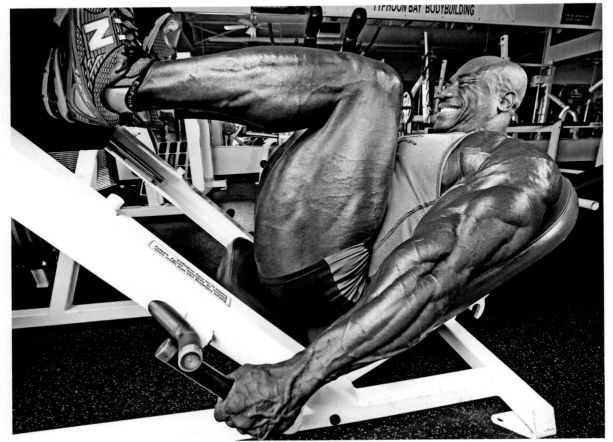

Photo by Paul Buceta
Model Joel Stubbs

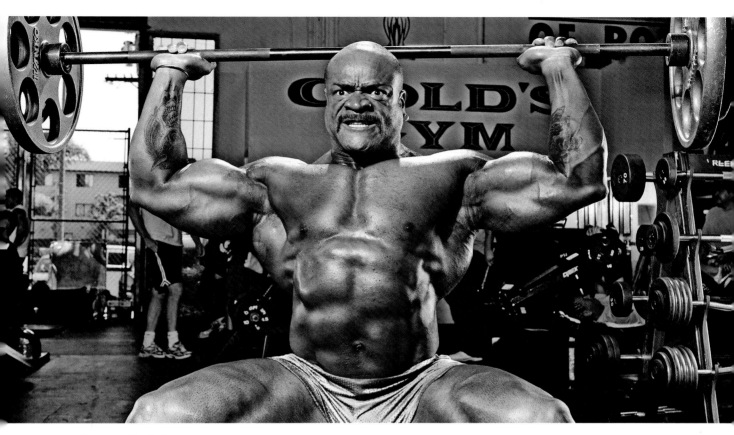

The seated barbell overhead press makes for a challenging and effective secondary back exercise.

Photo by Robert Reiff
Model Will Harris

SCHEDULE C PRIMARY WORKOUT — FRIDAY

BODYPARTS TRAINED: Back, Biceps

EXERCISE	SETS	REPS
Deadlift	4	6–8
Bent-Over Row	4	6–8
Barbell Curl	3	6–8

ECONO-TIME SECONDARY WORKOUT

BODYPARTS TRAINED: Back, Biceps

EXERCISE	SETS/REPS
Hack Squat	4-component set*
Donkey Calf Raise	1 set of 15–40 reps^
Incline Dumbbell Press	4-component set*
Barbell Overhead Press	4-component set*
EZ-Bar Triceps Extension (lying)	4-component set*
Seated Knee Pull-In	1 set of 15–40 reps

*The 4-component set should consist of 1 set of 8 reps to positive failure, 2 to 3 forced reps with a 10- to 20- second static hold on last forced rep and a 5- to 8-second negative.
^Do as many reps as possible with a training partner sitting on your back. When the extra weight becomes too challenging, continue just on your own to positive failure.

The exercises in this training schedule target every major muscle group (and some minor). When following this basic program, you don't have to add any supplementary exercises, as many of the movements are multi-joint and therefore call more than one muscle into play. If, however, you do have specific concerns with a lagging bodypart, you may consider incorporating a couple of specific moves to bring up the area(s); just be sure to schedule these extra exercises appropriately within the training split (so you're not overworking certain bodyparts). Remember, this workout plan is not designed to prepare you for a bodybuilding contest; the Modified Push/Pull System will activate your muscles in a new way, helping you overcome muscle stagnation or a training plateau so you can build a solid, massive physique.

Note: In the Modified Push/Pull System Chart (see p. 40-43), there are a number of anabolic "Core Growth" exercises listed in the Econo-Time Secondary Workouts. During the course of this program, if you notice your joints, ligaments, tendons and/or muscles become strained or sore, use a muscle-specific or isolation exercise (see Holistic Exercise Selection Chart/Group 2 on p. 480-484) for each affected muscle group.

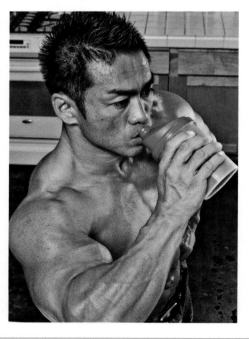

Your body is screaming for fuel right after training, so your best bet is to drink a protein shake within 30 minutes post-workout.

Muscle-wasting (catabolic) cortisol hormone levels are at their highest toward the end of a workout and then 30 minutes into the post-workout window. Therefore, for proper recovery and to promote muscle growth, it's crucial to consume the appropriate nutrients (a shake is ideal) within the first half hour after finishing your session. At this time, your best bet is to consume a shake with a 50:50 ratio of protein (e.g., whey) and complex carbs (e.g., maltodextrin, as it functions like a simple sugar and gets utilized rapidly by the body). Aim for 20 to 40 grams of each nutrient to promote anabolism, spare muscle wasting and limit negative side effects of intense training (i.e., rapid testosterone and growth hormone depletion, free radical overload, adrenal gland, adrenal gland exhaustion and central nervous system shock).

ANABOLIC "CORE GROWTH" EXERCISE SELECTION CHART

Most power bodybuilders will experience optimal muscle stimulation and will catapult their bodies into an anabolic environment with seven of the primary "Core Growth" exercises we have recommended (barbell squat, deadlift, bent-over row, bench press, upright row and curl and parallel bar dip). We realize, however, that every bodybuilder is different and individual genetics and body type will impact results. Other factors such as anatomical leverages (bone length, muscle origins and insertions) along with fast- and slow-twitch muscle fiber ratios will also impact a trainee's success on this basic program. In addition, certain exercises, no matter how anabolic in nature, just don't seem to work efficiently for some bodybuilders to stimulate the muscle-gain factor. A lack of mental focus and mind-muscle connection may also negatively affect a bodybuilder's performance of, and response to, a specific exercise.

For example, many power bodybuilders swear by the effectiveness of the flat bench press for piling slabs of new muscle on the pecs. But for every fan of this exercise, there's likely a hardgainer or other individual who has experienced very little or no pec stimulation from the standard bench press. This move in particular can also cause major strains or inju-

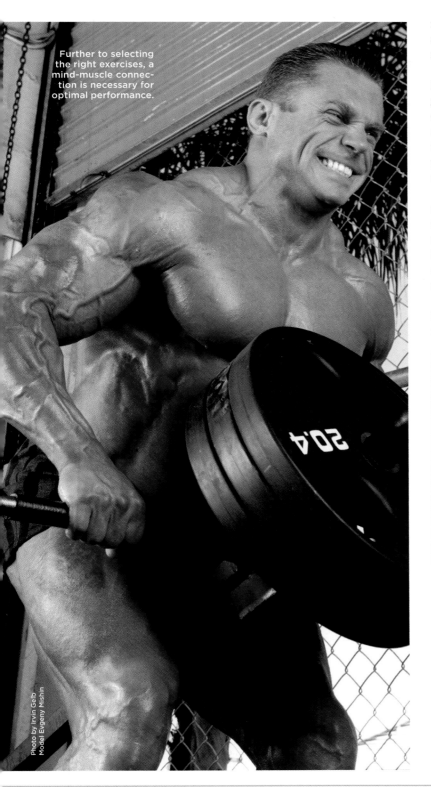

Further to selecting the right exercises, a mind-muscle connection is necessary for optimal performance.

Photo by Irvin Gelb
Model Evgeny Mishin

ries when not performed correctly or without an attentive spotter, and this can be a deterring factor for some trainees.

Therefore, exercise selection and variation is a critical part of any successful training program. You need to have a variety of choices in order to maximize each and every workout. By switching up exercise order or substituting certain moves to replace ones that aren't working, you're more likely to experience muscle growth and strength gains.

In order to determine which moves you respond to best, it's important you take the time to analyze your results, using trial and error to discover which primary exercises trigger anabolic growth. Once you've figured out your individual needs, your potential for gaining huge muscle and superior strength can be realized.

Try out the different exercises in the chart below to help you personalize your program for the primary and secondary workouts.

MUSCLE GROUP	EXERCISE OPTIONS
Thighs	Barbell Back Squat Leg Press Hack Squat Barbell Front Squat
Calves	Calf Raise Donkey Calf Raise (standing or seated)
Lower Back	Deadlift (conventional or semi-stiff leg)
Lats	Bent-Over Row Lat Pulldown Pull-Up (palms up or down) T-Bar Row
Traps	Shrug (barbell or dumbbell) Barbell Clean (from floor or dead hang)

Chest	Bench Press
	   (barbell or dumbbell)
	Bench Press
	   (flat, incline or decline)

Delts	Overhead Press
	   (barbell or dumbbell)
	Overhead Press
	   (seated or standing)
	Barbell Upright Row

Triceps	Parallel Bar Dip (close grip)
	EZ-Bar Triceps Extension
	   (lying, seated or standing)
	Barbell Bench Press
	   (close grip or reverse grip)

Biceps	Curl (barbell or dumbbell)
Abs	Reverse Crunch Leg Raise (lying or hanging)

CHAPTER 6

TRAINING SPLITS, OPTIONS, METHODS & TECHNIQUES

A workout extends far beyond the exercises you choose – it's the collection of approaches, strategies, philosophies and program specifics that fuel progress.

We've carefully designed the one-day-on / one-day-off split (except for weekends when you'll have to consecutive days off) to overload specific primary muscle groups on particular days and allow for adequate intervals of rest.

You can subject your body to maximum training stresses for a period of about 10 to 12 weeks. At the end of that time frame, your progress will come to a halt, and your overall performance may plateau or even regress. To prevent setbacks in your training, we recommend a seven- to ten-day complete layoff from heavy and intense workouts after using this program for about 12 weeks. This time away from serious gym sessions will help your muscles to fully recover from the stress

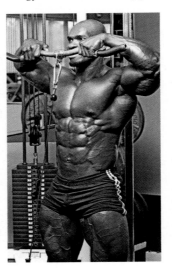

overloads placed on them over the course of the program. After the break, make sure you change up your regimen to shock your muscles, prevent stagnation and spark new muscle growth.

So after you've completed the *Huge & Freaky Muscle Mass and Strength* program and have rested for approximately one week, you should initiate a new plan. We suggest using a different variation of the every-other-day split. Here are three options you may consider:

Note: Option 1 is entirely a push/pull format, while Options 2 and 3 are derivatives of that approach.

Photos by Kevin Horton
Model Al Auguste

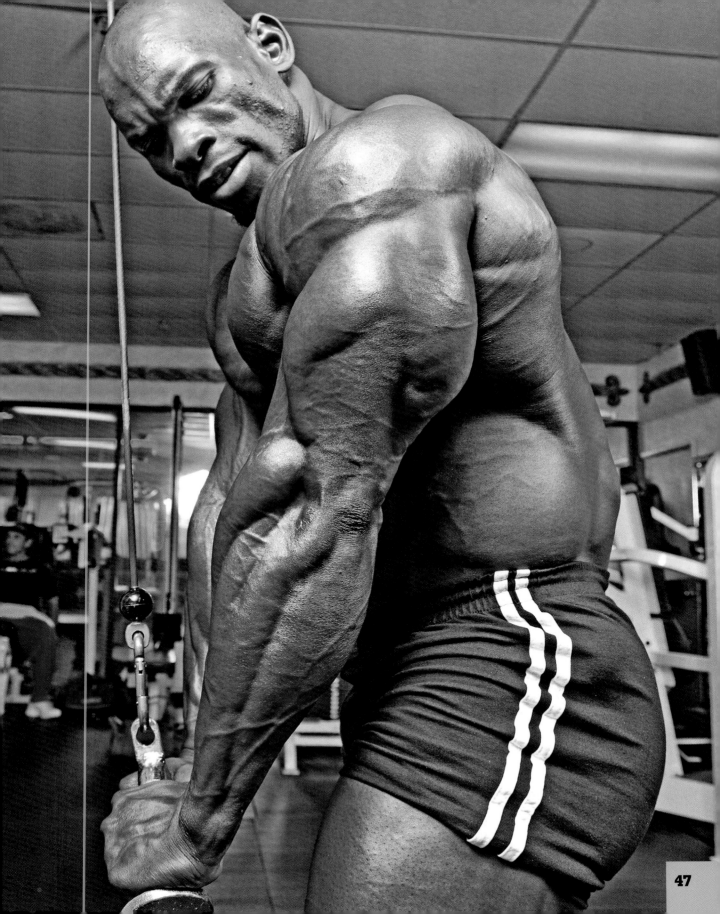

OPTION 1	
DAY	
1	Chest, Delts, Triceps
2	Off
3	Quads, Hams, Calves
4	Off
5	Back, Biceps
6	Off
7	Off

OPTION 2	
DAY	
1	Chest, Delts
2	Off
3	Quads, Hams, Calves, Triceps
4	Off
5	Back, Biceps
6	Off
7	Off

OPTION 3	
DAY	
1	Back, Chest
2	Off
3	Delts, Triceps, Biceps
4	Off
5	Quads, Hams, Calves
6	Off
7	Off

The barbell squat is an ideal exercise to use the intensity technique of drop sets.

There are, of course, many other training splits you can follow, and we realize your workout schedule needs to accommodate work and other commitments. We feel the every-other-day split is ideal from a physique standpoint, because it offers more in the way of rest and recuperation between workouts, which in turn translates to a higher intensity threshold during training.

For one training situation we suggest modifying the standard push/pull format. If you consider your chest strength to be an area of concern and want to prioritize that bodypart, you can specifically target the chest on its own separate training day.

DAY*	
1 (Monday)	Quads, Hams, Calves, Abs
2	Off
3 (Wednesday)	Chest
4	Off
5 (Friday)	Back, Biceps
6	Off
7	Off
8 (Monday)	Delts, Triceps

*Because this split incorporates four different training days, after Day 8 (Monday of week two) you would repeat Day 1 on Wednesday, Day 3 on Friday and so on.

PRIMARY WORKOUT TRAINING OPTIONS

Instead of doing three or four size- and strength-enhancing sets for each Core Growth exercise in the primary workouts, you can change up the pace with either the multi-poundage principle or the 1-6 method.

MULTI-POUNDAGE PRINCIPLE

This training concept has been successfully used by bodybuilders for decades and is similar to the drop sets technique. You can use it with a number of exercises – the barbell front squat, for example. Begin by warming up for 10 reps with a relatively light weight. After your warm-up, add enough weight so you can complete only one to three reps with proper form. Once you've done those reps, slide a 10-pound plate off each side of the bar and do

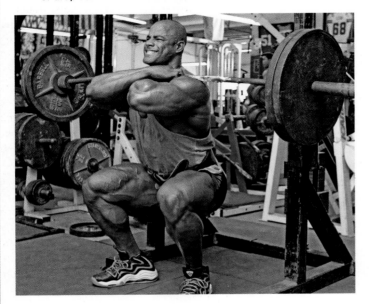

Photo by Paul Buceta
Model Manuel Romero

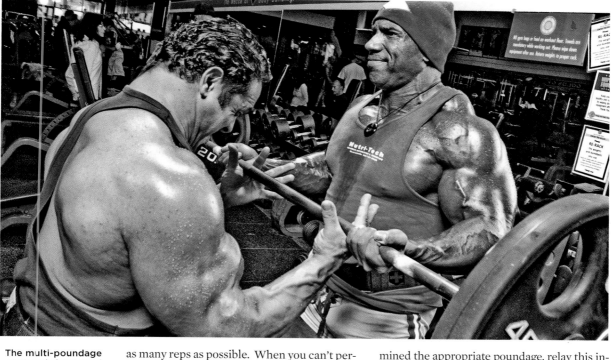

The multi-poundage system is best used with a training partner, as he can quickly offload plates between sets.

Photo by Michael Butler
Models David Hughes and Kevin Reeves

as many reps as possible. When you can't perform another rep, decrease the poundage a second time and rep out to failure again. Continue in this pattern until you have done a total of 25 to 30 reps.

To make this system 100 percent effective, you need a training partner who can remove the weights after each set so you can continue without much rest between sets. Having a spotter or training partner is beneficial for all the primary Core Growth exercises in this program. If a spotter isn't available, you can still use this method if you set up the equipment you'll need beforehand. For example, you could lay all the barbells out for, say, regular barbell curls if you didn't have a partner that day. Of course, this may not be possible if you work out at a busy gym or your space or equipment is limited. (You might also not be very popular if you hoard multiple barbells to yourself!) But if it's a slow day at the gym and there are enough weights, go ahead and put them to use.

Before utilizing this approach, you'll need to experiment and find the correct starting poundage and subsequent weight decreases that work best for you. Once you have deter-

mined the appropriate poundage, relay this information to your partner or set up the equipment ahead of time if you're training solo.

As a rule of thumb, the poundage decreases should be roughly 10 pounds on exercises such as the squat, bench press, deadlift and leg press. Drops of approximately five pounds per set generally work well for movements such as curls, overhead presses and triceps extensions. Note: Remove this weight (ten or five pounds) from each side of the bar.

The obvious advantage of this system is that you will be using maximum poundage for each set of reps, and with very minimal rest periods you will build sustainable strength. After you complete 25 to 30 reps for an exercise, move on to another primary Core Growth movement and perform it in the same fashion.

The following workout log illustrates some sample starting weights and subsequent drops for various exercises. Use this as a guide when determining your ideal weights for each move when incorporating the multi-poundage principle. Keep in mind that your level of ability, body type and exercise order will affect the weights you can handle.

EXERCISE	
Barbell Back Squat	300, 280, 260, 240, 220, 200, 150
	305, 285, 265, 245, 225, 205, 185, 100
	310, 290, 270, 250, 230, 150
Flat-Bench Press	255, 235, 215, 195, 155, 135, 95
	270, 250, 230, 220, 200, 180, 140
	280, 260, 240, 210, 190, 180, 160, 140
Leg Press	330, 280, 230
	350, 330, 280
	370, 350, 280
Barbell Overhead Press	170, 150, 130
	180, 170, 150, 140, 130, 110, 100
	180, 170, 150, 140, 120, 110, 100, 90
Standing Barbell Curl	150, 140, 130, 110, 90, 80, 70
	150, 140, 130, 110, 100, 90
	150, 140, 130, 120, 110, 100, 90

THE 1-6 METHOD

In 1991, strength-training guru Charles Poliquin was introduced to the 1-6 method at the National Strength and Conditioning Association Convention in San Diego. The system is based on a central nervous system phenomenon, or neurological preparedness, first discussed in strength-training circles by a German strength physiologist from the University of Freiburg. With this approach, if you do a six-rep max set within three or four minutes (up to 10 minutes at most) of doing a single-rep max, you can use a greater amount of weight than you could have if you hadn't done the single-rep max. The basic premise is to use maximum loads to potentiate your nervous system. By doing the single-rep max, you increase the efficiency of the central nervous system output, and, as a result, you are able to muster more explosiveness when doing a six-rep max set.

For example, say you can do 225 pounds for six reps on the bench press. You should be able to start with a single-rep max of approximately 270 pounds. This number can be computed using the three-percent rep max formula.

THREE-PERCENT REP MAX FORMULA

Poundage x .03 x number of reps (6) + poundage = one-rep max

So if you use 225 pounds for six reps, you would get this result

225 (poundage) x 0.03 = 6.75 (round upward to 7)

7 x 6 (number of reps) = 42

42 + 225 (poundage) = 267 (round upward to 270)

Using the formula, your next bench-press session might look like this with the 1-6 method. Note: Always do some specific warm-up sets prior to starting the 1-6 method, and always make sure you have a spotter on hand when doing the bench press or back squat.

SET*	
1	One rep with 270 pounds
2	Six reps with 225 pounds
3	One rep with 275 pounds
4	Six reps with 230 pounds
5	One rep with 277.5 pounds
6	Six reps with 235 pounds

*Rest approximately three of four minutes between sets. You can rest up to 10 minutes if necessary.

ADDITIONAL NOTES:

1. If you don't have a spotter on hand, avoid using the 1-6 approach. It cannot be done safely if you are training alone and will put you at risk for injury.
2. Refer to the article "The Mathematics for Determining a Single-Rep Max" for more information on figuring out your maximum weight loads. Visit www.dennisbweis.com.
3. The positive phase of each rep in every set should be completed as quickly as

possible (taking a maximum of two seconds) with perfect motion and precise form (without momentum). The negative phase should be two times slower than the positive portion. (If it takes you two seconds to raise the weight, take four seconds to lower it.)

ECONO-TIME SECONDARY WORKOUT OPTIONS

For this part of the program, instead of doing the four-component set, you can use either of these two techniques: One regular set plus fast doubles or the ten-speed pump.

ONE REGULAR SET PLUS FAST DOUBLES

We'll use the barbell curl as an example. Start out by doing a set of eight to ten reps. When you complete the 10th rep, put the barbell down. Rest for three seconds and then do two more reps. Take another three-second rest before doing two more reps. Rest yet again and then complete a final two reps.

In the secondary workout, you can perform barbell curls with one set plus fast doubles.

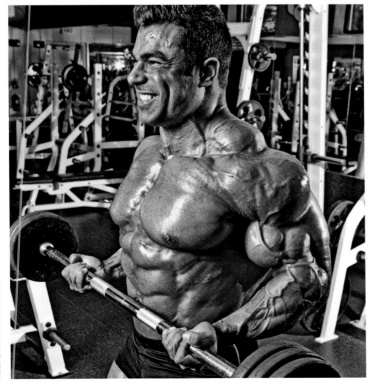

Photo by Paul Buceta
Model Eduardo Correa da Silva

TEN-SPEED PUMP

This advanced training technique was developed years ago by Denie Walter, former prolific sports magazine editor, photojournalist and the IFBB medical and press liaison. If you are going to incorporate this method, keep in mind that it can't be used for calves, abs and bodyweight movements.

The rep-by-rep explanation below outlines the 10 individual modes of specific performance in the standing barbell curl.

Rep 1: Complete one full-range-of-motion contraction with a moderate rep tempo.

Rep 2: Curl over the full range of motion, taking five seconds for the positive phase and five seconds for the negative phase.

Rep 3: Do a quarter-rep, holding at the top for three seconds. Lower your arms to full extension.

Rep 4: Do a half-rep, holding at peak contraction for three seconds. Lower your arms to full extension.

Rep 5: Do a three-quarter rep, holding at the top position for three seconds. Lower to full extension.

From this point, without pausing, reverse the action on the last five reps; now you'll be focusing on the negative (eccentric) portion of the reps.

Rep 6: Complete one full-range-of-motion contraction using a moderate rep speed.

Rep 7: Do one full-range-of-motion contraction, taking five seconds for the positive phase and five seconds for the negative phase.

Rep 8: Curl the bar up through the positive portion of the rep, then lower it one-quarter of the way down. Hold for three seconds and then curl the bar back up to peak contraction.

Rep 9: From the peak contraction of the previous rep, lower it one-half of the way down. Hold for three seconds and then curl back to peak contraction.

Rep 10: From the peak contraction position lower to three-quarters of the way down. Hold for three seconds, curl back to the top position and then slowly lower to full arm extension.

CHAPTER 7

HUGE & FREAKY MUSCLE MASS AND STRENGTH TRAINING SPECIFICS

To make the most gains in size and strength, you need to plot out everything from hand grip all the way to exercise poundage.

This workout program has been purposefully constructed with a basic framework to help you achieve massive gains in size and strength. However, throughout the course of the plan you will want to incorporate elements of variation to keep your momentum going and to further your progress. One way to accomplish these goals is by altering your exercise performance biomechanically.

HAND AND FOOT POSITION

If you are going to experiment with various hand or foot positions, you should limit your adjustments to no more than two inches' change per week. These small changes will help your muscles adapt to the new stress and will prevent injury and joint strain.

HAND SPACING

On barbell exercises you can vary your hand spacing to target the muscles in slightly different ways. Three basic options are a medium hand spacing (about shoulder width), a narrow grip (hands are six inches or less apart) and a wide hand placement (more than shoulder width and, in some cases, collar to collar on a regular exercise bar).

FOOT POSITION

The position of your feet will have importance when you do various forms of the squat and the deadlift. Medium spacing (between 12 and 14

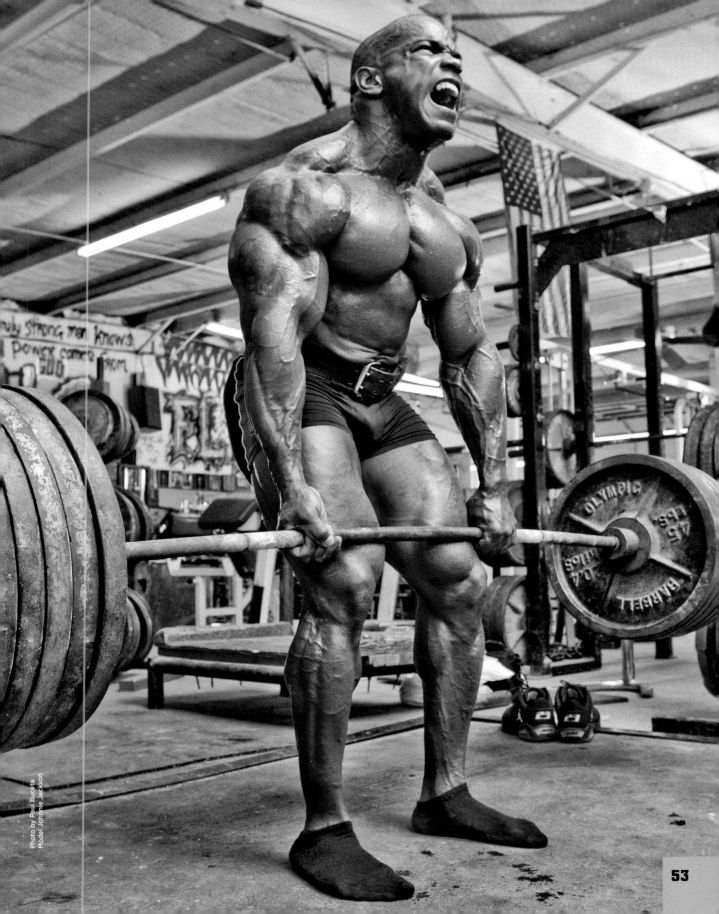

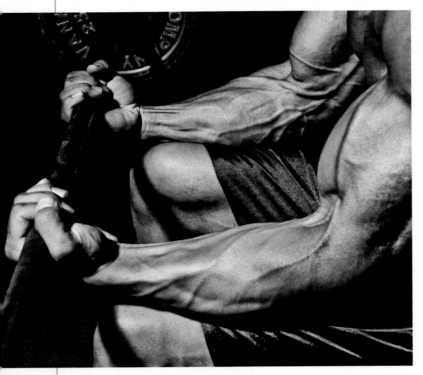

Two of the basic grips are overhand and underhand (shown here); each affects your muscles in a different way.

inches) from heel to heel is optimal for a bodybuilder with large thighs and small hips. A wide foot position (between 16 and 20 inches) is ideal for a bodybuilder who has larger hips and glutes. A narrow foot stance (six inches or less) will place more stress on the quads and hamstrings.

In general, the wider your stance, the farther outward your toes should be pointed. Angle your toes outward at 45 degrees using a 16- to 20-inch foot position. This placement gives more power to the muscles involved and helps you maintain balance.

HAND GRIP

The standard method is to place your thumbs around the bar and use either an overhand or underhand grip (or a mixed grip in which you use an underhand grip for one hand and an overhand grip for the other). If you want to develop a better grip on your deadlifts, you can use an overhand grip, wrapping your thumbs around the bar.

Another alternative you can try is the hook grip: You first grip the bar with your thumbs, but with this variation, you then wrap your

other fingers around the bar and overtop of your thumbs (instead of your thumbs overlapping your fingers). Some bodybuilders find this grip painful, but it will help with your grip strength when performing exercises such as deadlifts, barbell shrugs and pull-ups.

The thumbless grip (also called an open or false grip), where your thumbs are on the same side of the bar as the rest of your fingers, is a good variation for certain movements such as the palms-up wrist curl. It can also be used for triceps pushdown-type exercises and even the flat or incline bench press. This method relieves pressure and strain on the wrists and forearms, and the biomechanics of the grip will activate the triceps muscles at the back of your upper arms. The open grip generally isn't recommended for exercises such as the bench press, as the bar could more easily slip out of your hands.

Some strength experts believe the triceps account for 75 percent of an individual's bench press strength. When using the thumbless grip on the bench press, you are more at risk, as the bar can very easily roll out of your hands. So unless you have a capable spotter who can anticipate this situation, you should avoid this grip when bench pressing.

EXERCISE STARTING POINTS

Standard exercises such as the ones in this program can often be performed using a slightly different version: Standing, seated, lying, bent over, kneeling, and on an incline or decline. By incorporating different body positions you will work your muscles from various angles, therefore targeting more muscle fibers than you would if you used only one version of a particular movement.

When doing dumbbell, cable or certain machine exercises, you can switch up your routine by sometimes working unilaterally (one arm at a time) and other times using both arms simultaneously. The benefits of including unilateral training in your regimen include better muscle isolation, increased range of motion, built-in rest (for your nonworking limb), improved symmetry and stronger neuromuscular pathways.

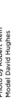

Photo by Robert Reiff
Model David Hughes

EXERCISE EQUIPMENT

Exercises involving a barbell (e.g., barbell curl) can generally be modified so you can replace that equipment with a different type of bar or dumbbells. You can better stimulate your muscles by regularly using a variety of training apparatus in your workouts. For example, switch to a cambered squat bar instead of using a straight bar for squatting. For your lat movements you might use a chinning V-bar in the place of a lat pulldown. On arms, you might choose an EZ-curl bar rather than a straight bar. Most commercial gyms offer a wide selection of weightlifting equipment or, if you can afford it, you can purchase an array of home gym equipment.

During weight training, make sure to focus on breathing through your mouth, not your nose.

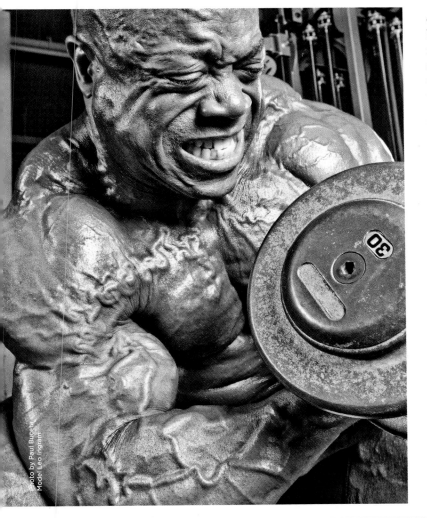

Photo by Paul Buceta
Model Leo Ingram

BREATHING PATTERNS

When performing the primary workout Core Growth exercises you should inhale with short, quick gasps of air between reps to build a reservoir of oxygen in the blood. Taking rapid breaths will also help you to quickly shift your mental focus back as you start each rep.

Always breathe through your mouth rather than your nose. This will allow more oxygen to reach your lungs. When you inhale, hold the air in your lungs as you begin each repetition. Then, start exhaling two-thirds of the way through the positive portion of the movement to relieve intrathoracic, or abdominal, pressure. Exhale fully when you reach lockout or the fully contracted position of the rep.

Never hold your breath for prolonged periods during training because doing so will impede blood flow. A backup of blood will cause too much pressure within the veins, which can result in dizziness or fainting from lack of oxygen. On secondary workout exercises, breathe rhythmically to the tempo of the movement pattern.

TRAINING POUNDAGE

You will find as you progress with your weightlifting that increasing training poundage can sometimes be a monumental task. The addition of even the smallest conventional barbell plate (1¼ pounds) to each side of a dumbbell or barbell can prove to be more difficult than you anticipated.

Some bodybuilders overcome this obstacle by adding one flat washer to each side of the bar in every workout. Although the process may be slower because the washers weigh just ounces, you will eventually work up to that seemingly impossible 1¼-pound increase on each side of the bar. You can purchase these flat washers at your local hardware store. Be sure to have a sales associate weigh one for you, so you will know how many you need to buy to make 2½ pounds (1¼ on each side).

Understanding these training specifics will help you go into each workout with the knowledge of how to get the most out of your session. By putting these recommendations into practice, you will maximize your potential for muscle growth and strength improvements.

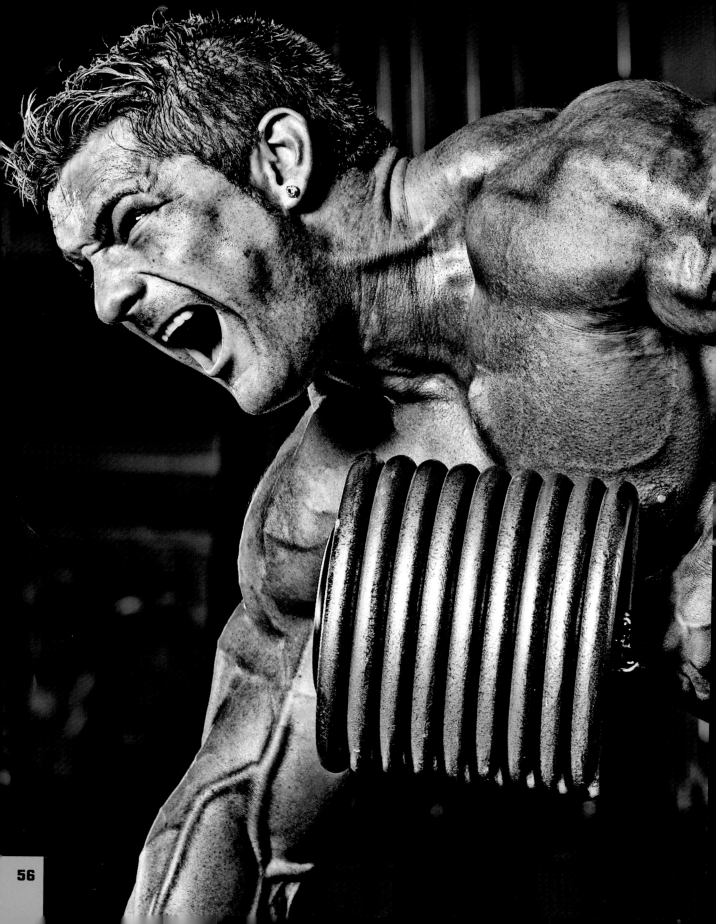

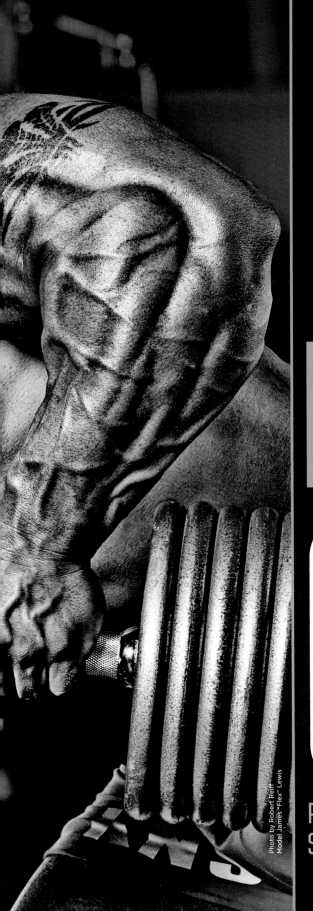

BOOK
02

Powerful Nutrition and
Supplementation Tactics

CHAPTER 8

PHASE 2: MUSCLE GAIN NUTRITIONAL PROGRAM OVERVIEW

While every bodybuilder has different individual nutritional needs, diet is a key part of the equation for anyone trying to gain mass and improve strength.

During your training career many of you have probably heard that "putting on muscle mass is at least 80 percent nutrition." If that statement is true, then intense workouts and heavy iron account for only 20 percent. Can this breakdown be accurate?

Larry Scott, the pioneer Mr. Olympia title holder, was probably the first pro bodybuilder who quoted this idea. Think about it this way: If nutrition really did constitute 80 percent of the muscle mass equation, why would anyone focus on regularly training hard when they could just chug a ton of creatine shakes every day? There are likely some naive rookie bodybuilders who have fallen victim to this type of thinking. When Larry said 80 percent, he did not mean it literally. His intention was to pick a figure sufficiently large that it would emphasize just how important proper nutrition is to building muscle – when combined with intense training. He and others who place a high value on their meal plans are in no way overlooking the importance of hard training. Leo Costa Jr. confirmed Larry Scott's point when he said: "Get the awesome muscle-building results of (anabolic) steroids ... with (nutrient-dense) food instead of drugs!"

In Book One we touched on the fact that every bodybuilder is different from every other, physiologically and metabolically. Some have a more difficult time finding a diet that works because their metabolic system interferes with the proper assimilation and use of food (nutrients) in the muscle-building process. Others have body chemistries prone to nutrient deficiencies or digestive issues that prevent proper

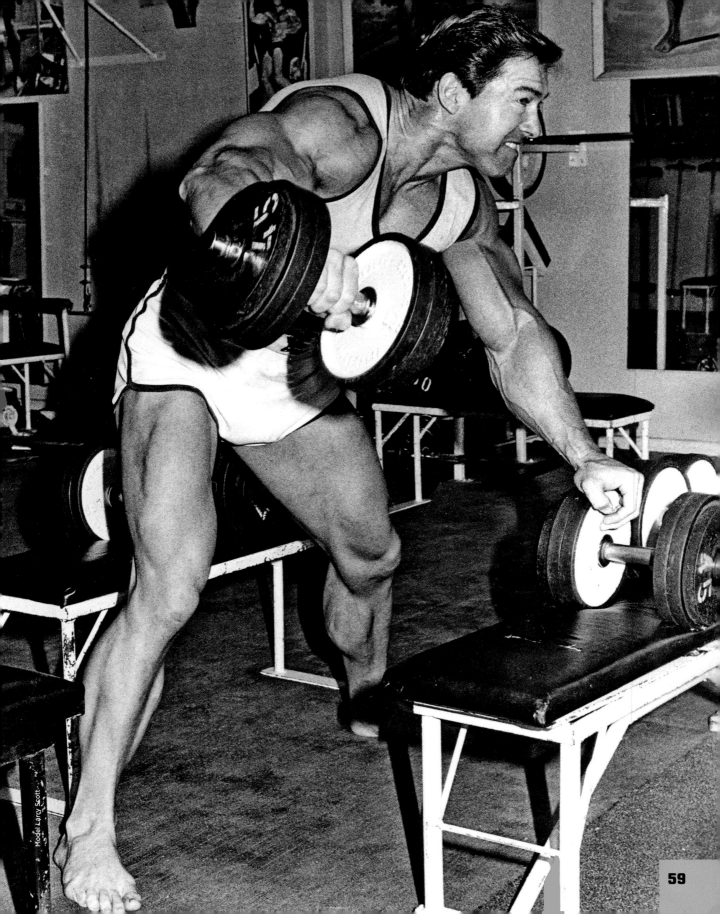

Model Larry Scott

absorption of key minerals and vitamins. Also, certain trainers do not take the time to devise a solid nutritional program and end up taking in the wrong quantities of foods or too many empty calories. Without proper meal planning specific to your body type and individual needs, you won't be able to reach your full muscle growth potential.

All of the top champions in competitive bodybuilding recognize the benefits associated with having Herculean muscle mass and power because those two traits coincide with gains in muscular bodyweight, measurements, strength and endurance. At this point, you may still be wondering whether adding huge and freaky muscle mass is good for your physique. Many bodybuilders, both pro and amateur, devote all their efforts to getting bigger and stronger as a strategy to be more competitive on bodybuilding stages. For example, Bill Pearl was beaten in the 1956 NABBA Mr. Universe by Jack Delinger. Shortly after this narrow defeat Bill decided to take his physique to a new level, and he did so by increasing his muscular bodyweight to 255 pounds. At his new bodyweight he had a 55-inch chest, a 60-inch shoulder circumference and 21-inch upper arms. Our good friend the late John Grimek, who was never defeated in any amateur or professional bodybuilding contest he entered, once increased his bodyweight to 250 pounds at a height of only 5'8½".

Some of the top physique champions from the '50s and '60s went to great extremes nutritionally to gain superior muscle mass (remember, this was before such a wide array of supplements and ergogenic enhancement was available). Bruce Randall, a former Mr. Universe winner, once reached a bodyweight of 400 pounds by following drastic dietary measures such as drinking eight to ten quarts of milk per day (claims have also been made that in one instance he actually drank 19 quarts of milk), 12 to 18 eggs each day, along with seven pounds of meat daily. Bruce's typical weight was around 220, but he gained this monstrous amount as a means to try and break some of Paul Anderson's lifting records. One of the ways he packed on so much mass was scoop

feeding (aka, the shovel method) where a bodybuilder gorges himself with gargantuan quantities of protein and other food calories in an effort to fuel remarkable growth and muscle gains. We do not recommend this approach, as it can be dangerous to your long-term and overall health, not to mention counterproductive to your physique goals.

NUTRITION PROGRAM OVERVIEW

Many individuals who train hard regularly, especially those with an ectomorph body type, will need to consume a minimum of 10 calories per pound of bodyweight just to meet their daily basal metabolic requirements. These trainers then need to consume additional calories based on daily activities (i.e., household tasks, walking, any task that requires movement) and focused exercise (i.e., weightlifting, jogging, cycling). If your day-to-day lifestyle is fairly busy and you train regularly, you will need to take in roughly an additional 10 calories per pound of bodyweight. For example, an individual who weighs 200 pounds, is moderately active throughout his daily life and who performs intense workouts routinely will need to consume approximately 4,000 calories a day just to maintain his weight (200 [weight] x 20 [10 calories for basal metabolic needs and 10 calories for activity level] = 4,000).

Your general goal should be to gain a half-pound to two pounds of muscle mass each week. To accomplish this weight increase you will need to gradually consume an extra 1,000 to 1,500 quality calories a day above your basal metabolic and activity exertion requirements. This additional caloric intake will promote faster muscle gains. A good strategy to ensure you're getting all the nutrients you need is to consume a total of five or six calorie-dense whole-food meals and muscle mass shakes each day. At first this may seem like a lot of surplus calories, but this amount is necessary to provide your body with the proper nutrition needed to facilitate muscle growth. You should try to eat every two-and-a-half or three hours. By doing so you will induce your body to continuously release insulin, which is important to

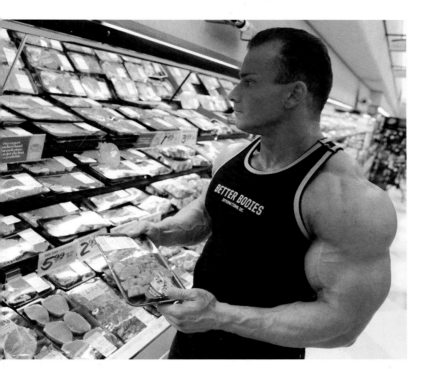

In general, you should aim to take in approximately 1.5 grams of protein for every pound of bodyweight each day.

growth because it transports amino acids into the muscle and keeps your body in a positive anabolic state. If possible, you should schedule your meals at the same times each day, as this will help your metabolic and digestive systems function optimally.

In the next chapter we outline a sample schedule for meal frequency and type (solid or liquid) throughout the day. The example provided is intended to be used as a guideline because, as we've discussed, your body has a unique set of dietary responses. Many bodybuilders will do well with a daily macronutrient calorie breakdown of 50 percent complete protein, 30 percent complex carbs and 20 percent fats. Others may find a different ratio works better for them. You will also have to adjust your serving sizes in order to meet your indi-

vidual macronutrient needs. Use your body and a mirror as your main guides – if you aren't happy with how you feel or what you're seeing in the mirror each week, make minor adjustments to your nutrient ratio and serving sizes until you find what works best for your body. A good secondary reference for determining appropriate serving sizes comes from Emeric Delczeg (an IFBB pro bodybuilder). Information on the Delczeg Training System can be found on the Internet or in his book, *The Delczeg Training System*.

To encourage muscle growth and strength gains you need to ingest sufficient amounts of high-quality protein along with enough complex carbs to fuel heavy and intense workouts. You should aim to take in 1.5 to 2 grams of protein per pound of bodyweight and 2 to 3 grams of carbs per pound of bodyweight each day. Pay attention to your body and how it responds to the ratio of protein and carbs you are eating – your individual needs will vary slightly, but we generally recommend closer to 2 grams of protein and closer to 2 grams of carbs per pound of bodyweight as a baseline.

Your dietary fat intake should account for no more than 20 percent of your total daily calories. When you are working toward adding lean mass, you should spread your intake of fats over the course of the day, consuming fats with each meal and snack because this macronutrient can be used as a long-lasting energy source. Energy is essential if creating gigantic muscles is your goal

The chart on the left includes a macronutrient formula designed by Gary Taylor, a former World's Strongest Man winner. Use this chart when devising your nutrition plan.

Always keep a daily food log to track the calories you consume in the form of proteins, carbs and fats. By logging your food intake you provide yourself with an accurate snapshot and ongoing reference guide of your nutrition. These notes are invaluable when figuring out the best macronutrient formula for your goals and personal needs. Since you can see everything laid out before you, you can easily see where you might need to make minor adjustments to your meal plans.

MACRO NUTRIENTS	MAINTAIN BODYWEIGHT	GAIN LEAN MUSCLE MASS
Complex Carbohydrates	8 grams per kilo of bodyweight	10 grams per kilo of bodyweight
Complete Proteins	2 grams per kilo of bodyweight	2.5 grams per kilo of bodyweight
Mono-Unsaturated Fats	0.65 grams per kilo of bodyweight	0.8 grams per kilo of bodyweight
To compute your bodyweight into kilos divide your weight in pounds by 2.2		

CHAPTER 9

MUSCLE MEAL BASICS: WHOLE FOODS & SHAKES

Consuming the right muscle-building foods at optimal intervals, five to six times a day, will have a major positive impact on your physique.

Eating five or six meals a day, every two or three hours, will help you get all the calories you need to add a substantial amount of muscle growth spread out evenly throughout the day. For example, six meals at 900 calories each would be easier to eat and digest than three larger meals of 1,800 calories each. By splitting the calories over several smaller meals you won't overload your digestive system and you'll provide a steady flow of nutrients into your body. Smaller meals will also limit indigestion, feelings of being overfull and stomach distention. No matter what your physique goals (lose fat, add lean mass, etc.) you should aim to eat six meals per day. You can adjust the fat, protein and carbs in each meal to fit your daily caloric needs and to consume the correct ratios depending on what you're trying to achieve with your body and muscle.

MEAL GUIDELINES
BREAKFAST

Taking the time to eat a quality breakfast each morning is crucial if you want to improve your physique. Bodybuilders and all athletes who train hard understand the importance of consuming a proper breakfast every day. When you subject your body to regular intense workouts, you need to replenish yourself with the nutrients necessary to support recovery and fuel growth. Starting your day without a nutritionally adequate breakfast would be like trying to drive your car on a long trip with only

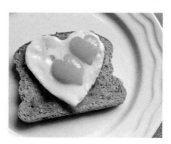

one gallon of gas in the tank – you will get a few miles, but the gas will run out before you get very far. If you begin your day with a poor breakfast, or worse, no breakfast, you won't give yourself enough energy to carry out the tasks ahead (i.e., high-intensity training) and your body will slip into a catabolic, or muscle-wasting, state.

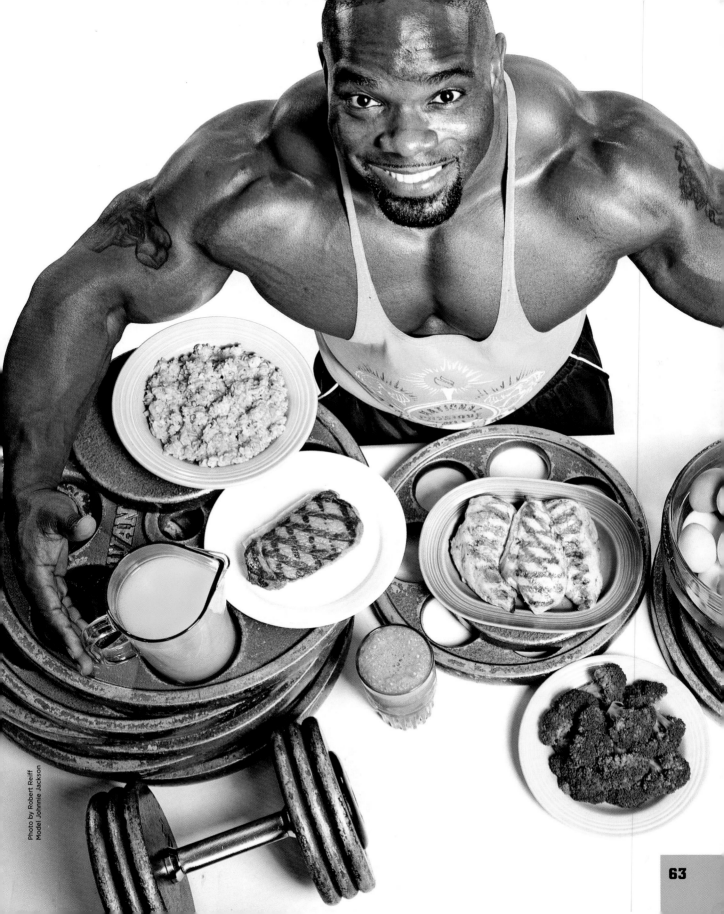

Here are some ideas for quality whole-food breakfasts:

OPTION 1

- 1 cup fresh-squeezed orange juice
- ½ cup whole-grain cereal (or oatmeal) with milk
- Omelet made with 5 eggs, 4 oz. lean beef patty, 2 cups nonfat dry milk and ¼ cup grated cheese

Note: If you are still hungry, have one slice of whole-wheat toast or twelve-grain bread with one to two tablespoons of natural peanut butter.

OPTION 2

- Omelet with 4 to 6 eggs, ¼ cup grated cheese, ¾ cup chopped tomatoes
- 1 whole papaya
- Chopped fresh pineapple
- 1 cup (dry measurement) three-grain cereal (brown rice, buckwheat and millet) with a pat of butter

Method: To make the cereal, add water and bring to a boil then let simmer for 10 minutes. Remove from heat and let stand until the extra moisture is absorbed. Add a pat of butter and you're ready for a delicious and healthy meal.

OPTION 3

- Fresh strawberries topped with certified raw cream and a dash of honey
- 4 to 5 whole eggs, scrambled in 1 tablespoon raw butter
- 1 or 2 slices whole-grain bread with natural peanut butter

OPTION 4
PROTEIN POWER PANCAKES

- 1 cup whole-wheat flour
- 1¼ cups milk
- 1½ cups whey protein powder
- 2 whole eggs
- 2 tablespoons cooking oil
- 2 tablespoons honey
- 1½ teaspoons baking powder
- ½ teaspoon sea salt
- Cooking spray

Method: Sift the dry ingredients. Add remaining ingredients and beat until batter is smooth. Thin with more milk, if necessary. Heat griddle to medium and lightly coat with cooking spray. Use a large spoon or ladle to pour the batter onto griddle. When edges are dry and the top begins to bubble, flip and cook the other side for approximately two minutes. Makes about twelve pancakes.

A healthy spin on the traditional pancake, this version is loaded with protein.

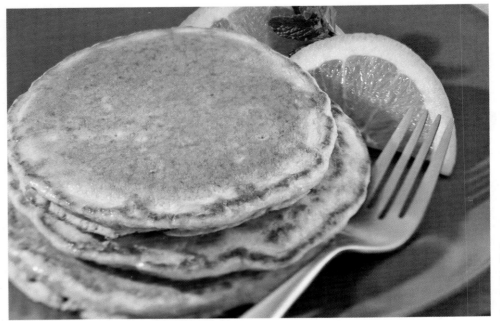

Photo by Michael Butler

Shakes are a good option when you're short on time.

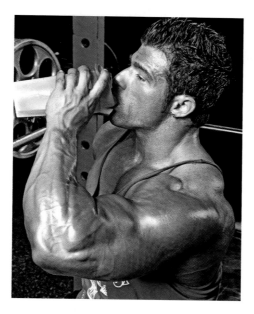

OPTION 5
SLOW-COOKED OATMEAL

To boost the protein and up the calcium content, cook your oatmeal with milk instead of water. About five minutes before the full cooking time add a half-cup of diced dates and one cup of cream. Stir in honey, one tablespoon of safflower oil and raw embryo wheat germ flakes. You can also spice up the oatmeal with nutmeg or cinnamon.

Tip: You can mix in a scoop of your favorite meal-replacement or protein powder to boost the protein content. You can also add fresh fruit or nuts of your choice.

OPTION 6
WHOLE (LONG-GRAIN) BROWN RICE

Cook as per the package directions. About five minutes before the full cooking time, stir in a half-cup of raisins and a half-cup of milk. Mix in some honey and wheat germ.

OPTION 7

- 1 large banana, sliced
- ½ cup chopped dates
- ½ cup raisins and figs
- Honey and plain yogurt

Method: Mix all ingredients together in a bowl.

OPTION 8

- 8 to 12 egg whites
- 2 cups oatmeal or grits (with honey, if desired)
- 2 scoops whey protein powder mixed with water

OPTION 9
GRAB-AND-GO SHAKE

Finding time to cook, sit down and eat a nutritious breakfast can be difficult, especially if you are rushed or tight for time in the morning. If you run out the door with nothing in your stomach, you immediately undermine your potential bodybuilding gains. If you find you're strapped for time in the morning, the best and fastest solution is to consume a protein or muscle mass shake. Here's a recipe for a hearty shake to start your day off right:

- 1 or 2 cups milk
- 2 raw eggs
- 2 scoops whey protein
- ½ banana
- 1 teaspoon honey
- 1 scoop natural ice cream
- Ice cubes (optional)

Method: Blend all ingredients on low speed until thoroughly mixed. For variety you can add flavorings such as extracts of coconut, banana, strawberry, etc.

If you are concerned about consuming raw eggs, boil them in the shell for about one minute before cracking and putting them in the blender.

OPTION 10
GRAB-AND-GO EGGS

Here's a quick grab-and-go solid breakfast that can be cooked in the microwave in just a few minutes.

- 2 or 3 whole eggs
- 1/3 cup milk
- 3 oz. cheese, grated
- 6 oz. sliced turkey breast, chopped into pieces

Method: Crack eggs into a bowl and whisk with milk. Place in microwave and cook for approximately three minutes, stopping the microwave every minute to beat the egg mix-

Photo by Robert Reiff
Model Tony Breznik

ture. When the eggs begin to fluff up, stop the cooking process and add the cheese and turkey pieces. Mix with a fork and continue cooking until the eggs are fully cooked (no remaining liquid and can be fluffed with a fork) and the cheese melted. Add pepper and any other seasonings to taste.

Tip: No matter what type of microwave egg recipe you use, always whip the raw eggs with a fork or whisk first. If you cook an egg in the microwave with the yolk and white still intact, it can explode under the heat.

MID-MORNING SNACK (TWO OR THREE HOURS AFTER BREAKFAST)

When you are attempting to add huge amounts of muscle mass and make appreciable strength gains, it is crucial that you never skip a meal or snack, even if you don't feel hungry at your scheduled time to eat.

If you haven't prepared a snack ahead of time, or you don't have access to high-quality whole-food snacks, a good alternative option is a protein shake. Here are three very popular and healthy muscle mass shake recipes:

AUSTRALIAN WEIGHT-GAIN DRINK

This eight-ingredient weight-gain shake, containing approximately 150 grams of complete protein (the recipe makes almost a gallon – store unused portion in fridge for a quick shake later), was created by the famous Australian bodybuilder Wayne Gallasch.

- ¼ cup natural honey
- Pure vanilla extract, to taste
- ½ cup safflower oil
- ¾ cup ovaltine
- 1 or 2 egg whites
- ½ cup brewer's yeast powder
- 1 cup whey protein powder
- 3 cups skim milk powder

Note: The various ingredients are measured by rough volume using a normal-sized tea cup, with one cup being roughly level with the top.

Mix the ingredients in a large bowl with a hand blender in the order listed, adding cold water as the mixture thickens until you have ap-

proximately three-and-a-half pints of liquid. To thicken the shake or add a bit more fat, you can add milk, yogurt, natural (sugarless) ice cream, powdered egg white, Knox gelatin or malt.

Store the shake in the refrigerator until you're ready to drink it. Make sure to stir well or re-blend before pouring a serving, as the ingredients tend to separate when sitting for a while. If you want to take some of this shake to go, use a stainless steel or other insulated thermos to keep the drink cool until your scheduled snack time.

Tip: This drink has a sweet, pleasant but very rich taste. Because of its thick consistency, you may want to have water on hand to wash it down with.

Wayne claimed that consuming two quarts of this drink over the course of one day would put additional bodyweight on all body types, even hard-gaining ectomorphs.

SERIOUS GROWTH MUSCLE MASS SHAKE

- 1½ cups whole milk
- 1 banana
- 4 strawberries
- 1 scoop of ice cream or flavored yogurt
- 3 scoops protein powder
- 1 tablespoon brewer's yeast

Note: Blend milk, banana, strawberries and ice cream/yogurt in a blender. Pour the protein and yeast into the center of the mixture. (This will keep the powdered ingredients from caking on the sides of the blender.)

VINCE GIRONDA'S EURO-BLAST MUSCLE MASS DRINK SECRET

In the 1960s Vince Gironda, the Iron Guru, revealed a secret to North American trainers that European muscle monsters had been using for years to gain muscle density. Vince began having his students use this secret food as a strategy to help them increase their bodyweight and muscle.

Though it may sound unorthodox or slightly unappetizing, the secret strategy used by the European athletes was simply drinking eight ounces of half-and-half or certified raw cream mixed with eight ounces of ginger ale. To trig-

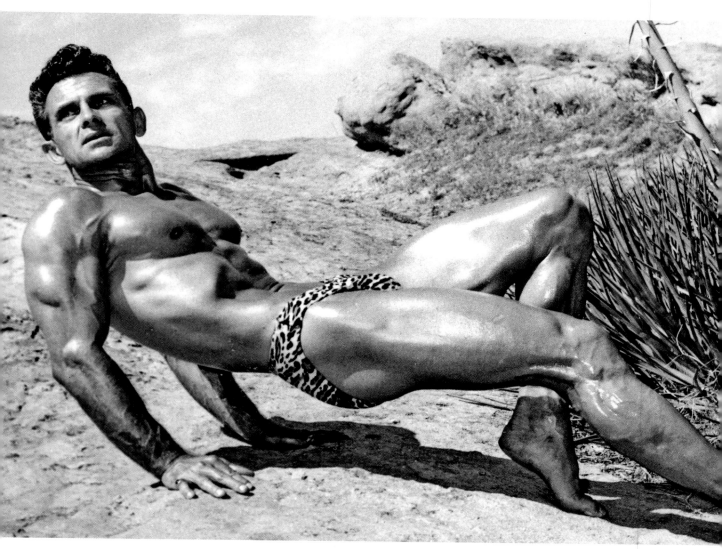

Vince Gironda certainly knew a thing or two about bodybuilding nutrition.

Model Vince Gironda

ger further anabolism in the body, Vince would sometimes advise his followers to add two tablespoons of a milk-and- egg protein powder.

The students at Vince's Gym in Ventura, California, consumed this drink as a daily between-meal pickup at 10 a.m., 2 p.m. and 4 p.m.

DAIRY AND MILK PRODUCTS

Some of the muscle mass meals and shakes in this chapter contain milk and other dairy ingredients. Milk is a popular food source among many bodybuilders because it contains all the essential amino acids and it mixes well with other ingredients to make tasty, nutritious pro-

tein shakes. Milk has an assimilability ratio of 60 to 90 percent, depending on whether it is pasteurized or raw. Raw milk has the highest assimilability ratio.

Some individuals, however, have a hard time enjoying the benefits of dairy products because of lactose intolerance. This condition can cause bloating, gas, diarrhea and stomach pains from an inability to digest the sugar lactose. If this is a health issue you're facing, you don't have to avoid dairy altogether. Two alternative options are purchasing an over-the-counter lactose enzyme (which helps you digest the lactose in milk), or you can find lactose-re-

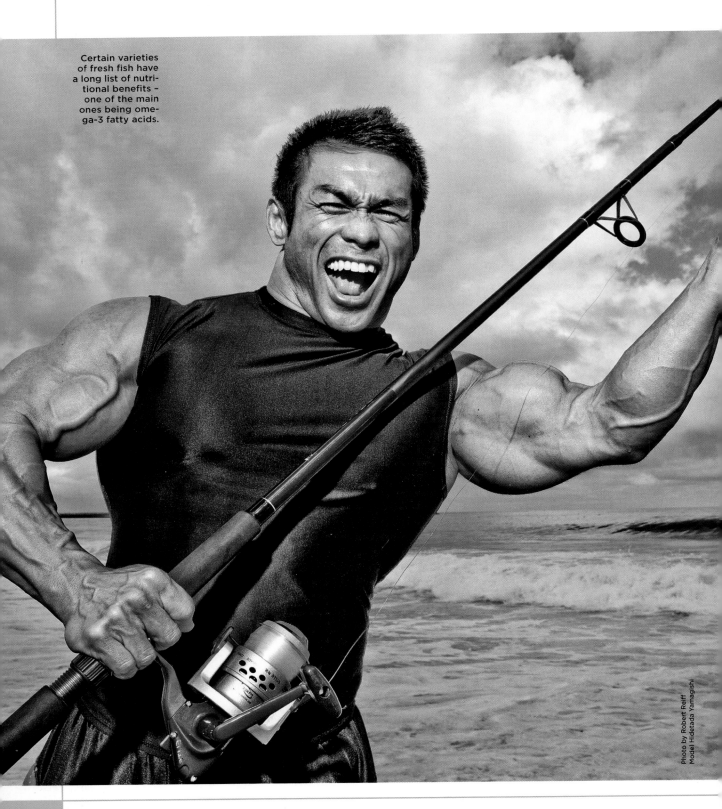

Certain varieties of fresh fish have a long list of nutritional benefits – one of the main ones being omega-3 fatty acids.

Photo by Robert Reiff
Model Hidetada Yamagishi

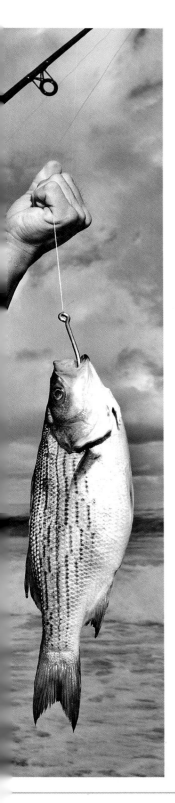

duced or lactose-free products in the dairy section in your grocery store. Whenever you are drinking milk, keep in mind that it is meant to be sipped, not chugged. A general rule of thumb is to consume one glass over a half-hour period. This recommendation may sound surprising, but when milk is consumed quickly or gulped down, the fat content gets digested poorly. Also, when using milk in a protein drink, avoid mixing it in a blender. Instead, blend the milk using a shaker container or simply stir in the milk with a spoon. If you must use a blender for a recipe with milk in it, blend the mixture with short bursts of power. If you do not have any intolerance or negative reactions to milk products, while on this mass-building program consider drinking one quart per day for two weeks, then increase to two quarts a day for another two weeks, then three quarts for two weeks and finally four quarts maximum per day. When you're shopping for milk at the supermarket, look for the freshest products – chemical reactions in milk take place quite rapidly. After a cow is milked, 10 percent of the vitamin A and 40 percent of the B-complex vitamin content in raw milk is destroyed within 24 hours. Pasteurization, oxygen and other environmental factors negatively affect many of the vitamins and protein in milk.

You'll notice that many of the shake recipes you come across when on a muscle-and-strength diet include powdered milk. Here's a little-known secret about how to get maximum flavor from it: The scientist who developed powdered milk decades ago went on record and suggested that a person should mix the milk at least four hours prior to use. Doing so evidently allows the flavor to develop maximally and the milk protein sufficient time to dehydrate.

LUNCH (TWO HOURS AFTER SNACK)

OPTION 1

- ½ pound fresh fish
- Tossed green salad
- 2 hard-boiled eggs
- 1 orange

OPTION 2

- 1 cup low-fat cottage cheese
- 1 omelet (made with two or three eggs, ¼ cup shredded cheese, chopped onions and tomatoes)
- 1 fresh vegetable (e.g., carrots, broccoli, celery) or 1 slice watermelon
- 1 cup apple juice

OPTION 3

- 2 orange roughy fillets, baked
- 1 or 2 cups pasta, cooked (plain or with a low-fat sauce)
- Fresh green salad (you can use low-fat dressing or lemon juice)

MID-AFTERNOON SNACK (TWO TO THREE HOURS AFTER LUNCH)

- 1 cheese or meat sandwich on whole-wheat bread
- 1 muscle mass shake (choose from mid-morning recipes)

DINNER (TWO TO THREE HOURS AFTER SNACK)

OPTION 1

G.L.O.P. MEAL

Steve Henneberry, who starred as "Tower" on "American Gladiators" (1991 to 1994), goes for peak performance in the kitchen by preparing one-step high-protein meals. One of his all-time favorites is called G.L.O.P. (Get Lots of Protein).

- 16 oz. fat-free ground turkey breast
- 2 packages boil-in-bag instant long-grain brown rice (e.g., Kraft, Uncle Ben's)
- 16-oz. jar picante sauce (mild, medium or hot)
- 8 oz. low-fat cottage cheese (small curd)
- Non-stick cooking spray (optional)

Note: Lightly coat the surface of a large skillet with cooking spray and place over a medium-high flame. Add ground turkey to skillet and cook until meat is no longer pink (about five minutes), stirring occasionally with a wooden spoon. Be careful not to overcook the meat, as it can lose moisture and become rubbery. Once the meat is browned, stir in the picante sauce. Turn heat to low and let simmer so the turkey picks up the flavor of the sauce.

While the meat and sauce are simmering, prepare rice according to package directions.

Remove meat mixture from skillet and scoop into a large glass mixing bowl. Add cooked rice and cottage cheese. Stir lightly just until combined and serve. Any leftover portions can be stored in a sealable container in the refrigerator for a couple of days.

Tips: G.L.O.P tastes as good cold as when just cooked, so it makes a good high-protein cooler meal on the go.

- You can make a shake while you are waiting for the turkey and rice to finish cooking. Pour two cups of cold distilled water (not spring or ionized) into a blender. Add one packet of meal replacement powder and two packages of sweetener. Blend contents (adding ice cubes, if desired) for approximately 45 seconds.
- You can use a wok instead of a skillet to cook the meal. Also, consider using a rice steamer/cooker for brown rice.

OPTION 2
DOC TILNEY'S MUSCLE-BUILDING NUT LOAF

If you are looking for a new recipe to try, Doc Tilney's nut loaf might be just the ticket. Though you won't recognize his name from pro bodybuilding, Doc was a good friend of those in the iron game. He was a famous lecturer and author on physical culture, and over the span of his life he wrote hundreds of articles on exercise and nutrition for the Weider publications and numerous other bodybuilding magazines. In addition to the articles, he authored several books, including *Young at 73* and a nutrition textbook for Oregon State University. Earlier in his life, Doc Tilney formed a partnership with Charles Atlas and wrote the famous Atlas course plus the dynamic ads and sales materials associated with it.

Doc Tilney rubbed shoulders with many elite members of the bodybuilding community and there was always an open invitation to stop off at the Tilney home for a nutritious dinner of Doc's famous nut loaf. This meal is tasty and hearty whether you are a meat eater or vegetarian. The recipe serves four or five people.

- 1 onion, chopped
- 1 cup American or cheddar cheese
- 1 cup shelled walnuts or pecans
- 2 cups whole-wheat, pumpernickel or rye bread crumbs (or a package of Pepperidge Farm Stuffing)
- 1 can Campbell's tomato soup
- 1 egg
- Milk (sufficient amount to make a thick, creamy batter)

Note: If you add too much milk, the loaf will be soft inside. If the oven temperature is too hot, the top and bottom crust will end up too thick.

Preheat the oven to 400 degrees F. Put the onion, cheese, nuts and finally the bread crumbs through a food processor in that order (you can also use a blender or meat grinder). In a bowl, mix together the blended ingredients with the tomato soup, egg and milk (add milk gradually until the batter is smooth). Pour batter into a glass baking dish. Cut thin slices of cheese and place on top of the batter. Bake for 45 minutes to one hour, until the loaf is golden brown. You can also place baking potatoes in the oven alongside the loaf to cook at the same time. Cook up some fresh or frozen peas, green beans, broccoli or other green vegetable to serve alongside.

Bodybuilding champions from years ago such as John Grimek, Reg Park and Charles Atlas have enjoyed this nut loaf at Doc Tilney's home. Many bodybuilders have asked for this recipe, and now you have it, too!

OPTION 3

- 6 oz. serving of chicken, fish or steak
- Large tossed green salad (alfalfa sprouts, sliced cucumbers, lettuce and radishes sprinkled with sesame seeds and sunflower seeds, topped with a mixture of lemon juice, olive oil and vinegar)
- 1 baked potato or 1 cup brown rice

OPTION 4

- 8 oz. ground beef patty or 6 oz. liver
- 1 glass tomato juice
- 1 or 2 pieces cheese (cheddar or other natural cheese)

- 1 piece fruit (1 cantaloupe or 1 banana, sliced), with cream poured over and a drizzle of honey

OPTION 5

- 2 skinless chicken breasts
- 1 cup brown rice
- 1 banana

OPTION 6

- 6 oz. turkey breast
- 2 sweet potatoes
- mass-builder shake

Trial and error with your diet plan is necessary to figure out what foods and nutrients ratios work best to keep bodyfat low.

OPTION 7

- 8 to 12 egg whites
- 1 skinless chicken breast
- 1 baked potato

BEDTIME SNACK (TWO OR THREE HOURS AFTER DINNER)

- 3 or 4 slices cheese, 1 or 2 pieces fresh fruit or 2 cups air-popped popcorn

Note: Make sure to go easy on the salt for the popcorn. For an extra treat, lightly sprinkle on some Parmesan cheese. You can also have a glass of grapefruit juice to wash down your popcorn.

Tip: Have a large bowl of soup with at least one of your daily meals; varieties like black bean, lentil, split pea or other mixed bean type are a great way to add some extra fiber to your diet. Top your soup with a spoonful of cream or raw wheat germ flakes.

If you want to try out some new, innovative recipes, check out www.trulyhuge.com for a good cooking resource for bodybuilders.

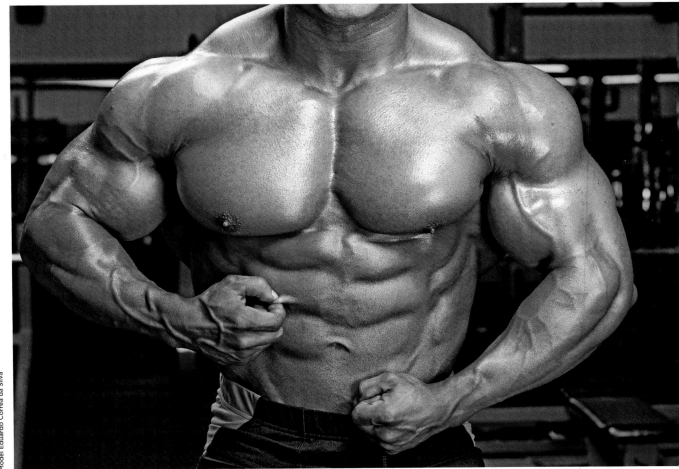

Photo by Kevin Horton
Model Eduardo Correa da Silva

CHAPTER 10

ELEVEN SUPERFOODS

Typical grocery stores house thousands upon thousands of food items, but there are a certain few that absolutely need to be in your grocery cart.

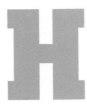ere's a quick, aisle-by-aisle, grocery store tour of what the majority of amateur and professional bodybuilders consider the 11 superfoods for getting huge and freaky muscle mass and strength.

1. BANANAS

Bananas are one of America's most popular fruits. They taste great, are easy to eat and they're available year round. Bananas contain 23 grams of carbohydrates per 3 ½ ounces and have a low amount of protein with less than 1 gram of fat. They contain healthy amounts of potassium, vitamin B6, vitamin C and magnesium.

2. BEANS

Beans are almost 25 percent protein and contain nearly no fat. They are very high in vitamin B6 and B12, potassium, zinc, calcium, iron and magnesium. Beans are also a great source of carbohydrates, are digested very slowly and provide you with a steady stream of energy throughout the day.

3. BROCCOLI

Broccoli contains about 30 calories, 1 gram of fat, 5 grams of carbohydrates and 3 grams of protein per 3 ½ ounce serving. It also contains vitamin C, calcium, folate, vitamin B6, manganese, potassium and beta-carotene.

4. CARROTS

Carrots are good for your eyesight since they're very high in vitamin A, which is responsible for proper functioning of the retina. They contain very little fat and a modest amount of protein, but they're very rich in carbohydrates, vitamin C and potassium. If you enjoy eating them raw, remember to always wash (clean) your carrots thoroughly with a vegetable brush because they have a lot of potential places for bacteria to buildup.

5. EGG WHITES

Egg whites are packed with pure protein. They're considered nearly perfect because of their sublime blend of amino acids. The white of one egg contains 4 grams of pure protein. This is the cheapest and best protein you could ever consume.

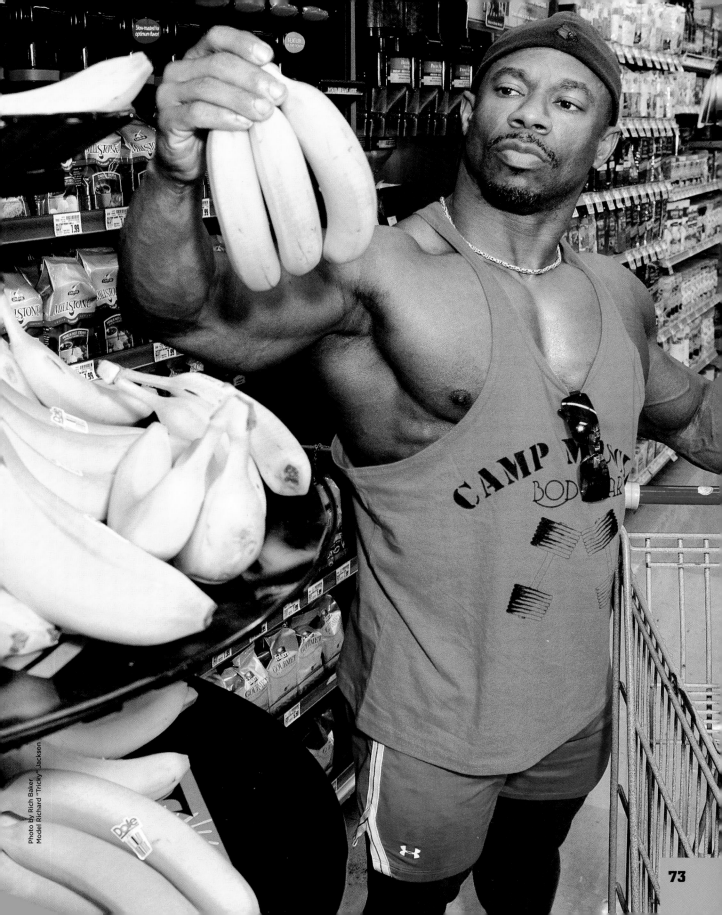

6. OATMEAL

Oatmeal is a tremendous source of high-quality carbohydrates. It has more protein than wheat, twice as much as brown rice, and is very low in fat. The total amount of fat is less than 2 grams per serving, which is hardly enough fat intake to worry about. Oatmeal is a good source of iron and manganese, and has high amounts of vitamin E, copper, folate and zinc. It's a great source of dietary fiber and it helps lower cholesterol. As an inexpensive pre-workout meal ingested one hour before training, oatmeal also makes a superior energy source for a tough workout.

7. PASTA

Pasta is virtually fat free if eaten by itself, so forget about the fat-filled sauces, sausages and meatballs. Use vegetable-rich tomato-based sauces instead. Pasta contains less than 1 gram of fat and about 2 grams of protein for every 3

½ ounces. It's rich in vitamin B6, magnesium and copper. Go for a whole-grain variety.

8. SWEET POTATOES

Most people assume that because of their sweet taste, sweet potatoes are higher in calories than regular potatoes. This isn't true. An enzyme in sweet potatoes converts starches into sugars and this adds to the deliciously sweet taste. Every 3 ½ ounces contains 2 grams of protein, 24 grams of carbohydrates, an adequate amount of dietary fiber and less than 1 gram of fat. They're also rich in vitamin A, vitamin C and vitamin B6 along with traces of copper and magnesium.

9. TOFU

Along with liver, Brussels sprouts and prunes, tofu is one of the foods most people hate. Still, over a billion people use this soybean product. Many brands of tofu come in water-filled plas-

Save a page or two in your training journal to make your weekly shopping list.

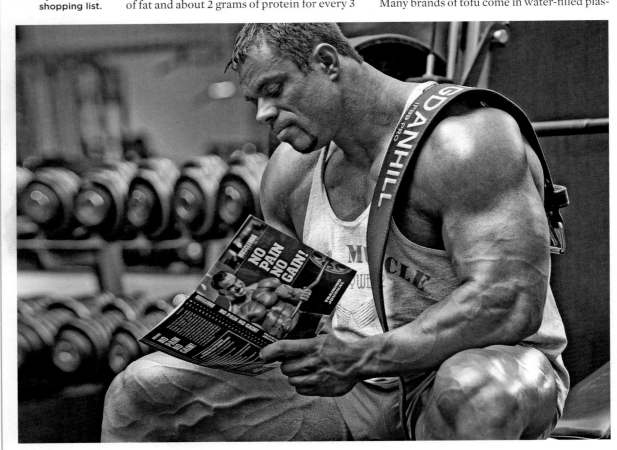

tic tubs and look like a lard omelet gone bad, so it's easy to see how it gets on people's most hated lists. Tofu is high in iron and calcium and contains 8 grams of protein in every 3 ½ ounces. It's also cholesterol-free and low in saturated fats and sodium. Regardless of its taste, it should be a staple on your grocery list.

Note: Soy products contain a natural chemical called a phyto-estrogen, which mimics the female hormone estrogen. This chemical sends a negative feedback signal to the pituitary gland to lower testosterone levels in the body. As good as Tofu is, don't make it your main protein source.

10. TUNA

The best canned tuna is packed in water. Forget about tuna packed in oil, as it has double the calories and 10 times the fat. Tuna is particularly convenient and very high in protein with 30 grams of protein per 3 ½ ounce serving and less than 1 gram of fat. Tuna also contains 100 percent of the RDA for B12, and is a rich source of niacin, phosphorus, vitamin B6, magnesium and potassium. Albacore, bluefin and yellowfin are the three types of tuna most commonly found fresh or canned.

11. TURKEY BREAST

Turkey breast is the leanest of any meat (without the skin of course). A 3 ½ ounce serving contains 1 gram of fat and 30 grams of protein. It contains high amounts of vitamin B12 and B6, copper, iron, niacin, phosphorus, riboflavin and zinc. Turkey can be roasted, broiled or sautéed. You can also buy ground turkey from the grocery store. Look for ground turkey breast with the lowest fat content. You can use ground turkey anywhere you would normally use ground beef.

SIDE EFFECTS

Please keep in mind that any one or a combination of these superfoods may in some cases cause side effects or hypersensitive reactions (food allergies). It's a good idea to keep a food and symptom diary, writing down everything you eat and any side effects you experience (diarrhea, fatigue, gas, joint soreness, sinus irritations, water retention and any other feeling you experience).

SHOPPING LIST FOR QUICK AND EASY NUTRITION

PROTEIN (LOW TO MEDIUM FAT)

Eggs
Cheese
Ground Beef (10% or less fat)
Nonfat Milk or Lactaid
Fresh Turkey
Fresh Fish
Tuna in Water
Fresh Chicken Breast
Top Sirloin Steak
Canadian Bacon
Cottage Cheese (low fat)

CARBOHYDRATES (HIGH TO MODERATE)

Oatmeal
Whole Grain Bread
Pitas
Rice (brown/long cook)
Pasta
Yams
Apples
Grapefruit
Grapes
Cantaloupe
Strawberries
Plums
Spring Mix Salad
Mushrooms
Green Peppers
Broccoli
Tomatoes
Asparagus

FAT (FRIENDLY FATS)

Raw Nuts
Vegetable Oils
Peanut Butter (all natural)
Avocado
Olive Oil
Sour Cream (low fat)
Guacomole
Fish Fat
Flax Seed Oil

CHAPTER 11

FOOD SUBSTITUTES, COOKING METHODS AND FOOD TOXICITY

There are a lot of dos and don'ts when it comes to bodybuilding foods and cooking.

Hitting the gym and training hard is only one part to the puzzle on the quest for massive muscle mass. Another important factor is watching your diet. If you're finding it difficult to get out of your bad eating habits, rest assured, you're not alone. One of the reasons that some people find it so difficult to eat healthy is because they simply don't know or understand what foods fit into a clean-eating lifestyle. Don't worry, we've got you covered. The following three charts are specifically designed to give you a brief, crash course in healthy eating. More specifically, you'll find the foods to avoid, reasons to avoid them and the ideal substitutes all conveniently interconnected through an easy-to-follow numbering system.

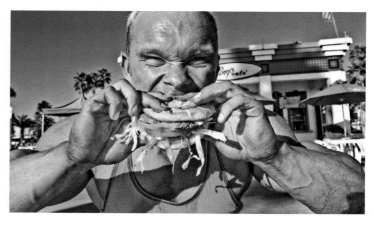

Photos by Robert Reiff
Model Ben Pakulski

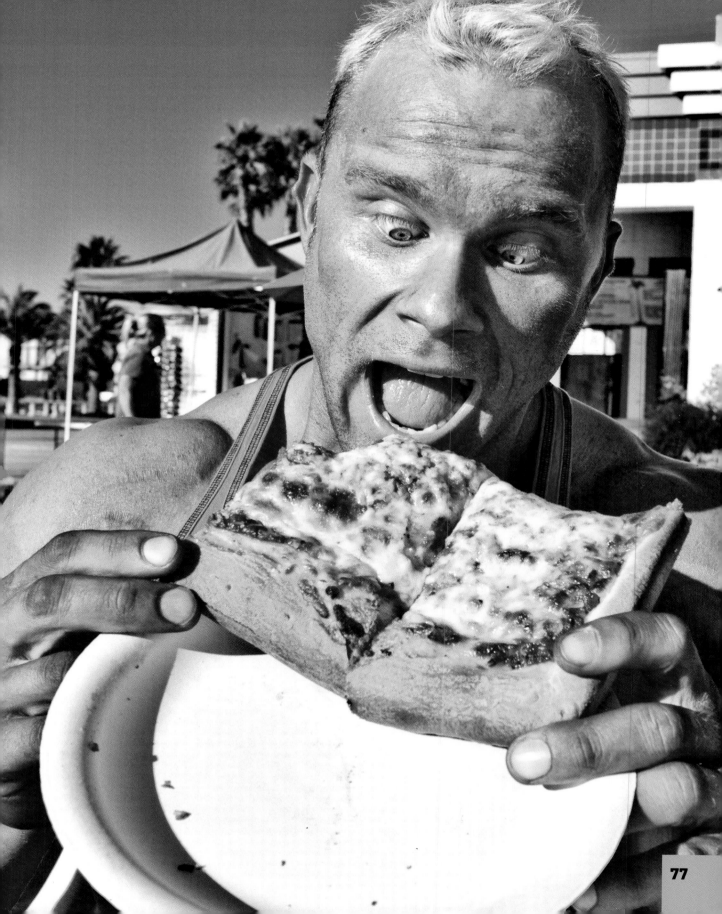

FOODS TO AVOID AND SUBSTITUTES

AVOID THESE FOODS

1. Commercial candies.
2. Chocolate products.
3. Commercial cereals.
4. Canned fruits.
5. Desserts and pastries (butterhorns, cakes, cookies, chesse cakes, cream puffs, doughnuts, Twinkies, sweet rolls, etc.)
6. Ice cream products.
7. Juice drinks and soda pops, including diet varieties.
8. White sugars.
9. White flour products (breads, macaroni, muffins, rolls, spaghetti, etc.)
10. Butter substitutes (margarines) and prepared hydrogenated fats.
11. Coffee and tea.
12. Alcoholic beverages (beer and wine, etc.)
13. Rich sauces.
14. Corn chips, potato chips, etc.
15. Pork products (bacon, ham, sausage links and cold cuts.)
16. Airline food.
17. Fast food.
18. Table salt.
19. Canned vegetables.
20. Chemical laxatives (Lasix, etc.)
21. Commercial salad dressings and sandwich spreads.
22. Canned meats packed in oil.

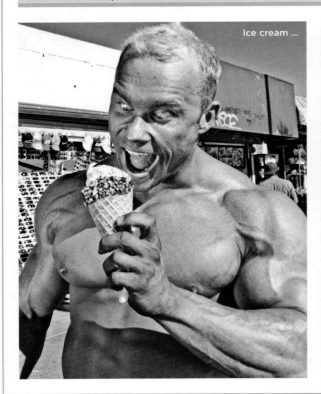

Ice cream ...

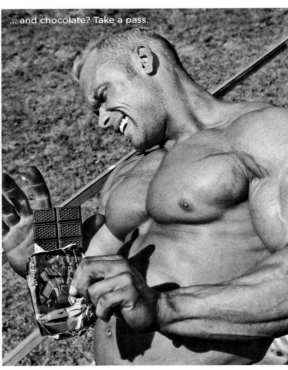

... and chocolate? Take a pass.

Photos by Robert Reiff
Model Ben Pakulski

REASONS TO AVOID

1. Concentrated sugar.
2. Excess sugar/salt; presweetened with white sugar and synthetic glucose.
3. Loaded with excess sugars and heavy syrups.
4. Excess sugar and white flour.
5. Excess sugar and chemicals.
6. Excess sugar (12 teaspoons per 12 ounce can). Diet colas contain excess sodium.
7. Mucus-forming, accelerates mineral loss and is bleached in sulphuric acid.
8. Contains "empty calories" and is usually bleached, chemically treated and synthetically fortified.
9. Causes a cholesterol buildup.
10. Causes fluctuating blood sugar levels, which in turn results in overeating. It's also loaded with caffeine, which can interfere with certain vitamin nutrient assimilation by up to 45 percent.
11. Contains caffeine and tannic acid and causes some of the same problems as coffee.
12. Promotes overeating where calories from food are stored as fat and your body uses the calories from the alcohol for energy. Worsens flight-related dehydration.
13. High in saturated fat, which contributes to elevated cholesterol levels.
14. Excess saturated fats and sodium.
15. Loaded with sodium. Proteins can't be fully utilized, which results in overworked kidneys and toxins entering your bloodstream. Deli meats contain excess chemicals.
16. Loaded with sodium.
17. Loaded with sodium, excess fat and empty calories.
18. Salt is a water retainer. One extra teaspoon of table salt could cause retention of as much as 1/2 pound of water.
19. Loaded with salt and sugar.
20. Damage to the intestinal tract and a cause of potassium loss.
21. Contains sugar and salt and includes a food additive that inhibits the use of iron and causes hunger.
22. Too much oil and excess calories.

SUBSTITUTES

1. Dried fruit.
2. Carob and Cara Coa.
3. Whole-grain cereals such as oatmeal, multigrain hot cereal, homemade meusli and granola.
NOTE: Soak all natural grains overnight in distilled water (less salt) to expand the grain to its maximum or original size. This helps to eliminate gas and gas pains.
4. Canned fruits packed in natural juices or water.
5. Dried and fresh fruit.
6. Yogurt and other dairy products made with natural ingredients.
7. Water and fresh-squeezed juices.
8. Simple sugars listed earlier in this book.
9. Whole wheat products.
10. Butter, canola and olive oils.
11. Herbal teas and tisanes.
12. Water, juices, mineral water.
13. Herbs and spices.
14. Low-fat and low-sodium brands found in health sections and specialty shops.
15. Products that are low in fat and cholesterol, including vegetarian foods.
16. For long flights, prepare your own meals ahead of time.
17. Order a salad.
18. Dulse, Irish moss (carrageen) and kelp powder.
19. Low-sodium vegetables and those in the vegetables and fruits group listed earlier in the book.
20. Natural and organic diuretics such as cucumbers (and its juices), pitted prunes (or unsweetened prune juice) and natural bran. As a last resort, perform an enema.
21. Oil with vinegar and lemon juice.
22. Water-packed variety (including fish products like tuna, sardines, etc.)

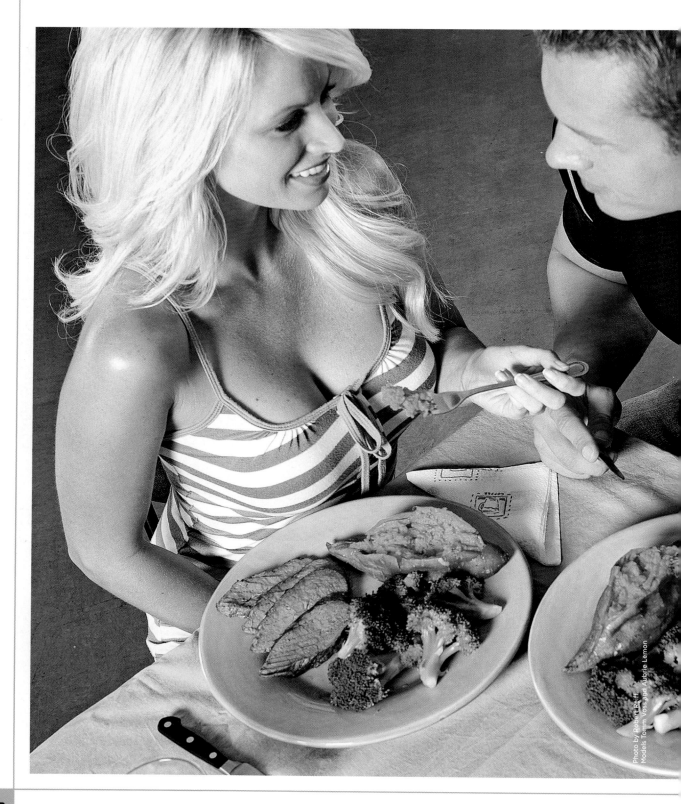

Photo by Robert Reiff
Models Tomm Voss and Aubrie Lemon

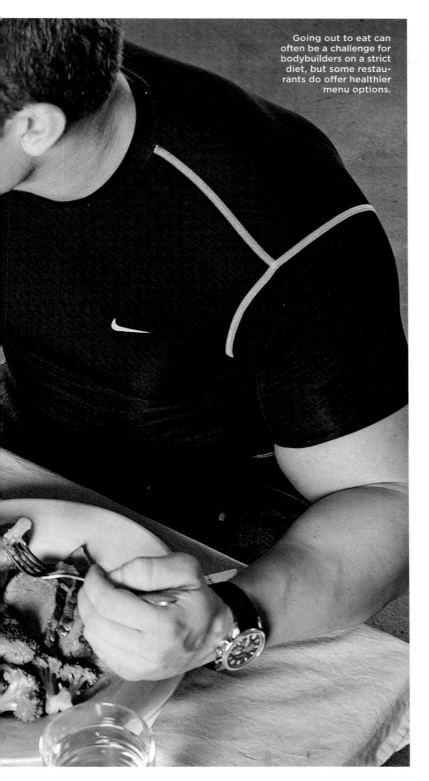

Going out to eat can often be a challenge for bodybuilders on a strict diet, but some restaurants do offer healthier menu options.

COOKING METHODS TO AVOID & ALTERNATIVES

WRONG CHOICE

1. Deep-fried fish and fried beef (hamburger, steak).
2. Fried eggs.
3. Boiled vegetables.

DRAWBACKS INVOLVED

1. Alters fat which, over time, accumulates on the walls of your arteries.
2. See above.
3. Loss of vital nutrients.

BEST CHOICE

1. Bake or broil. With light fish such as halibut, you could also steam.
2. Poach, hard-boil or soft-boil. If you like raw eggs, but don't like avidin's destruction of the B vitamin biotin, boil the egg for no more than 10 seconds.
   NOTE: If you have difficulty swallowing raw eggs, here's a unique way: Find two small glasses. Drop the yolks into one glass. Fill the other with mineral water. Chug the raw egg yolks and then immediately drink the mineral water to wash away the taste.
3. It's best to eat them raw. To ease the digestion process, steam your vegetables, as the cellulose fiber otherwise makes the process difficult.

A SECRET FOR DETERMINING FOOD TOXICITY

Take your pulse 30 minutes prior to eating a meal, then take it three more times 30 minutes apart, starting at the beginning of your meal. If your pulse doesn't increase more than 10 beats per minute, then the meal is nontoxic to your digestive system. If your pulse increases more than 15 beats, avoid those foods in the future. Since you'll probably be eating from all the basic food groups at each meal, it may take a little trial and error to identify which food is toxic. You may have to eliminate one food at a time.

Remember, always bake, grill, broil or microwave your meat. Never fry! Meats should be obtained fresh, not processed, prepackaged or canned. Fruits and vegetables should be fresh or frozen, not canned. For the sake of your health, always try to eat foods in the most natural and least chemically-altered state possible.

TWELVE-WEEK CALORIE BLITZ & ANABOLIC STIMULATORS

Adding quality mass means more than just consuming extra calories; you need to consider how many calories and which foods are the best choices.

On your quest to reach your muscular best, you'll be consuming a lot of food. It's important that you remember to do some type of aerobic activity (running, biking or walking) at least two times per week for about 30 minutes each session. If you find you aren't gaining muscle mass, increase your calories, but don't decrease your aerobic activity. On the other hand, if you're gaining fat, increase your cardio by an additional session, but don't decrease your food intake.

12-WEEK CALORIE BLITZ CYCLE

Here's an excellent way to increase your muscle mass by gradually adding up to 1,200 extra calories (consisting of low-fat, complete proteins and complex carbs) to your daily meals.

In the following table, we've provided an example of a subject weighing 200 pounds and consuming 4,000 calories with a goal of gaining 3.5 to 14 pounds of muscle mass.

WEEK	EXTRA CALORIES PER DAY	DAILY CALORIC INTAKE
1–2	1 X body weight = 200	4,200
3–4	2 X body weight = 400	4,400
5–6	3 X body weight = 600	4,600
7–8	4 X body weight = 800	4,800
9–10	5 X body weight = 1,000	5,000
11–12	6 X body weight = 1,200	5,200

Many ectomorphic bodybuilders will do well to consume the calories listed above (consuming one extra calorie for every pound you weigh, every day for two weeks and then bumping your caloric intake accordingly as detailed in the chart) on training and non-training days

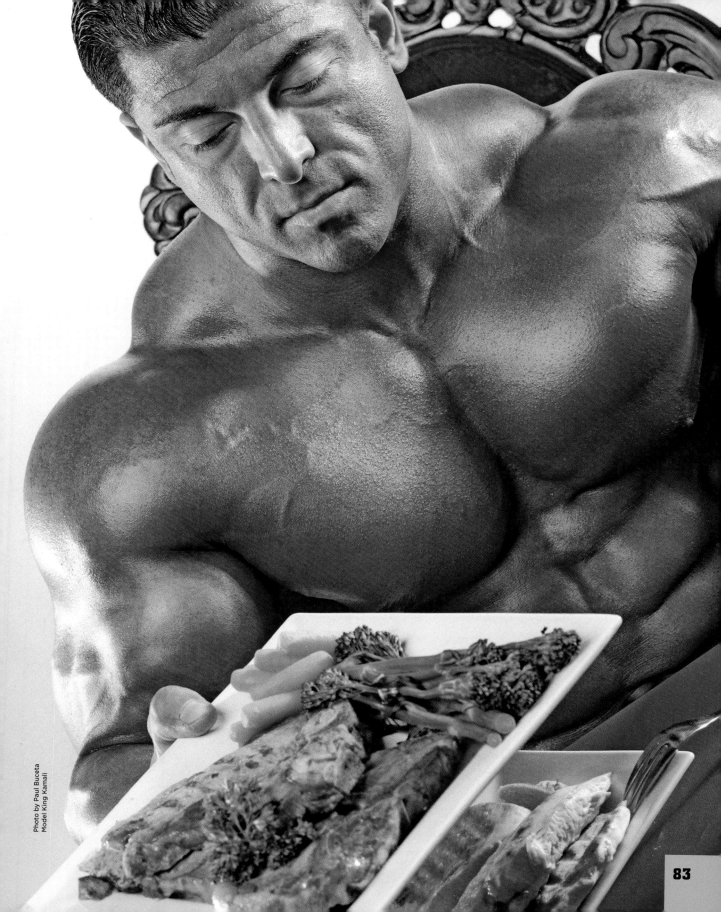

Some bodybuilders find it effective to take in extra calories only on days when they're doing high-intensity training.

alike. Others may find it more beneficial to consume extra calories only on high-intensity training days, especially if they experience signs of quickly gaining weight in the form of bodyfat. Increased fatigue, shortness of breath, lack of energy and excessive sweating are all signs of gaining more bodyfat than muscle mass. To avoid this, you may have to back off the bi-weekly increment of an additional calorie per pound of bodyweight and instead multiply your bodyweight by 0.75 to determine your caloric increase. The six-meal plan mentioned earlier includes a couple of mus-

cle-mass shakes. You can even go one step further by setting up an early morning rising at around 2:00 A.M. to have a third muscle-mass shake before getting back to sleep as quickly as possible. You might also want to try a medium-chain triglyceride product to increase your calories. Be sure to follow the directions carefully to avoid stomach problems. Once you've reached your desired additional muscle bodyweight, discontinue the Calorie Blitz Cycle and gradually decrease your daily caloric intake to a level that will help you maintain your new body.

Photo by Paul Buceta
Model Paul Dillett

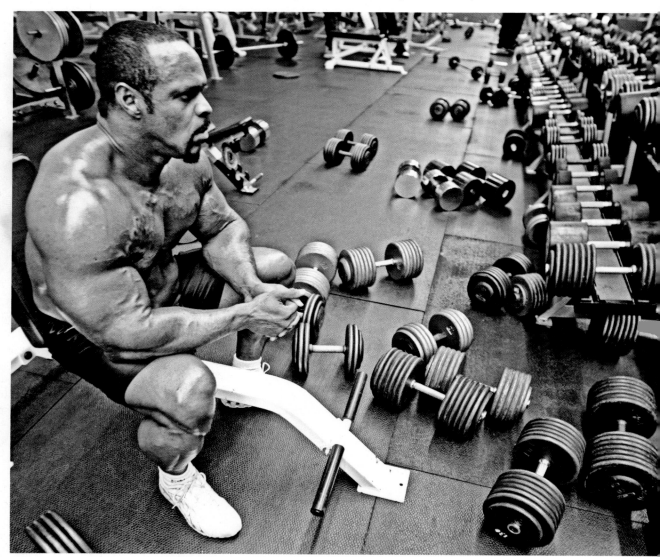

Studies have shown that amino acid capsules can help produce a natural hormone precursor effect.

NATURAL ANABOLIC STIMULATORS FOR INCREASING MUSCLE MASS

Natural methods do exist to help you create a positive nitrogen (protein) balance in your body. Anabolic steroids are not your only option. The method we recommend is cell regeneration through protein and amino acid feedings. Recent research reveals that certain combinations of amino acid capsules, desiccated liver tablets and eggs can create a natural hormone precursor effect that has, in some cases, nearly equaled the results of tissue-building anabolic steroids but without the devastating side effects. The basic plan is to take 10 amino acid tablets (these should contain 20 free-form L amino acids) and 10 desiccated liver tablets (10 ½ grain) every three hours.

Liver contains a red protein pigment called cytochrome P-450, which accounts for the increased endurance that many hard-training bodybuilders experience when taking it. Back in the 1960s, '70s and '80s it was common to see bodybuilding competitors take as many as 60 liver tablets a day in the off-season and increase to 100 tablets a day in the last few weeks prior to a competition. Free-form amino acid tablets and defatted desiccated liver tablets are very good supplements to carry with you as an extra protein source.

Eat one egg every hour until three hours prior to bedtime (boiled eggs are most convenient). Before you go to sleep, take an amino acid combination known in bodybuilding circles as human growth hormone releasers (HGH), consisting of arginine, ornithine and tryptophan.

A ratio of two parts arginine (not to exceed 1,200 mg) to one part ornithine and one part tryptophan seems to provide the best results. When taken as directed on an empty stomach, these amino acids will cause the pituitary gland to secrete more somatropin (human growth hormone). Research has shown that, when taken under these conditions, this combination produces an increase in muscle size, as well as a loss in bodyfat.

You may wonder why the three-hour intervals are an important condition. The reason for this schedule is that you don't want to take sup-

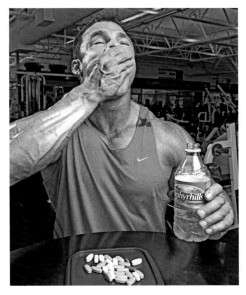

plements until your digestive system has absorbed all the nutrients from the main meals. The metabolic and digestive system has an efficiency rate of nearly 98 percent in breaking down animal protein foods and this can't be improved on very much. We recommend that you eat four to six meals a day. Usually the stomach can hold a maximum of two cups of food at a time, so it is foolish to overload it. Following this practice, along with using some additional digestive supports that we will comment on later, will result in more complete digestion, less uric acid and less waste matter.

While these supplements and any other we refer to in this chapter are not drugs or chemicals, they are concentrated food. We recommend caution when using these powerful supplements. Start out with just a few each day and increase the amounts slowly while you observe the results. You may not have to go to the extremes mentioned to obtain maximum results for your body type.

THE EGG: THE NATURAL ANABOLIC STEROID

Many years ago, nutritional scientists made a startling discovery that would have a major impact on bodybuilding for decades to come. They discovered that activity takes place in human cell tissue every microsecond. For ex-

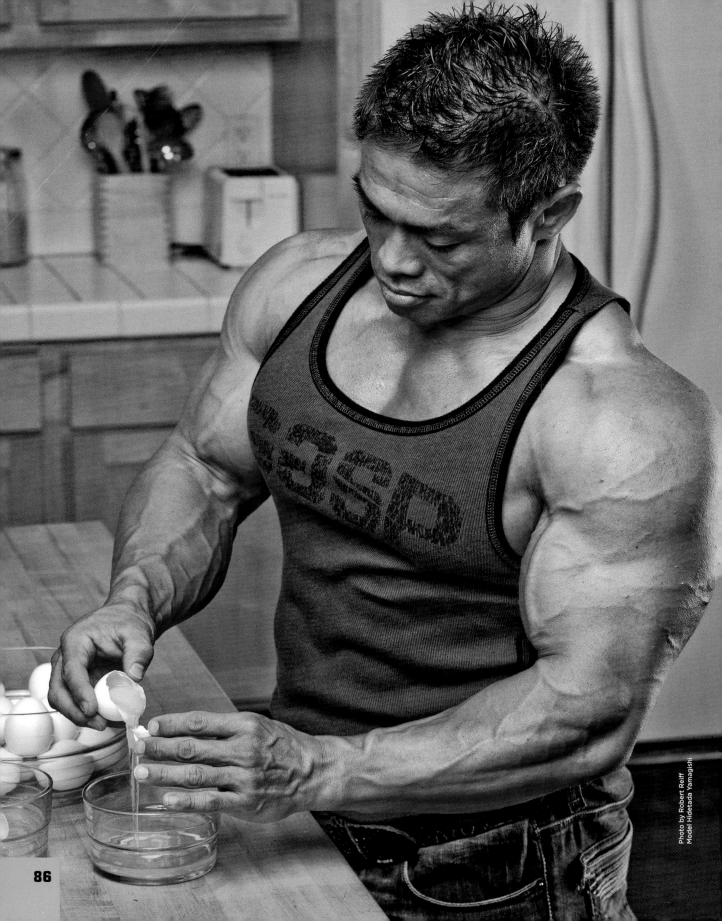

ample, every protein molecule in a healthy human body breaks down and is replaced every 160 days. If you live to be 70, you will have replaced the body's stores of protein molecules approximately 160 times. This revelation led nutritional scientists into extensive research to find natural complete protein sources that would be suitable in the regeneration and continued rebuilding of muscle tissue.

Many natural and complete protein sources were tested. Mother's milk was found to be 98 percent biological in its protein structure when compared to human tissue. With a biological value of 95 percent, the egg was recognized by nutritional scientists as being the next best complete protein. Remember that the biological value does not indicate the amount of protein contained in the egg, but is a term nutritional scientists use to determine just how much of the protein from a specific food is used by your body. The egg is therefore 95 percent usable in the rebuilding of human muscle tissue, something particularly noteworthy to a bodybuilder because it's one of nature's most nearly perfect foods for creating maximum muscle tissue. Because of its dramatic impact on the ability to create muscle size, top bodybuilders around the world call the egg a natural steroid.

The main ingredients in an egg that cause anabolism (the chemical process in the body where nutrients are used to build up muscle tissue) are fat or cholesterol along with lecithin. If you suffer from high cholesterol levels, you should eat eggs only occasionally. If you suffer from hypertension, you must be very careful about how many egg whites you eat because the white of the egg contains a great deal of salt.

Be mindful how you include eggs in your diet. You should never eat eggs raw because raw egg whites can be toxic to the point where your body won't accept them thoroughly and efficiently. The white of an egg contains the amino acid avidin, which destroys the function of the biotin vitamin and suspends the absorption of vitamin B12 and iron. Also, eat natural or fertile eggs only. Never eat egg substitutes such as heat-dried egg yolk powders. These egg substitutes contain oxidized cholesterol and can cause artery wall damage. The best way to

eat eggs is to poach egg whites and scramble them with bits of chopped onions and fresh mushrooms or simply make an egg-white omelet with bits of fresh fruit.

If you're following the guidelines of super nutrition and abstaining from animal fats (meats), you could eat quite a few whole cooked eggs per day without any worry of elevated cholesterol levels. The whites contain no fat, 3.3 grams of protein and only 16 calories. A whole medium raw egg contains 5.5 grams of fat (cholesterol), 3 grams of carbohydrates and 6.1 grams of complete protein. The white of a medium egg contains a fat emulsifier (lecithin containing choline, which prevents the accumulation of fatty acids in the liver) that will break down the fat content of the egg yolk. As a matter of fact, there is enough lecithin in one medium egg white to break down the fat content in eight medium eggs.

Eating eggs will cause a natural anabolic effect in your body and will help push your muscles to new size and strength plateaus. Many pro bodybuilders eat as many as 36 or more egg whites daily. Because eggs are a natural steroid, we suggest that you eat up to 12 to 20 poached egg whites per day. Follow this regimen for a period of six to eight weeks; then go back to eating six or seven eggs daily (with four of the yolks removed). This advice should not be followed by individuals whose LDL cholesterol level is moderately high (160-189) or high-risk (greater than 190).

In addition to the suggestions of consuming amino acid tablets, desiccated liver tablets and eggs, we feel it would be a good idea to also take one or two high-potency B-complex vitamin capsules every couple of hours throughout the day when in a muscle-mass building phase. These vitamins stimulate the appetite and help to increase muscle building following a hard workout.

ALFALFA AND CHLOROPHYLL SECRET

By combining five alfalfa tablets and five chlorophyll tablets with your breakfast, lunch and dinner, a natural anabolic effect occurs that results in an increase of your bodyweight and strength.

Whole eggs have a biological value of 95 percent, meaning that percentage can be used by the body to rebuild muscle tissue.

CHAPTER 13

OVERVIEW OF BODYBUILDING SUPPLEMENTS

Along with a calculated nutrition plan, your supplement regimen plays a key role in furthering your muscular progress.

You only have to look at the hundreds of advertisements in bodybuilding publications to realize that the age of supplementation has been upon us for quite some time. Hardly a magazine issue passes without a new and better product being heralded. All of these advertisements revolve around a few key claims – developing mass, increasing strength, enhancing peak performance – and some even go so far as to say that a certain product is a substitute for pharmaceutical anabolic steroids.

In their attempt to separate fact from fantasy, many up-and-coming bodybuilders turn to their favorite superstar in the iron game to see what he or she personally recommends in supplementation. Lo and behold, they find that for every product advertised, there's a top champion endorsing it. This also carries over into the selection of training equipment and training procedures. To further complicate matters, rumors soon begin to circulate that these bodybuilding superstars have made all their progress by using anabolic steroids.

So here we stand, totally confused. Is it the supplements, the training equipment, the special training procedures or the anabolic steroids that helped the superstar achieve his lofty status? Frank Zane, three-time Mr. Olympia, has stated "There is no one thing that does it! It isn't the supplements or the training equipment or even a special training procedure. It's none of that, but all of it. You can't rely on any one thing as the secret to bodybuilding success. Something by itself may add a little extra boost in the way of results to your training, or it may not." Maybe that hope of finding a new supplement that provides that little extra boost is the reason why some bodybuilders decide to load up on every new supplement. We've spoken to some bodybuilders who tell us they're taking as many as 10 to 15 different supplements each day. When you ask them which supplement, or combination of supplements, is most beneficial, they appear unsure and can't give you much of an answer. No doubt, you've experienced the same sort of reaction when you've asked your friends at the local gym. That's where we come in. This chapter will help eliminate any further confusion.

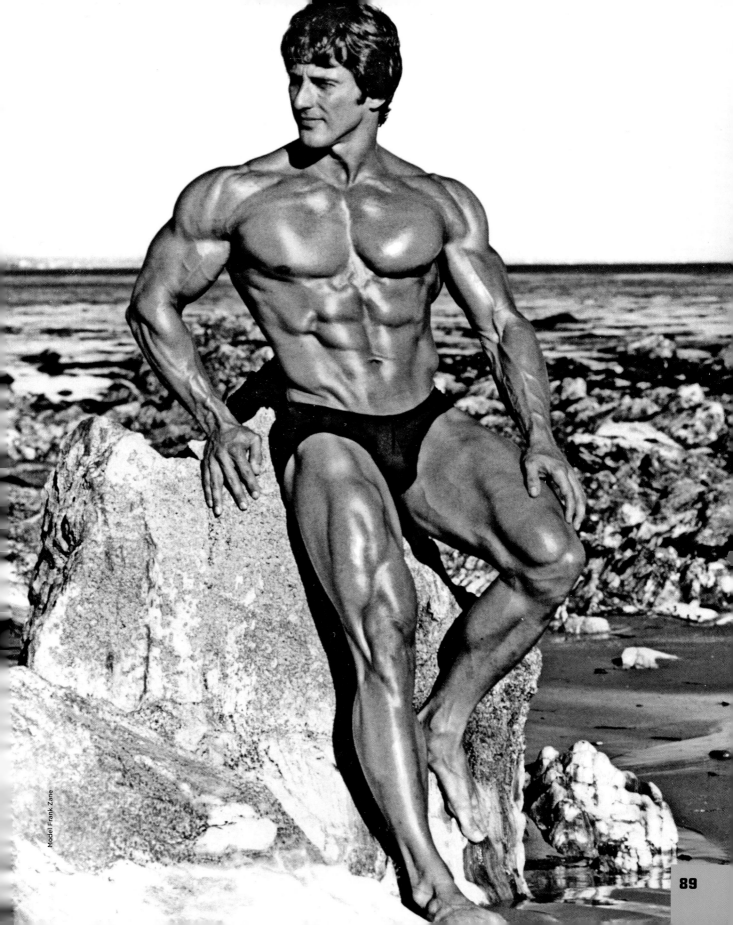

Model Frank Zane

THE 72-HOUR SUPPLEMENT PLAN

Throughout most of his nutritional writings and personal consultations, the late Vince Gironda advocated taking supplements during a 72-hour period and then going off them completely for the same time period. He believed if you were to glut the endocrine system you would cause toxemia. Vince trained many physique champions over the last four decades, so he was very familiar with their excesses in using supplements. His plan gives the body a rest from the megadoses of vitamin and mineral supplements many would-be champions take.

This principle is sound because a lot of bodybuilders consume supplements in such quantities that they overtax their system's ability to utilize and store these nutrients. On a long-term basis, this habit can present a real problem with the fat-soluble vitamins A, D, E and K, which can be potentially dangerous to your health if your body becomes oversaturated with them. Iron might also cause you to experience some problems. Some people take in so much of this mineral that their blood can't release oxygen efficiently because of the binding of the iron components.

When you aren't taking vitamin supplements, your body experiences the glut/famine syndrome so it goes through adaptive responses. If you allow 72 hours to pass before introducing your body to more supplementation, you're often able to turn these adaptive responses into something beneficial. How? Assuming your usual diet is lacking in vitamins and minerals, your body will become more prone to absorbing these supplements following the 72 hour period of non-consumption.

However, you must also be aware that if you're deprived of any of the water-soluble vitamins for up to 72 hours, your water-soluble storage pool will become depleted, and serious metabolic consequences will occur. Another consideration is that your system may "adapt" to receiving larger than normal amounts of vitamin C and may come to require them; once this supplement is discontinued, deficiency symptoms may occur. The fat-soluble vitamins aren't subject to temporary inadequacies or deficiencies in the daily diet. However, this does assume normal nutrition status.

Our final word on supplementation is to approach it with caution and common sense. No matter how long you have been taking some of these vitamins and minerals, some of them can be toxic to your system. You must be careful not to take too many supplements that you may not need. Always remember that your vitamin and mineral supplements should always be taken with food because the many nutrient factors in food assist in the transport and absorption of the vitamins and minerals. Minerals must be chelated by your body (using protein and carbohydrates as the chelating agents) before they can be utilized. Food-type supplements such as desiccated liver, bone meal and wheat germ oil can be taken without food because they have their own unique carriers built in.

ONE ON ONE WITH DENNIS WEIS

Neither Bob Kennedy nor I are big advocates of taking a large variety of supplements. Back in the '70s when I competed in powerlifting, bodybuilding and arm-wrestling competitions (usually all on the same day), nutritional protocol consisted of 50 to 100 desiccated liver tablets, a good combination of vitamins and minerals (there weren't vitamin packs back then), Rheo H. Blair's protein, brewer's yeast powder (mixed with a fruit-flavored drink) and some wheat germ capsules.

I learned early on from my bodybuilding mentor Donne Hale, more isn't always better when it comes to variety and daily dosages of nutritional supplements. Donne advised me to experiment and find the least amount of supplements and dosages that would provide the absolute maximum nutritional results.

For example, I mentioned that I took 50 to 100 desiccated liver tablets daily. I didn't just start taking that many tablets from day one. I started out taking 10 desiccated liver tablets, and each day thereafter I would take one or two tablets more than the previous day. From there, I worked my way up to what I determined was most beneficial to me (nutrition-wise and from the standpoint of assisted recovery), which was 50 to 100 tablets a day.

Supplementation in your daily diet is an important issue, but not as complicated as you might think. Bob Kennedy and I would suggest you consider using the following supplements on a daily basis: One or two multi-vitamin/mineral super packs (which contain major antioxidant properties such as vitamin C, vita-

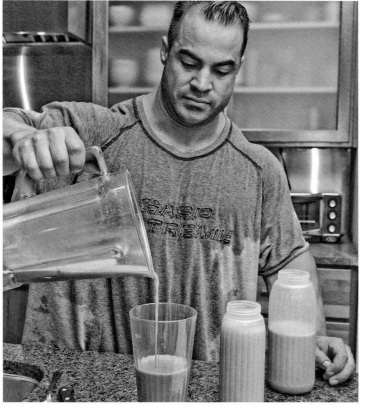

Many supplements come in powder form and can be easily mixed into a shake.

min E, beta-carotene, selenium), a good protein powder or perhaps two or three meal-replacement packets and some desiccated liver tablets. As well, we suggest you take two to four bromelain (digestive enzyme) tablets after each meal or snack, eaten with two tablespoons per day of wheat germ or other blended germ oils.

You should also consider incorporating a time-tested creatine monohydrate plan. Creatine monohydrate is well known for its effects on muscular gains, and it also helps to buffer lactic acid.

CREATINE SUPPLEMENTATION PLAN

The following sample of major meals/snacks, workouts, and creatine supplementation is for a power bodybuilder who rises at 6:30 A.M. and performs a high-intensity workout at 6:00 P.M.

Phase I: Consume 5-gram doses of creatine as scheduled on workout and non-workout days alike.

Phase II: Consume 5 grams of creatine at two separate intervals on non-workout days, preferably after a main meal. Though not listed above, another strategy is to consume 3 grams of creatine after breakfast and lunch and 8 grams of creatine after your workout.

Phase III: During the first two weeks of this phase, consume two doses of 4 grams of creatine every other day, including workout days if possible. In the next two weeks, consume just two 4-gram doses of creatine once every seven days. Schedule this on a heavy-duty training day.

TIME	PHASE I (5–7 DAYS)	PHASE II 30–45 DAYS	PHASE III 15–30 DAYS
6:30 A.M.	Breakfast	Breakfast	Breakfast
8:30 A.M.	5g creatine	5g creatine	4g creatine
9:30 A.M.	Midmorning snack	Midmorning snack	Midmorning snack
11:30 A.M.	5g creatine		
12:30 P.M.	Lunch	Lunch	Lunch
2:30 P.M.	5g creatine	5g creatine	
3:30 P.M.	Midafternoon snack	Midafternoon snack	Midafternoon snack
5:30 P.M.	5g creatine		
6:00 P.M.	70 minute workout	70 minute workout	70 minute workout
7:30 P.M.	5g creatine	5g creatine	4g creatine
8:30 P.M.	Supper	Supper	Supper
10:00 P.M.	Bedtime snack	Bedtime snack	Bedtime snack

Photo by Michael Butler
Model Mark Dugdale

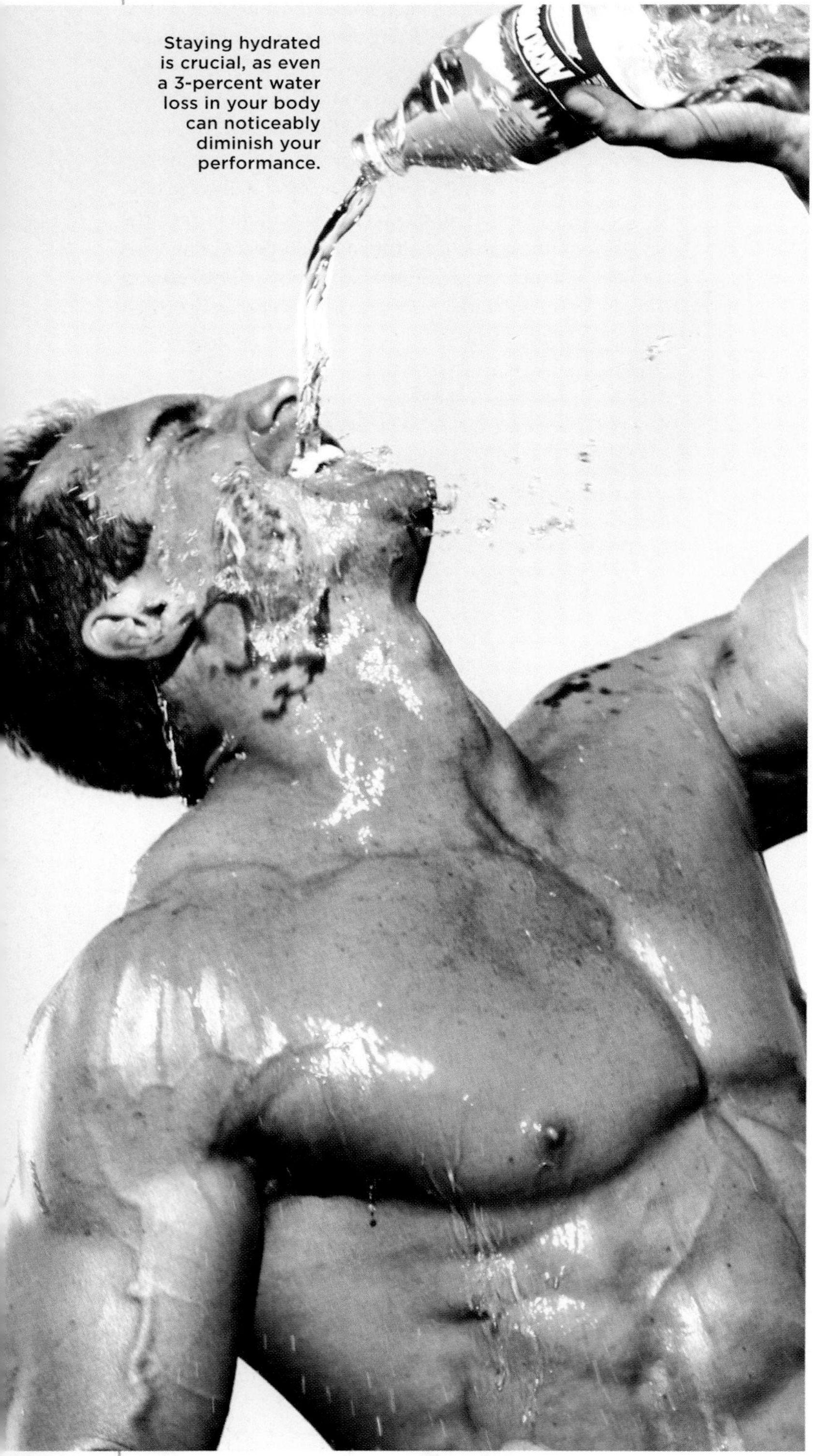

Staying hydrated is crucial, as even a 3-percent water loss in your body can noticeably diminish your performance.

SUPERHYDRATE YOUR SYSTEM

Drinking copious amounts of water throughout the day is essential to your physical well being and the success of this creatine program. We suggest that a person who doesn't have a kidney disorder and isn't taking diuretics drink at least 0.66 times their bodyweight in ounces of cold (45 to 50 degrees Fahrenheit) water daily. For example, if you weigh 200 pounds multiply that number by 0.66 and it totals 132 ounces of cold water.

Hydration is also very important when you are breaking a good sweat during a workout. A water loss of as little as 3 percent of your bodyweight can cause a 15 percent deficit in performance. For example, a 200 pound power-bodybuilder who loses 6 pounds of water weight during a workout will significantly lower his ability to perform physical tasks. We recommend drinking water before, during and after your workout. Drink at least 2 pints of water prior to a workout and 3 to 6 ounces every 15 minutes during the workout. After a workout, consume at least one pint of water for every pound of water weight lost.

Old-school bodybuilders used to prevent fluid loss by sipping on the following water-weight-stabilizer cocktail during a routine:

- 1 quart warm water
- Juice of two fresh lemons
- 6 tablespoons honey

3 TIPS FOR BOOSTING MUSCLE GAIN

1. Slow down your basal metabolic rate by doing absolutely nothing beyond your daily obligations such as your job or family activities. Don't participate in any extra sports activities.

2. Avoid overtraining, poor nutrition, not enough rest, emotional stress and any other negative influences because they upset the nervous system, burn up valuable calories and create a catabolic (muscle-robbing) effect on the muscles.

   The positive influences for staying in the anabolic (muscle gain) environment include: Proper training, nutrition, rest

Photo by Alex Ardenti
Model Tony Morris

and a positive mental attitude. Eliminate anger, anxiety, fear, frustration and the like, whenever possible. Put them in the driveway and back over them with your car as you leave for the gym. Work at developing mental and physical ease and positive energy.

3. Never smoke cigarettes or any tobacco products because they constrict the blood capillary beds in your body, which, in turn, has a debilitating effect on oxygen-carrying enzymes in your body. Smoking also triggers a risk in blood sugar levels, which depresses your appetite. It also destroys vitamin C at the rate of 35 milligrams (one

orange) per cigarette and could cause cancer. Try adding muscle mass with that.

POWERFUL NUTRITION AND SUPPLEMENTATION TACTICS CLOSING COMMENTS

We'll admit that the eating regime we've talked about is unbalanced for normal living. It's intended for adding muscle mass to your physique and will do exactly that; it is not recommended for use throughout the entire year. Use the nutritional concepts provided in this chapter along with the other five phases detailed in this book, and you'll get those additional pounds of muscle mass.

Photo by Paul Buceta
Model Steve Kuclo

Be careful to avoid overtraining and any other cause of extra stress to your nervous system.

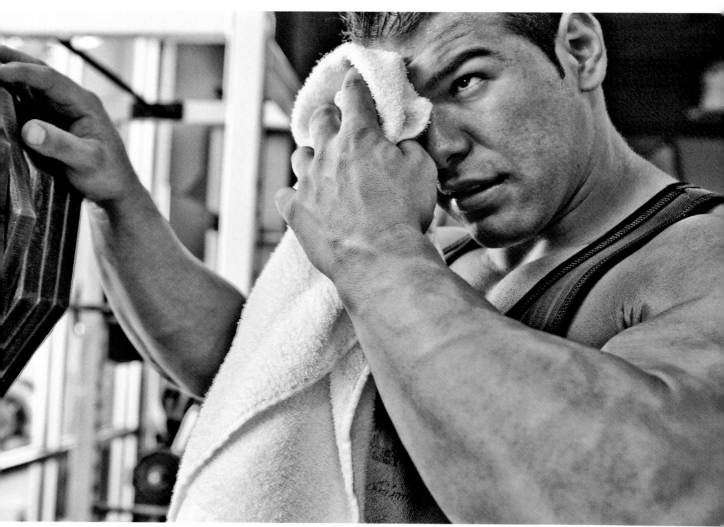

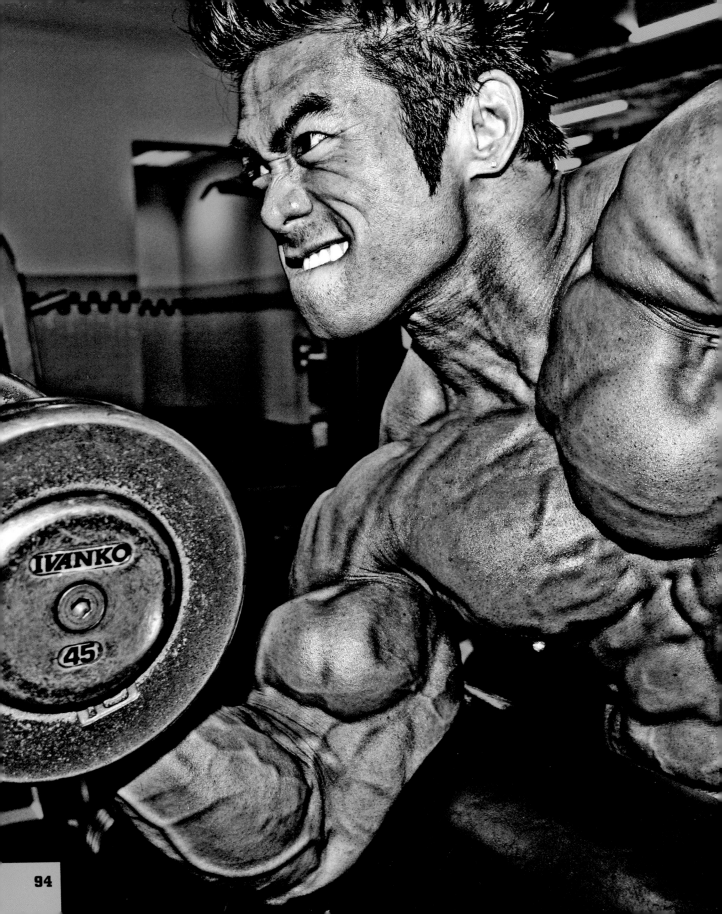

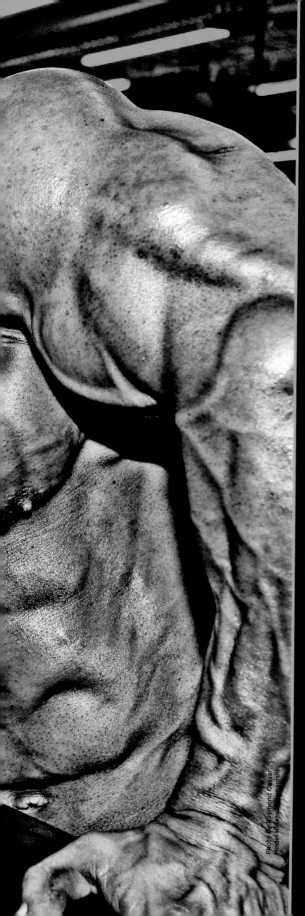

Photo by Raymond Cassar
Model Hidetada Yamagishi

BOOK 03

Sleep and Recovery

CHAPTER 14

SLEEP STAGES & QUALITY SLEEP

Adequate rest and appropriate recovery are of paramount importance to muscle repair and growth.

Rest between workouts, and especially on non-training days (i.e. "muscle-growth days"), is essential. This will allow your muscles and central nervous system to recover completely. Also, get a good night's sleep – a minimum of eight hours – every night of the week. Growth hormone release occurs during these rest cycles and the results come in the form of the massive muscle mass and strength gains you want.

Few bodybuilders or powerlifters relax enough. With the tempo of life stepped up so high, it's easy to fall into a pattern of fast living. And this doesn't necessarily mean the fast lane of nightclubs, drinking, and parties. Television, movies, sporting events or any other activity can keep you up much later than is optimal. As a result, you might try to sleep a little later in the morning, and then it's a race against time. Rushing all day with nerves on edge, eating fast meals and hurrying through your workout (where the weights feel much heavier than they are, but you push yourself to continue) is more exhausting than beneficial, and you end up with no gains to show for your efforts.

Kick back and slow down your pace. Get to bed early so you can wake up with plenty of time to take care of your morning hygiene and eat a sound breakfast. Leave for work or school early enough that you don't have to hurry. Arrange your workouts so they fit into your daily routine and you won't have to rush through them.

Get rid of the fast pace and make an effort to relax several times a day. Reading is a good way to relax, as are power naps. Ted Arcidi, the first man to officially bench press 700 pounds, used to take a 1½-hour nap each afternoon when he was in training for those monumental world-record bench-press assaults.

Avoid "sleep debt" by making it a point to get to bed by 9:30 or 10:00 P.M. so you can get at least eight hours of sleep (but never more than nine, as that would make you sluggish). This suggested bedtime works quite well if you work an 8 A.M. to 5 P.M. weekday job with weekends off. If you work a different time schedule, adjust your sleep schedule accordingly.

FIVE STAGES OF SLEEP

The five stages of sleep recur on a regular pattern throughout the night. The first four stages are classified as non-REM (Rapid Eye Movement) sleep. The most important stage is stage 5, known as REM (Rapid Eye

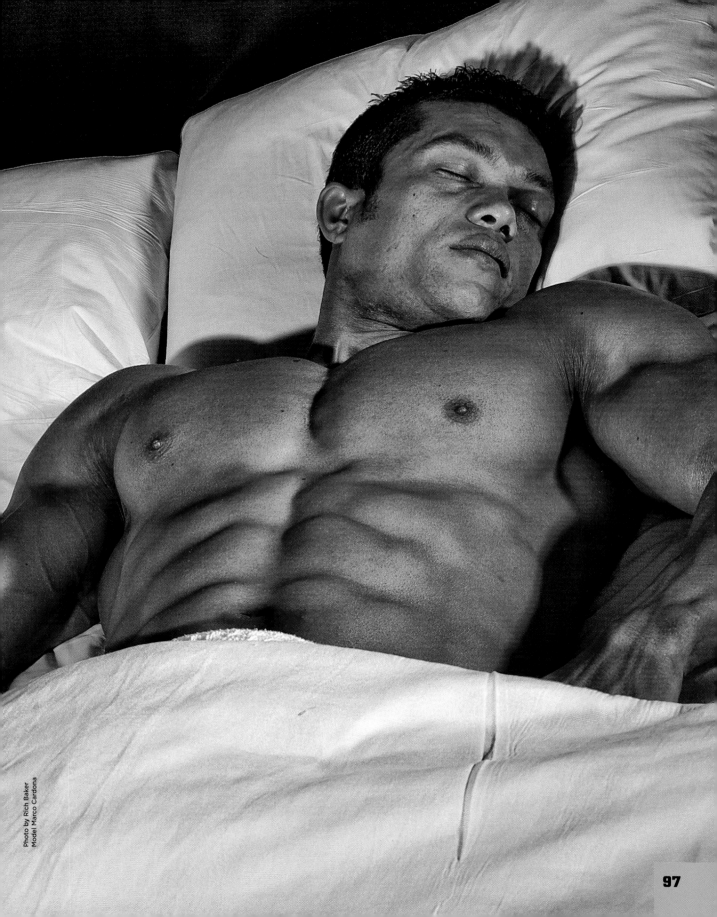

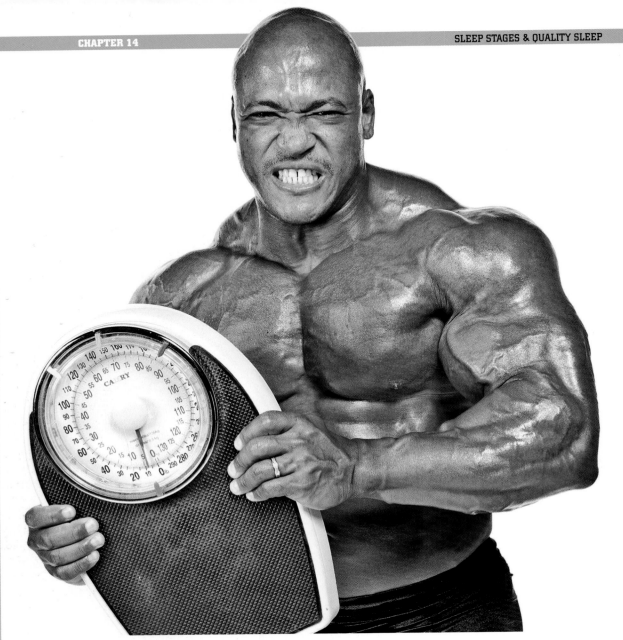

Proper sleep can, in fact, help you conquer the scale – sleep promotes GH release, and GH is involved with fat loss and growth of lean muscle.

Movement) sleep, which accounts for 25 percent of total sleep time and occurs every 1½ hours.

The first four hours of sleep are vital because it's during this time that a substance called growth hormone (GH) is released from the pituitary gland. This hormone is essential for protein synthesis, as well as for the repair and growth of muscle tissue. Many factors will increase GH production and secretion. The release of GH increases during short-term fasting (e.g. Immediately before a bodybuilding competition). Other ways to increase your GH levels include reducing intercellular bodyfat

levels and elevating your body temperatures (as you do when spending time in a sauna).

During a continuous eight-hour sleep pattern, you can't program an increase in the very important REM-sleep stage. However, some pro bodybuilders have found by breaking their normal eight- to nine-hour period of sleep into two different four- to five-hour naps, the proportion of time spent in stage 5 (the stage most associated with GH release) inexplicably increases. When GH levels are increased naturally, they enhance muscle growth and directly impact on fat loss.

Photo by Jason Breeze
Model Craig Richardson

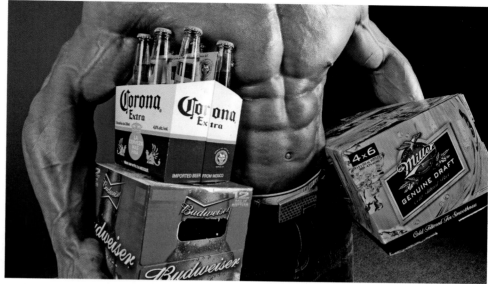

Your hours spent in the gym will be all-for-naught if your evenings or weekends involve polishing off a six-pack (and not the ab variety).

SIX STEPS TO GUARANTEE QUALITY SLEEP

ONE: Avoid consuming caffeinated beverages (coffee, sodas, tea) and fat-burning combos containing ephedrine or caffeine at least five hours prior to bedtime. These substances will suppress stage 5, REM-Sleep.

TWO: Avoid alcoholic beverages at least five hours prior to sleep because alcohol can strongly interfere with "pattern sleeping" by reducing the quality and quantity and, as a result, minimize muscle recovery. It also inhibits the enzymes involved in energy production for upcoming workouts. A Friday evening of alcohol bingeing at the local pub can derail pattern sleeping and decrease testosterone production until the following Tuesday. You must abstain from hanging around with Jack Daniels or Jim Beam.

THREE: Make sure the last couple of meals of your day contain a protein source high in the amino acid tryptophan (which is good for relaxation and inducing sleep). Turkey and milk products are good sources.

FOUR: Reduce any activity that might produce stress, especially before bedtime. Don't get involved with any issues requiring deep concentration such as personal finances, relationship problems or any other personal conflicts. It's a good idea to shut off the phone, TV or anything else that could distract you. You could also try some behavior-calming techniques such as light reading, taking a nice warm shower or using a sound therapy system that encompasses your room with relaxing sounds.

FIVE: Melatonin is produced in the pineal gland of your brain and improves sleep patterns. Take 1 to 3 milligrams 30 minutes before your bedtime.

SIX: Open your bedroom window slightly so you can breathe a free and uninterrupted supply of cool air (but keep your bedroom as pitch black and noise-proof as possible). Avoid a severe draft, a freezing atmosphere or a hot bedroom. If possible, keep the temperature in your bedroom (and other rooms of the house) between 60 and 70 degrees.

Make sure your mattress is an ideal sleeping surface. It should distribute your weight evenly and, in doing so, it should reduce stress on your shoulders, hips and legs. Whether you sleep on your back, stomach or side, your spine should remain in a neutral position without sagging. Use a light pillow for head support.

In our discussion of sleep, we talked about GH release and its contribution to protein synthesis, as well as repair and growth of muscle tissue. Whenever the subject of growth hormones comes up, it always presents an opportunity to discuss the topic of our next chapter – anabolic steroids.

Photo by Rich Baker
Model Matthew Roberts

CHAPTER 15

IMPACT OF STEROIDS

There's no denying that anabolic steroids are an extremely potent substance – the question is, at what cost?

Over the years, we've received many questions on the subject of anabolic steroids. Those questions usually center on their potential side effects and how to take them correctly. These questions often come from people who consider themselves serious bodybuilders, but feel they've reached a crossroads in their training. They've been training hard and consistently, four or five days a week and for a number of years, but feel as though they've reached a plateau because they aren't seeing the results they had always envisioned. Like a mirage, the desired results appear within grasp but are forever just a little too far away. Unfortunately, these bodybuilders have come to the conclusion that without some kind of external assistance, they'll never realize their dream. As a result, they begin to wonder about experimenting with the drug they've heard will yield great muscle gains: Anabolic steroids.

As all-natural bodybuilders, we don't even like discussing the topic of anabolic steroids. It's our opinion that taking anabolic steroids at any stage of your training is a mistake. Gaining muscle mass takes time. Many guys expect to look like a bodybuilding champion after four or five years of training. In any other sport, would you expect to become a world champion that quickly? No way. It takes great patience, hard work and sometimes even a lifetime of dedication to attain great success in any walk of life. Bodybuilding is no different.

Most bodybuilders who use anabolic steroids will tell you they feel the drugs are a necessary tool to compete with other national and pro-level athletes, but they'd really rather not take them. These guys feel they've gone as far as genetics will take them and they need that extra push to get to the next level. They begin to believe that the risks of taking anabolic steroids are outweighed by the rewards. This misguided belief leads them to making the mistake of experimenting with anabolic steroids. Once on the juice (anabolic steroids), they begin to accomplish their muscle-gaining goals, but they soon discover that this road is full of perils. They become dependant on steroids and find they must continually increase their dosages to get the same results, and this habit often spirals out of control. The side effects include the very real possibility of a failure of key bodily functions including kidney and liver.

Years of use can leave their once awe-inspiring physiques looking quite different from their stunning earlier forms. They become nothing

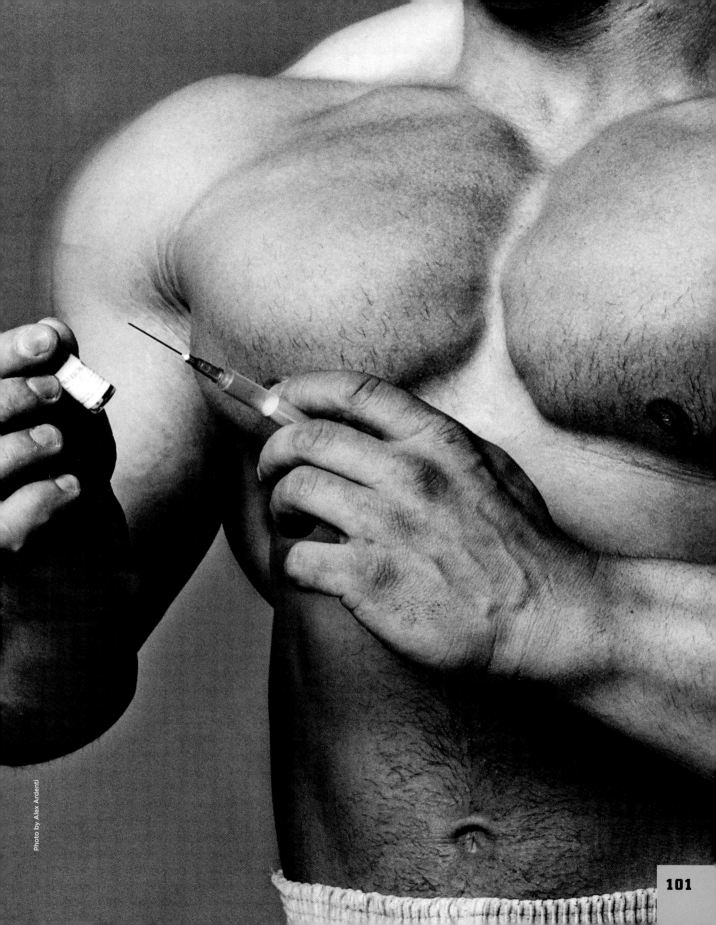

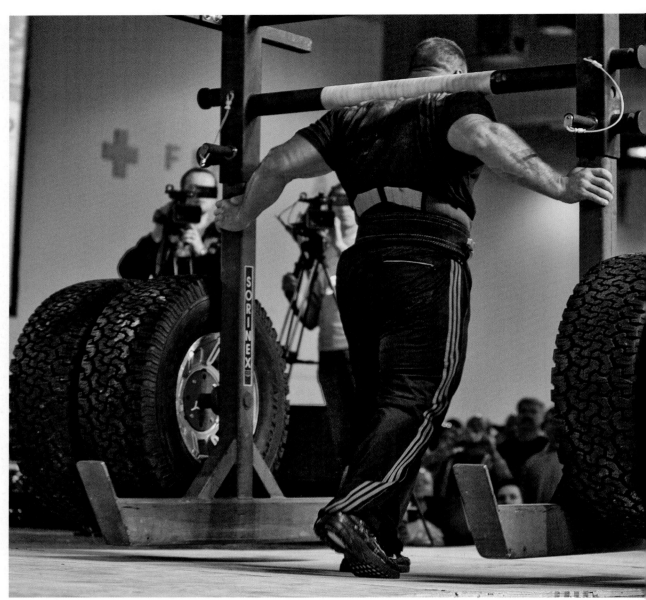

Illegal substances like anabolic steroids have infiltrated many sports, but it's powerlifting and bodybuilding that have gotten the bad rap.

but pathetic shells of their former selves, with little muscle and a host of health problems. We've seen this cycle occur in powerlifters within mere months. While training for competitions, they take enough doses of anabolic steroids that they very quickly increase their deadlift and squat totals by roughly 100 pounds. After they come off the juice, those totals come crashing down almost as quickly as the weights hit the floor following an impressive lift.

With all the negative news that's been generated of late about anabolic steroid abuse, and with law-enforcement officials cracking down, we recommend you don't even think about asking around. Like cocaine and heroin, anabolic steroids are a controlled substance. Anabolic steroids are a prescription for serving hard time. Don't run the risk of being forced to wear government-issued casual wear. The life you know and love will cease to exist.

Photos by Rich Baker
Model Derek Poundstone

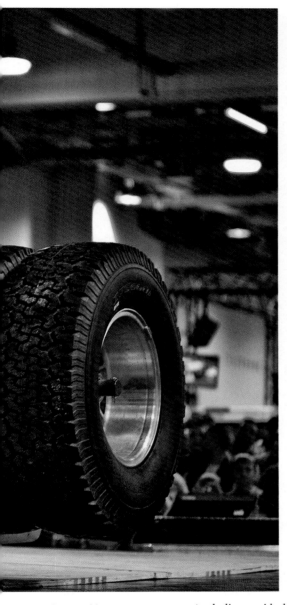

Some athletes turn to steroids because they think they've maxed out their natural genetic potential.

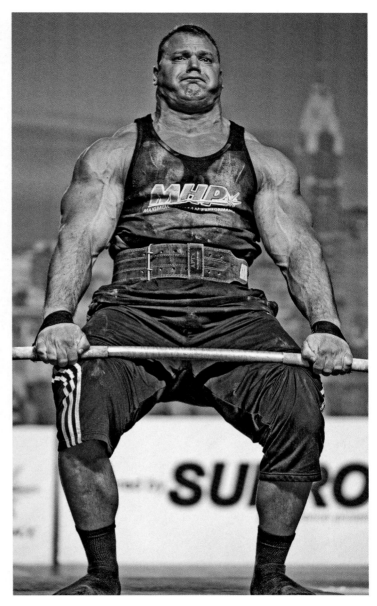

Anabolic steroids do work, but at what cost? Are the risks really worth the rewards? Don't make the mistake of thinking that just because you know someone who looks great while on the gear, that it somehow indicates anabolic steroids are safe. They aren't. Healthier, natural alternatives to anabolic steroids do exist, and they'll give you a far greater chance to live your life to its fullest. If you want another opinion, you might also consider checking out Chris Bell's captivating documentary, *Bigger, Stronger, Faster*. At the very least, it will give you some ideas to ponder regarding the subject of anabolic steroids.

We recommend you take the safe approach. A steroid-free bodybuilder will be healthier, have greater longevity and a more consistent physique. Best of all, your loved ones won't have to prematurely contact an undertaker about your funeral arrangements.

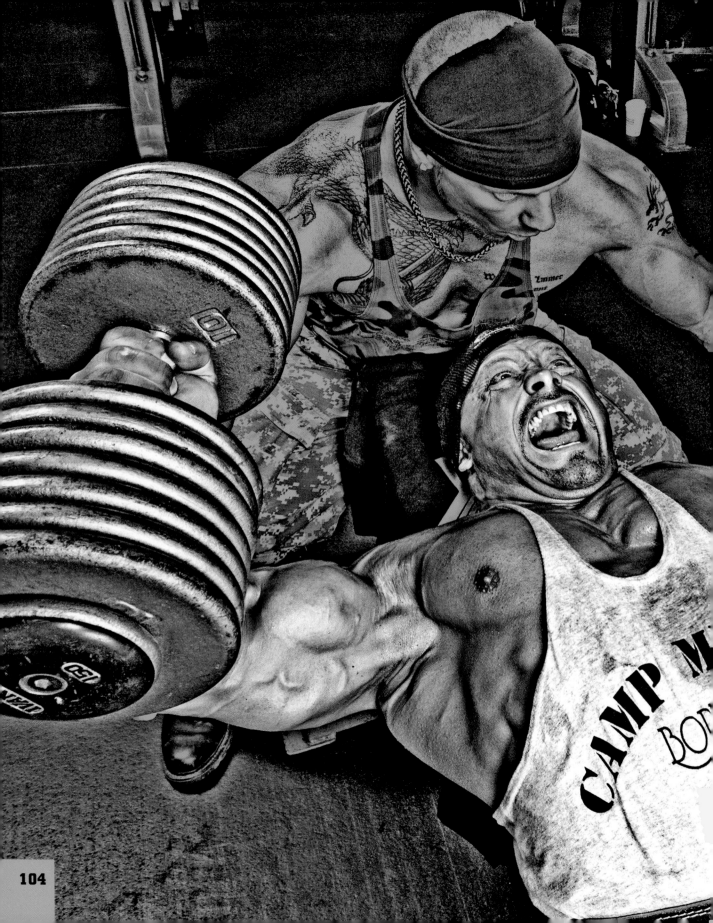

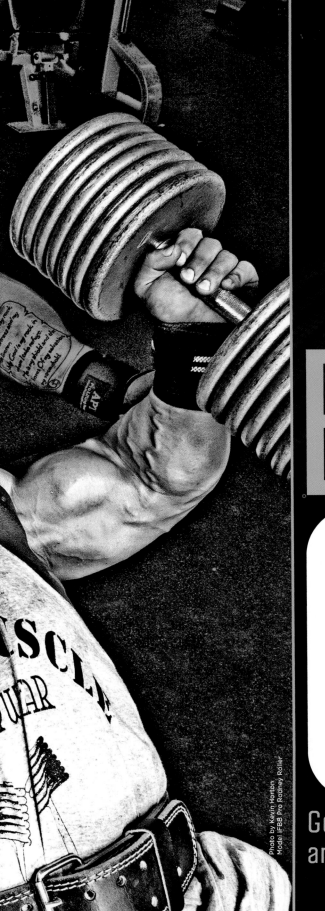

BOOK
04

Genetic Potential, Motivation and Goal Setting

CHAPTER 16

THE "PERFECT" TRAINING PROGRAM

Your individual physiology, genetics and lifestyle are main determining factors for what program will work best for you.

Genetic potential plays a major role in gaining massive muscle size and strength, but even with superior genetics, developing a championship physique will require a great deal of effort. Desire, discipline and the motivation to succeed are also imperative to success, and many bodybuilders are lacking in these areas. There is only one Jay Cutler and few others rival him. And even with his superior genetics, he works harder than probably any other bodybuilder out there. You must work with what you have, and strive for new and better ways to pile on the muscle mass. In the end, you'll mold yourself to be the best you can be, and that is the essence of being a superior bodybuilder.

We've all seen guys in the gym with great genetics who train once or twice a week, if that often, and who often train more with their mouth than they do with their body. On the other end of the spectrum, some guys train hard and consistently but will never have great bodies because of the hand they were dealt. It's a shame because while they will never be great bodybuilders or powerlifters, they have awesome desire and discipline. Another group of trainers believes there is one big bodybuilding secret and they are constantly in search of the perfect training program. We're not too proud to admit that we have spent our many years in the iron game seeking the perfect training program for developing muscle mass and strength. We still haven't found the perfect program, and we're certainly old enough to know we probably won't, but we're also young enough to keep on searching.

Bodybuilding for muscle mass and strength is not a cookie-cutter process and you shouldn't be misled by the methods of genetically superior bodybuilders, powerlifters and strongman competitors. These pros, almost regardless of what they eat or how they train, will devel-

Photo by Robert Reiff
Models Darrell Terrell / Joel Stubbs

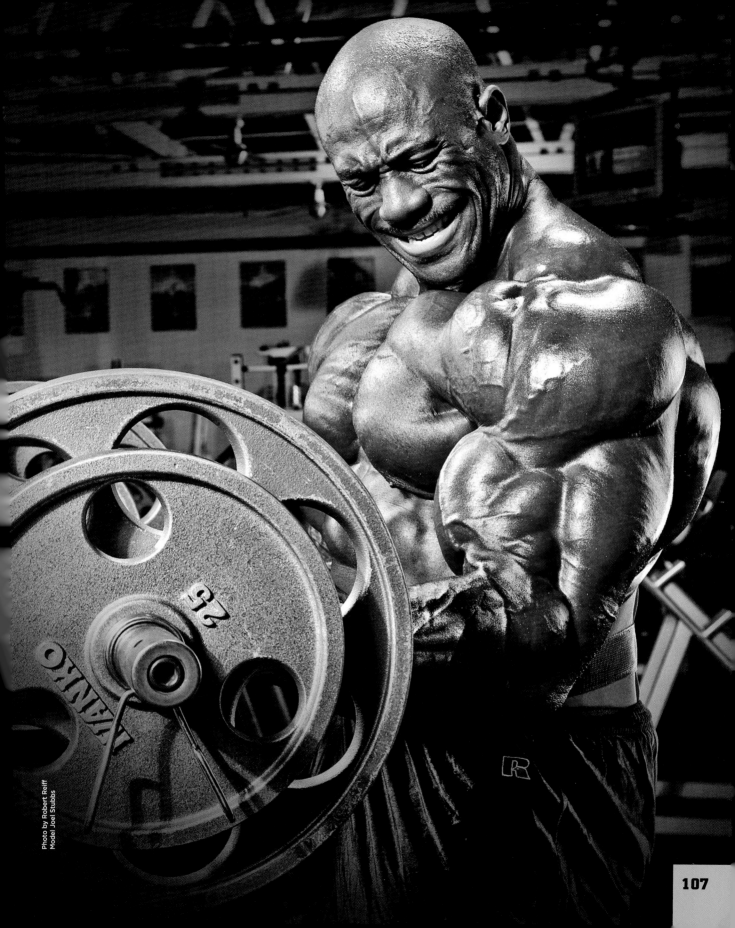

107

Your natural body type will impact your training and nutritional needs.

op outstanding physiques of muscle mass and strength and win bodybuilding contests. The average bodybuilder will not achieve the same results by following the training and eating methods of these lucky few.

Your body evolves through many physiological changes during your life. As a result, you'll discover that pretty much every training program works to some degree, but some will work better for you than others, whereas some will work fine for a while and then stop working.

10 PERFECT TRAINING PROGRAM REQUIREMENTS

The perfect training program for you has to take into account the discovery process. Here are our thoughts regarding the requirements necessary for a perfect training program.

1. AGE FACTOR

This consideration is a biggie, especially for the two of us these days! On average, stamina or endurance peaks in your mid 30s and then declines at a rate of about one percent per year. Strength, on the other hand, develops well into your 20s, 30s and 40s and then begins to decline at a little less than one percent a year from then on. During this time, we lose muscle at a rate of about 11 ounces a year and gain fat at 1½ pounds per year.

The body's natural testosterone levels also decline as a person ages. For the average male this decline begins in his 40s, although an aggressive nutrition and exercise program with a healthy lifestyle can slow it down. In essence, the training you do in your 20s and 30s won't be anywhere near as effective in your 40s and 50s because of physiological changes. Over the years, the ratios of fast- and slow-twitch muscle fibers change.

2. RECUPERATION

Regardless of whether or not you're following a solid nutritional regimen, recuperation changes with age. When we were in our 20s, 30s and 40s, we might have recovered from a certain workout in only two or three days. Now, even with a solid nutritional regimen, recovery can take five or six days.

3. TRAINING EXPERIENCE

Training intensity is often directly related to your iron-pumping experience. Of course, there are exceptions to the rule. We've seen some very experienced people in the gym who look as if they've been training for only a few months. We've also seen the opposite.

4. BODY TYPES

In the 1940s, William Sheldon came up with biological identification tags (somatotypes) describing the different body types. The somatotypes – endomorphs, ectomorphs and mesomorphs – have unique training and nutritional considerations. Which of these body types best describes you and its respective considerations need to be accounted for when mapping out your training program. The following is a brief overview of the training and nutritional needs of each somatotype.

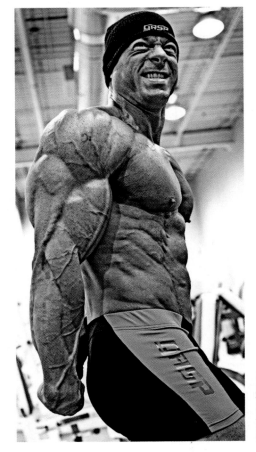

Photo by Paul Buceta
Model Adam Headland

Advanced body-builders have years of experience under their belts, and that skill level is typically reflected in routines of high intensity.

An endomorph consumes large portions of food and has the ability to gain muscle or fat quite easily. Unfortunately, an endomorph typically has a great deal of excess bodyfat with little evidence of any muscle definition.

1. Train four times per week using the push/pull system.
2. Do two or three exercises (three sets of 12 to 15 reps) per bodypart.
3. Do the exercises in a superset or tri-set fashion and rest only 30 to 45 seconds between sets.
4. Eat low-calorie, low-fat foods every 3½ hours. Remember, if you eat more than a certain level of calories you will gain fat. You must find that level.
5. Use thermogenic (fat-burning) agents.
6. Do an aerobic session (early morning before breakfast or immediately after your weight workout) of 40 to 50 minutes per day.

An ectomorph tends to be a hard gainer and is usually tall and almost rail thin. On the bright side, the ectomorph can lose weight on a high-calorie diet of pizza, cheeseburgers and ice cream, however, he will have a tough time gaining muscle.

1. Do a total-body workout, twice per week on non-consecutive days.
2. Do five to seven basic exercises such as squats, bench presses, deadlifts, bent-over rows, overhead presses and curls.
3. Do three or four sets of five to eight reps. High reps are counterproductive except when targeting abs (15 to 40 reps is ideal) and calves (15 to 40 reps).
4. Eat at least six to eight small meals (natural unprocessed foods) every two to two-and-a-half hours.
5. Get lots of rest between sets and exercises (four to six minutes in some cases).

Photo by Jeremy Maurer
Model Jon Andersen

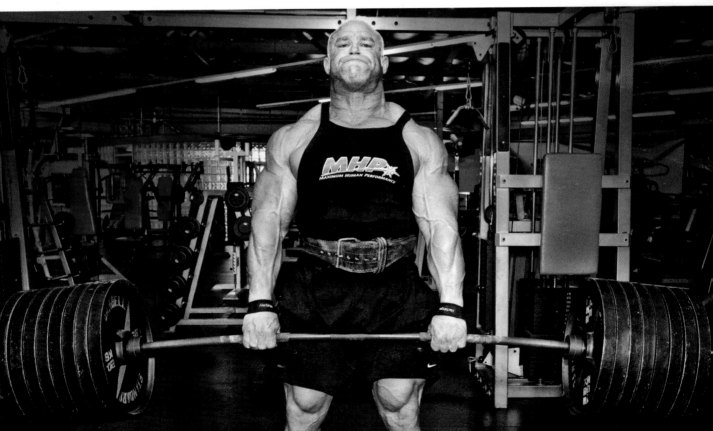

A mesomorph is a naturally athletic type, muscular and powerful. He has to watch his bodyfat levels, but can gain muscle easily.

1. Do total-body workouts, two or three times per week on non-consecutive days.
2. Do 10 to 12 exercises.
3. Do four or five sets of 8 to 10 reps each, except for abs and calves.
4. Do an aerobic session of 20 to 30 minutes, two or three days per week.

Very few people, if any, fall completely into any one somatotype. Most are a combination of two or even three. Somatotyping is considered outdated and of little value to many in the iron community, but we think it's helpful.

5. MUSCLE AND TENDON INJURIES

Past or present training injuries may not allow you to perform certain exercises in an otherwise perfect training program. Some common examples include: Barbell bench press or barbell behind-the-neck press (rotator cuff); barbell preacher curl (elbow tendons); barbell back squat (low back and knee joints).

Training injuries require immediate attention – they can shorten your career. Act now to be injury-free for the rest of your life. It's highly possible that you'll experience some type of muscle injury in your bodybuilding career. To prevent that from happening, this chapter will help you become more aware of the causes and types of injuries, as well as preventive measures and treatments.

Overtraining and physical fatigue will increase your chances of suffering an injury.

CAUSES OF MUSCLE INJURY

THE FATIGUE FACTOR

The more physically fatigued you become during a workout, the more susceptible you are to injuring yourself. Fatigue is usually the result of performing more sets than are necessary in an effort to focus on a specific bodypart. Injuries can occur in any of the three important muscles (prime movers, synergists and stabilizers, which are necessary to the force and stability of exercise movement).

A prime mover in one exercise may very well be the synergist in another exercise; a stabilizer may become a prime mover in a following move and so forth. Injuries can occur as a result of inadequate technique, not warming up properly, or, in the case of a specific exercise, going too heavy and placing too much stress on either the muscle or the tendon.

Injury to a muscle can also occur when the prime mover muscle in one exercise (e.g., overhead press with the anterior delt as prime mover) was functioning earlier in the workout as a synergist (e.g., bench press with anterior delt as synergist). In this case, the anterior delts were already fatigued slightly in the bench press, and once you began doing overhead presses, fatigue in the delts accelerated and an injury resulted.

When a muscle is suddenly forced to switch roles between being a prime mover and a synergist, or vice versa, fatigue increases. You must perform just the right number of sets and ex-

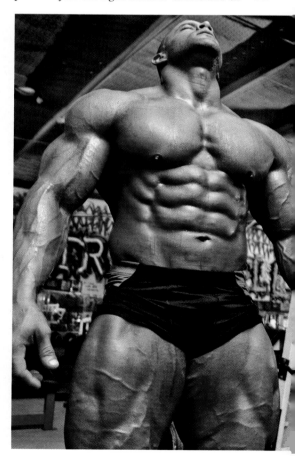

Photo by Paul Buceta
Model Manuel Romero

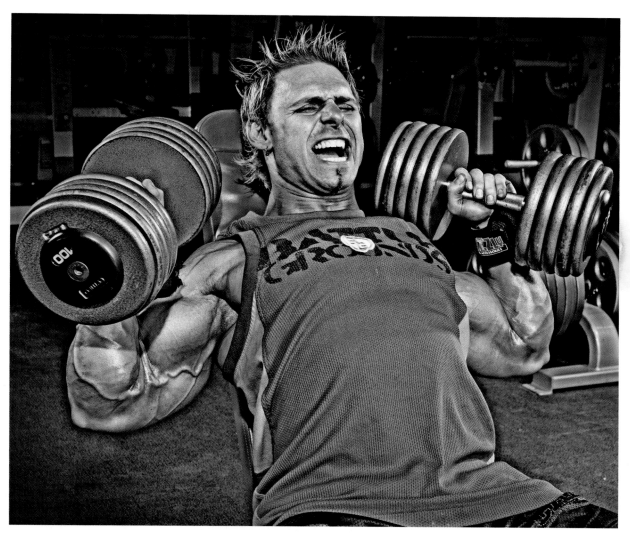

Photo by Jason Breeze
Model Andre Rzazewski

Tall bodybuilders use more energy during their workouts because they have to push and pull the weights over a greater range of motion.

ercises for each bodypart. Follow the advice of experienced bodybuilders who, through trial and error as well as scientific research, have discovered the ideal number of sets and exercises that promote size and strength gains with minimal injuries.

FATIGUE AND THE TALL BODYBUILDER

Fatigue is a common problem for tall bodybuilders. A taller bodybuilder must push or pull the weights a greater distance than a shorter bodybuilder. As a result, the taller lifter must expend a great deal more energy, especially near the completion of each rep. Under these conditions,

injuries can occur, and, for that reason, it's very important that taller bodybuilders take more time to recover between workouts than their shorter counterparts.

LACK OF FLEXIBILITY

Injury can also be caused by forcing a muscle through an unfamiliar range of movement. We frequently hear about the potential of a knee injury when performing squats. But when performed properly, squats actually improve the muscle stability around your knee joints. The best method for introducing a muscle to a new range of movement is to inch your way gradually into that new depth.

ADDING POUNDAGES TOO RAPIDLY

Injuries can result when you add poundages far exceeding those previously used in training. Increase your poundages slowly.

UNBALANCED STRENGTHS

Injury can also result when muscles and supporting tissues are developed disproportionately. For example, you might injure your lower back while performing some heavy parallel squats because the supporting strength of the lower back is not in proportion to the strength of the thigh muscles. Equal training is an absolute necessity for development around the joints of the body, especially since many of these muscles work in pairs, as shown in the following table.

Triceps and Biceps
Anterior Delts and Traps and Posterior Delts
Pectorals and Lats
Quadriceps and Hamstrings
Spinae Erectors and Abdominals
Calves and Tibialis Anterior

Of all the muscle groups depicted in the table, the two that are most often treated unevenly in training are the quadriceps and hamstrings, as well as the spinae erectors and abdominals. If you focus exclusively on any one area, you're inviting injury. To prevent such injuries, train sensibly by applying equal effort to opposing pairs of the various muscle groups.

If you're like most people, your quadriceps are stronger than your hamstrings by a ratio of nearly four to one. Your goal should be to give equal training time to your hamstrings and work at achieving a quad-to-hamstring strength ratio of at least three to one. The ideal would be a two-to-one ratio.

Likewise, lower-body specialists who train their legs with little regard to training the spinae erectors and abdominals in the upper body are headed for some major injuries. If you're one of these bodybuilders, you risk blowing out your lower back or groin due to the unbalanced strength ratio between the weaker undeveloped erectors/abs and the stronger quad/hamstring muscles. To prevent injuries, train your upper and lower body equally.

Muscular proportion through equal training for muscle pairs, like biceps and triceps, is very important to prevent injury.

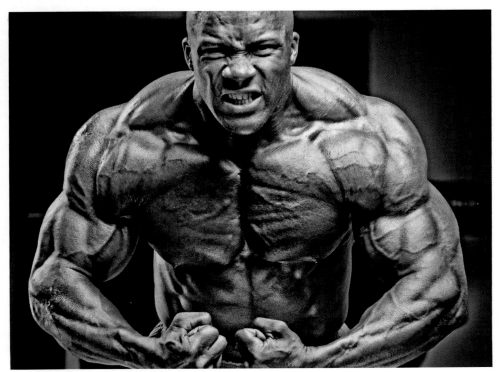

Photo by Kevin Horton
Model Jonathan Rowe

Connective tissue doesn't get stronger at the same rate your muscles do, so it can't handle the same weight the muscles can.

TENDON AND LIGAMENT INJURY

Ligaments and tendons are connective tissues. Tendons attach muscle to bone and ligaments connect bone to bone. Ligament and tendon injuries usually occur when a joint is bent further than its existing range of movement. The three particular situations most associated with these injuries include:

1. Over-enthusiastic beginners who over-tax their inflexible and previously unused muscles will suffer strains in the connective tissues of the joints.
2. Advanced bodybuilders experience the same problems as these beginners, especially when coming off an extended training layoff.
3. Lack of flexibility can result in sprains.

Strength in the connective tissue doesn't increase in proportion to an increase in muscle strength. As a result, the connective tissue may not be ready to handle the weight the muscle can, and is therefore very susceptible to injury. Remember: A minor tendon strain can take months to heal and a sprained ligament can take even longer.

TREATMENT AND PREVENTATIVE MEASURES

It's vitally important that you apply ice packs within 10 to 15 minutes of the injury taking place. You may use a cold pack (made of crushed ice in a zip lock with a squirt of water) or the frozen gel pack variety. Regarding the latter, it's important to realize that, depending on the temperature of the freezer unit they're stored in, these gel packs may be significantly below zero and could cause a mild form of frostbite. You can prevent this by wrapping the ice pack in a thin cloth before applying. Chemical ice packs usually won't keep your injury cold enough for long enough periods. They also have the reputation of causing chemical burns on your body.

If your injury is to a limb, elevate your injured muscle six to ten inches above heart level. Place the ice application on your injured area with an even compression. Secure the ice

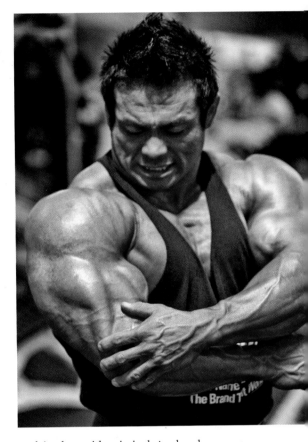

pack in place with a six-inch Ace bandage wrap. Apply ice treatments for 15 to 20 minutes at a time, with a $1\frac{1}{2}$- to 2-hour lapse between applications. To control your swelling, be sure to follow these directions for the 24 hours immediately following the injury (only during the hours that you're awake). To help control your pain, take an anti-inflammatory drug every four to six hours (read directions). Consult a doctor if the pain doesn't subside.

If you remove the ice pack application, remember to immediately reapply the Ace bandage. You should wear the wrap at all times, even when you sleep. Use a sling for arm injuries and crutches for leg injuries as this will lessen the pain and hasten recuperation.

After the initial 24 hours of ice therapy, you should begin applying the packs intermittently. When these procedures are not possible, such as during sleep or work, use an analgesic sports cream. It's also a good idea to take strong

Photo by Paul Buceta
Model Hidetada Yamagishi

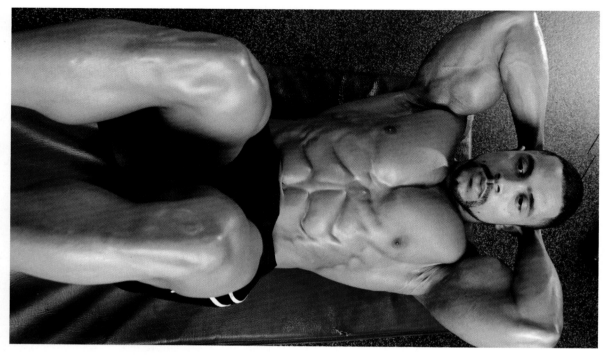

Healing can only take place with rest, but depending on the injury, you can often train around the injured bodypart.

doses of calcium (phosphorus-free), magnesium and especially manganese in chelated forms, every three hours, for three to ten days.

Resting your injured bodypart is of the utmost importance, but that doesn't mean you should cease all workout activity. Train around your injury. For example, if you have a shoulder injury, train around this by performing crunches and lying leg raises for the abdominals and leg extensions and leg curls for the quads and hamstrings. Options for the legs include Roman-chair squats, sissy squats and one-leg squats, all of which can be done with just your own body weight. Do one-arm exercises and movements for your upper body utilizing a Universal machine.

Injuries that don't respond to the treatments suggested are in need of more intense therapy such as ultrasound or diathermy and a good anti-inflammatory agent. If your injury reaches this critical point, you'll most definitely want to consult a knowledgeable sports medicine doctor, chiropractor or physical therapist. These professionals will assist you on your road to recovery by helping you renew your flexibility and strengthening your injured muscle.

Some of the best exercises that will provide an exceptional degree of stretching are full squats, stiff-leg deadlifts, shrugs, parallel bar dips, barbell wrist curls (performed on a slight decline) and heel raises.

Elbows deserve additional attention. If you're training with sore elbows, follow the guidelines:

DON'T:

• Perform any type of lockouts or full-extension movements either overhead or in the supine position. Stay away from performing any of the various pressing movements for your chest, deltoids and triceps.

• Perform any exercises with a wide grip that would cause the elbows to extend away from the sides of your body including exercises such as the wide-grip bench presses or wide-grip Gironda body drag curls, wide-grip upright rows, etc. These exercises cause the muscles and tendons to be stretched tight and this won't assist you as you recover from sore elbows.

DO:

• Moves such as pushdowns and dumbbell kickbacks for your triceps and thumbs-up lateral raises for your deltoids.

• Only those exercise movements where your arms remain close to the sides of your body.

Photo by David Ford
Model Tim Liggins

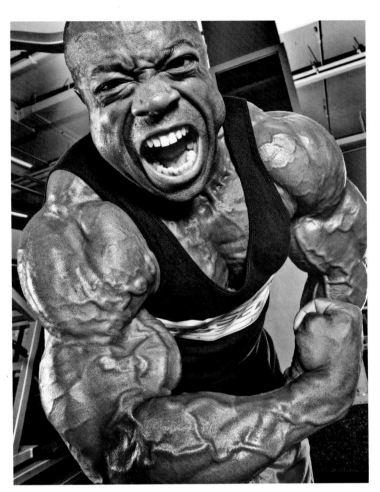

Motivation can be a real driving force in your training.

Photo by Paul Buceta
Model Leo Ingram

A final note on prevention: The best way to prevent injuries altogether is to follow the proper exercise procedure, as detailed throughout this book.

6. EXERCISE EQUIPMENT

Some perfect training programs call for a plethora of training equipment that you'd only have access to at a commercial gym. Unfortunately, you may not live near one of these gyms and only have free weights available, or at the very least you have less equipment than the program suggests. What do you do then?

7. LIFESTYLE

Obviously a 17-year-old bodybuilder living at home and working part time can train virtually any time he likes. Some of the perfect training programs suggest training more than once per day, which doesn't take into consideration the possibility of having a 12-hour shift or two part-time jobs. The end result of maintaining such a training schedule is that you'll end up losing your job, your spouse or your social life.

8. TRAINING PLATEAUS

As we've mentioned on many occasions, your body evolves through many physiological changes during your lifetime. As a result, you'll discover that almost any training program will work, some better than others, but not all the time. With this in mind, you should alter training programs every few weeks.

Our philosophy regarding the perfect training program is that a good training plan today is better than a perfect training plan tomorrow, because tomorrow never comes. Ultimately if there's a secret at all, it's that proper training is brutally hard and maintaining a regular and consistent schedule (preferably at the same time each day) is absolutely necessary to keep a bodybuilder's physiological clock in a positive mode.

The only way to get truly huge and strong is to push past the pain threshold. The last two or three reps of a really hard set aren't called the golden reps for nothing. We have spent plenty of time in the pain zone. Being able to do reps when your muscles are screaming at you to stop is when you'll make truly magnificent and massive muscle gains.

9. TEMPERAMENT

Some people enjoy heavy-duty, screamfest, push-it-to-the-limit training. Others thrive on building muscle in a more quiet and thoughtful fashion.

10. MOTIVATION

Highly-motivated bodybuilders like being pushed and have a better success rate training in a home-gym environment than those who are only moderately motivated. If you're not highly motivated, train in a commercial gym. You might also consider hiring a personal bodybuilding coach.

CHAPTER 17

TEN MOTIVATIONAL TOOLS

High levels of motivation will better your chances of success with your physique goals.

Here are 10 tools and suggestions that should help you maintain a high level of motivation.

1 If you train alone, find a training partner. He or she can spur you on to greater efforts through words of encouragement or friendly competition. Just be careful the training sessions don't turn into social hours. If you can't find yourself a training partner, then load up your iPod with your favorite energetic music. It'll help you maintain a vigorous tempo from rep to rep and set to set – plus it'll make your training time appear to go by a little bit faster.

2 Attending or entering drug-tested physique and powerlifting contests can be excellent for ramping up motivation. You'll certainly come away with some ideals with regard to physique and strength standards. Also, entering a physique transformation challenge can really supercharge you to train and eat correctly. Motivation should always be intrinsic (to satisfy yourself) and not extrinsic (doing it for someone else).

3 Many well-produced motivational training DVDs are currently on the market. Use these for tips on training, nutrition and discipline and learn such information as how the top pros keep their diets on track.

4 Another major motivational monitoring tool is a non-shrinkable nylon tape measure. It's important to take circumference measurements when the muscle is cold and not pumped. Be honest and accurate.

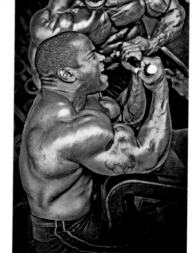

Photo Rich Baker
Modes Joel Stubbs / Johnnie Jackson

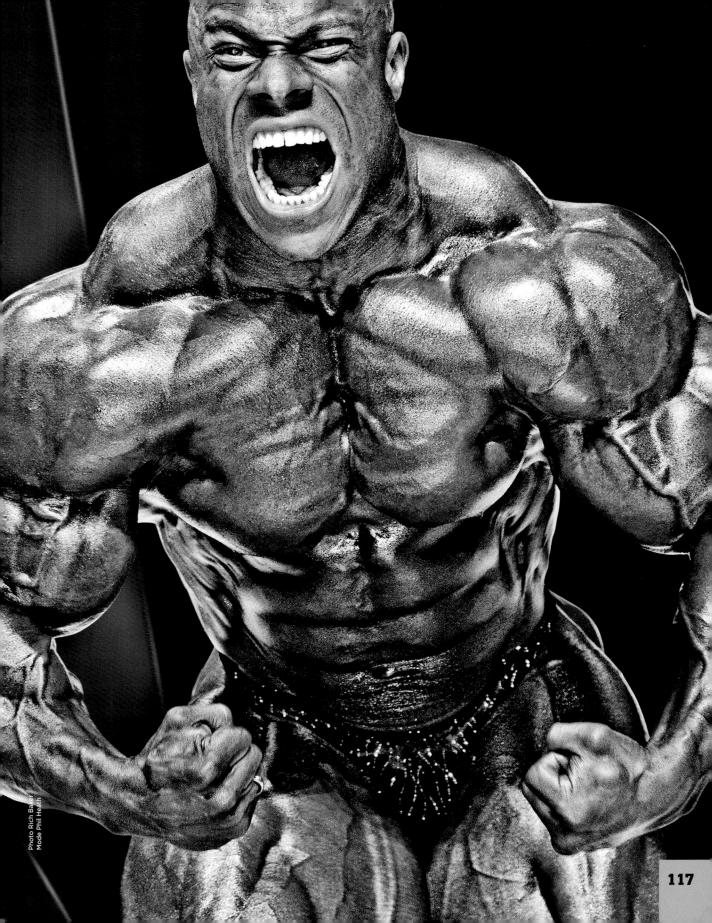

HOW TO TAKE ACCURATE CIRCUMFERENCE MEASUREMENTS

Neck – Measure just above your Adam's apple.

Shoulders – Have someone else measure at the widest portion of your deltoids with your arms hanging and your palms resting flat on the sides of your thighs.

Chest – After exhaling, measure under arms across your chest at nipple level.

Biceps – Contract the biceps and with the upper arm parallel to the floor, measure to its peak.

Forearms – With elbow straight, make a fist and bend wrist. Measure the largest portion below elbow.

Wrist – With your palm open, measure around the bones of your wrist.

Abdomen – After a deep breath, gently exhale and measure around waist at navel level.

Hips – Measure at largest point around buttocks with heels together.

Thighs – Measure just below buttocks, high on thigh and feet shoulder-width apart.

Calf – Measure around largest portion with feet flat and knee straight.

5 Here's some nifty little motivational bodyweight, measurement and training poundage guidelines:

Measurements aren't the criterion of bodybuilding perfection because they don't take into account symmetry and proportion.

HEIGHT	WEIGHT	ARMS	NECK	CHEST	WAIST	THIGHS	CALVES
5' 4"	155 lbs.	16"	16"	44"	30"	22½"	15½"
5' 6"	175 lbs.	16½"	16½"	46"	31"	23"	15¾"
5' 8"	185 lbs.	17"	16¾"	47"	31½"	23½"	16"
5' 10"	200 lbs.	17½"	17"	48"	32½"	24½"	16½"
6' 0"	210 lbs.	17¾"	17½"	49"	33"	25"	17¼"
6' 2"	220 lbs.	18"	18"	50"	33½"	26½"	18"

To accurately measure your chest, exhale and then measure under your arms across your chest around nipple level.

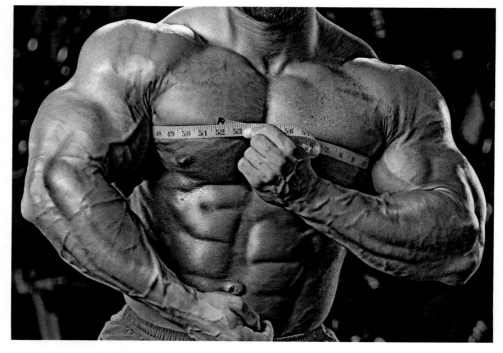

Photo by Robert Reiff
Model Santana Anderson

For example, you might have 18 inch upper arms, but what the tape measure doesn't reveal is perhaps a short biceps or high triceps muscle fault.

TRAINING POUNDAGE CONSIDERATIONS

There's another measurement guide at www.dennisbweis.com/charts.html that covers a wide range of bodyweights and what's considered a fair, good and excellent one-rep max (one rep) for most healthy, anabolic-drug-free power bodybuilders in their 20s, 30s and early 40s. Our very good friend, bodybuilding writer Nelson Montana, also developed a useful system for calculating the ratio of poundage to bodyweight that an adult male bodybuilder might wish to use on select compound exercises for a scheduled number of sets and reps. The chart on the right is an encapsulated look at the system he mathematically blueprinted featuring six different exercises, which target every major muscle group in your body and, if followed properly is guaranteed to generate results.

On moves like the barbell bench press, it's important to use a weight you can handle and always have a spotter on hand for safety.

HEAVY BARBELL BACK SQUATS (TO PARALLEL)

Work up to using 100 pounds in excess of bodyweight.
2-4 sets x 8-12 reps

FLAT BARBELL BENCH PRESS

Use a minimum of 25 pounds over bodyweight.
3-4 sets x 6-10 reps

STIFF-LEG BARBELL DEADLIFT

Employ a minimum of 50 pounds over bodyweight.
3-4 sets x 10-15 reps

BENT-OVER ROW

Work up to using at least 15 pounds over bodyweight.
3-4 sets x 8-12 reps

BEHIND THE NECK BARBELL PRESS

Work up to a minimum of 35 to 40 pounds under bodyweight.
4-5 sets x 5-8 reps

STANDING BARBELL CURL

Work up to using 60 pounds under bodyweight.
3-4 sets x 6-8 reps

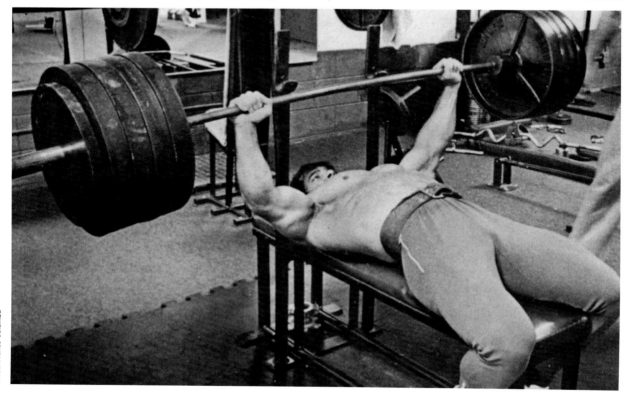

Model Franco Columbu

A training journal is an important tool that allows you to log every detail of your efforts that can be analyzed to see what's working and what's not.

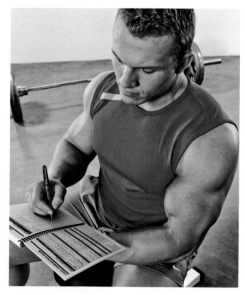

6 The visual feedback of a full-length mirror in a well-lit room (training quarters) can be a tremendous source of motivation, especially as you begin to notice the ever-increasing musculature, proportion and symmetry of your body. While the mirror will be one of your best sources for motivation, don't get so vain that you overdo it, as the mirror is only a means to an end, not the end itself.

7 The bathroom scale can be an excellent source of inspiration and motivation, especially when, at the end of the week, the weight indicator displays a muscle mass gain of a half pound to two pounds.

8 From time to time, have someone take plenty of high-quality and focused "before" and "after" photos of you. Have shots taken from all angles (front-back-side) and using different lighting schemes. For example, have some relaxed shots taken from the front and back, with your arms hanging by your sides. Also get some posed shots featuring front and back double-biceps pose, front-lat-spread pose, front most-muscular pose, side-chest and side-triceps pose. When you do your follow-up photo shoots, you should always use the same lighting scheme and background as you did in the previous sessions.

9 Another terrific motivational tool is a training log diary. It should become a diary of everything concerned with your systematic bodybuilding efforts. Writing training notes on scrap paper, as some do, is not a good idea because the notes can become lost or you can simply forget to transfer the notes to a permanent, inexpensive notebook, such as the *MuscleMag No Pain No Gain Training Journal*. The journal will prove to be an invaluable tool that will help you track important workout information. Rest assured, the information contained in the training log will be most helpful in analyzing your previous training efforts and how to develop a better systematic training plan for the future.

10 Specific goal setting is yet another motivational tool for helping you to reach your genetic potential as you strive to build your massive muscle mass and strength. Set, achieve and reset realistic goals to provide yourself with a roadmap to success. Evaluate your present conditioning levels and genetic potential. Based on your findings, choose several reasonable short-term goals, and one long-term goal. Rather than just thinking about the goals, it's better to write them down in a section of your training log diary. This stimulates a filtering part of your brain called the reticular activating system, which creates an acute goal-setting awareness in the subconscious portion of your mind.

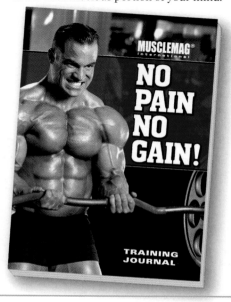

Photo by Robert Reiff
Model Tomm Voss

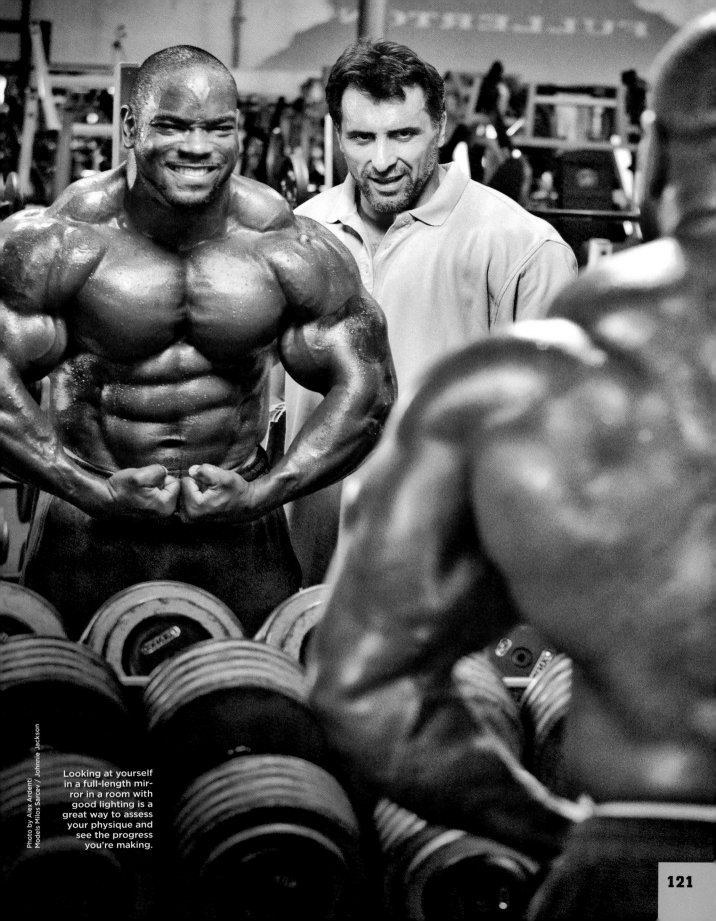

Looking at yourself in a full-length mirror in a room with good lighting is a great way to assess your physique and see the progress you're making.

CHAPTER 18

GOAL SETTING

Bodybuilding is process; growth and improvements start with making specific goals and creating a strategy to achieve those goals.

In order to achieve any goal, you have to address obstacles, formulate a strategy, set deadline dates and continually evaluate your progress. Setting specific short-term goals will bring you closer to achieving a long-term goal.

Setting a long-term goal should be easy. Long-term goals are made up of several short-term goals, which can serve as benchmarks. Your first step will be to address any obstacles in your way. Are you not eating right? Are you not training with a plan? These are the types of questions you have to ask yourself. Second, you need to formulate a strategy. Are you looking to add 15, 20 or 30 pounds of solid muscle? From there, you need to set deadline dates. Do you want to achieve your best body in 90 days? You'll need to set short-term goals of adding anywhere from half a pound to 2½ pounds of muscle per week and monitor your progress. In the long run, setting these short-term goals and deadlines will help you meet your long-term objective.

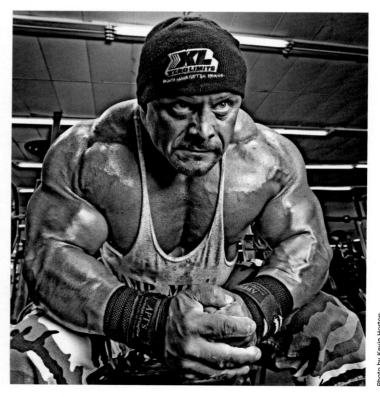

Photo by Kevin Horton
Model Rodney Roller

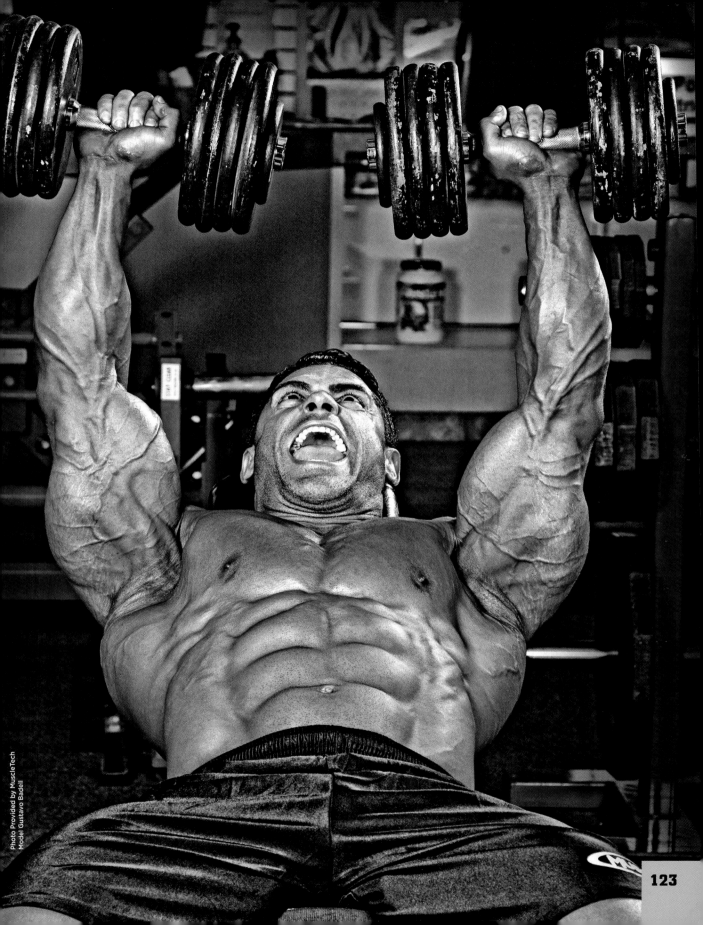

Assume your all-time best in the barbell back squat is 275 pounds for one set of 12 reps and your long-term goal is to be able to do 20 reps. Set a short-term goal of adding one additional rep in every third workout. This may seem insignificant, but it will point you in the right direction to meet your long-term goal. Some very successful competitive bodybuilders set 52 weekly short-term goals to reach one long-term goal per year. Other potential strategies include:

- Maintain a constant workout and nutrition program during the next 10 to 12 weeks.
- Eat eight small meals each day rather than the usual six, as a way to ensure you stay in a positive anabolic balance.
- Regularly use a variety of sauna and massage muscle-recovery techniques.
- Set an annual long-term goal and subdivide it into 12 short-term monthly goals.
- Record your progress in a training journal, making sure to check it for added motivation.

Setting short-term goals for yourself, even daily ones, is a very effective step-by-step strategy that will help you stay motivated and on track to reach your long-term goals.

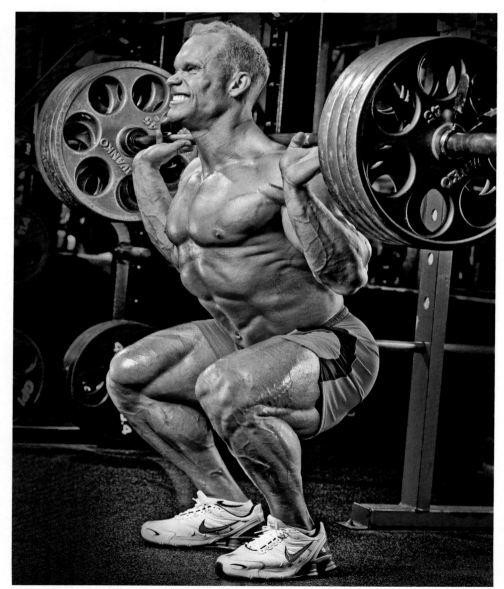

Photo by Robert Reiff
Model Ben Pakulski

Some tangible motivation can go a long way to help you achieve your goals. The $500 Goal Guarantee is one example of a reward system you can use in your training.

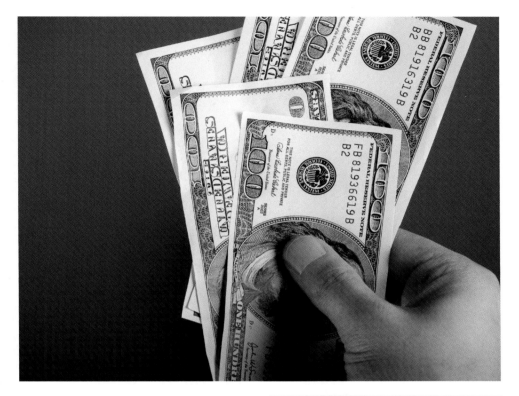

A lot of people, including bodybuilders, set their goals at the start of a new year. Sadly, few follow through on their resolutions. We won't get into all the excuses and reasons for their failure. Instead we're simply going to reveal a unique and somewhat radical method to achieving your goals of attaining a great physique.

THE $500 GOAL GUARANTEE

Put a $100 bill into five envelopes and address each envelope to an organization you dislike intensely. Give these envelopes to a trusted friend and tell him or her to mail the first envelope if you fail to meet your first short-term training goal on schedule (barring injury, sickness, a death in the family or any other reasonable excuse). If you meet your objective, your friend simply gives you back the envelope. Keep this going until you've either succeeded or failed in your quest to reach all of your goals. If you want to make sure you get all five of those envelopes back, you should create a list like the one that follows.

GOAL-SETTING CHART

Name
Area Needing Improvement
Statement of Goal
Obstacles
Solutions
Target Date
Short-Term Goals
Long-Term Goals
Rewards / Benefits
Evaluation Date Progress

A FINAL THOUGHT ON MOTIVATION

If you aren't motivated to train, you simply won't achieve the type of results you crave. When you're motivated to train and take it as seriously as an IRS tax auditor does his job, you'll achieve tremendous bodybuilding results. The bottom line is that you can successfully improve your existing size and strength, no matter who you are, by following the training recommendations in this book.

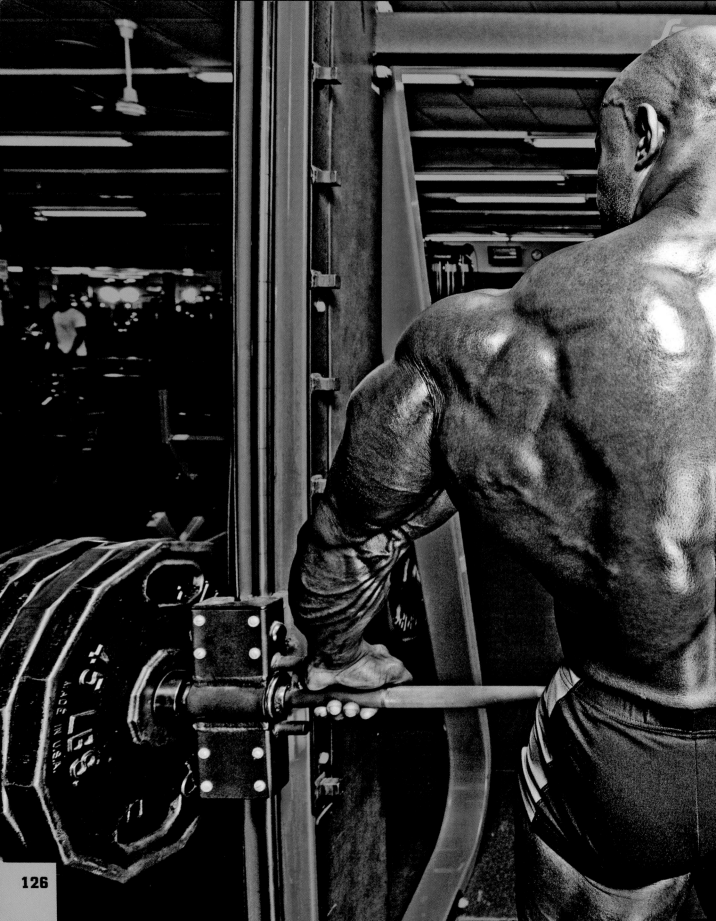

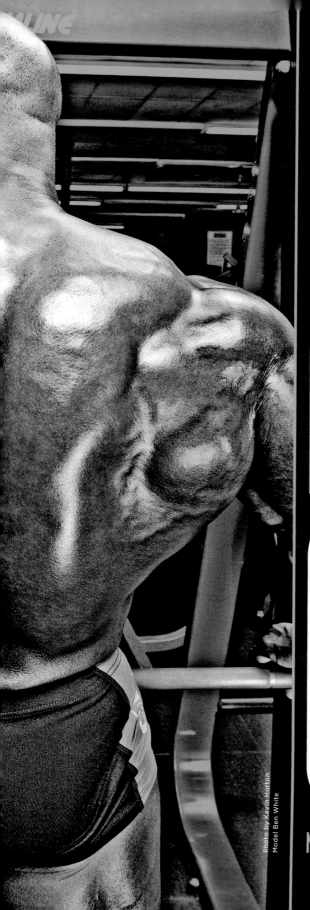

BOOK 05

Mental Power

CHAPTER 19

MIND-MUSCLE IMAGERY

Establishing a concentrated mind-muscle connection when you train will have a positive impact on your muscle growth and strength improvements.

Bill Pearl, former four-time Mr. Universe, once said, "A proper mental attitude plays a large role in your efforts to build size and strength. When thinking positive thoughts, one has a happy outlook on life. You should think positively about all your daily activities – physical, mental and moral. It will aid you in your training in the gym as well as your personal life. A healthy, positive attitude will improve your body and help make you a better person."
– *Bill Pearl, former four-time Mr. Universe*

"The mind controls everything when it comes to adding quality muscle. How you program the mind determines your success rate. It's a real trip to kick back and imagine yourself looking 10 pounds heavier, to visualize yourself possessing much improved muscle density."
– *Rich Gaspari, 1989 IFBB Arnold Classic winner*

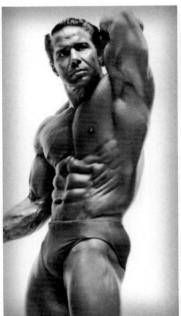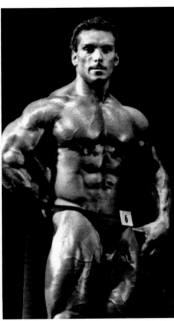

Models (left to right) Bill Pearl / Rich Gaspari

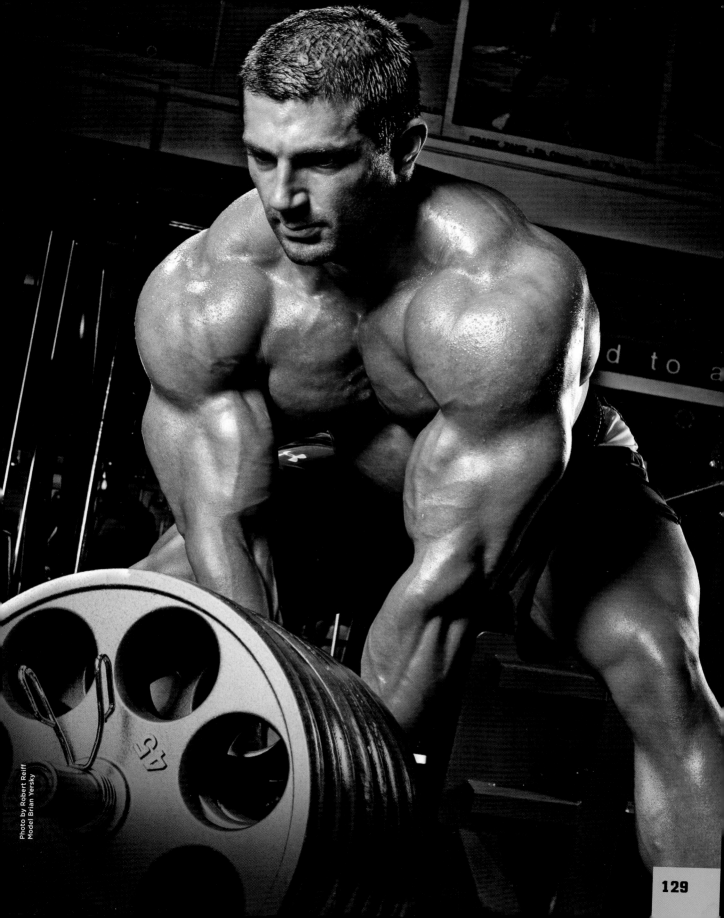

THE REHEARSAL

To the iron athlete, mental-muscle imagery rehearsal and its application is a thoughtful and intelligent two-stage event consisting of pre-workout and one-set interval preparation. Here's a brief look at each.

STAGE 1: PRE-WORKOUT IMAGERY REHEARSAL

Simply stated, you will visualize. It should seem like you're watching your workout on a movie screen before it even happens.

REQUISITES TO EFFECTIVE VISUALIZATION

About 15 to 30 minutes before your workout, go to a place of solitude. Ideally, go to a dark room, void of ringing telephones, ticking clocks, people talking and bright lights, and sit in a comfortable chair. Close your eyes. Breathe in and out through your nose, slowly and deeply, (called relaxed breathing) and just relax.

Now empty your mind of all the thoughts that do not pertain to the workout. A troublesome remark someone made might pop into your head, but don't let it. Keep any intruding thoughts out. Drive away the nagging negative voice that's telling you to skip your workout because you have to wash the car. Visualize yourself well rested, recovered and stronger from your last workout.

As you progress into a more relaxed state, picture the collective training energy being generated by the other iron warriors in the gym. Feel this sensation. Feel the energy giving you a special power to dominate the heavy iron. Become a master of training by mentally reproducing the tracking patterns of the exercises rep for rep, set for set. Repeat this process several times in your mind. Finally, see yourself at the conclusion of the workout with a bone-deep, growth-producing, vein-choked pump in the muscles of your upper arms. When the mental pictures and related sensations are clear and vivid, open your eyes. You should now have an unyielding commitment, intense desire, determination and a powerful will to succeed flowing, pulsing and surging through your veins. It's now time to get up out of your chair and step into the hardcore trenches of the gym.

STAGE 2: ONE-SET MENTAL-MUSCLE REHEARSAL

This stage of mental-muscle imagery is conducted approximately 10 to 15 seconds before each set of an exercise. Close your eyes. Inhale and exhale deeply as you prepare for the moment at hand. Go to that place in your consciousness where there's no pain, no negative influences and no fear. It's a state of mind where only positive forces dwell and your goals can be attained by capitalizing on this mindset.

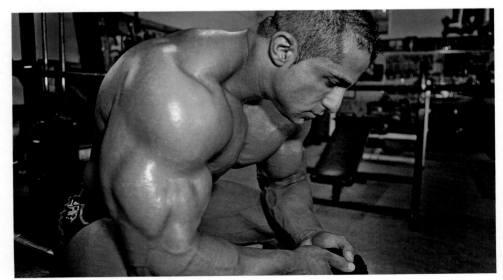

Right before each set of an exercise take a few moments to mentally prepare with deep breathing and visualization.

Photo by Jason Breeze
Model Fouad Abiad

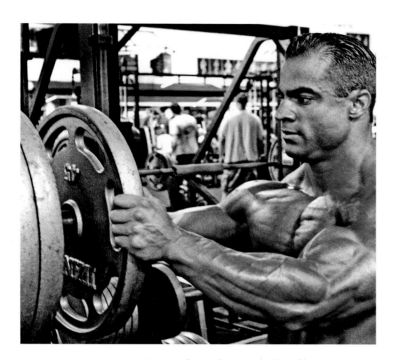

Even at the end of each set you should also focus your mind on the muscle reaction.

It's not only important to focus on the muscle action of every rep of each set prior to the beginning of your workout, you must also tune your mind into the muscle reaction at the conclusion of every set. Stand still for roughly 10 seconds and visualize how that set has worked the muscle. Feel the nutrient-rich blood being forced into your muscle, causing it to swell until it feels like it will burst through your skin. You can silently will the muscle to stunning and dramatic growth. Fine tuning the mind-to-body connection through mental training is one of the obvious alternatives to using drugs to achieve peak performance.

All of the champion bodybuilders back in the day would tell you that the right mental attitude is perhaps the most important factor in achieving your desired massive muscles and strength. Everything else is secondary to having the correct mental attitude. The late Chuck H. Sipes, 1968 IFBB Mr. World, taught the key elements to achieving a proper mental attitude. Sipes said: "The most important thing to remember in training for strength is that deep concentration is necessary to get the best results." As you progress, the poundages you'll be lifting will require the correct attitude as much as it requires physical energy

Training methods are focused entirely on getting results. When you train, you want to apply every bit of concentration you can gather to the application of the energy and effort needed for the movements of the exercises. You want to feel every muscle fiber, tendon and ligament swell and contract through every inch of the movement.

The use of concentration when exercising sounds simple enough. You might think paying attention to what you're doing is all this means, but that isn't the case. You have to link your mind as well as your muscles to the weight. Every physical movement you make must be thoroughly guided by your thoughts. As the strength builds up in your body, you have to feel it. There must be a deep sense of involvement between the physical and mental parts of your body. If you think big, you will be big.

When you're in a training session, you don't want to be interrupted. You must keep

To avoid a mediocre training effort, your mind must be locked with your muscles as you prepare to go to battle with the heavy iron. Begin by seeing clearly in your mind's eye the bench, the bar and the plates. Imagine this so intensely that you can smell the sweat, feel the knurling on the bar, hear the plates rattle and so forth. Whatever exercise you're about to perform, recreate all the techniques necessary for the masterful completion of each gut-wrenching rep of the set. Feel every muscle coming to life and then moving the weight with a great force. The more detailed and clear you make this ritual of mentally focusing on your sets, the better chance you will have for training to the outer limits of muscular size and strength.

As your mental-muscle rehearsal becomes more and more vivid, you'll begin to feel torrents of unleashed fury. Your heart will beat in a manner that reflects your ability to dominate. Open your eyes. You are now 100 percent mentally focused and psyched. Go for it! It's time to lift the heavy iron!

Tip: During your workout, play your favorite high-energy music to trigger strong energy responses.

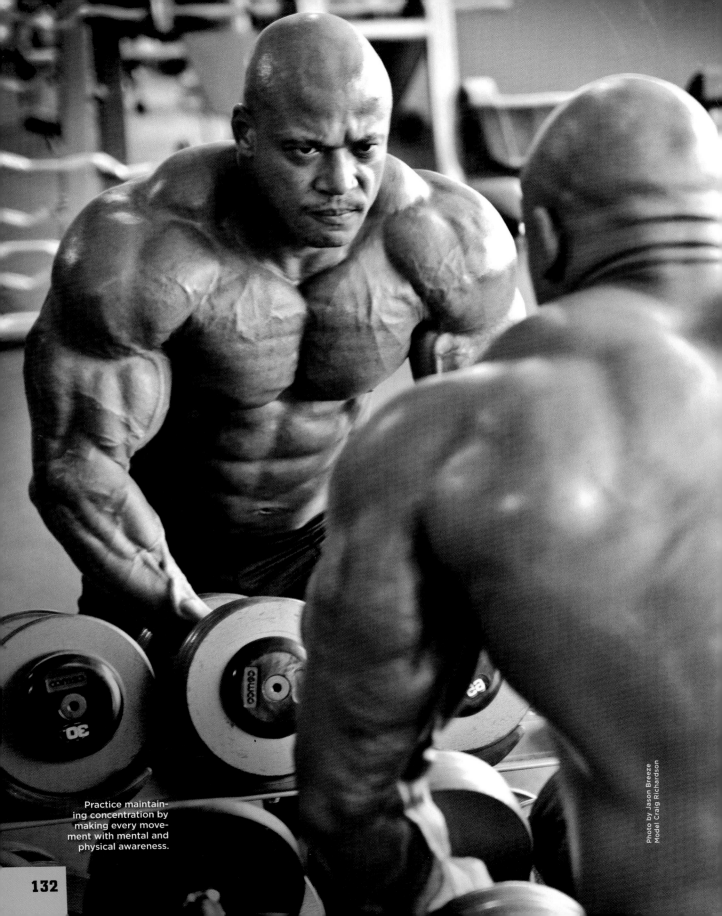

Practice maintaining concentration by making every movement with mental and physical awareness.

your concentration or lose the momentum you've built up. Teach yourself to concentrate. Pick up the barbell and put everything else out of your mind. Try it next time you work out and odds are you'll be able to go through your exercises much faster and more easily. You will also undoubtedly be able to increase the poundages you're using.

8 MENTAL-MUSCLE POINTERS

To aid you in your efforts of maintaining good concentration during your training sessions, here are eight mental muscle pointers:

1. Plan your workout so you won't be interrupted in any way.
2. Don't make excuses to miss any workout sessions.
3. Set a goal for each session.
4. Stay focused on your training. Don't let your thoughts wander off to other things.
5. Make every movement mentally as well as physically. Don't let weak mental focus keep you from exerting maximum muscle strength.
6. Totally rest between sets (but remember to limit the time).
7. Pick a training partner who thinks and trains like you.
8. Be pleasant to others, but make it clear that you're there to train and nothing must interfere.

When you're finished your workout, let your mind relax. Talk about other things and put all your thoughts of training aside until your next workout. Much of your effort has been channeled through your body mentally and there's a need for rest. You can lose interest in anything if you overdo it. Take the time to enjoy other things that interest to you. Your life will become fuller with this attitude, and you'll be able to approach your training sessions with more enthusiasm each time.

Adopt the attitude of a champion, not only in your bodybuilding endeavors, but in your day-to-day life. Develop a positive self-image. The positive self worth or image of professional bodybuilding champions such as multitime Mr. Olympia winner Jay Cutler, WNBF

Pro World champion Dave Goodin, Natural Mr. Olympia John Hansen and six-time IFBB Mr. Olympia Dorian Yates doesn't revolve around the gym-rat mentality. These competitors have a wonderful sense of well-being that isn't dictated by their reflection in a mirror or how another person perceives them. They simply ignore criticism, or at most use constructive criticism to improve.

Negative comments almost always come from those who don't feel good about themselves. Such criticisms are never helpful. Constructive criticism, on the other hand, might help you improve in your bodybuilding endeavors. This type of feedback should never confuse you or make you feel bad. Of course, it should also come from someone you respect who has more bodybuilding expertise than yourself. You'll instantly recognize constructive criticism because its application will move your bodybuilding progress forward in a new, energized way.

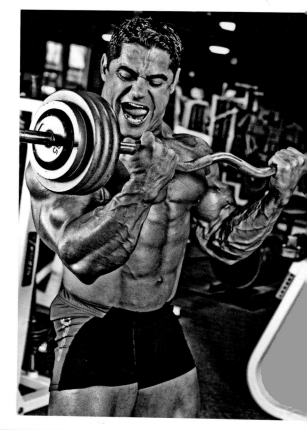

CHAPTER 20

ALPHA-ZONE CONCEPT

The power of visualization for mind-muscle rehearsal can catapult you to new levels in your workouts.

When discussing the perfect set, Dennis Tinerino, former AAU Mr. America and NABBA Mr. Universe, once said, "It's where I can handle a weight above my usual maximum, and do the full number of reps very easily. It's the culmination of your whole body and all of its physiological processes. The weight goes up as if only your mind were lifting it. It's like the perfect dive – poetry in motion, an aesthetic feeling, the perfect natural bodybuilding high."

– Dennis Tinerino
Former AAU Mr. America and NABBA Mr. Universe, discussing the perfect set

Earlier we cited an example of how short- and long-term goals might be approached for a bodybuilder wanting to increase his reps in the barbell back squat from 12 to 20. If you take our advice, your gains should go as planned ... that is, unless a metaphysical event takes place.

ONE ON ONE WITH WEIS

I was home alone and training in my gym. I loaded up the bar for some flat barbell bench presses with what I thought was 250 pounds. My plan was to do 10 reps, but instead I ground out 11 reps, which I thought was exceptional since it was one rep more than I had ever performed unassisted. The bar felt real light, just like warm-up poundage.

What took place next shocked me beyond belief. For some reason I happened to count the weight on the bar and it came out to 270 pounds! I was in disbelief, so I counted the poundage twice more and, sure enough, it was still 270. I was numb with shock because I had never done more than five reps with 270 pounds, and that was on a good day. I had just slightly more than doubled my rep output – without even meaning to. I managed this only once and then it was back to business as usual with 270 pounds for only five reps.

METAPHYSICAL EVENTS

The late "Iron Guru," Vince Gironda, once had a similar experience. He was able to do 24 reps in the preacher barbell curl with a weight that would usually allow him only 12 reps. Those results were nearly miracu-

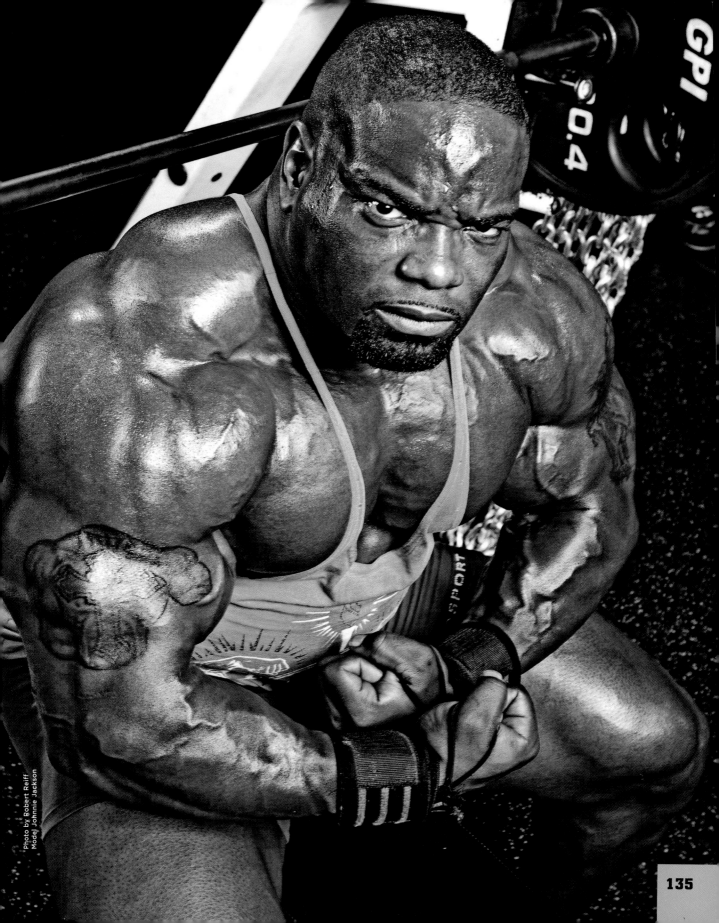

lous! How had he managed it? He did it with the secret we're just about to teach you: Mind-muscle rehearsal via visualization.

Just before starting the exercise, Vince concentrated on the ideal set of preacher barbell curls. In his mind's eye he saw the perfect muscle tension, rep tempo and range of motion. He concentrated for over two minutes this way, completing every set one after another in his mind. At that point, he was in a total state of meditation. As a result, his body somehow disregarded the fact that 12 reps were his maximum. He then performed 24 reps with no more effort than when he had done 12 reps.

Vince believed that in order to perform in this desirable state, which he referred to as the "alpha zone," a bodybuilder must train almost immediately upon waking up in the morning. According to Vince, a bodybuilder will find his strength might be 50 percent higher in the morning than at any other time of the day. Plus, the sense of satisfaction achieved by early-morning workouts is unequalled at any other time of the day.

The alpha-zone concept and its obvious potential to have a tremendous impact on training quickly captivated our attention. Could we find a way to harness the elements of the alpha-zone concept to create a powerful training tool that would allow bodybuilders to achieve these incredible sets on a more regular basis?

Our research indicated that the alpha-zone concept depends on three factors. The first factor we discovered was muscle fatigue and recovery. Before your muscles can grow, you must give yourself adequate periods of rest and relaxation. Muscle memory also plays a significant role in the alpha-zone concept. Your muscles can remember past gains and you can achieve nearly the same level several months or even years later through neurological pathways. The final factor is autogenic hypnosis, which helps develop a positive attitude to overcome physiological barriers to growth.

THE THREE ALPHA-ZONE CONCEPT FACTORS EXPOSED

FACTOR 1: MUSCLE FATIGUE AND RECOVERY:

Make Sure Your Muscles Aren't in a State of Fatigue from a Previous Workout

Muscle biopsies confirm that you need anywhere from 24 to 72 hours of rest between workouts for the same bodypart in order for

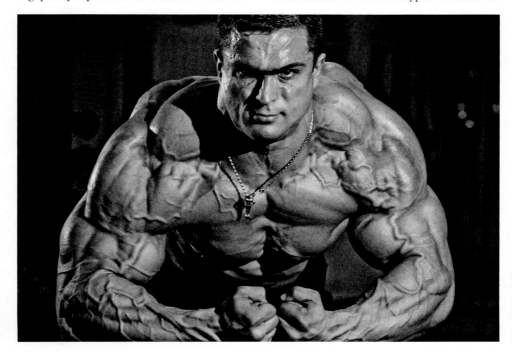

Muscle growth can only occur with adequate periods of rest and recovery.

Photo by Irvin Gelb
Model Alexander Fedorov

muscle restoration and growth to take place. The chemical and reserve chemical (necessary for muscular contraction) levels in your localized muscle tissue return to normal very quickly after a workout. However, there's a certain altered chemical energy that can be replenished only through periods of rest and relaxation. Recovery always precedes growth.

cused on some of the late Arthur Jones' (former owner of Nautilus Sports Industries) discoveries in weight training. Jones performed some short-term exercise tolerance experiments on over 600 test subjects. He found that some subjects who were least tolerant to exercise had a recovery rate of eight percent after two hours of rest. The subjects took two to

One sign that you're not giving your body enough recuperation time is a drop in measurements, such as your arms.

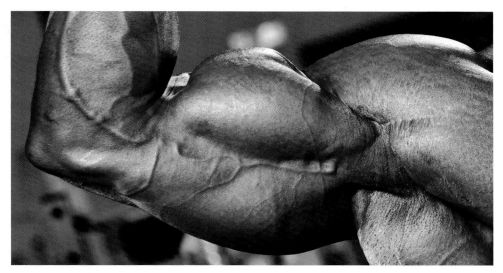

You may experience four pitfalls when you don't allow sufficient recovery time:

- You no longer enjoy your workouts and, as a result, you experience unusual physical strain during a routine that used to be a pleasant challenge.
- Your muscles don't achieve the desired pump, which prompts you to perform more sets to achieve the proper burn.
- You notice a drop in your overall body measurements (though a decrease in bodyweight without overtraining can also produce this condition).
- You experience an unexplained performance decrease in training poundages.

All of these are signs of overtraining. You should consider having an exhaustive blood workup conducted by a sports-medicine doctor who will be able to monitor your blood enzyme and hemoglobin levels, as well as other chemical productions.

In an article published in the August 1987 issue of *Muscle & Fitness*, Fred C. Hatfield fo-

three days to fully recover, which is in line with our previous knowledge of recovery time. Jones also discovered that some of the subjects were able to recover a full 106 percent of their strength after only one hour of rest! It's quite possible that the 106 percent recovery was in the eccentric or negative phase of the exercise, where the motor nerve pathways to the muscle had been established a little better.

Intermediate to advanced bodybuilders are the most likely groups to experience this recovery phenomenon, which is a function of reestablishing glucose/glycogen supplies. Studies have shown that athletes who exhaustively train over a period of two or three successive days will deplete their muscle and liver glycogen. Diet is important, and complex carbohydrates should make up at least 55 percent of your daily intake. By consuming complex carbohydrates, you will experience less fatigue and you will recuperate more quickly. If you're expecting full recuperation, however, it may take you anywhere from two to four days of carbing up and rest.

THE 96-HOURS MYTH

Some studies have shown that size and strength will decrease after as little as 96 hours of inactivity. Your body is in a constant state of flux. Your muscles can't maintain their pumped-up condition indefinitely. They're constantly adjusting to whatever exercise you're doing. It would seem logical that taking 96 hours of rest for certain bodyparts could be as devastating to your bodybuilding progress as not having enough rest. Some exercise physiologists have stated that after 96 hours of inactivity, oxygen efficiency significantly decreases, strength levels decline and muscles go into a state of atrophy.

If this were the case, you could never take a needed layoff from training without the risk of losing your hard-earned gains, which is simply not the case. These exercise physiologists fail to tell you that the 96-hour figure is based on enzyme studies. After an intense workout, some enzymes are being replaced and others are in the phase of building muscle. Therefore, it makes sense that the readings of enzyme and chemical by-products aren't normal. It may take you even longer than 96 hours to fully adapt to a hard workout.

It will take you a lot more than four days off before you experience any decrease in size or strength. In fact, one Soviet study indicated that the decrease may be as little as 10 percent after a whole year off training. The study was conducted on athletes who were performing generalized movements such as the squat and military press and had taken a one-year layoff from training due to a non-weightlifting condition (either illness or injury unrelated to the specific muscle area being tested). It was discovered that these athletes were still within 10 percent of their previous maximums. Some bodybuilders have confirmed this. One iron-game enthusiast who hadn't touched a barbell in over 2½ years went into a gym and performed 21 reps of 225 pounds in the flat barbell bench press with a pause. He actually felt as if he could have done eight or nine additional reps. His previous all-time best was 36 or 37 reps of the same poundage with a pause, so even with a 2½-year layoff he was down only 20 percent from his previous best. Everybody is different. You may find that the bodypart you're using loses size and strength more quickly than perhaps another bodypart that genetically holds the majority of its form re-

A layoff from the gym won't destroy all your hard work in the gym. Many bodybuilders incorrectly think they lose mass faster than they actually do.

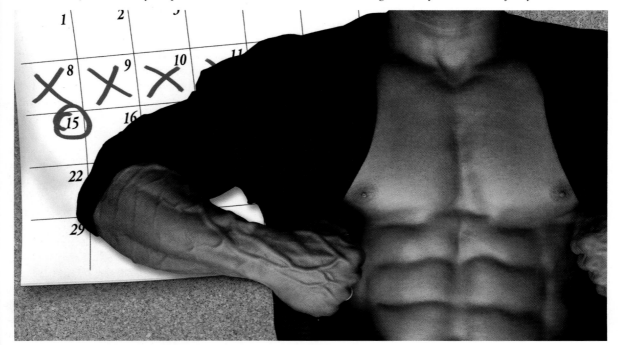

Photo by Rich Baker
Model Marco Cardona

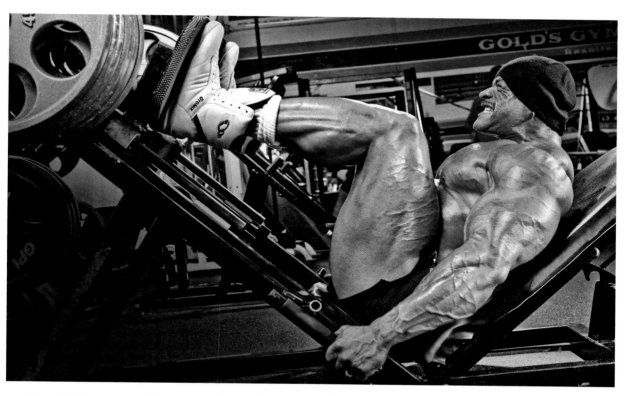

More isn't always better – it's that type of thinking that causes some bodybuilders to overtrain.

gardless of exercise. The bottom line is that bodybuilders often think they lose muscle mass at a greater rate than they actually do.

A common mistake in bodybuilding is following the tenet that if a little is good, more must be better. As a result, many of us tend to push ourselves a little too hard in our workouts. To prevent this from causing overtraining, use workouts that allow for a recovery period of 96 hours or more. One of the most popular methods of training that allows for a recovery time of nearly 96 hours is the five-day training cycle (four days on, one day off, or four-way split training). Many professional bodybuilders use this method of training to quickly get into contest shape. You train your entire body over a period of four days. The key is that generally you are working only two muscle groups per workout. For example, you train your thighs and calves on Monday; back, traps, neck and abs on Tuesday; chest and deltoids on Wednesday; and your arm (biceps, triceps and forearms) on Thursday. You then rest on Friday and Saturday and then begin the cycle again, com-

mencing with your thighs and calves. Depending on your training needs, your calves and abs can be worked more often.

Another method of training that allows even more than 96 hours of rest between workouts is the six-day training cycle. You don't have to save your energy for other muscle groups, so it's much easier to motivate yourself to train with more intensity. Many competitors use this method of training successfully. Below is the ideal six-day training cycle.

THE SIX-DAY TRAINING CYCLE

Monday	Legs (quads, hamstrings and calves: gastrocnemius and soleus)
Tuesday	Chest (pecs and rib cage)
Wednesday	Back (erectors, traps and lats)
Thursday	Deltoids (all three heads)
Friday	Biceps (includes forearm work)
Saturday	Triceps
Sunday	Total rest and recuperative sleep

A FINAL COMMENT ON SIX-DAY TRAINING

When using the six-day training cycle, always do one "flush set" for a routine done three days earlier. For example, after you've completed your delt work on Thursday, perform one set of 15 reps of an exercise for your legs (Monday's program). Work your abdominals, calves and neck every other workout day.

A FINAL WORD ON RECOVERY

Ted Arcidi once said he did his last heavy bench press (650 pounds for two solid reps) 10 days before accomplishing a world record-shattering bench press of 705½ pounds in March 1985 at the Hawaiian International Powerlifting Championships. Obviously this debunks the 96-hour myth. Granted, if you lay off for too long, you'll experience some decreases in the functional output of a muscle, but that takes a lot longer than 96 hours.

Remember, an indirect effect occurs on other bodyparts from exercises such as squats and deadlifts, and there's also a synergist carryover. But many advanced bodybuilders believe their potential to gain will decrease dramatically after taking 96 hours off. Rest assured, most powerlifters take anywhere from seven to ten days off prior to a competition and they usually come into a contest at their strongest.

If you're like most bodybuilders, you are compulsive. You have a tendency to overwork and don't know when to rest or back off ... or you're afraid to. Again, there's nothing wrong

There's something to be said for how powerlifters view rest; leading up to a contest they take seven to ten days off and usually come into the event at their strongest.

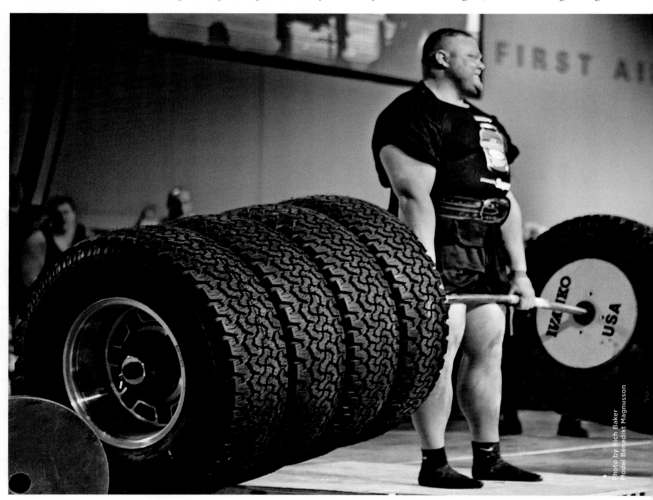

Photo by Rich Baker
Model Benedikt Magnusson

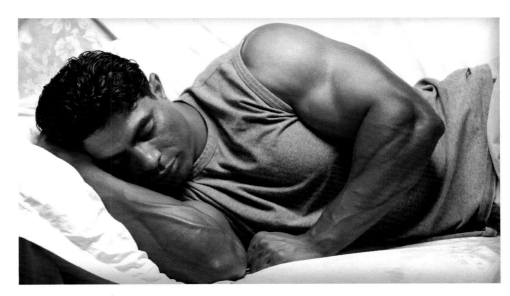

Getting enough sleep on a regular basis is very important to your overall muscle growth and strength goals, as this is the time when your muscle tissue recuperates and regenerates.

Photo by Alex Ardenti
Model Tamer El Shahat

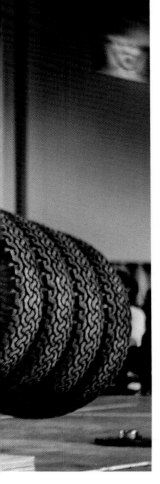

with taking a layoff for a month or two if you've been lifting for three to four years. In fact, many trainers believe you should take at least one week off for every couple of months' training. Take this time to get active rest (cycling, speed walking, etc.) – it's one of the best things you can do to prevent burnout.

FACTOR 2: MUSCLE MEMORY

ESTABLISH THE NEUROLOGICAL PATHWAYS

Your motor-nerve pathways link your mind to your muscles. When we recommended a layoff at the end of the previous factor, you probably couldn't help but wonder how long it would take to regain your pre-layoff fitness and strength levels. Your ability to return to your previous best depends on how long you've been training. Your training experience affects your muscle memory recall rate. After years of training, some bodybuilders have taken layoffs much longer than two months and were able to return to their peak following only 12 to 14 weeks of training.

Bodybuilders were making massive gains of 25 to 30 pounds in a month or less as far back as the 1930s. Joseph Curtis Hise and Buck Reed were the most famous of the era. In the 1950s, the late "Monarch of Muscledom" John C.

Grimek had the ability to vary his weight by roughly 30 pounds (either up or down) in as little as two weeks. In 1975, when Arnold Schwarzenegger completed the movie *Pumping Iron*, he weighed 210 pounds. He quickly gained 25 pounds and won the IFBB Mr. Olympia in that same year. He had had those 25 pounds once already, so it was just a matter of his muscles "remembering." Other examples of muscle memory recall include the "Colorado Experiment" in 1973, showcasing the 1971 AAU Mr. America, Casey Viator. Casey gained more than 45 pounds in 28 days. He performed only 12 to 14 high-intensity workouts, each of which lasted less than 33.6 minutes.

An experienced and healthy bodybuilder will have better established motor nerve pathways to his muscles than a rookie bodybuilder. The reason is simple: His muscle memory recall rate is far superior. When you start performing a new exercise, it will take you at least six to ten weeks of continuous training before muscular or physiological adaptation takes place. During that period, the reps you perform essentially train and condition your muscles into a more efficient response. This is when the neurological pathways are developing. Once established, these pathways remain established for years unless your body as a whole greatly declines.

UNDERSTANDING MUSCLE OUTPUT

Watch a champion bodybuilder train and you'll notice that he's a lot more efficient in his training movements than a novice. He can achieve an incredible pump and blood-choked vascularity from a given exercise, but when you try the very same exercise, it just doesn't seem to work your muscles in the same way. The first thing you should determine is whether or not the exercise is putting your muscle into a position of maximum tension over the entire range of movement.

At the beginning of your press off the chest in the bench press, your pectorals are the prime movers. Toward the mid-range of your movement (six to eight inches off your chest) your smaller deltoid muscles take over and assume the primary function of moving the weight. When approaching the lockout phase, your triceps begin to take most of the load. Bodybuilders often think the smallest muscle of the muscle group moving the poundage is the limiting factor determining whether they can complete the rep. Very few guys seem to miss a bench press off their chest. They seem to miss it more of-

Arnold is a prime example of a bodybuilder who mastered every aspect of his training.

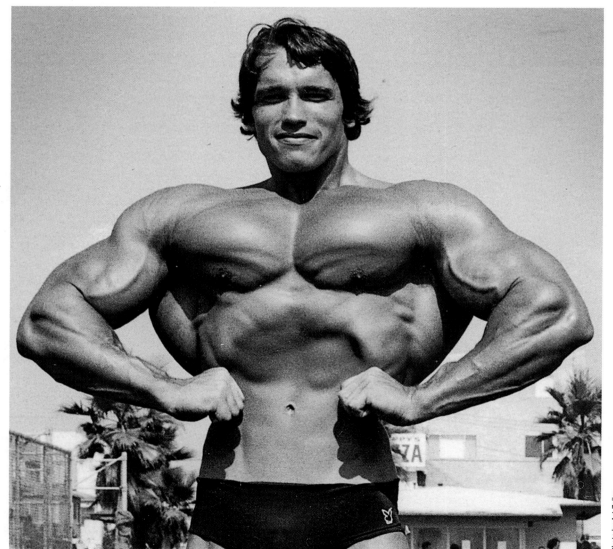

Photo by Art Zeller
Model Arnold Schwarzenegger

ten near the middle (deltoid function) or near the lockout phase (triceps function) of the movement. But these problems aren't necessarily a function of muscle output; rather, they could come about because of leverage. At specific ranges of an exercise, certain muscles are placed in a poor mechanical position and, as a result, can't exert the force necessary to complete the lift. Your limiting factors could be as much a function of the specific origins and insertions of your muscles as simple muscle output.

To overcome these problems, you must attack the limiting point (sticking point) of your movement with specific exercises and isometric work. If you're one of those rare few who experience a poor mechanical advantage off your chest, you'll want to do exercises that take the movement well below the level of your chest, such as flat dumbbell bench presses. You can also try using the cambered bench press bar for seated shrugs for your traps as well as prone bench rowing and half bench presses for mid-back density. All three of these exercises require the cambered portion of the bar to be facing down.

For the mid-range area of the bench press where weak deltoids might be a problem, you could try doing bench presses using a moderate or wide grip. Lower the bar to your chest. Then pause before pressing the bar to 90 percent of lockout. Return the bar to your chest, and so on. For the lockout phase of the bench press where your triceps may be weak, try doing narrow-grip bench presses with an EZ-curl bar. This exercise will help increase your inner pec line development.

To help you increase your lifting ability at a sticking point, include the barbell squat, bench press and deadlift or any of the Olympic lifts. Any of these assistance exercises will improve your performance dramatically (your narrow-grip bench press could go from 125 pounds to 210 pounds for 8 to 10 reps, for example), but you won't develop any increase in your lockout ability in the actual bench press. All muscles involved in the bench press, not just your triceps, must make a coordinated effort to produce the strength necessary to blast through a sticking point.

If the assistance exercise does help you blast through a sticking point, that's all the help you'll need. If it doesn't, you might want to try pure isometric contractions (using an empty exercise bar and exerting cumulative tension against an immovable object such as a set of holding rods in a power rack), or you can use a more advanced form of isometrics called isometronics. Isometronics is the term for isometric contractions done using various poundages and positions within the range of an isotonic exercise. You need to use a power rack and a barbell. With a power rack, you can work through every inch of a normal exercise range performed in isometronic style. Best of all, you can vary the exercise poundages to suit your strong or weak points.

Assume your sticking point in the supine bench press is six inches off your chest. Position one set of starting pins about one inch from where the barbell would normally touch your chest, which will allow you to position yourself under the barbell resting on the support rods. A second set of power rack rods should be positioned at the exact joint angle of your sticking point. You are now ready to begin your bench press in this short-range movement by pressing the barbell off the starting pins and up to the holding pins. As the barbell makes contact with the holding rods, employ the sustained contraction technique (explained in Book 11, entitled Super Muscle and Strength Specialization) for a total of three consecutive reps.

If you wish to increase the intensity of this triple-repetition scheme, incorporate pauses in the following systematic manner. As you lower the barbell during the descent (negative phase) of the first rep, stop one inch short of touching the power rack pins in the starting position on your chest. Hold this pause for ten seconds; for the second rep, pause five seconds; and on your third and final rep, pause three seconds. Once or twice per week you can perform one more set of three reps (pauses included) for a particular sticking point. Do not continue this past a two-month period or you'll burn out, resulting in an often very-difficult rut to get out of for any bodybuilder.

LEARNING THE CORRECT MOVEMENT

If you're having a problem just getting the feel of a certain exercise and the problem doesn't involve one of the two mechanical factors, you might not be performing the exercise correctly. Increasing the poundage and then cheating your way through the movement will not give you the best results, because you won't be working the muscle as it should be worked. If you cheat through all your reps, you will be depending upon momentum to some degree rather than stressing the muscle you are trying to target. Along with momentum, synergist muscles come into play to a greater degree than normal, to help you move the weight. As a result, while you are adding more weight you aren't increasing the load on the muscle group you're trying to work! Former eight-time IFBB Mr. Olympia Lee Haney once said: "I'd rather work for a pump than do heavy weights in poor style." If you don't use the muscles you're supposed to be attacking directly, all you'll accomplish is using some other group of muscles for support. As a result, the neurological pathways to your muscles won't be properly established. You will gain very little until you finally establish these pathways to the muscles you're trying to attack.

Once you learn to properly perform an exercise, you'll become efficient at the movement. One of the secrets shared by contest training champions is that when you perform an exercise efficiently, the energy requirements actually decrease. Consequently, a champion bodybuilder can make gains with much less effort and food.

If you're an advanced bodybuilder, establishing the neurological pathways to your muscles is one of the most important factors in the alpha-zone concept. It's primarily a mental function and it can actually increase your maximum strength output by as much as 20 percent over your average amount.

FACTOR 3: AUTOGENETIC HYPNOSIS AND BODYBUILDERS

One factor that separates a champion bodybuilder from a wannabe is the subconscious. You can train in the best-equipped gym, take the most expensive supplements and have the best workout partner, but if you don't train your subconscious, you won't achieve your best. Your thoughts nourish your mind. Autogenic hypnosis is self-induced meditation and employs techniques of mental imagery to overcome inhibitions that limit bodybuilding progress, and promote a muscle-building mindset.

Eight-time Mr. Olympia Lee Haney never compromised proper form for heavier weights.

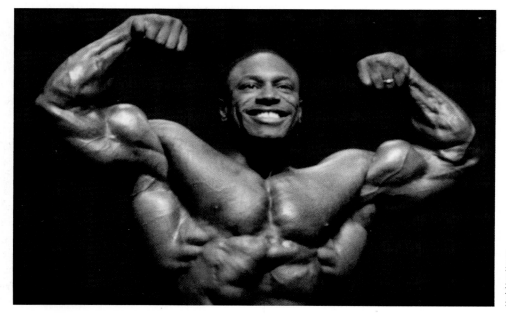

Model Lee Haney

It's rather ironic that our search for effective ways to develop muscular size and strength has always revolved around the physical aspects of training. We are overeducated on the physical, but totally uneducated on training the mind. We've all rattled off clichés such as "It's all in the mind," but how many of us program our mind to sustain motivation? We must learn how to train our subconscious because it's one of the most powerful training tools we have. With proper mental training, bodybuilders can learn to control muscle contractions, which in turn creates muscle growth.

Every bodybuilding champion actually sees himself winning before it happens. Win-ners make it happen. Physiological barriers aren't even a consideration. Even the top champions are using only 85 to 90 percent of their full potential, so it's of the utmost importance that the rest of us tap into our subconscious.

The subconscious cannot distinguish between what is real and what isn't. When you train to fatigue, your conscious mind places limits on your pain-barrier threshold. Your muscles still have a lot of energy. If you can cue your subconscious to accept no pain barriers (within reason), as the champions do, the power will astound you. Just as picturing yourself winning helps you win, thinking positive thoughts produces positive results. Bill

During his competitive years, Tom Platz was known for his intense visualization and mental rehearsals before his training sessions.

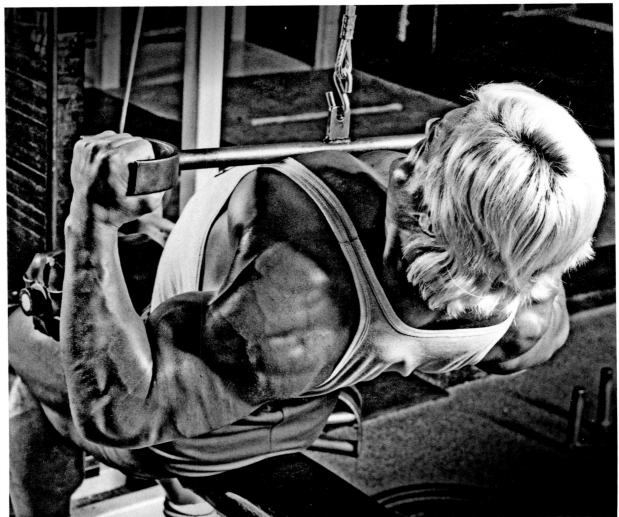

Model Tom Platz

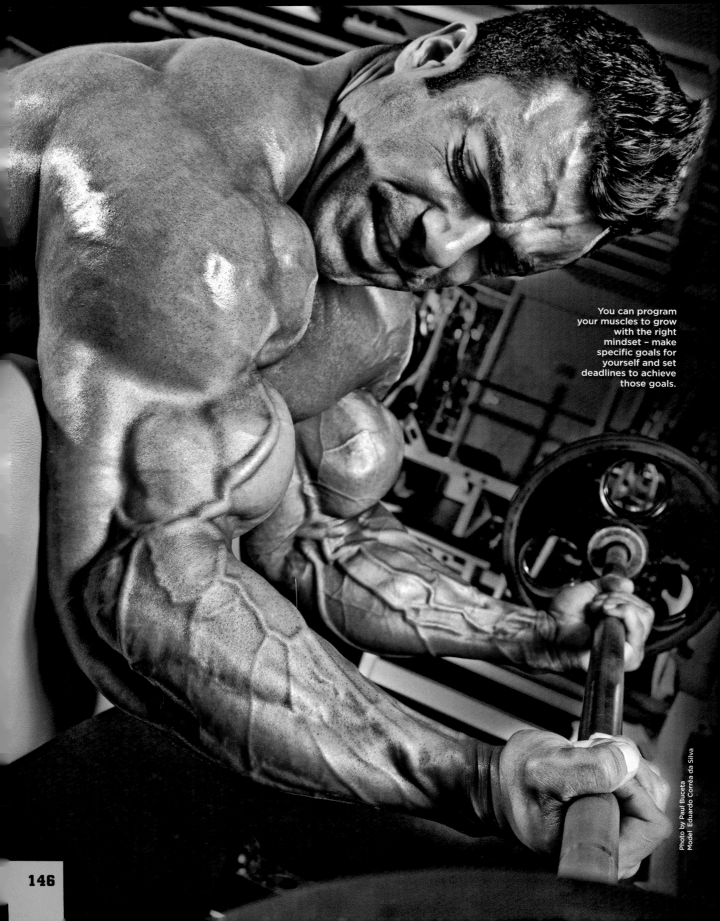

You can program your muscles to grow with the right mindset – make specific goals for yourself and set deadlines to achieve those goals.

Pearl says: "You can't take anything negative you are doing in the sport of bodybuilding and turn it into positive results. It won't happen." You must condition your subconscious to think that you're getting bigger and training with more intensity. Your body will be forced to respond accordingly.

Every time you do a barbell curl or a squat and say "my arms or my legs won't grow," you are literally programming these muscles (and your body in general) to not grow. You have to change your mindset by creating some specific training goals and establishing when you're going to reach those goals. Remember: Your brain controls your muscles; your muscles don't control your brain. When you properly motivate yourself by maintaining a positive attitude about everything you do, you'll be capable of doubling your usual output.

One characteristic the top champions share is the ability to focus all their available energy and strength on the task at hand. This extreme concentration is a semi-hypnotic state, which is one of the many effective ways to train your subconscious. To harness the power of this near-hypnotic state at every workout, you must increase your awareness to the point at which you're conscious of only three factors: Yourself, the equipment and your objective. Watch yourself performing exercises in a mirror. Concentrate fully on each rep and the effect it has on the particular muscle or even muscle section you wish to develop as you take your set to (or close to) positive rep failure. Also concentrate on the negative half of your movement. Your training tempo during and between exercises, as well as the proper rep selection, play equally important roles in developing optimal awareness.

There are some who subscribe to the theory that if you're training for strength, you should spend two to three seconds in the positive phase of the movement and four to six seconds in the negative phase, which places maximum tension on all aspects of the muscle belly (as much as leverages will allow). Spending two to three seconds in the positive phase of an exercise rep makes sense, but spending four to six seconds in the negative phase doesn't.

Physical testing standards are generally determined by your increased capacity in the positive phase output of a muscle or group of muscles. No conclusive evidence exists suggesting that the negative phase of a rep can significantly influence the positive phase of a movement. A better guideline would be two to three seconds in the positive phase, one to two seconds in the isometronic or lockout phase, and two to three seconds in the negative phase (but no less, because you don't want to lose control of your rep tempo over any given range of the movement). The one to two second pause generally applies when using moderate exercise poundages in excess of 75 to 80 percent and heavy poundages in excess of 85 percent of your current one rep maximum. Light poundages of 50 to 70 percent require no pauses or contractions in the lockout phase. A five- to eight-second count may seem slow, but experimentation has shown that if you do your reps slowly and correctly, you'll realize maximum benefits. Training tempo and proper rep selection are only parts of a total training package.

Exercises that require a lot of energy and oxygen also demand greater skill, speed and coordination. And you will need sufficient recovery time between sets to avoid fatigue. Battling fatigue will prevent you from using the poundages necessary to develop maximum size and strength. The Holistic Training Guide in this book will serve you well in determining the appropriate rest periods between sets to avoid fatigue.

Other causes of fatigue include doing too many warm-up sets before your initial strength-building sets, which can reduce your exercise efficiency through the buildup of lactic acid waste. A normal lactic acid level in the bloodstream is 10 milligrams per 100 milliliters of blood. During certain types of exercise, the level can increase to 20 times that, but it will return to normal after a three-minute rest following a set. Doing too many reps can also fatigue a muscle, which will obviously detract from the skill, speed and coordination that you exhibit while performing an exercise. A muscle cannot learn when it's overworked or in a state of fatigue.

CHAPTER 21

THE MENTAL ATTITUDE OF A CHAMPION

Make your workouts mentally productive by breaking down each exercise step-by-step.

Building a championship physique requires great workouts that are only possible with confidence. Champions always have a sharp mental image of their specific short-term and long-term training goals, which gives the stimulus necessary to mold a top-caliber physique. Without that image, workouts aren't productive.

If you're like most people, you need to be motivated when you're training. When you're motivated by an upcoming physique or power-lifting competition, you'll find it very easy to have a series of outstanding workouts. However, when you aren't training for a competition, it's very easy to occasionally fall into the trap of thinking: "What difference does it make if I'm only doing Olympic-style squats with 300 pounds for 25 reps when I used to lift 400 pounds for more than 20 reps? No one will know the difference except me."

SELF-ACTUALIZATION RESOURCES

Self-actualization is an invaluable mind-power technique. If your mind can see, then your body can achieve. A helpful tool for practicing the mental rehearsal of your exercises would be to read all the kinesiology columns in the mainstream bodybuilding magazines. You'll get a detailed explanation of the correct and incorrect execution of the selected exercise along with detailed illustrations. Mind-muscle rehearsal via visualizationand its application is a thoughtful and intelligent two-stage event consisting of pre-workout and one-set interval preparation.

DEVELOPING A PRECISION TECHNIQUE THROUGH MIND-MUSCLE REHEARSAL VIA VISUALIZATION

To give you a general idea of how you might apply mind-muscle rehearsal via visualization to your training, we're going to take you through three of the most important core growth exercises you'll ever do as a bodybuilder: the barbell back squat, flat bench press and conventional deadlift.

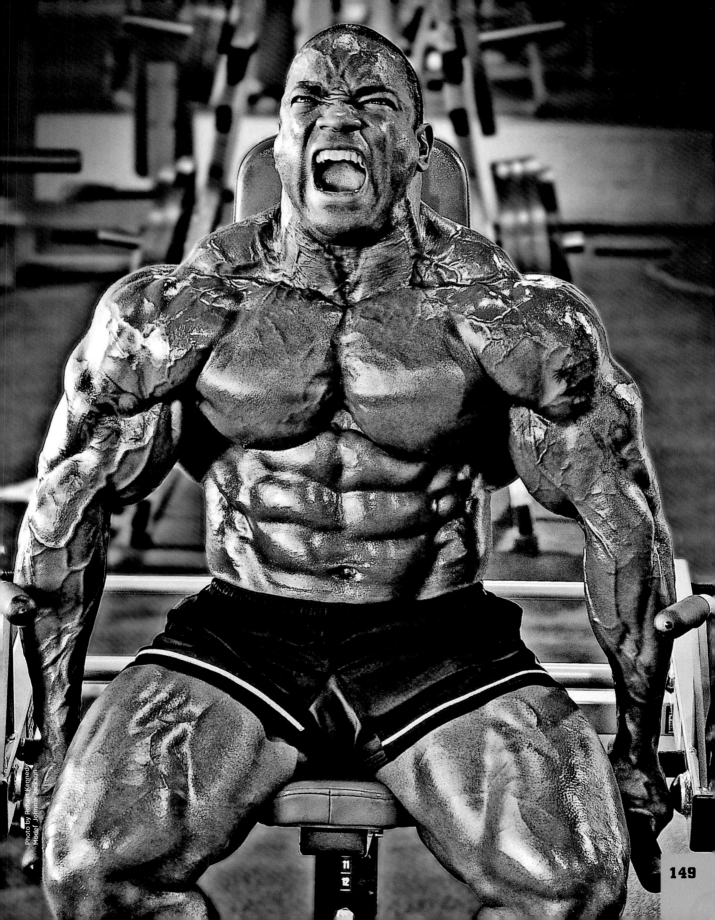

For safety and to help prevent injury, always secure your hand position before you unrack from the squat rack.

BARBELL BACK SQUAT
HAND POSITIONING

Grip the bar in a place where your hands are most comfortable. Settle on your hand position before you back out of the squat rack and never change your position during the lift, regardless of whether you're doing a one-rep max or a multiple-rep set. Some bodybuilders come out of the squat rack with one type of hand positioning and then adjust it prior to the squat descent. Doing this is very dangerous and invites injury because the tremendous poundages place great demand on your spine and back muscles. The mechanics of this exercise suggest that any additional shifting of your hands after you have unracked the barbell could put your spine into a non-supporting position of weakness, thus causing injury.

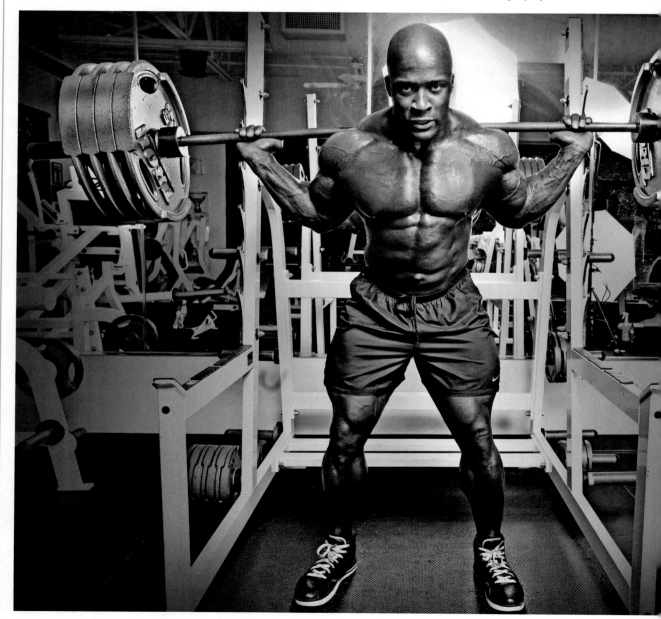

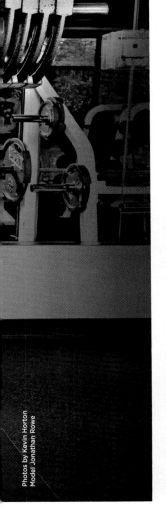

To ensure even weight distribution over your back, the barbell is usually positioned about one inch below the top of your shoulders, across the traps.

A hand position of three to six inches wider than shoulder width will act as a tripod support system, with your two arms and back sharing the stress load. A grip that's too narrow, however, can cause an elbow injury. If you find your grip is too narrow, gradually work your hands out wider, but never to a collar-to-collar grip.

You may experience severe stiffness in the wrist as you squat, especially when the bar is positioned low on the traps. One of the best things you can do to prevent this is to warm up with some PNF (Proprioceptive Neuro-Muscular Facilitation) stretching and flexibility exercises for your wrists.

Remember to push up hard with your hands (which are squeezing the bar with a vise-like grip) on the bar, as if you were trying to do a press behind the neck, during the ascent phase of the squat. You'll find that this will help you push through a sticking point.

BAR POSITIONING

The placement of the bar as it relates to your shoulders before you unrack it is called the bar positioning. The weight is positioned across the trapezius muscles approximately one inch below the top of your shoulders, with the load evenly distributed over the multiple muscles of your back. When the bar is in this position, and you have the proper foot placement, you'll be able to promote the development of your stronger quad muscles. If you have a long upper torso, you may find this position awkward. In that case, consider placing the bar slightly lower. Positioning the bar in this manner will give you better vertebral leverage and explosion when you're coming out of the bottom position of the squat, because your back and legs will be in a more favorable mechanical position. Conventional squatting methods place the weight a full four to five inches behind your body's center of gravity, which causes you to lean forward. Your best bet is to use a Hoagland Safety Squat Bar, as it perfectly aligns itself to your body's center of gravity.

Now that your hand and bar positions are set, stand up with the weight, step back and establish an upright position. The idea is to conserve your energy for the performance of the rep scheme, so take only a couple of steps to clear the rack while compensating for any leaning you might do during the exercise. If you find the bar gradually slides down your back, rub some magnesium carbonate chalk across your shirt in the area where you'll be placing the bar.

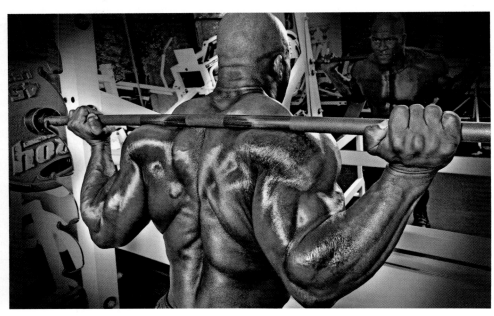

HEAD AND BACK ALIGNMENT

Always keep your chin parallel to the ground during all phases of the squat descent and ascent. Doing so will help your back and spine to stay flat and discourage you from leaning forward, thereby ensuring proper squatting stability and position. When your upper torso is upright, your shoulders and hips are almost in line. Your legs are stronger than your spine, so it's very important that the weight be directly over the spinal column. It's a good idea to arch (not round) your back to eliminate lower back or erector soreness. Keep in mind that an incorrect arch could create trauma or pressure on your spinal discs and various vertebrae, which could then lead to a herniated disc.

When your back is crooked, it absorbs additional pressure just trying to counterbalance the misaligned weight. If you discover that your upright squatting stability is a weakness, you may need to do some additional training on your abdominals and lower back stabilizers.

To keep your back flat and discourage a forward lean, make sure your chin is parallel to the ground at all points during the squat.

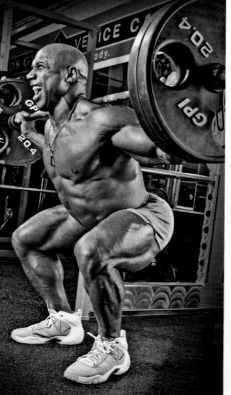

FOOT PLACEMENT

If you have large thighs and small hips, place your feet 12 to 14 inches apart. If you have large hips and glutes, try a distance of 16 to 20 inches. The wider your stance, the more you should turn your feet outward (30 to 45 degrees). Doing so rotates your hips, thereby positioning them more directly under the bar for added power. If you're going to experiment with even wider foot placements, increase the width of your stance by no more than two inches a week to avoid muscle and joint sprains.

If you could view your squatting posture from the side, you'd notice that the bar is not only directly over your hips, but also lined up with the instep, or middle of your foot. It's important to maintain this because the bar will be following a perpendicular path during the descent and ascent. However, if your ankles are somewhat inflexible (your heels will begin to come up off the floor), you might not be able to hold this rather rigid posture. The bar will then become misaligned over your toes rather than the instep, with your hips drifting up and to the rear, consequently placing a tremendous amount of additional stress on your back and hips.

There are three ways around this problem. First, you can do your squats on your toes with your back against a door-jamb post or any stationary object where you'll be able to slide your back up and down. This exercise will stress the quads almost exclusively, with very little pressure on the back. Your calves will also receive some benefit from being up on your toes. Another way around the problem would be to place a block beneath your heels. Or you can purchase a pair of high-top weightlifting shoes with an elevated 1½-inch tapered heel to support your ankles. You are now ready to begin.

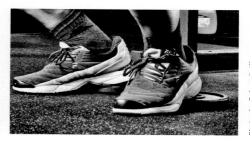

Photos by Robert Reiff
Model Darrell Terrell / Tarek Elsetouhi

THE DESCENT

Begin your descent by unlocking and bending your knees. With a controlled moderate speed, descend to a parallel or slightly lower position, where the surface of your thighs at the hip joints are an inch or so lower than your knees. The descent should take approximately two to three seconds. During the descent, your shins remain vertical with your knees extending slightly forward.

Maintain control and descend at a moderate speed until you reach parallel or slightly below.

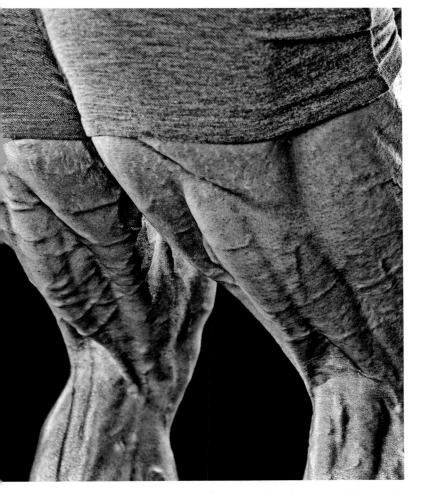

Photo by Robert Reiff
Model Monty Rogers

Begin gearing for the ascent when you're about two to three inches above the parallel position. You should never employ speed or a ballistic-type movement during the descent because it can create a bouncing effect. Bouncing can lead to all sorts of problems, including loss of balance and control as well as over-stretched tendons and ligaments in your knee area. You could end up with a knee joint separation (the femur in the upper thigh and the tibia in the lower leg open up). Maintain absolute muscle tension throughout the squatting movement to build up your connective tissues, ligaments and tendons. Consider this the golden rule of training: You control the weight; never let the weight control you.

If you have difficulty hitting the pocket (the parallel position), you'll find that a competent spotter along with a mirror are invaluable aids. A video camera can also be helpful. Lacking any of these, you can simply place your lifting belt lower around your waist region so it will dig into your hip area sooner. Doing so will help you identify the approximate parallel position, especially if you feel you have been descending too low. If you aren't squatting low enough, then raise the belt position higher.

PRESTRETCH FOR EXPLOSIVENESS

Prestretching involves pulling a muscle into a position of increased intramuscular tension prior to the positive or concentric contraction. When prestretching is initiated, muscle fibers called spindles pick up the sensation of the stretch. These muscle spindles then send out neurological impulses to other associated muscles and your brain in a coordinated effort to involve a greater number of muscle fibers during the contraction. The end result is the ability to use heavier weights, which, in turn, increases muscular size and strength.

Prestretching in the squat is best done during the descent or negative phase. Follow through in the controlled manner described earlier to within one to two inches of your final position and at this point rapidly drop into your final position. Then immediately begin your explosion out of the bottom position. Another method that creates the effect of prestretching is to squat to your normal depth using 20 percent over your best current one-rep max. Hold this position of tension for four or five seconds, and then have a spotter or training partner take off enough poundage (generally a 40 percent reduction) so you can explode to lockout position. If you don't have a spotter, the only other alternative is to get your hands on a safety squat bar. (This bar was the secret weapon in "Dr. Squat" Fred Hatfield's leg-training arsenal when he was squatting more than 1000 pounds.) The safety bar is great for when you are lacking a partner because it frees your hands to push off the thighs after the four- or five-second pause in the parallel position. Perform this move with a safety squat bar at 80 percent of your maximum weight.

THE ASCENT

Now that you're in the parallel or lower position of the squat, explode out of this position with all your muscle contractile force. Developing explosiveness is a key to blasting through your sticking point. For most bodybuilders, this will be approximately 30 degrees out of the bottom position, though this will depend on unique leverage factors, muscle origins and insertions, slow- and fast-twitch muscle fiber recruitment and other factors. The main idea is to keep the weight moving as fast as possible through all the various leverage ranges of the positive contraction movement to just short of your actual lockout, where you'll want to slow it down to avoid hyperextension of your knee joints and possible loss of balance.

A few things to remember when squatting: Don't lift your hips too fast when coming out of your sticking point or the weight will tip you forward. In fact, make a conscious effort to pull or thrust your hips forward under the bar. Never allow the upper torso to lean forward, as it places too much stress on your back and abdominals. Don't allow your back to bow to the point at which your chest is collapsed. At your sticking point, it's sometimes helpful to look upwards, while maintaining your form. The knees of some bodybuilders turn in toward each other when the adductor muscles of the inner thighs are stronger than the abductors, which can place a lot of stress on the surrounding knee joint and lead to injury. Follow the squatting procedures outlined and do some strength-building exercises for your muscles to develop an improved strength balance. Two-thirds of the way through your ascent, release air from your lungs. The positive contraction

process should take you approximately two to three seconds. At the lockout position, contract your glutes isometrically for one to two seconds before beginning another rep. If you have any doubts as to the proper ascent-versus-descent technique, simply follow the exact descent procedure in reverse. Consider filming your precision squatting technique and then watch the video to see your ascent technique.

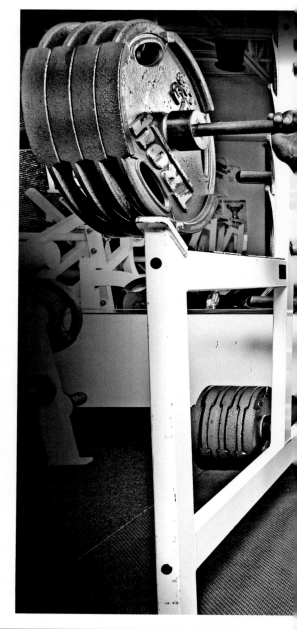

Photo by Kevin Horton
Model Jonathan Rowe

The ascent on the squat is all about exploding out of the bottom position with full muscle contractile force.

SQUATTING MYTH

The following information doesn't have a direct effect on your mental preparation for the squat, but it does have an indirect impact because believing any of these myths may discourage you from including squats in your program (which will mean missing out on some great gains). The "squats will make you musclebound" myth suggests that squats decrease the speed of muscle movement. Exercise physiologists tell us that the stronger a muscle is, the faster it can contract. If you use full contractions and extensions on each and every rep, you'll develop the ultimate in muscular size and strength, as well as agility, endurance and flexibility. Endurance and flexibility are keys to enjoying a healthy and productive life. Don't let the myths steer you wrong.

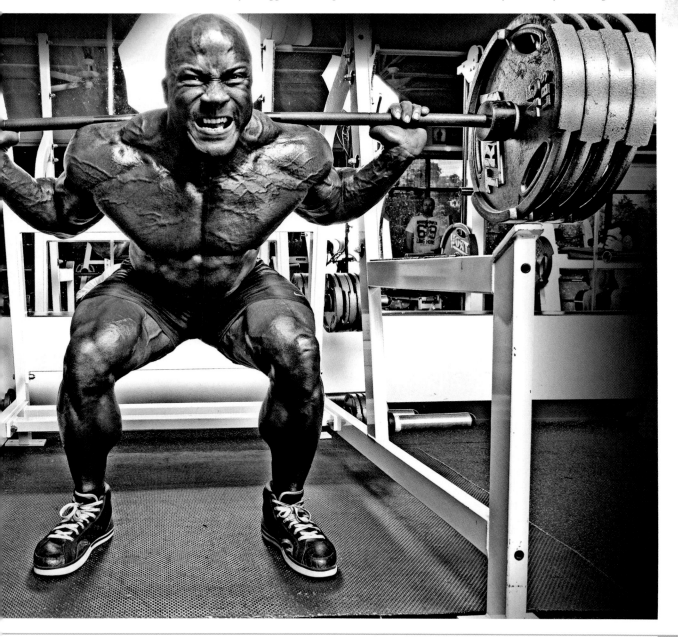

Your control center on the bench press consists of three key elements: grip, hand spacing and elbow angle.

FLAT BARBELL BENCH PRESS
BODY ALIGNMENT

Lie down on the bench in a supine position, with your head, shoulders and glutes in full contact with the bench, and your feet planted firmly on the floor. For the maximum amount of leverage advantage in bench pressing, it's a good idea to try to bring your shoulders as close to your hips as possible. You can accomplish this by arching your back during the concentric (lifting) phase, but remember to keep your shoulders and glutes in contact with the bench at all times.

THE CONTROL CENTER

Three fundamentals constitute the control center: Grip, hand spacing and elbow angle.

Very little has to be said regarding your grip; the safest method is the conventional thumbs-under-the-bar grip. Some bodybuilders use what's called a thumb-less or false grip, where the thumb is not wrapped around the bar. They believe this is necessary to fully activate the strong triceps muscles on the back of the upper arm, as well as to relieve some of the pain and pressure in the wrists and forearms resulting from holding very heavy poundage. The real danger in this method is that it's very easy

Photos by Paul Buceta
Model Fouad Abiad

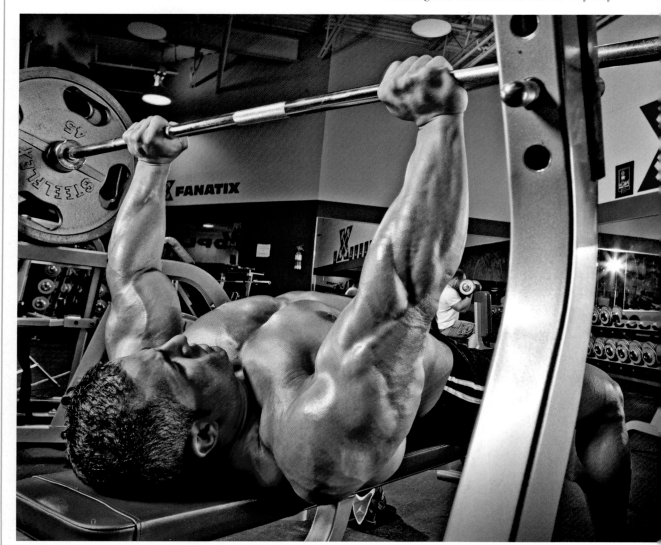

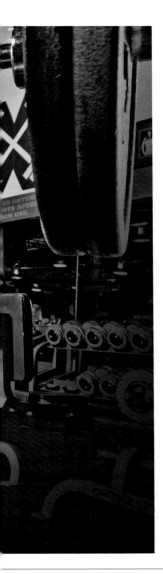

Lowering the bar too fast is ineffective for your muscles and dangerous overall.

for the bar to roll out of your hands, even when they are heavily chalked. Our theme throughout this book is to train smart, and if you are diligent in doing this you will use the conventional grip.

For hand spacing, follow the rules of powerlifting – no more than 32 inches between the forefingers – and at the same time make sure your hand spacing allows you to use the muscle leverages you were born with to your best advantage. Your hand spacing can vary from around 22 inches (which will generate maximum triceps recruitment) to 32 inches (which should stimulate pectoralis growth). Deltoid strength will be built with any grip in between.

As you gain more muscular size and density, your hand spacing may change. For example, if you are 6 feet tall and weigh 150 pounds with 14-inch arms and a 36-inch chest, you'll use a slightly different technique than if you weighed 225 pounds and had 17½- to 18-inch arms with a 50-inch chest. The average bodybuilder uses 28- to 30-inch hand spacing. When the bar is resting just above your sternum, your forearms should approximate a vertical position, giving you the best leverage advantage in bench pressing when coordinated with your elbow angle.

Your elbow angle determines which muscle groups will be the major contributing force during a particular range of movement. When the bar is resting on your chest, your elbows will normally be at a 90-degree angle to your body and will activate the pectoralis muscles for a strong drive off the chest. During the transition of power from your pectoralis muscles to your deltoids (approximately six inches from your chest), your elbows may be at a 70-degree angle to your body. In the final power assault, where the triceps take over from the deltoids to the completed lockout, the angle of your elbows to your body may be 45 degrees.

THE HANDOFF

The handoff occurs when you lift the barbell off the uprights of the bench to a locked-arms position over your chest, before beginning the actual bench press descent. Ideally you should have a training partner who can help you lift

the bar off the uprights. Most uprights are non-adjustable and seem to accommodate bodybuilders who are less than 5'10", which means taller bodybuilders can lose considerable energy in simply lifting the barbell off the uprights. A training partner can spare you this cost and also help you with some forced reps and negatives, thereby allowing you to handle heavier poundages as you progress in your workouts. Note that one training partner is usually more efficient than two, because no matter how experienced they are, they always seem to lift the bar off unevenly.

A final word of caution: Never bench press without a spotter. We've seen some incredible accidents befall lifters who decided to go it alone. Take two or three deep breaths, holding the last one. Your training partner will then help you with a coordinated handoff with the barbell at a locked-arms position over your shoulders.

THE DESCENT

Unlock your arms and, over a period of two to three seconds, lower the barbell to just above the sternum on your ribcage. That time frame seems to be the perfect tempo – allowing enough energy to blast through the sticking point off your chest while preventing injury. Lowering the bar faster could make it crash or bounce off your chest, which could not only injure your ribcage or tear a pec at its origin or insertion, but would also cause you to depend on momentum rather than strength recruitment.

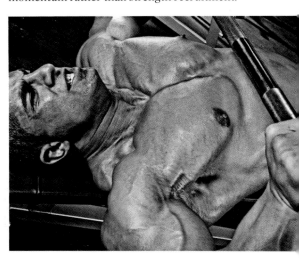

Note that bodybuilders who have deep chests and short arms may be able to keep their elbows from dipping below a parallel position to the floor when the bar is touching their chest. (This is like doing a parallel squat as opposed to doing Olympic full squats.) The less distance the bar has to travel, the better your chances of blasting through any sticking points, all because of a shorter stroke through improved leverages.

THE EXPLOSION

As the bar touches your chest, channel the strength of all the muscle fibers necessary for blasting that weight off the area. The muscles involved – pecs, delts and triceps – should be tensed to the absolute maximum. Your lungs should be full of air and your back should be well arched, as this will shorten the actual distance the bar has to travel during the positive phase of the movement. To initiate the blast off your chest, follow the pre-stretching technique mentioned under "The Squat," accelerating the downward speed of the bar until the final one to two inches before contact with your chest, and being careful not to bounce the weight when it does come in contact with your chest. At that point, summon all your muscle fibers to instantly explode the weight off.

As you apply continued and maximal pressure throughout the range of the movement, don't press the weight straight up from your chest. Instead, when you hit the sticking point, press the bar back and up simultaneously so it lines up over your shoulders at the completion of the rep. Applying maximal pressure or steady effort all the way to lockout will not only blast you through the sticking point in the lift, but it will also help to eliminate oscillation of the bar (the vibration of the plates catching up to the springy bar).

Most bodybuilders experience uneven arm lag during sets with poundages in excess of 84 percent of their current one-rep maximum. In that case, try looking at the center of the bar during the press off your chest and to lockout. If this helps but does not completely solve the problem, try off-setting the hand spacing on your weaker lagging arm an inch or two to the inside or outside (if your right arm lags, move it to the right to put more resistance on the stronger left arm, and vice versa).

Expel all the air from your lungs about two-thirds of the way toward completing the lockout. As you lock the weight out at arms' length, squeeze your pecs for one to two seconds and then take one or two deep breaths, holding the last breath, before beginning your next rep.

At the bottom position, your pecs, delts and triceps should be maximally tensed to explode the weight upward.

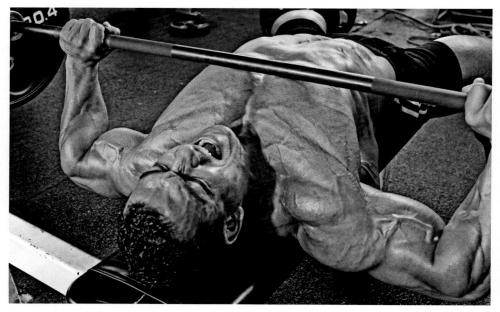

Photo by Robert Reiff
Model Tarek Elsetouhi

Proper foot placement for the conventional deadlift is six to seven inches apart.

Photo by Jason Breeze
Model Andre Rzazewski

CONVENTIONAL BARBELL DEADLIFT
FOOT PLACEMENT

Position the barbell horizontally in front of your feet, with your shins barely touching the bar. Place your feet as you do for the squat. To develop leg strength, your heels should be six to seven inches apart. Your balance may suffer doing this, but there is an increase in leg drive, especially if your feet are parallel and pointed straight ahead.

WEIGHTLIFTING SHOES

To achieve the best mechanical position in the deadlift, wear a shoe that has virtually no heel but has a non-skid sole. If you were to use the shoes we recommended for squatting during your deadlifts, you'd find your body tilting forward, putting you at an immediate leverage disadvantage. When lifting weights, you don't want to leave any room for error. One mistake created by improper footwear could be costly, sometimes resulting in a serious injury.

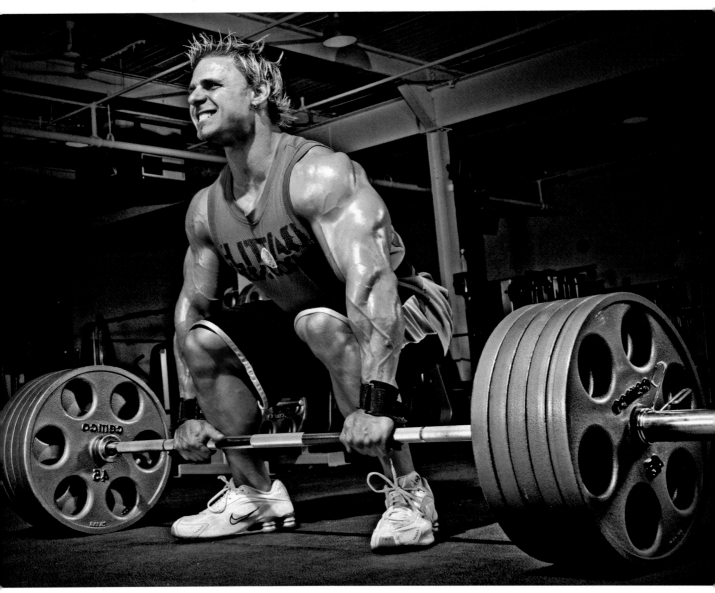

HAND SPACING AND GRIP

Your hand spacing should be two inches outside of the lateral portion of your ankle. You never want to extend your arms out very far from the sides of your body. Doing so would not only create a leverage weakness in your grip, but it would also force you to bend over further and thus pull the bar farther from the floor. You would also find it more difficult to lock your shoulders back at the completion of the lift.

Using varying grip positions – overhand versus underhand – will target the muscles in slightly different ways.

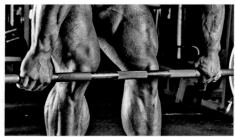

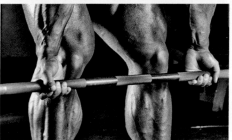

With your hands chalked, bend at the hips and knees and grasp the bar with a viselike, alternating grip (one hand is pronated or palm down while the opposite is supinated or palm up). The bar should ride as close to the fleshy part of your palms as possible, and you should wrap your thumb over the index finger as far as possible. Get your grip set by making sure the wrist in the pronated, or overhand, grip is directly over the bar. On the supinated, or underhand, grip, extend your wrist back so that it's momentarily behind the bar.

When you get ready to pull the bar, rotate your wrist until it's directly over the bar. This bit of wrist action will tighten the skin in the palm of your hand and will give you that added bit of gripping power you need to complete your reps without having to worry about the bar literally hanging off the tips of your fingers in the final sets. Using this maneuver just

once prior to the beginning of your set should ensure that you'll sustain a solid grip through to your last rep. Another alternative is to use a hook grip with your thumbs around the bar, and your index and middle fingers wrapped tightly around the top of your thumbs. It's a very good idea to alternate your grip from workout to workout. This practice alone will balance out any strength and body torque imbalances that may result from using one style for extended periods. We know of one lifter who didn't bother to change his style for years; this practice caught up with him in the form of an injury to the adductor muscles in his thighs.

The increased torque that results from using the mixed overhand and underhand grip can almost turn your body sideways in corkscrew fashion at the completion of a deadlift. This happened to our good friend Roger Mc-Whorter at the North Carolina State Powerlifting Championships when he was completing a deadlift with nearly 630 pounds. At the lockout position his upper torso was in a corkscrew position. Using a double overhand grip probably would have eliminated the excess torque, but it also likely would have decreased his deadlift by 100 pounds or more, so that wouldn't have been the best solution during a competition.

The solution to the problem was right there in an old issue of *Powerlifting USA* magazine. In his article entitled "Fix Up Your Grip," Roger Benjamin explained that improper hand spacing magnifies the torque experienced from the overhand and underhand method. Apparently the middle line of pull or force occurs between the joints of your index and middle fingers on each hand. Your measured grip from the center of the bar is not really centered at all. The line of pull or force of the underhand is approximately two inches farther away from the center of the bar than the pulling line of force on the overhand. When the bar is off center, the force or pull on the underhand grip begins to transfer, causing the body to drift up and out, which can cause you to lose your grip and even tear a biceps muscle in the process. The solution is to place your hands far enough apart to compensate for any transfer of force that might occur.

Photos by Ralph DeHaan
Model Mark Dugdale

Keep your back slightly arched, shoulders squared and chest in front of the bar at the start position.

Photo by Jason Breeze
Model Andre Rzazewski

BODY POSITION

Your legs should be bent so that you're in a quarter-squat position (though this will vary, depending on the height of the bar from the floor). If you're using an Olympic barbell with 45-pound plates, the depth you squat will be quite different from that when doing deadifts with a conventional bar and 25-pound plates (with your knees slightly in front of the bar). Your hips should be down but slightly higher than your knees, which will give your glutes a more direct advantage in helping your powerful quad muscles get the weight moving off the floor. Your back should be slightly arched with your lats and spinae erector muscles tensed, and your shoulders squared (but not pulled back) and slightly ahead of the knees. Your chest should be in front of the bar. Your arms should be completely straight and serve as hooks throughout each repetition. The position of your head should be at approximately 45 degrees (between looking straight ahead and straight up). When your shins are slightly touching the bar, the barbell should be directly over the center of your feet so that the repetition or lift can be done through the center of your legs. If the weight is positioned out on your toes, your back will become rounded and this will cause your hips to rise too high. It will double the pressure on your spine and put excess and undue pressure on the spinae erectors, which could result in a serious injury.

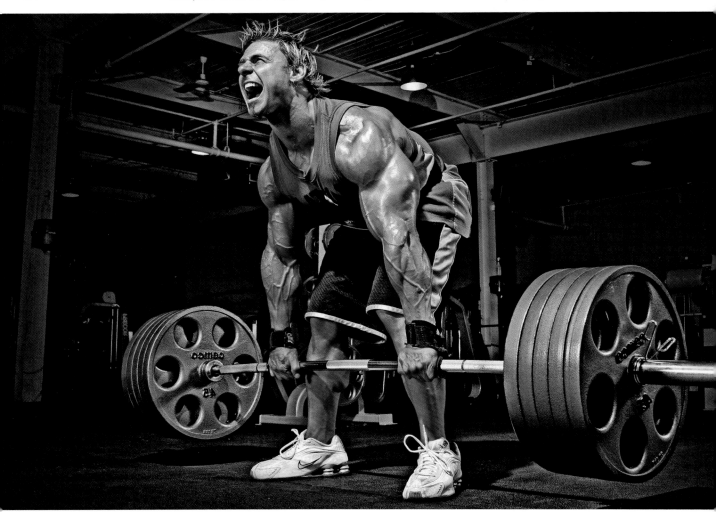

TECHNICAL PULL

Take three deep breaths, holding the last one. Begin with a powerful leg drive, remembering that your legs shouldn't straighten completely until your shoulders and traps are locked back at the completion of the lift. This action will keep your hips from coming up faster than they should. If you lift your hips too fast, you're apt to lose the lift at the sticking point around your knee area. Be sure the bar is lightly touching your shins and thighs during the appropriate aspect of the pull. Be careful not to slide or hitch the weight at any point of the lift.

As the bar begins to approach your knee area, you may notice a slowing down as the deadlift is being pulled away from your leg and glute strength. At that point tilt your head back completely so you are looking up at the ceiling. At the same time bring your hips as close to the bar as possible, keeping them in line with your shoulders, which should have remained in a fixed vertical path in front of the bar throughout the lift.

THE LOCKOUT

At this point your knees and hips finally lock out and you lock your shoulders back (this is where the frontal delts pass the frontal part of the hips). Align them with the torso as if you are in a natural upright posture.

When you're about two-thirds of the way toward completing the lockout of your deadlift, exhale the air from your lungs. Lower the barbell to the floor in the reverse manner in which you lifted it. Take one deep breath and begin your next rep. Never rest the bar on the floor any longer than it takes for one deep breath.

DEVELOPING DEADLIFT EXPLOSION: EXTENDED DEADLIFTS

If you really want to develop your explosive pull off the floor, you should try executing your deadlifts while standing on a platform or something stable and elevated (something three feet long by two feet wide is ideal). The best elevation is completely dependent on the barbell plate diameter. Be sure to allow the bar to touch the instep of your foot when you are standing on the block. Not only will you develop your explosive pull-off-the-floor abilities, when you go back to your regular deadlifts on the floor, the bar will cruise past any former sticking points.

A bodybuilder will occasionally have difficulty locking the shoulders back during the completion of the deadlift and well-meaning gym buddies often advocate extra trapezius work to compensate for the problem. It sounds like good advice because the primary function of the trapezius muscles is to pull the shoulders down and back. As a result, the bodybuilder begins an enthusiastic campaign of shoulder shrugs. The weeks pass and soon his poundages in the shrugs exceed his poundages in the regular deadlift. Yet still he experiences improvement because the whole approach is based on a misconception of anatomy. The scapulae must pull together, or rotate inward, to help stabilize the shoulders. If this doesn't happen, your shoulders move forward rather than going into a locked-back position. The rhomboid muscle causes the scapulae to pull together, and it's the rhomboid that needs to be worked with some bent-over rowing with a barbell, using a palms-up grip such as in a barbell curl (a training tip from the late Reg Park, and popularized in the '90s by six-time IFBB Mr. Olympia, Dorian Yates).

CONCLUSION

If you want to further your understanding of mind-muscle rehearsal via visualization read all the bodybuilding magazines and books you can get your hands on. Continually tell yourself that you're going to build more muscle and become stronger. You'll never experience failure or bad workouts. You'll only experience success.

Concentration during the actual workout is also very important. Think of whatever muscle group you're training and do anything possible to focus your mental powers on that group. Try to get the maximum amount of feeling in the muscle in relation to the amount of weight used, tension and pumping effect. Make your mind work for you, and you'll begin to get results you never imagined possible.

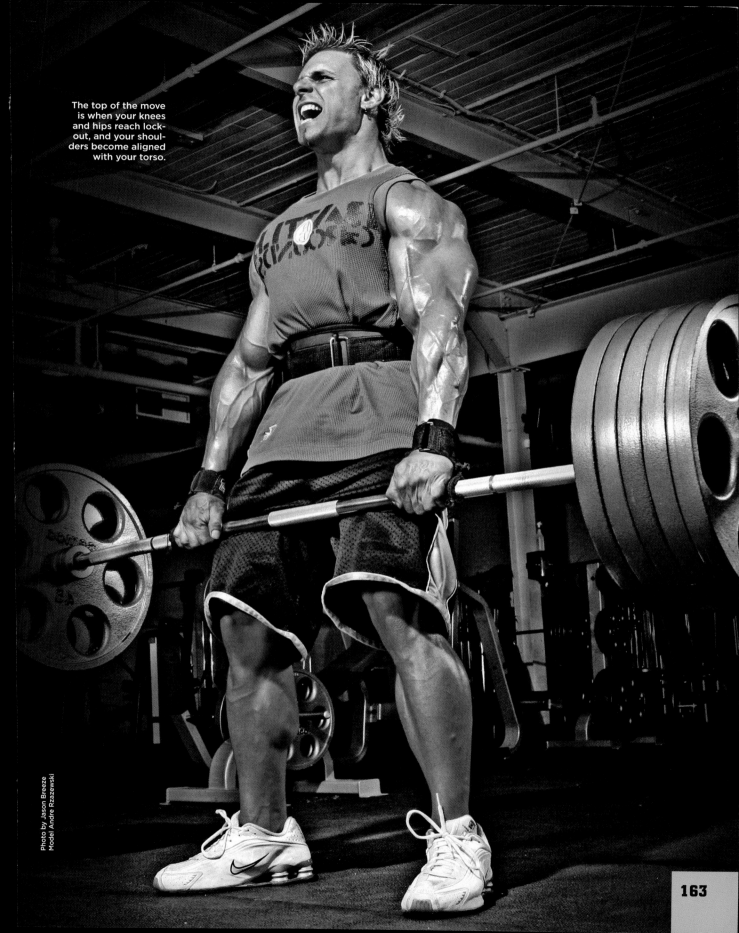

The top of the move is when your knees and hips reach lock-out, and your shoulders become aligned with your torso.

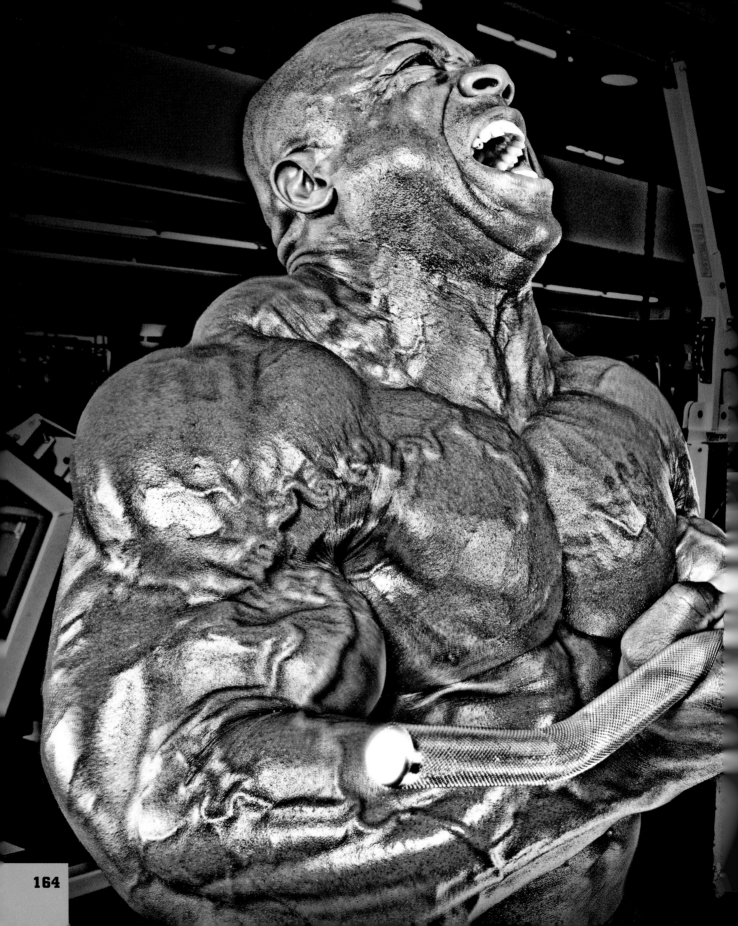

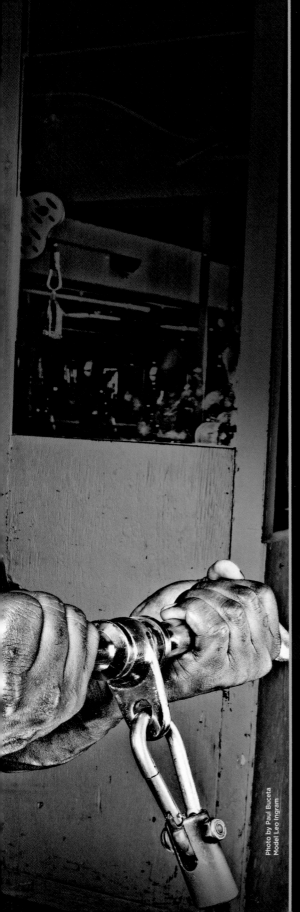

BOOK
06

Physical and Mechanical
Restorative Modalities

CHAPTER 22

PHYSICAL RESTORATIVE ACTIVITIES

There are many treatment methods you can employ to prevent injury and soreness and encourage muscle growth.

To really open up the muscle growth zone it's important to employ the elements of physical and mechanical restorative activities during and after any other exercise protocol.

The following activities are used to accelerate the essential physical, chemical and metabolic responses in the body, and for the release and reduction of toxic metabolites and residual fatigue. This allows for the maximum recovery of the muscles and central nervous system.

ANALGESIC BALM MASSAGE

To achieve an increase of hyper-circulation in the muscles, apply a liberal coat of analgesic balm to the muscle to be worked, before you begin exercising – for example, you would apply to your thighs before doing the barbell back squat. Massage it into each leg for 2 to 2½ minutes each, approximately 5 minutes before each set. Be sure to rub the cream into the muscles with a stroking action. You could also try a vibrator massage unit for a one-minute period on each bodypart.

CRYOKINETIC ICE MASSAGE

Cryokinetics means combining cold treatment with exercise movement. Before beginning, apply a thin coat of baby oil to your muscles to reduce the shock effect that occurs when first touching the ice. Begin the massage by applying ice directly to your muscles, and then moving it over your skin surface in circular motions. In the case of elongated muscles such as the biceps or triceps, simply move the ice up and down the length of the muscle rather than in circular motions.

You can perform ice massage before and after a daily workout session for eight to ten minutes (three times daily) or until the muscle goes numb. Be careful not to get frostbite. Ice massage seems to promote more fresh blood to the muscle area. For smaller muscles (biceps, triceps and calves), ice cubes and ice sticks are helpful. With larger muscles such as the abdominals or quads, use ice packs or bags. Have your materials in an easy-to-find area and apply as necessary.

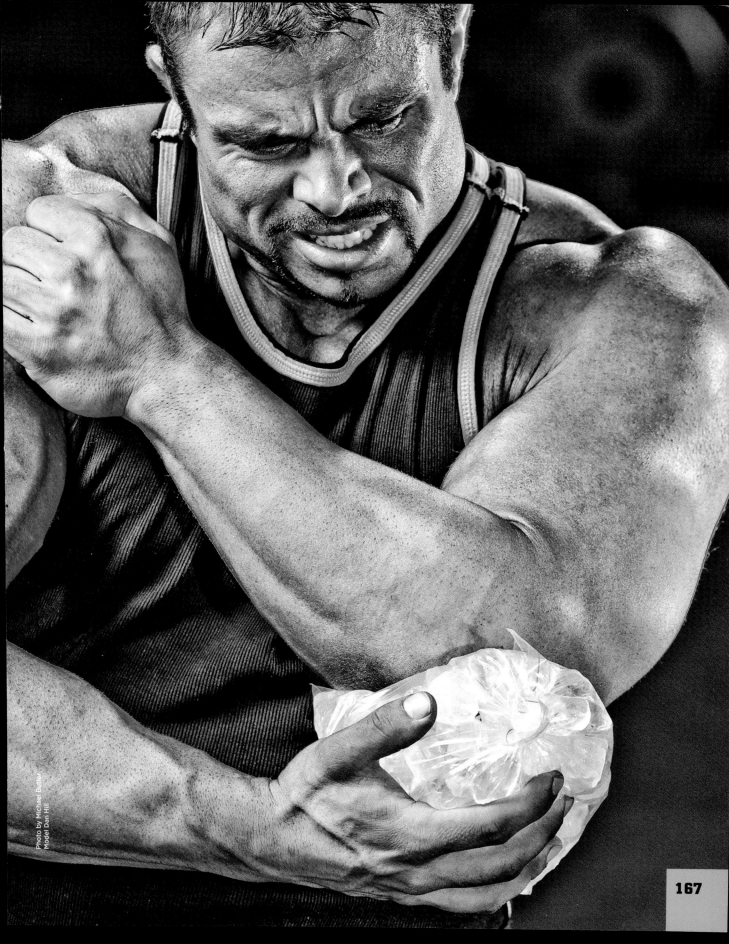

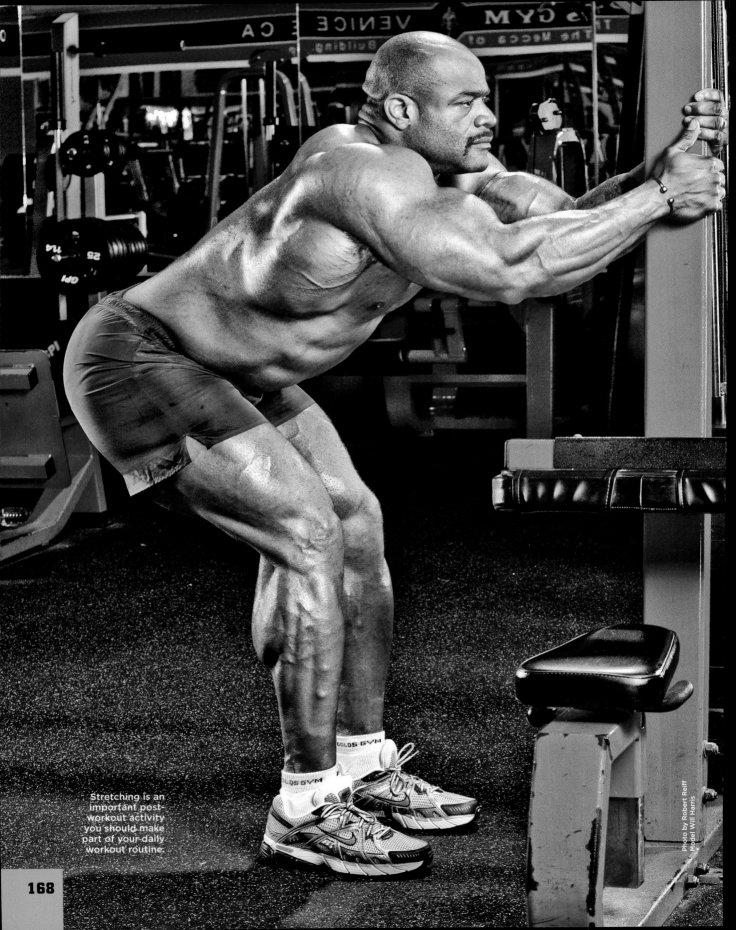

Stretching is an important post-workout activity you should make part of your daily workout routine.

POST (MICRO) WORKOUT MASSAGE

After your workout, get a few minutes worth of superficial massage on your body followed by some fascial stretching (unique self- or partner-assisted stretches that help open up the muscle growth zone). You might consider talking your significant other into helping you.

SPORT RECOVERY MASSAGE

Partial or full-body massage manipulations from certified massage therapists are a terrific idea if you want to assure maximum recovery. The massage sessions can last anywhere from five to sixty minutes, depending on the type of massage and size of the bodybuilder. For example, partial body massages are most dependent upon particular workout intensities. Light training requires five to ten minutes of massage; medium requires 10 to 15 minutes; hard, 15 to 20 minutes; maximal training requires 20 to 25 minutes of partial body massage. For a full body massage to be most effective, individual bodyweight is the main factor: Those weighing 135 pounds or less require 40 minutes of deep massage; 136 to 150 pounds, 50 minutes; 151 to 200 pounds, 60 minutes; 200 pounds and beyond require over 60 minutes of total body massage.

After training, a brief superficial massage can be of extreme benefit to your muscles – this is something even your wife or girlfriend could do.

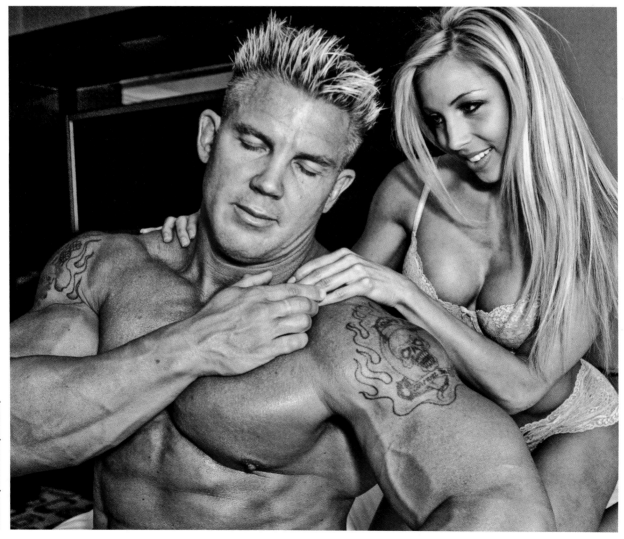

Photo by Rich Baker
Models Andy Haman and Taylor Matheny

CHAPTER 23

MECHANICAL RESTORATIVE TREATMENTS

Speed up recovery time with proven forms of water, heat, electro and movement therapies.

Mechanical restorative treatments are used to accelerate the recovery of your muscles and central nervous system. In the following pages you'll find some of the best, time-tested treatments, including sauna, electro muscle stimulators, hydrotherapy showers and power walking.

POWER WALKING

Power walking is an aerobic activity that improves circulation and helps in the removal of residual metabolites. To power walk, you walk as fast as you can (within 60 to 85 percent of your working target heart rate) and take as many long strides as possible while breathing in and out in cadence with your strides. Time, distance traveled, degree of incline of walking terrain and the amount of resistance carried, if any, also contribute to your results. Try using a weight belt or wrist and ankle weights for added intensity. Work up to approximately 20 percent of your bodyweight.

HYDROTHERAPY SHOWERS

Using a pulsating showerhead, alternate between cold (50 to 55 degrees Fahrenheit) and hot (115 degrees) showers. The cold segment should last 30 seconds followed by two minutes of hot water. Complete this cycle four to six times and then follow it with a cold shower. You could also take a warm shower for 15 minutes and then follow that up with a cold shower lasting one or two minutes. The late IFBB bodybuilding superstar Chuck Sipes considered this one of his favorite post-recovery treatments.

ELECTRO MUSCLE STIMULATORS (EMS)

Electrotherapy of this type is simply micro-currents of alternating frequencies (10 to 15 pps at 30 micro-amps daily). Doing this will strengthen muscles, while at the same time increasing circulation and speeding up the recovery process of your muscles and central nervous system.

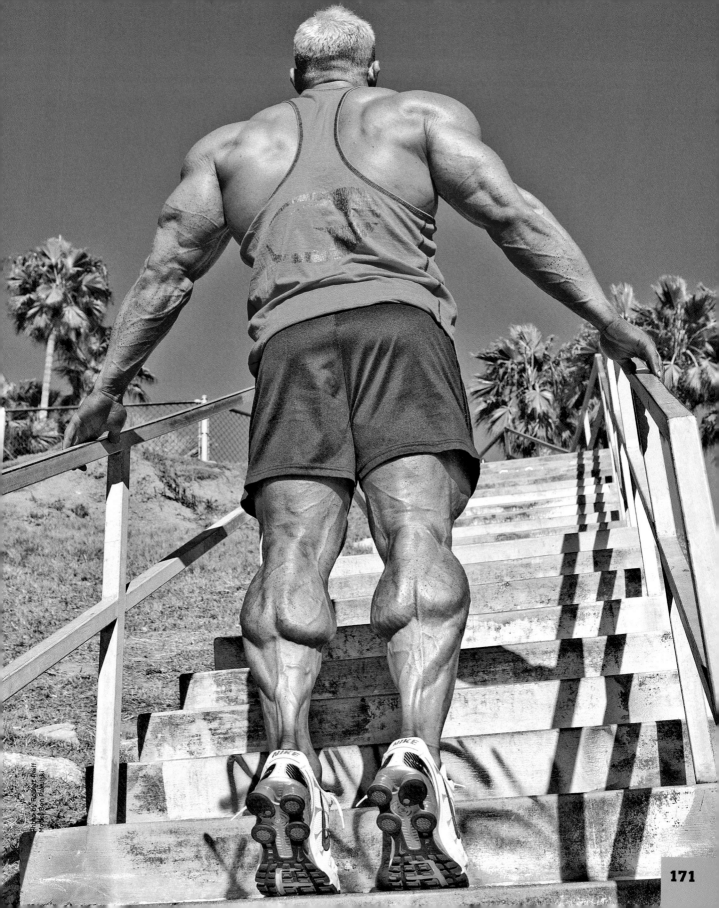

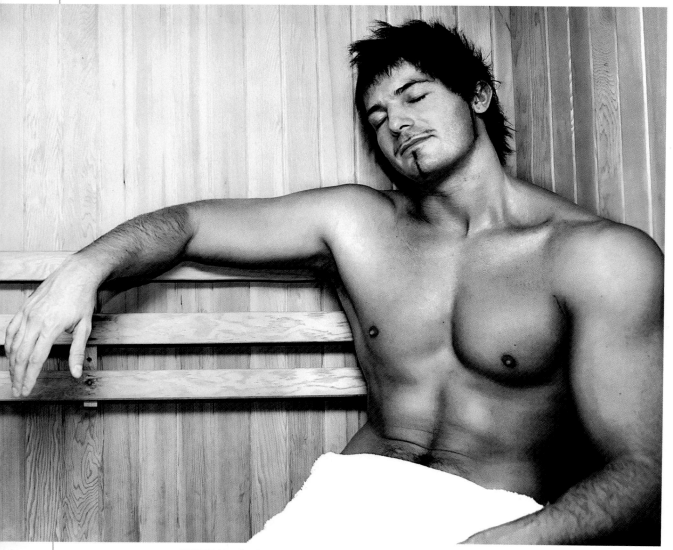

A dry heat sauna, when used correctly, can improve circulation and alleviate lactic acid buildup.

SAUNA (DRY HEAT)

Used once or twice a week, a sauna is an excellent environment for increasing circulation and assisting in the removal of irritant lactic acids and residual metabolic intermediates. In the past, Olympic lifters from many of the Eastern Bloc countries used the dry sauna on a weekly basis to accelerate their bodies' necessary physical, chemical and metabolic responses. Here are some valuable tips for getting the most expedient use out of a dry heat sauna:

• Prior to entering the sauna, drink some water and then take a warm shower (100 to 110 degrees). Don't get your head wet, and be sure to dry yourself immediately following your shower.

• To help prevent dizziness in the sauna, wrap a cool, damp towel around your head.

• Take a dry towel to sit on when you enter the sauna. Sit on the bottom level of the sauna to get your body used to the high temperatures (165 to 175 degrees). After two or three minutes, move to a higher level where the temperature should be between 195 to 205 degrees. Avoid moving around, remain calm and lie on your back, if possible. Above all else, never exercise in the sauna.

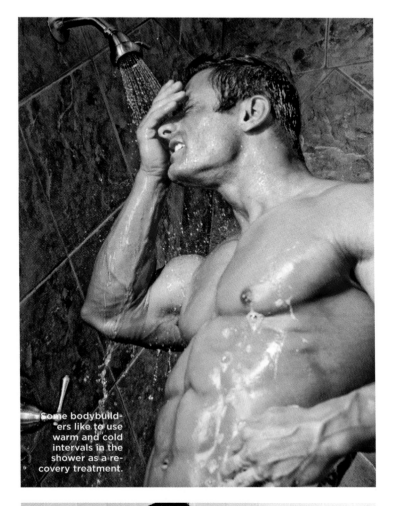

Some bodybuild-ers like to use warm and cold intervals in the shower as a recovery treatment.

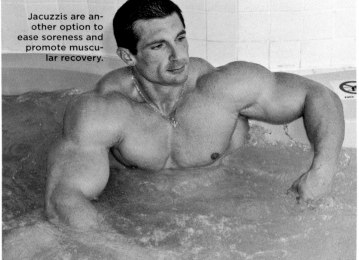

Jacuzzis are an-other option to ease soreness and promote muscu-lar recovery.

Photos by Robert Reiff / Rich Baker
Model Dan Decker / Brian Yersky

• Stay in the sauna for a maximum of six to ten minutes, then leave the sauna and quickly take a cool shower (50 to 55 degrees) for 20 to 40 seconds. Follow that up with a warm shower (about 100 degrees) for one or two minutes. Alternate the cool shower with the warm shower sequences for three or four more series. Remember: Don't get your head wet. Towel off and take a 15-minute break before reentering the sauna. In that time your body will have a chance to rehydrate. Slowly drink an 8- to 12-ounce glass of cool juice or an electrolyte drink. Continue this practice for one to two hours following your sauna use.

• Re-enter the sauna and repeat the prior tips.

• Never enter a sauna while intoxicated, overly fatigued, dehydrated or sick.

• According to former IFBB Mr. Olympia Larry D. Scott, you can increase your growth hormone release just by spending time in a dry heat sauna before working out and three or four more times during the workout. Larry recommends staying in the sauna just long enough to get warm and leaving just before breaking a sweat.

Some other mechanical restorative treatments include:

• Pulsed ultrasound is an effective way to improve muscle tonus when used for 8 to 15 minutes and pulsed in a 1:4 ratio at .8-1.0 watts/cm with a frequency of 1.0 MHZ.

• Jacuzzis and tanning beds can aid in the recovery from a maximum overload on a muscle group.

• Vitamins are very effective in combating muscle soreness. One of the most effective remedies for decreasing post-workout soreness after a workout is to consume 500 mg of Vitamin C (with bioflavonoids) prior to your workout and 400 mg immediately upon completion of your workout. You might also want to consider a mega dose of Vitamin C. In the three hours prior to and immediately following your scheduled workout, consume three 500 mg dosages of Vitamin C. Be sure to take each Vitamin C dosage one hour apart. Vitamin E supplementation may also be helpful in preventing muscle soreness. Both vitamins are easy to find.

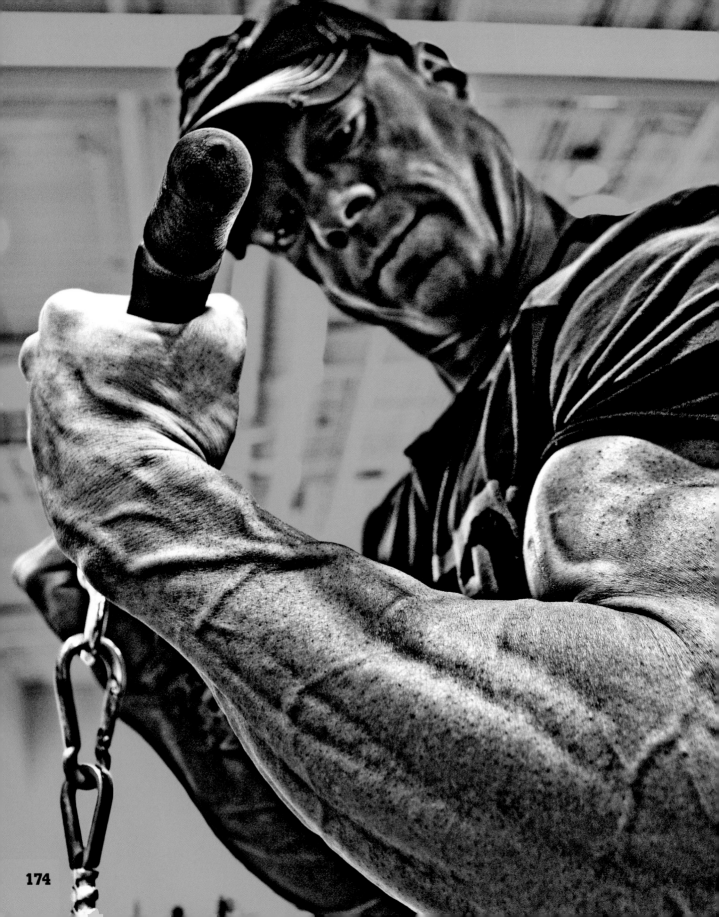

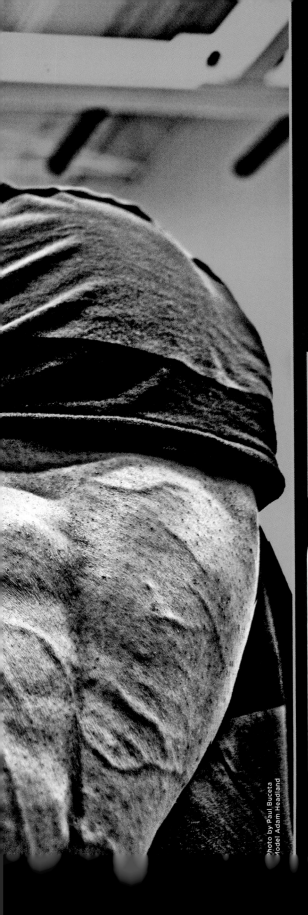

BOOK 07

Realistic Training Expectations

CHAPTER 24

WHAT TO EXPECT FROM TRAINING

Results won't happen overnight, but if you stay dedicated and disciplined, you can expect to see substantial long-term gains in size, strength and lean bodyweight.

If you're like most people, you're probably wondering what type of results you should expect from your training efforts. Somatotyping is an excellent way for you to measure your potential. But if you're not very dedicated or disciplined in your training, you might be displeased with your results.

If you follow the time-tested programs we describe in this book, then within the first two to three years of training you can expect to gain as much as 4½ to 5¼ inches on each upper arm, 7½ to 10 inches on your chest, 3½ to 4¼ inches on each thigh and 1½ to 2¼ inches on each calf. You should experience muscle gain of around seven to twelve pounds in your first year of bodybuilding, five to ten pounds in the following year and an additional four to eight pounds in your third year. After this initial burst of growth, your rate of progress will slow down.

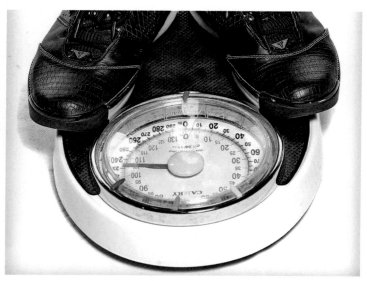

Photo by Jason Breeze
Model Craig Richardson

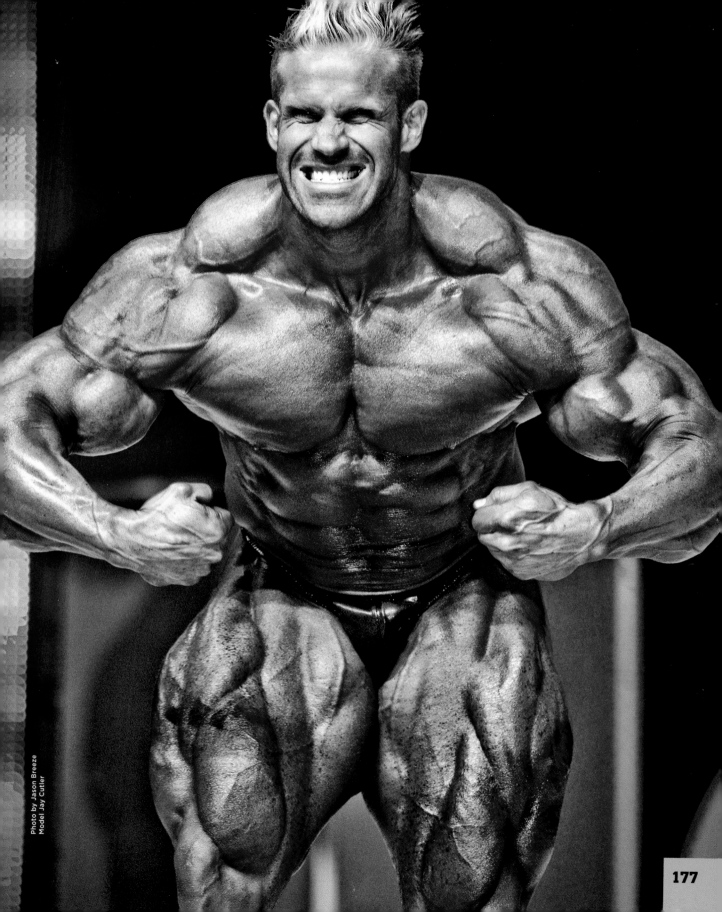

Photo by Jason Breeze
Model Jay Cutler

177

Essentially, the more muscle you've gained, the tougher it is to gain more.

You might think our projection of a first-year muscle mass weight gain of seven to twelve pounds is conservative. Sure some bodybuilders with high caloric intake and determination have made gains of more than 30 pounds in much less than a year, but you can bet for almost all of them only a third of that is pure muscle.

Gaining 10 pounds of muscle in a year, as most steroid-free bodybuilders will experience, amounts to adding .027 pounds per day or less than one pound of muscle mass a month. Many pro bodybuilders who go on the juice reach their genetic potential in as little as two or three years and then struggle to add even two or three pounds of muscle in each of the following years. If you're already in your 40s or beyond, your testosterone levels aren't the same as when you were younger. Although you will make some decent gains in muscle size and strength, you'll likely make only 60 percent of the gains you would have made when you were younger.

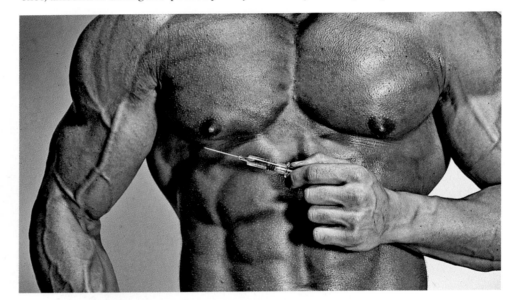

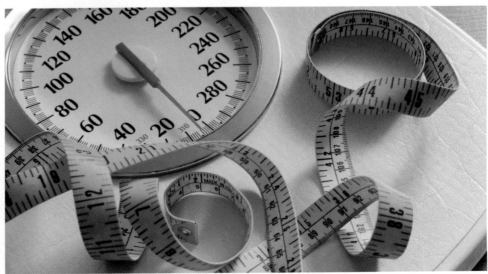

A scale and tape measure will give you accurate numeric readings of your gains in pounds and inches, but remember that the mirror can also act as a useful guide.

ACQUIRING MASSIVE MUSCLE

Your mind creates your body. It crafts your body's potential and cultivates its urges and feelings. If you're looking to build massive muscle mass and incredible strength, you must accept that success is every bit as much mental as it is physical. Stay patient. Keep your eyes on the prize and remember that if you believe it, you can achieve it. Train intelligently and train hard. In time, you'll build the body you always dreamed about, as long as you maintain your courage and character and never give up on the challenge. Remember, you've earned every hard-training inch and pound of muscle mass you've created. In this book, you'll find all the advanced training techniques and secrets for keeping that muscle mass and building on it. You'll still have to work hard and pay attention to your nutrition, but the good news is that it's not as hard to keep your muscle mass once you've already built it as it is to build it in the first place. Books 8–15 reveal some advanced training techniques and secrets for maintaining the previous gains in muscle mass and strength.

Achieving success with your physique is both a mental and physical endeavor – train smart and train hard.

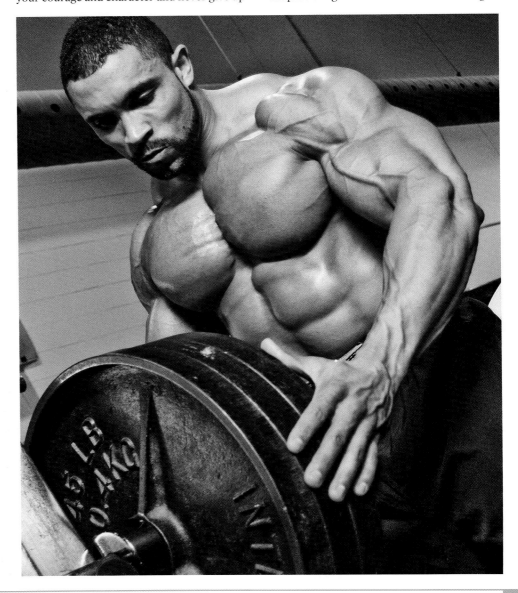

Photo by David Ford
Model Tim Liggins

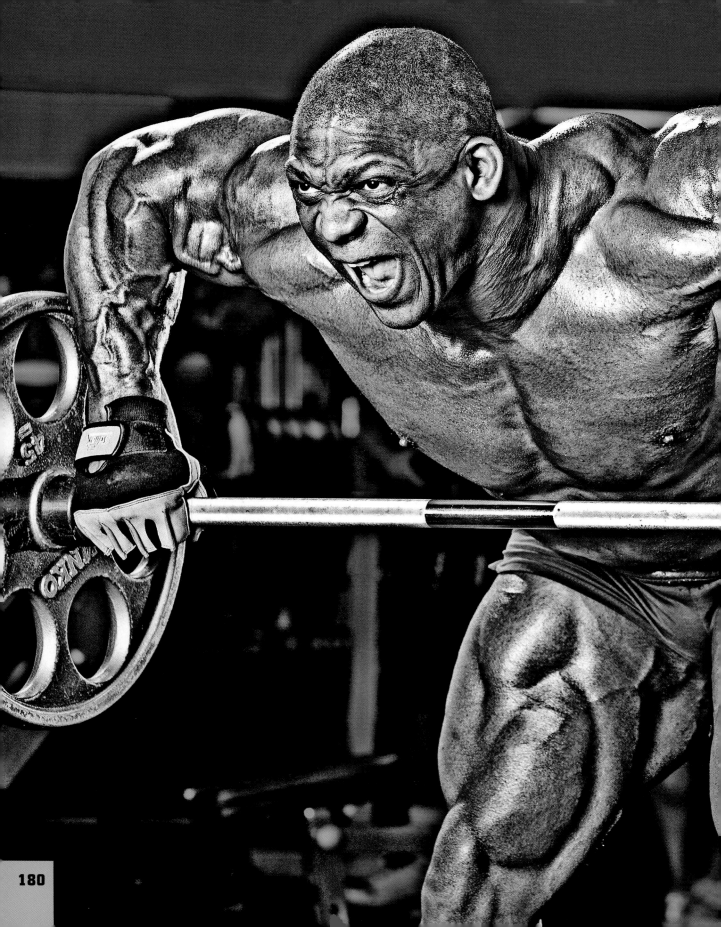

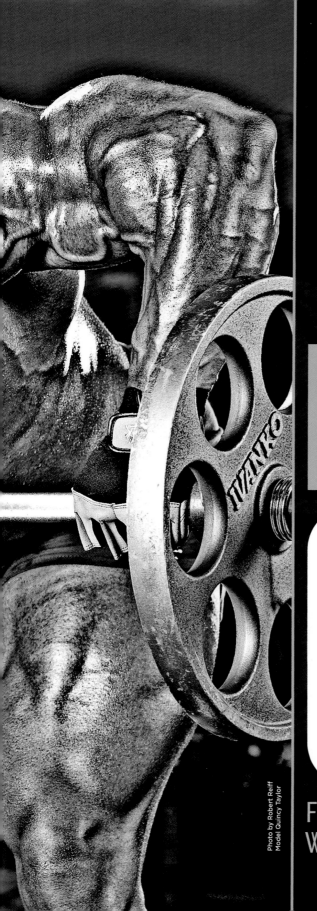

BOOK
08

Four Signature Training
Winning-Edge Workouts

CHAPTER 25

BODY CONTRACT SYSTEM

Preserve and protect your hard-earned muscle and strength with a signature program created by Dan Duchaine.

If you're fairly new to bodybuilding, it's very easy to make the mistake of following someone else's workout schedule. Just because a bodybuilding champion sets his program up a certain way doesn't necessarily mean you'll look like him if you follow it. His routines might not be suitable for you. You could even lose muscle size, especially if his program causes you to overtrain. The best approach is to simply pick up a tip here and there, incorporate those tips into your own schedule and pay close attention to how your body reacts. Just remember that you have to work within the limits of your fitness level and recuperative abilities.

For decades, top champions have endorsed everything from specific equipment to supplement programs, and the bodybuilding public is quick to plunk their dollars down in an attempt to look like their heroes. Countless beginning and even seasoned bodybuilders have attempted the routines of these greats without taking into consideration that these professionals have generally spent years of regular training to reach their present level of tolerance for lengthy, high-intensity workouts. In addition, the top bodybuilding champions tend to be genetically blessed with a superior skeletal structure consisting of wide clavicles, narrow hips and good muscle shape, in addition to the innate ability to gain muscle fast.

Of course, some approved workouts are logical to follow if you're trying to protect hard-earned muscle mass and strength. Why? They're time tested to produce eye-opening, second-to-none results where it matters most: The gym. In order to gain ultimate credibility these workouts must have a proven track record in the form of results. An excellent indication of proven results is when bodybuilders around the world use a particular program and consistently see amazing results. This is what we refer to when we say "signature training."

Simply stated, signature training is any rational, winning-edge workout, any advanced muscle-pumping technique or any particular exercise developed by, accredited to and synonymous with a well-known and respected bodybuilding authority. A few examples include: Dan Duchaine's Body Contract Workout, Bob Kennedy's Pre-Exhaust Principle and Larry Scott's Preacher Bench Barbell Curl. Signature training can also be equated with a specific muscle factory or gym. The Bulgarian Leg Workout obviously comes from the muscle factories in Bulgaria, while an exercise such

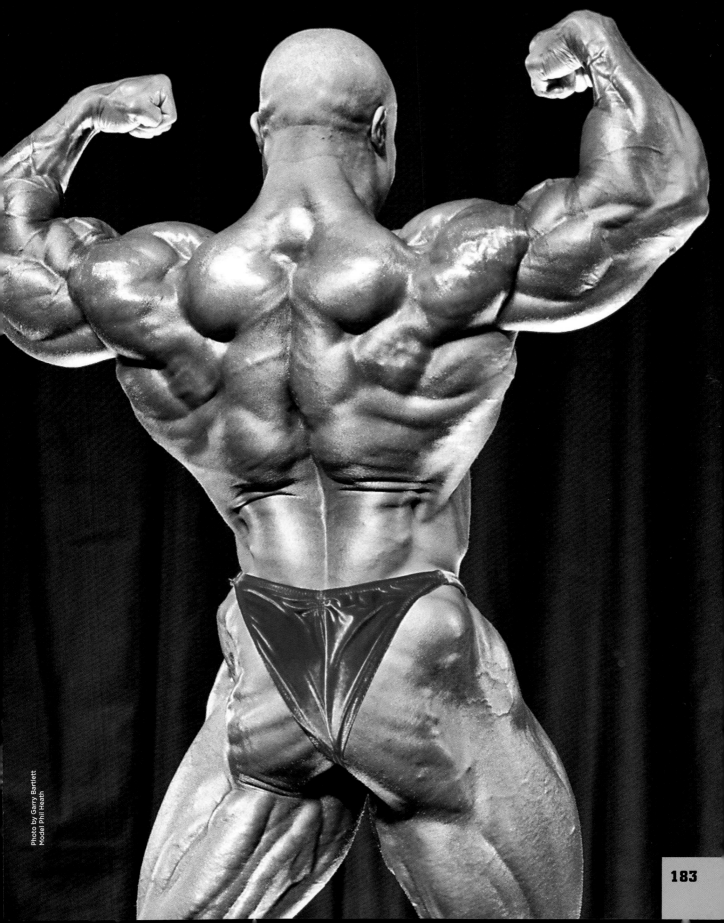

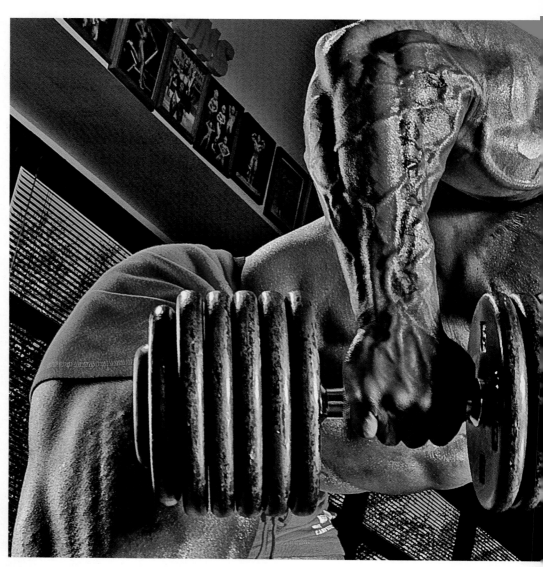

The one-arm dumbbell row is an effective move to engage a high number of muscle fibers in your back.

Photo by Michael Butler
Model Marcus Haley

as the sissy squat was developed and popularized in the muscle factories of Muscle Beach.

Signature training advanced muscle-pumping techniques can be used to avoid or break through a training plateau and to jumpstart the muscle gain factor. Some of these include Leo Costa's Muscle Rounds, Charles Poliquin's German Volume Training, Vince Gironda's Four Sides to A Muscle and IFBB pro bodybuilder Emeric Delczeg's Training System.

If you're looking to protect hard-earned muscle mass and strength, here are four excellent programs: Larry Scott's Four-Day Definition Workout, Rotation for Recuperation, Size Alive Training Program and the Body Contract System.

The Body Contract System was the brainchild of the late "Steroid Guru" Dan Duchaine. The name Body Contract is a play on words. Contract has a dual meaning of a binding agreement (between a person's body and the heavy iron) and a muscle contraction. Dan was probably one of the most interesting and knowledgeable characters in the bodybuilding world and he described the Body Contract System as the strangest workout he ever came across. Beyond being an expert on anabolic pharmacology, he

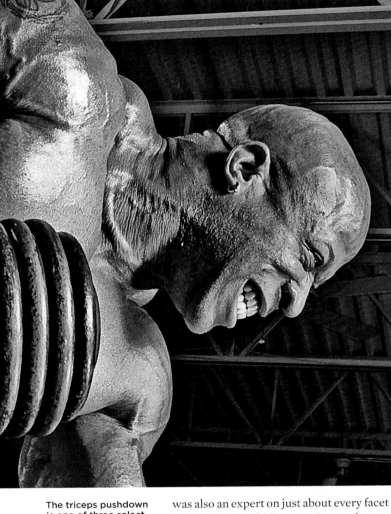

The triceps pushdown is one of three selected moves for that bodypart in the Body Contract System.

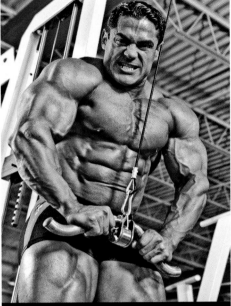

BODY CONTRACT EXERCISE SELECTION

Delts	Overhead Barbell Press, Dumbbell Lateral Raise, Bent-Over Rear Dumbbell Lateral Raise and Barbell Shoulder Shrug
Biceps	Seated Incline Dumbbell Hammer Curl and EZ-Bar Preacher Bench Curl
Triceps	Triceps Pushdown (from a High Pulley Cable), Single-Dumbbell Triceps Extension Overhead and Bench Dip
Quads	Front Barbell Squat or Hack Squat, Leg Press and Leg Extension
Hamstrings	Stiff-Leg Deadlift and Lying Leg Curl
Calves	Standing Calf Raise, Seated Calf Raise
Abs	Quarter-Crunch and Reverse Crunch (on an Incline Bench)
Chest	30-Degree Incline Barbell Press, Flat Dumbbell Flye, Parallel Bar Dip or Decline Barbell Press
Back	Lower Power Rack Half-Barbell Deadlift (pull the bar from the knees upward), One-Dumbbell Pullover, Upper-Lat Pulldown (pull bar to nose/chin area) and One-Arm Dumbbell Row

Note: Dan Duchaine determined through magnetic resonance images of the muscles worked that these exercises would engage the maximum number of muscle fibers for each particular muscle group.

was also an expert on just about every facet of bodybuilding including creating workout programs. Here's an overview of the Body Contract System schedule:

Day 1 (Monday): Delts, biceps and triceps
Day 2 (Tuesday): Quads, hamstrings, calves and abs
Days 3 and 4 (Wednesday and Thursday): Rest and recuperation
Day 5 (Friday): Chest and back
Days 6 and 7 (Saturday and Sunday): Rest and recuperation

Dan put a lot of thought into this workout schedule. Upon the completion of a maximum overload on the major muscle groups (days two and five) are two full days reserved for rest and recuperation. Repeat this seven-day plan for three weeks and then take an entire week off from training.

BODY CONTRACT POUNDAGE, SETS, REPS AND REST-PAUSES

For each exercise (with the exception of the ab exercises, which can be done for two or three sets of 15 to 40 reps) use 70 percent of your one-rep max (1RM) for a maximum of three sets of 12 reps in the first exercise of a muscle group. Then, perform one set of 12 reps in the remaining exercises. Immediately following the one set, increase the poundage to 85 percent and, with the assistance of one or two competent training partners, do three slow negative reps. According to Dan, each set of 12 regular reps along with three negative reps should take approximately 40 seconds. Upon the completion of each set (and between muscle groups as well) be sure you rest for three minutes.

With this system of training, your poundage should start at 70 percent of your 1RM.

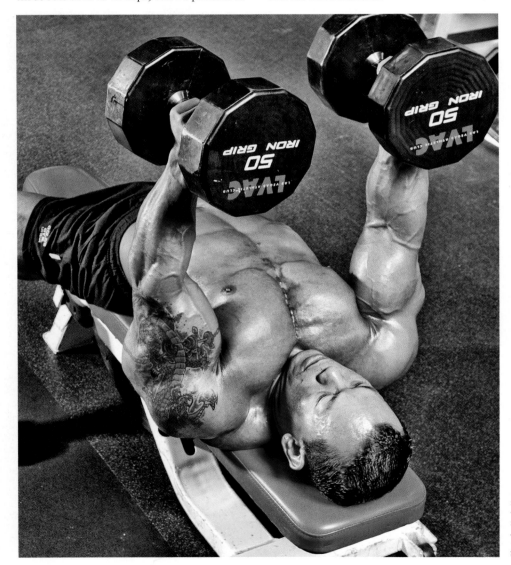

Photo by Kevin Horton
Model Chris Dim

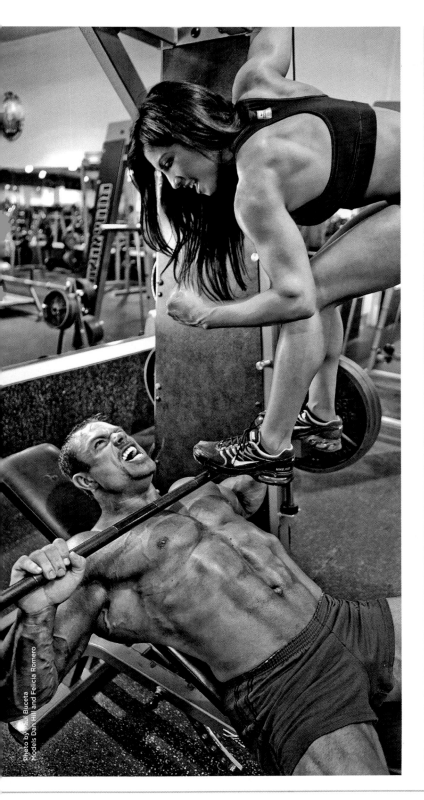

Photo by Paul Buceta
Models Dan Hill and Felicia Romero

BODY CONTRACT WORKOUT SEVEN-POINT SUMMARY

1. If 300 pounds is your 1RM, do two specific warm-up sets of 12 reps, each at 35 percent (.35 x 300 = 135 lbs) of 1RM. Then, do a third and final warm-up set for eight reps at 60 percent (.60 x 300 = 180 lbs) of your 1RM. This warm-up procedure is for the first exercise of each muscle group only. No warm-ups are necessary for the second and third exercises of a selected muscle group.

2. Increase the poundage to 70 percent of your 1RM (.70 x 300 = 210 lbs) and in the first exercise for a specific muscle group, perform
   Set 1: 210 x 1 set of 12 reps
   Sets 2 and 3: 210 x 1 set of 12 reps plus three negatives with 85% of your 1RM (.85% x 300 = 255 lbs)

In the second and third exercises for a muscle group, do only one set of 12 reps at 70 percent of your 1RM and then put the weight down while one or two training partners immediately increase the poundage to 85 percent of max. Be sure your training partners assist you when you perform the three slow negatives – don't do it alone.

3. A set of 12 reps should be accomplished in rapid fire and last only 40 seconds. You should then take another five to eight seconds for each negative rep. Dan also directs you to take no pause between reps, even for a split second.

4. Rest for three minutes between each set, exercise and muscle group.

5. Don't add exercises to those already listed or you may become overworked. Substitute an exercise only if the one you're doing is causing some type of muscle strain or injury.

6. Don't perform more than a half-hour of cardio in three non-consecutive days per week.

7. Perform the Body Contract Workout three days per week. Rest and recuperate the other four days. Each daily workout should last an hour. Follow this schedule for three weeks and then take a week off from any kind of training.

Keep in mind the suggested 70 percent of a one-rep max is not written in stone. If you find 12 reps at 70 percent of a maximum single rep too difficult, then find the appropriate weight that will allow you to perform 12 reps per set.

If you want a workout that offers more anabolism and less catabolism, then the Body Contract Workout is your ticket to massive gains. We know this to be a fact because, along with many of our friends, we have used it with great success. Good luck!

CHAPTER 26

LARRY SCOTT'S FOUR-DAY DEFINITION WORKOUT

The first IFBB Mr. Olympia offered a wealth of knowledge and experience through his workout program.

As the name would suggest, this signature training winning-edge workout program comes from our good friend Larry Scott, the first IFBB Mr. Olympia. Larry is adamant: When performed cautiously and intelligently, this program will not only burn stored fat, but also force your muscles to grow – simultaneously.

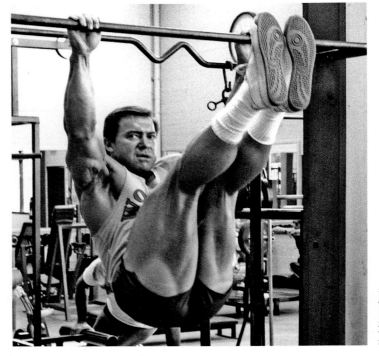

Model Larry Scott

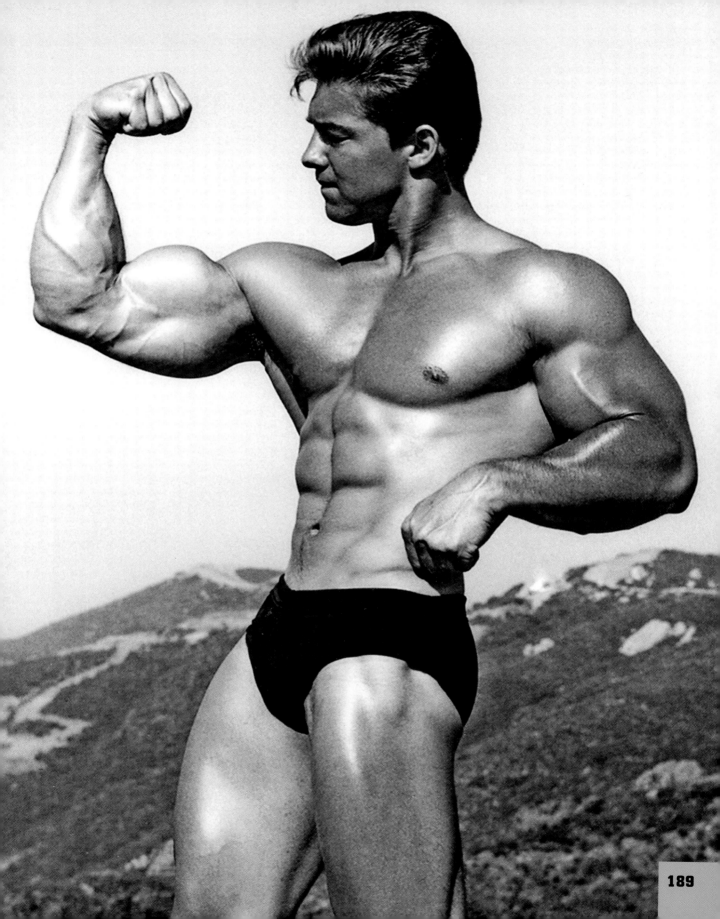

MONDAY AND THURSDAY

CHEST

Bench Press	Do three series of four sets with 10 reps of the bench press. Don't rest between sets.
Parallel Bar Dip / Incline Dumbbell Press	Alternate between dips and incline presses for three series of two sets (10 reps each). Don't rest between sets.
One-Dumbbell Pullover (across bench)	Perform four sets of 12 reps of the dumbbell pullover. Use all the weight you can handle.

LATS

Pull-Up (to nose on chin-up bar)	Alternate all three of these exercises for five series of three sets with 12 reps. Don't rest between sets, only between each series. The long pull is performed by pulling the bar to your waist with the pulley in front of you set about five feet high.
Pulldown (on lat machine)	
Long Pull (on lat machine)	

QUADS AND HAMSTRINGS

Barbell Back Squat	Perform six sets of 12 reps. Work up to your maximum weight and down again with little rest between sets. Your fourth set should be the heaviest.
Leg Curl	Using the leg curl machine, be sure to alternate between each of these exercises. Do three series of two sets of 12 reps.
Leg Extension	

ABS

Sit-Up	Alternate between these exercises and perform four series of two sets with 8 reps (8 sets in all). Don't rest between sets or series. Do sit-ups with your feet flat on the floor. Stop when your feet start to come off the floor.
Leg Raise	

Warm up on each exercise with a light weight. You will be using a heavy weight from your first set, so it's important that you warm up properly.

Series Training: Start the first set with the maximum weight you can handle and complete all the reps. Don't rest and then drop 10 or 20 pounds off the weight and do the next set. Continue until you have done all your sets in the series. Rest and start the next series as soon as possible.

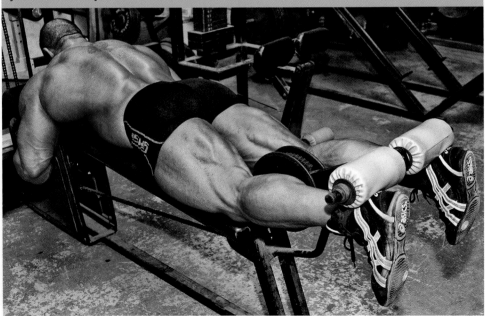

On this program, bodybuilders should alternate sets of leg curls and extensions.

Photo by Jason Breeze
Model Fouad Abiad

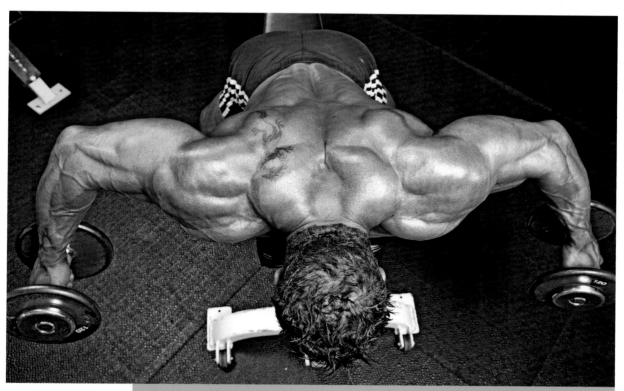

There are three delt exercises in the four-day definition work-out, one of which is the bent-over dumb-bell lateral raise.

TUESDAY AND FRIDAY

DELTOIDS

Barbell Press (behind neck)	Warm up with a light weight, then do six sets of 10 reps. No resting between sets.
Standing Dumbbell Lateral Raise	Alternate these exercises for four series of two sets (12 reps).
Bent-Over Dumbbell Lateral Raise	

BICEPS

Preacher Bench Barbell Curl	Alternate between these exercises for four or five se-ries of two sets. Do eight reps for each set with three small-movement burns* at the top. No rest between sets, but you can rest between each series.
Preacher Bench Dumbbell Curl	

TRICEPS

Supine Triceps Barbell Press	Alternate between these exercises for five series of two sets. Do 10 reps and three small burns at the top of each set. No resting between sets.
Triceps Pushdown (on lat machine)	

CALVES

Donkey Calf Raise	With your feet on a four-inch platform, and while holding onto something or leaning on a bench, do five sets of 25 reps. Start with fewer reps and work up to 25.

*Burns: If you've completed your required number of sets, whatever muscle you have been work-ing should be exhausted to the point that no more complete reps are possible. However, you may still have sufficient strength to perform small partial reps that will burn out the muscle completely. These small burns will greatly speed up your gains by increasing the intensity of your workouts.

Be aware of yourself, your goals and your capabilities. Rather than worrying about how much you can lift, concentrate. Become more in tune with the purpose of your movements. Don't forget that your mental attitude will determine whether you're successful in reaching your goals.

HUGE & FREAKY MUSCLE MASS AND STRENGTH SECRETS

CHAPTER 27

ROTATION FOR RECUPERATION

Using an every-other-day training split will help keep your muscles guessing to prevent quick adaptation and conditioning.

How frequently should you train? We get asked this question all the time. There's really no single answer. The correct amount of training frequency varies greatly, from person to person and even for one person at different times of his life. Genetics, recuperation, age, experience, goals and diet will all have a direct impact on how often you hit the gym. By taking a good look at these factors, you should be able to determine the best training frequency and program for you.

Ideally, your training should consist of a solid combination of cardio, muscle-building exercises and adequate rest. While you're building muscle and strength through intense and progressive resistance, cardio training will focus on your heart. You must also allow sufficient time for complete recuperation and make sure you don't train with too much intensity too often, because overtraining could actually do more harm than good.

Performing the same exercises on a daily basis may be one of the worst ways of training. According to Arthur Jones, if you're a beginner you'll find the best results are generated with a full-body workout on three non-consecutive days per week (e.g. Monday, Wednesday and Friday) and adapting two exercises for every bodypart in each workout session. After roughly six weeks, as your body adjusts and becomes conditioned, four sessions per week working each muscle group twice a week is generally the best result-producing split. The one drawback with this method is that you'll be training two consecutive days, which impacts on the various chemical and muscle recovery abilities of your body.

After six to eight weeks using this training scheme, many bodybuilders will split their workouts into one day for the upper body and the next day for the lower body (a six-day split training Monday through Saturday, resting only on Sundays, for about two months). At the conclusion of this stage, if you're a dedicated bodybuilder, you've adjusted to training and have numerous options when setting up your next workout schedule.

At this point, individualism comes into play. A much better alternative to the upper-body/lower-body training scheme would be to use the Rotation-for-Recuperation workout (Every-Other-Day Split Routine). Here's how it looks:

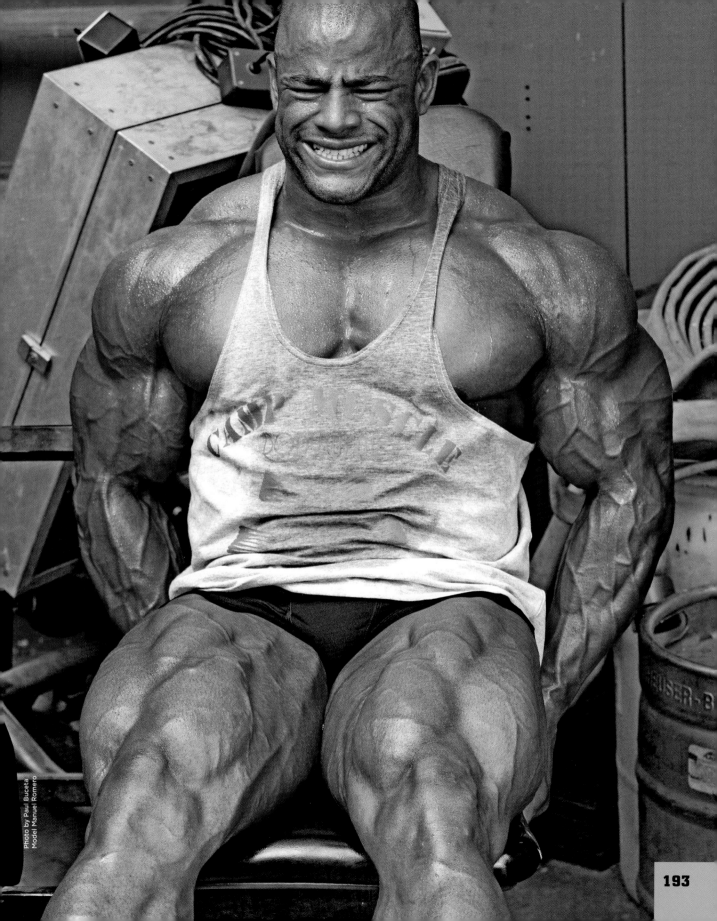

Photo by Paul Buceta
Model Manuel Romero

193

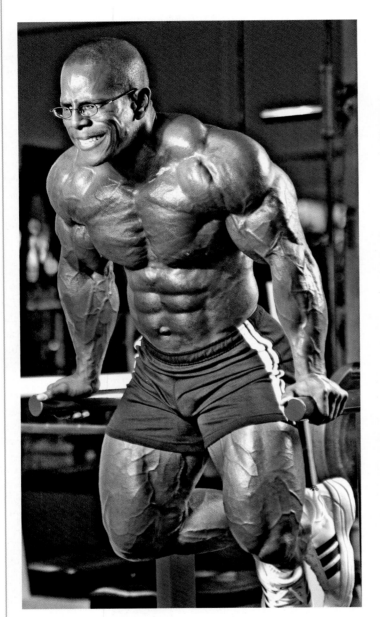

The parallel bar dip is part of Workout B – Day 1, 3 and 5 of the split.

After the first week, you'll begin a 10-to-12-week period of exclusively doing Workout B. Here's a sample Rotation for Recuperation, or Every-Other-Day Split:

WORKOUT A	SETS/REPS
THIGHS	
Barbell Back Squat	4 x 6
45-Degree (non-lock) Leg Press	2 x 6-8
Machine Leg Curl	2 x 8
Leg Extension	2 x 8
CALVES	
Standing Calf Raise	3 x 6-8
Seated Calf Raise	2 x 6-8
Donkey Calf Raise	2 x 6-8
BACK	
Semi-Stiff Leg Barbell Deadlift	3 x 6-8
Wide-Grip Pull-Up	3 x 6-8
Seated Long-Cable Pulley Row	2 x 6-8
BICEPS	
Standing Barbell Curl	3 x 6-8
Preacher Bench Dumbbell Curl	2 x 6-8
FOREARMS	
Standing EZ-Bar Reverse Curl	2 x 6-8
Seated Barbell Wrist Curl (palms up)	2 x 6-8
Seated Barbell Wrist Curl (palms down)	2 x 6-8
WORKOUT B	**SETS/REPS**
CHEST	
Barbell Bench Press	3 x 6-8
Incline Dumbbell Flye	2 x 6-8
Incline Dumbbell (non-lock) Press	2 x 6-8
Dumbbell Pullover (across bench)	2 x 6-8
DELTS	
Standing Barbell Press Overhead	3 x 6-8
Standing Dumbbell Lateral Raise	2 x 6-8
Standing Barbell Upright Row	2 x 6-8
TRICEPS	
Close-Grip EZ-Bar Bench Press	3 x 6-8
Triceps (non-lock) Pushdown	2 x 6-8
Parallel Bar Dip	2 x 6-8
ABDOMINALS	
Hanging Knee Pull-In (holding a dumbbell between your feet)	2 x 6-8
Incline Bench Bent-Knee Sit-Up (holding a barbell plate on your chest)	3 x 6-8
Abdominal Floor Crunch (holding a barbell plate on your chest)	2 x 6-8

Day 1: Workout A: Thighs, calves, back, biceps and forearms

Day 2: Rest

Day 3: Workout B: Chest, delts, triceps and abs

Day 4: Rest

Day 5: Workout A: Thighs, calves, back, biceps and forearms

Day 6: Rest

Day 7: Rest

12 POINTS TO REMEMBER ABOUT THE ROTATION-FOR-RECUPERATION ROUTINE

1. Use three or four exercises per muscle group (in order to blitz the muscles from a variety of stress angles). Perform at least one compound movement first and then do isolation exercises. Over the course of 10 to 12 weeks, use as many pieces of exercise equipment for any particular muscle group (nautilus machines, barbells, dumbbells, pulley and expander cables, etc.) as you have at your disposal.

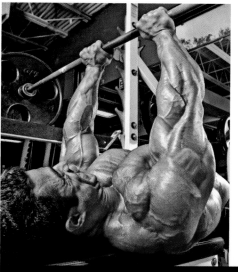

At the peak of certain moves, like the bench press, contracting your muscles maximally for a few seconds creates iso-tension.

2. Do a total of eight to ten sets for the larger muscle groups (legs, back and chest) and five to seven sets for all of the other muscle groups. Always perform a warm-up set of the first exercise of a muscle group. The warm-up set doesn't count as a regular set.

3. Use a weight heavy enough to restrict your reps per set to a minimum of six and a maximum of eight. If you're striving for eight reps, make sure that the eighth rep is so intense that you couldn't possibly do a ninth.

4. Do your reps at a moderate speed and always lower the weight twice as slowly as you lifted it. If you took two seconds to lift the weight, then take four seconds to lower it.

5. Rest for one minute between each set. In the 10 to 15 seconds before your next set, close your eyes and visualize all the exercise mastery techniques that will be necessary for the successful completion of each gut-wrenching rep.

6. Using the iso-tension technique, contract your muscles as hard as possible for two seconds at the peak of the movement. This technique works well for such exercises included in the following Iso-Tension Technique chart seen below.

ISO-TENSION TECHNIQUE

MUSCLE GROUPS	EXERCISES THAT PROVIDE RESISTANCE IN THE CONTRACTED POSITION
Quads	Barbell Back and Front Squat, Leg Extension, Leg Press and Smith Machine Squat
Hams	Machine Leg Curl (standing/lying)
Calves	Seated/Standing Calf Raise
Traps	Barbell High Pull, Barbell Shrug/Row
Lats	Barbell or Dumbbell Row, Lat Pulldown, Seated Low-Pulley Cable Row and Pull-Up (palms facing forward)
Pecs	Barbell or Dumbbell Bench Press, Pulley Cable Crossover, Parallel Bar Dip and Pec Deck
Delts	Overhead Barbell Press, Dumbbell Lateral Raise (front/side/rear) and Low Pulley Cable Lateral Raise
Biceps	Barbell Curl, Chin-Up, Dumbbell Concentration Curl, Incline Dumbbell Curl and Low-/High-Pulley Cable Curl
Triceps	Close-Grip Barbell Bench Press, Lat-Machine Triceps Pressdown, Parallel Bar Dip and Barbell/Dumbbell Triceps Extension
Forearms	Barbell (palms up) Wrist Curl
Abs	Crunch and Swiss-Ball Crunch

7. Occasionally do a couple of forced or negative reps at the end of a set to stimulate a muscle that might need a little jolt. Don't make a habit out of it. Stay away from supersets, tri-sets and giant sets.

8. You need to get your rest. Try to get at least eight hours of sleep each night. Never get more than nine hours or you'll become sluggish.

9. Relaxation is as important as sleep. Three hours of total relaxation can replace hours of sleep.

10. The Rotation-for-Recuperation Routine has been designed to overload specific muscle groups on particular days, with adequate intervals of rest provided. Unless otherwise advised, don't change this routine or you may become overtrained and possibly injure yourself.

11. Take a seven-day layoff following every 10 to 12 weeks of hard training.

12. Begin a new Rotation-for-Recuperation Routine as follows:

Day 1: Workout A: Chest, back, biceps and forearms

Day 2: Complete rest

Day 3: Workout B: Thighs, calves, shoulders, triceps and abs

Day 4: Complete rest

Day 5: Workout A: Chest, back, biceps and forearms

Day 6: Complete rest

Day 7: Complete rest

Note: For a change of pace, you could take some of the exercises out of the previous routine and include some new ones. For example, when working your back, you might take out seated long-pulley cable rows and replace it with the barbell shrug. In the case of the biceps, you could consider adding the one-dumbbell concentration curl as a finishing exercise for two sets of six to eight reps.

MIND & MUSCLE LEARNING CURVE

Your mind and body must learn form and technique, and that's why, in the fourth point, we briefly mentioned to always lower a weight twice as slowly as you lifted it. Lifting and lowering the weight with a slow and steady pace is an excellent method to prevent bouncing and jerking, which can result in injury. It's also important to gradually work your muscles and coax them into learning how they should respond to an exercise. This response changes as one becomes more advanced. An advanced bodybuilder constantly tries to avoid having a set pattern, where his muscles are so aware of a movement that they'll actually fail to respond. Once you reach the advanced stages of training you'll notice that your muscles demand constant change.

If you aren't genetically gifted, working each muscle group only one time per week is sufficient. You may experience success with training each bodypart twice a week, but that should be the maximum number of sessions if you're trying to add mass and strength. Most bodybuilders at some point will fall into the trap of thinking more is better. This is definitively not the case.

Perhaps one of the very best suggestions we can make is to leave each workout session while you still have some fuel left in your tank. If you train each session to total failure and complete exhaustion, you can't expect to gain. It's impossible. You simply can't run your body into a negative zone each and every session and expect to see results. As the eight-time Mr. Olympia Lee Haney once said: "Stimulate, not annihilate!" Larger muscles can be worked more often, longer and harder than smaller muscles. By larger muscles we're referring to your back, legs and chest. Smaller muscles consist of biceps, triceps and delts. The exception to this rule are your calves, abs and forearms, which can be worked with more frequency than has been listed in the Rotation for Recuperation Routines; they're high-density, or slow-twitch, muscles. Your forearms and calves are used constantly and they're accustomed to work. In order for them to respond, you need to provide more stimuli than you do for your other muscle groups. You can increase both frequency and intensity.

Most people give their abs more training than is necessary. If you simply follow a good total-body training program and watch your diet, you'll find that you can train your abs less often. Just following these rules will put you on the road to having a well-defined mid-section while training your abs only three or four times per week.

The late Mike Mentzer stated many times that recovery always precedes muscle growth. Your central nervous system requires 48 to 96 hours of rest to fully recover after exercising. Muscle recovery can occur more quickly. If you're even slightly sore, that bodypart is not ready to train again. Since there's no solid rule as to frequency that applies to all bodybuilders, you'll have to experiment. Everyone is different. You probably don't want to go more than 96 hours without attacking the same muscle group again, since that amount of time is a little outside the recovery zone (although Mike Mentzer had some of his clients training once every seven to eleven days). Train, but don't train too much or too often because it could result in less-than-desired muscle gains or even no gains at all.

Frequency of training can best be determined when you learn what is ideal for you through experimentation. Not everyone is the same. Recuperation is the most important gauge in determining your training frequency. If you don't recuperate, you can't build muscle. It's that simple.

Finding the right balance between exercise and recuperation time takes a great deal of trial and error. Once you determine what works best for you, however, the doors open for progress.

Photo by Rich Baker
Model Jay Cutler

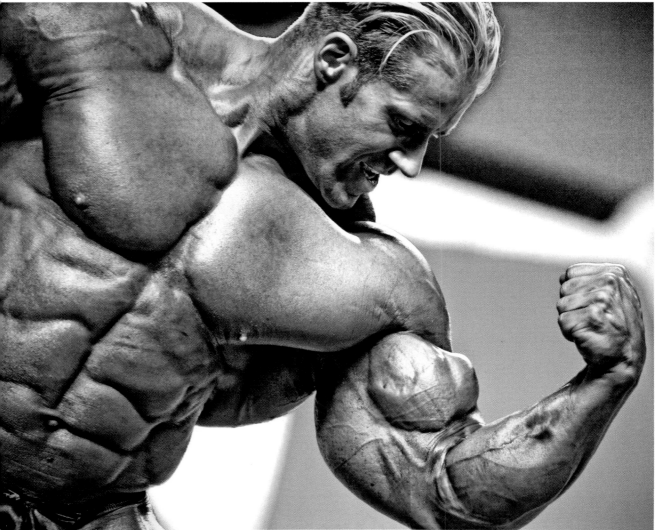

CHAPTER 28

SIZE ALIVE TRAINING PROGRAM

A 13-day split with nine days of intense, strictly sequenced training equals maximal stimulation, one muscle group at a time.

The Size Alive Training Program was designed by the late Steven J. Allgeyer, exercise physiologist and a recognized expert in bodybuilding and powerlifting. His program (which he preferred to call the Structured Instinctive Training program) consists of nine days of precisely sequenced workouts. This program does not allow for any alteration of the sequence or skipped days. During this training, you'll be maximally stimulating muscle growth in one group of muscles at a time. By focusing exclusively on one group of muscles, you'll greatly reduce your risk of overtraining and yet continue to stimulate your other muscles. You should be able to do this program in virtually any well-equipped gym. It will take about two cycles to adapt to this program.

13-DAY INTENSITY MANIPULATION WORKOUT CYCLE

Perform the 13-Day Intensity Manipulation Workout Cycle using a three-day-on and one-day-off sequence. Train on days one through three and rest on day four. Resume training on days five through seven, and rest on day eight. Start training again on days 9 through 11, and use days 12 and 13 to rest. Begin a new 13-day cycle and follow this procedure for seven cycles.

You will have to determine what weight you're able to lift for the designated number of sets and reps ahead of time. If you're able to comfortably perform your workout twice, you should add weight. Doing so will provide you the opportunity to continue making progress. Going through the motions won't help you improve. Always warm up by doing two light sets before starting each muscle group (but not before each exercise).

(100 PERCENT OF ONE-REP MAX - POUNDAGE THAT CAN BE USED FOR THE GIVEN NUMBER OF SETS AND REPS)

Day 1:	Chest / triceps / biceps
Day 2:	Back / shoulders
Day 3:	Quads / hams / calves
Day 4:	Off

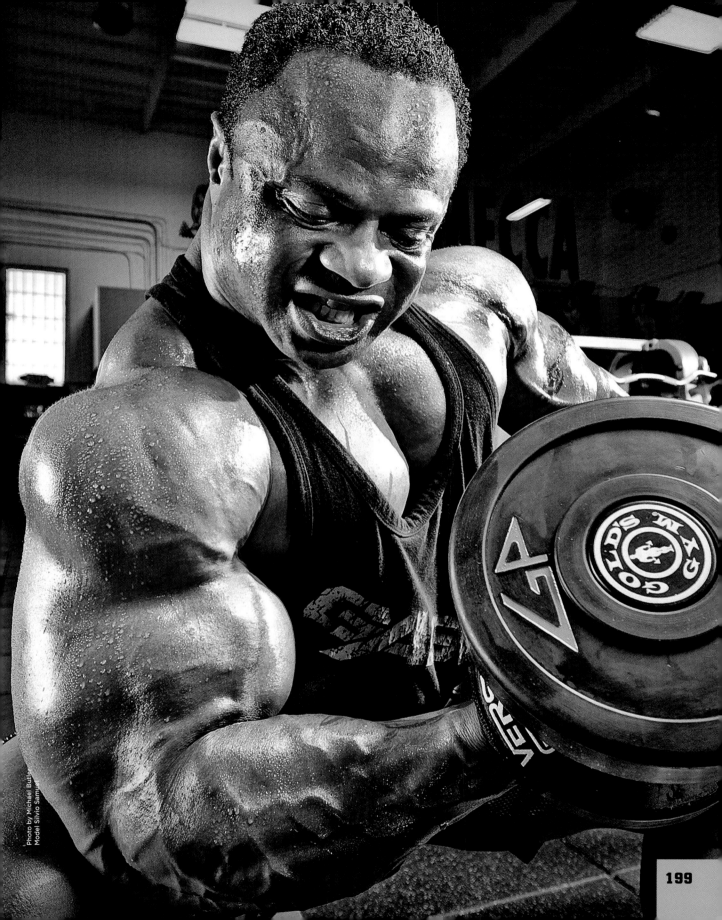

(75 PERCENT OF ONE-REP MAX - POUNDAGE THAT CAN BE USED FOR THE GIVEN NUMBER OF SETS AND REPS)

Day 5:   Chest / biceps / triceps
Day 6:   Shoulders / back
Day 7:   Quads / hams / calves
Day 8:   Off

(85 PERCENT OF ONE-REP MAX - POUNDAGE THAT CAN BE USED FOR THE GIVEN NUMBER OF SETS AND REPS)

Day 9:   Chest (triceps / biceps superset)
Day 10:   Back / shoulders
Day 11:   Quads / hams / calves
Day 12-13: Off

Note: The 100 percent maximal training days provide the necessary overloading of your muscle groups involved, while the 75 to 85 percent sub-maximal training days aid in recuperation, energy rejuvenation and the prevention of muscle atrophy.

The flat-bench dumbbell flye is move No. 2 in the chest workout.

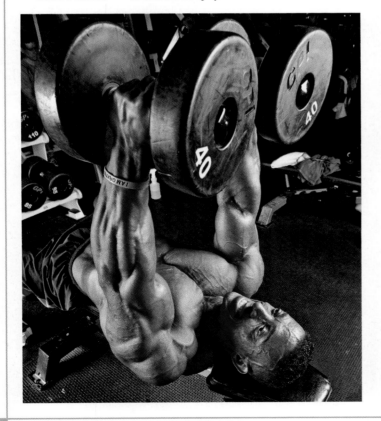

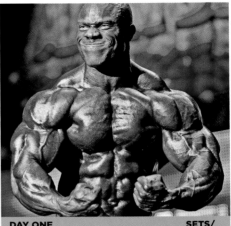

DAY ONE	SETS/REPS*
CHEST	
Flat-Bench Barbell Press	5 x 6
Flat-Bench Dumbbell Flye	6 x 12
Incline-Bench Barbell Press	4 x 8
Parallel Bar Dip or Pec Dec	3 x max 3 x 15
TRICEPS	
Dumbbell Kickback	3 x 12
Cable Pressdown	3 x 12
Two-Arm Dumbbell French Press	3 x 10
Close-Grip Bench Press	3 x 8
BICEPS	
Concentration Curl	3 x 15
Seated Alternate Dumbbell Curl	3 x 8
Close-Grip EZ-Bar Preacher Curl	3 x 12
Standing Barbell Cheat Curl	3 x 8
DAY TWO	**SETS/REPS***
BACK	
Straight-Arm Narrow-Grip High-Pulley Cable Pulldown (serratus)	4 x 12
Wide-Grip Behind-The-Neck Pulldown	4 x 12
Dumbbell Cross-Bench Pullover (lats)	3 x 12
Underhand Narrow-Grip Pulldown (front)	3 x 12
Low-Pulley Cable Rows (narrow or medium grip)	3 x 8
SHOULDERS	
Bent-Over Dumbbell Rear Lateral Raise	4 x 10
Standing Dumbbell Lateral Raise	4 x 8
Seated Dumbbell Press or Behind-The-Neck Barbell Press	4 x 10
Lee Haney Barbell Shrug (behind back)	4 x 12

Photos (left to right) by Ralph DeHaan / Gordon Smith
Models Troy Alves / Phil Heath

DAY THREE	SETS/REPS*
LEGS	
Medium-Stance Barbell Squat	3 x 10
Dumbbell or Barbell Lunge	3 x 10
Leg Extension	4 x 10
Barbell Front Squat or Smith-Machine Sissy Squat	3 x 12
Leg Curl	4 x 8
Seated Calf Raise	3 x 15

DAY FIVE	SETS/REPS*
CHEST	
Incline Barbell Bench Press	4 x 12
Decline Dumbbell Flye	4 x 8
Incline Dumbbell Press	4 x 8
Pec Deck or Flat Dumbbell Flye	3 x 10
Flat Bench Press	2 x 12
BICEPS	
Cheat Barbell Curl	6 x 6
Seated Alternate Dumbbell Curl	3 x 15
Close-Grip Preacher Curl (21s – 7 full range, 7 bottom half of motion and 7 top half of motion)	3 x 21
TRICEPS	
Skullcrusher (finish each set with 4 Close-Grip Presses)	3 x 8 (plus)
Two-Arm Seated Dumbbell French Press	3 x 15
Cable Pressdown	3 x 8
Close-Grip Barbell Bench Press	3 x 15

DAY SIX	SETS/REPS*
SHOULDERS	
Behind-The-Neck Barbell Press or Dumbbell Press	4 x 20
Dumbbell Bent-Over Lateral Raise (heavy)	4 x 5
Standing One-Arm Dumbbell Lateral Raise (light)	3 x 12
Barbell Upright Row	3 x 10
Dumbbell or Barbell Shrug (full range, good trap squeeze)	3 x 15
BACK	
Deadlift	3 x 8
Bent-Over Row	4 x 5
Narrow-Grip Low-Pulley Cable Row	4 x 12
T-Bar Row	3 x 8
Pulldown (front of neck, medium or wide grip in perfect form)	3 x 15

DAY SEVEN	SETS/REPS*
QUADS & HAMS	
Medium-Stance Deep Power Squat (do 3 or 4 warm-up sets)	3 x 5
Leg Extension	3 x 6–8
Single Leg Curl or Barbell Lunge	3 x 10
Lying Leg Curl	3 x 10
Stiff-Leg Barbell Deadlift	3 x 10
CALVES	
Standing Calf Raise	3 x 12
Seated Calf Raise	3 x 8

On day five, you should be using 75 percent of your 1RM during the chest session.

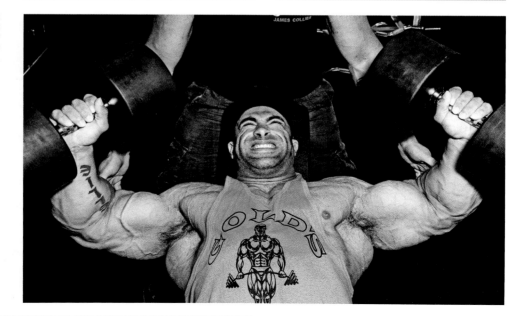

JAMES COLLIER

Photo by Rich Baker
Model Darren Ball

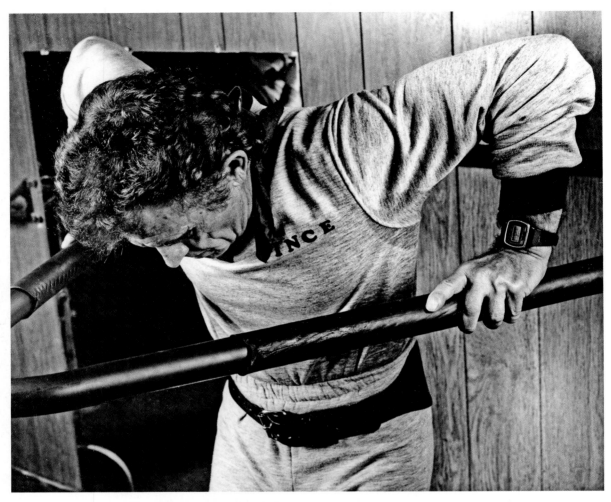

Vince Gironda performing his signature V-bar dip.

DAY NINE	SETS/REPS*
CHEST (SUPERSETS)	
Flat-Bench Barbell Press	5 x 3
Incline-Bench Barbell Press	3 x 6
Flat-Bench Dumbbell Press	3 x 6
Flat Dumbbell Flye	3 x 12
Vince Gironda V-Bar Dip	3 x max reps
BICEPS & TRICEPS (SUPERSETS)	
Close-Grip Barbell Bench Press with Barbell Curl	3 x 15 each
EZ-Bar Skullcrusher with Preacher Bench Barbell Curl	3 x 10
Dumbbell Triceps Kickback with Dumbbell Concentration Curl	3 x 21
Triceps Pressdown using Underhand Grip with EZ-Bar or Low Pulley Cable Reverse Curl	3 x 12

DAY TEN	SETS/REPS*
SHOULDERS	
Seated Dumbbell Shoulder Press or Barbell Front Press on High Incline	3 x 6

Perform 5 trisets of 10 reps / exercise. Do triset: A,B,C,A,B ...

A) Bent-Over Dumbbell Lateral Raise
   Dumbbell Lateral Raise
   Alternate Dumbbell Front Raise

B) Dumbbell Lateral Raise
   Alternate Dumbbell Front Raise
   Bent-Over Dumbbell Lateral Raise

C) Alternate Dumbbell Front Raise
   Bent-Over Dumbbell Lateral Raise
   Dumbbell Lateral Raise

	SETS/REPS*
Barbell Upright Row (superset with) Lee Haney Behind Back Barbell Shrug	3 x 12

Model Vince Gironda

Day 11 leg extensions should be four sets of ten reps.

BACK	
Wide-Grip Pulldowns (behind neck)	3 x 8
Wide-Grip Pulldowns (in front)	3 x 12
Standing Narrow-Grip Low-Pulley Cable Row	4 x 10
Seated Medium- or Wide-Grip Low-Pulley Cable Row	3 x 8
Serratus High-Pulley Cable Straight-Arm Pulldown	3 x 10
DAY ELEVEN	**SETS/REPS***
THIGHS	
45-Degree Leg Press or Hack Squat (with toes at bottom of the platform)	4 x 10
Barbell Front Squat (heel on board)	3 x 6
Triset next three movements – no rest between exercises – two minutes between trisets	
Leg Extension	4 x 10
Leg Curl	4 x 10
Stiff-Leg Barbell Deadlift	4 x 8
Smith-Machine or Sissy Squat	2 x 15
Regular Full-Depth Barbell Squat	2 x 10
CALVES	
Standing Calf Raise	4 x 8

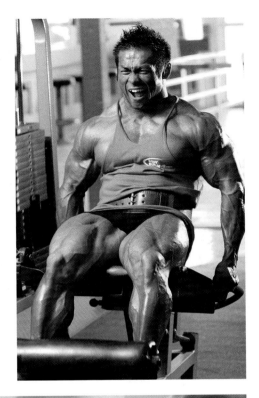

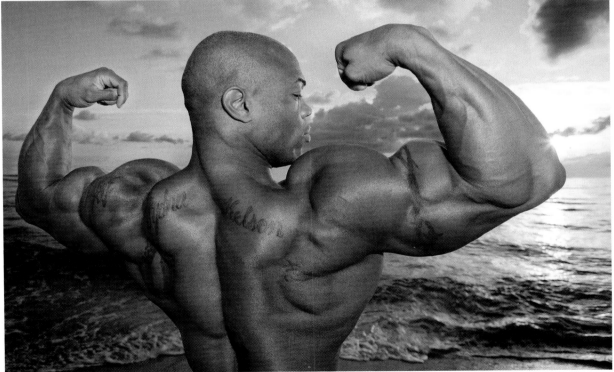

Photos (top to bottom) by Jason Mathas / Rich Baker
Models Hidetada Yamagishi / Dennis Hopson

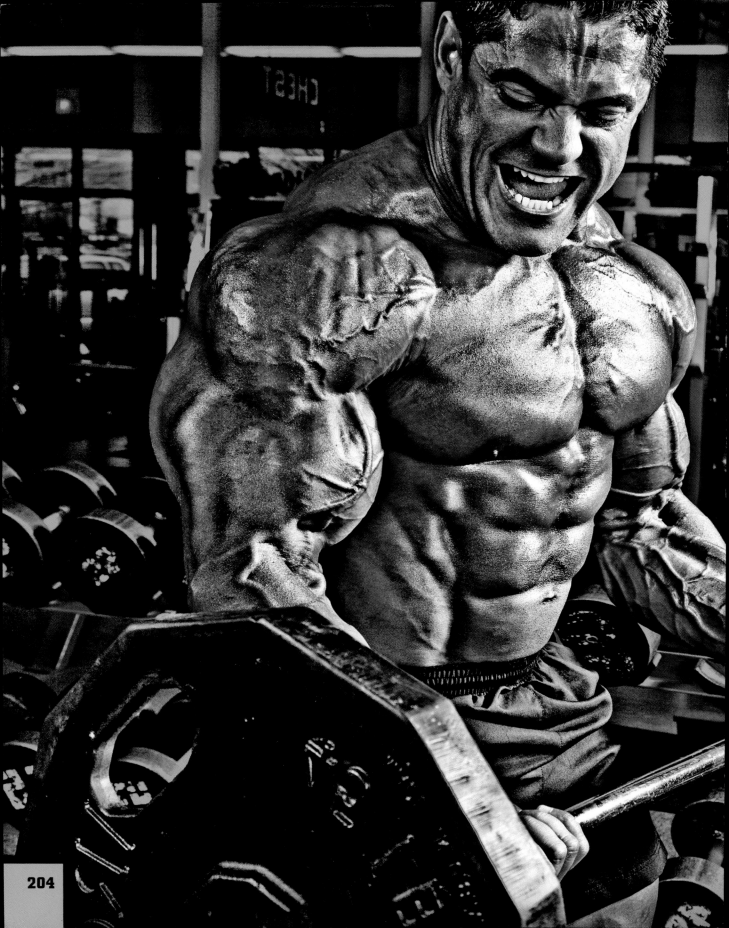

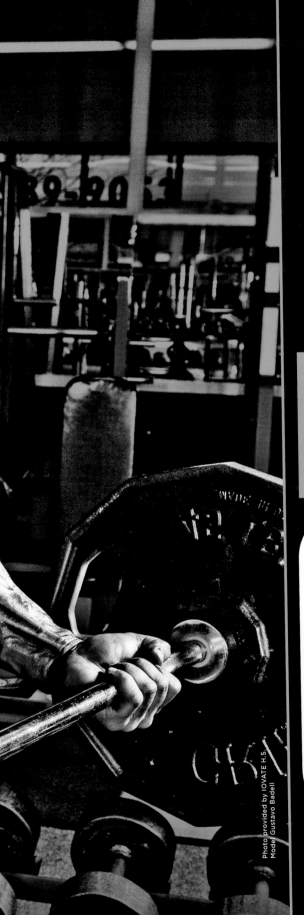

BOOK
09

Phase Training

CHAPTER 29

PHASE TRAINING OVERVIEW

Periodic changes to training volume, intensity and methods will stimulate more gains in size and strength.

Many of the world's strongest and best-developed men and women use phase training to achieve their goals of acquiring superhuman strength or molding a superior physique. Phase training is commonly known in the bodybuilding community as periodization (or cycle training) where each scheduled training block builds on a prior phase. It's aimed at stimulating the ultimate in size and strength through the periodic alteration of training volume, intensity and methods. Successful phase training requires certain exercises, specific sets and reps and corresponding poundage percentages to be performed for a minimum of three weeks.

Steve Colescott, former editor of *Peak Training Journal*, explains that in periodization training "Microcycles are grouped together in one- to eight-week segments or phases. Each phase focuses on one primary goal, such as increased muscle size, definition or strength. These phases are sometimes called mesocycles." Steve relates that in periodization training, "intensity refers to the poundage used, as a percentage of your one-

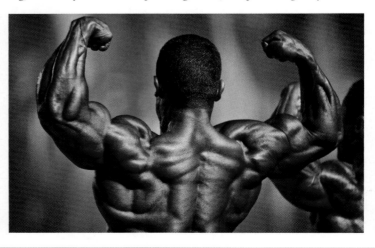

Photo by Rich Baker

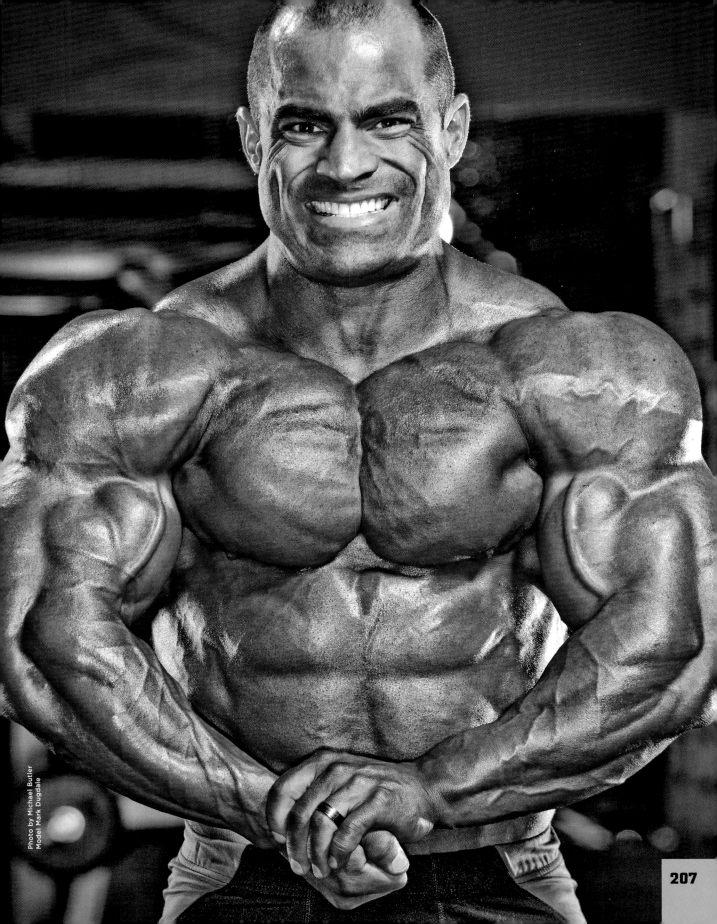

Your body may occasionally respond to particular exercises, such as the bench press, with decreases in performance level. If it persists for more than three workouts in a row, you're experiencing a plateau.

rep maximum (1-RM) in a particular exercise. If you can squat 345 for an all-out single, then 345 is your 1-RM and a squat set with 345 would have an intensity of 100 percent." If you're looking to set up a periodization program, Steve adds that the following factors should also be considered: "Exercise selection, order of the exercises, rest between sets, workout frequency, rep tempo and special training techniques (such as forced reps, accentuated negatives, cheat reps, etc.). Nutrition and supplement intake will also be adjusted to reflect the different goals and requirements of these phases."

If you were to review your training on a month-to-month basis (as you should), you would likely find occasional plateaus or de-

creases in performance level as your body reacts to particular exercises. Your central nervous system, mind and muscles work together as a unit to produce the necessary, natural chemical changes in your body. These changes create your strength, endurance and physical development. Your central nervous system and muscles adapt to whatever stress you place on them. When this happens, there's usually a temporary termination of gains. For example, you might encounter a plateau while attempting to bench press a particular poundage. If you experience this only once, it's probably not a plateau. A plateau occurs when in three or more workouts you don't experience any gains in either poundage or reps.

Photo by Jeremy Maurer
Model Jon Andersen

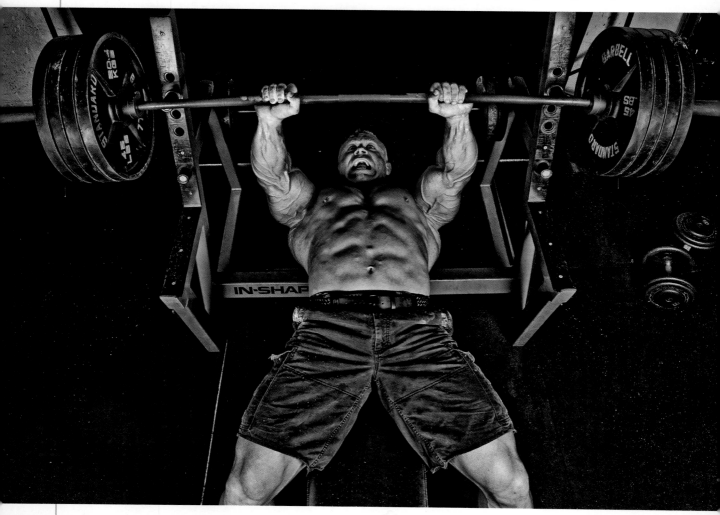

If you don't allow yourself enough recovery time between workouts, you can set yourself up to hit a training plateau.

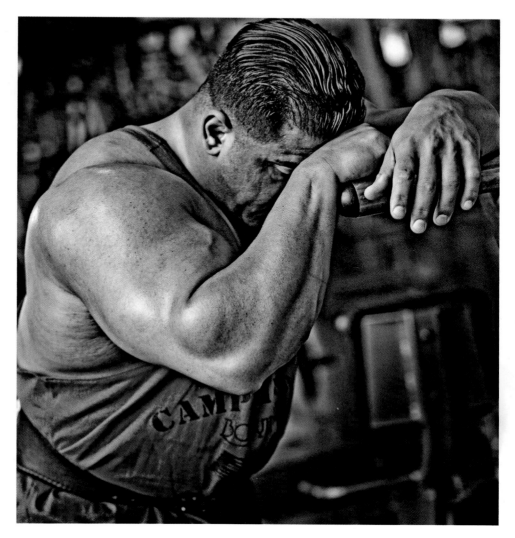

Photo by Paul Buceta
Model King Kamali

Training plateaus can also occur when your body isn't able to regain its prior energy levels by the time you start your next workout session. For larger bodyparts, you must allow for more recovery time between workouts than you would for smaller parts. Larger body-parts such as your thighs and lower back need about five days of rest between workouts that include conventional squats and deadlifts. You must give your chest three or four days of rest when performing bench press movements.

When squatting and deadlifting, you are using many of the same muscles. Do these exercises one after another on the same workout day to have the speediest recovery possible.

Schedule your bench press workout at least one day before or after your squat/deadlift workout. You might think it's okay to do these on the same day because the bench press works different muscles, but your energy levels will be severely depleted. Deltoid and shoulder strength also tend to be somewhat depleted following a deadlift workout, and you'll need this strength for synergistic and stabilizer functions in the bench press. If possible, separate these sessions by roughly 36 hours to give yourself ample recovery time. By now your should be well aware of the fact that rest and recovery are essential elements of the muscle-building process. Whatever you do, don't skip out on rest.

CHAPTER 30

BRITISH POWERLIFTING SYSTEM

Organize your training and conveniently plan your workouts to allow for adequate recovery time.

The rest periods for deadlifting and squatting are different than for bench presses. Unfortunately, this can create a conflict for you. The British Powerlifting System can clear up that confusion and make it convenient for you to plan your training around these exercises. If adequate recovery time between workouts is important to you, then this method of training is likely your best choice.

BARBELL BACK SQUATS FIRST

Your thigh area has more muscle mass than any other in your body and requires the greatest output of energy. Therefore, squats should be your first exercise. Squats typically force very heavy deep breathing, which results in overall body stimulation.

The best rep scheme for powerlifting workouts is three to five reps per set. Aim for three and work up to your maximum poundage often. Here is a sample routine:

Warm up:	Do one set of eight to ten reps with a light weight.
Working up:	Perform three sets of three to five reps using a weight near your maximum poundage.
Maximum:	Complete one set of three reps with as much weight as possible, then do one set of one rep (yes, only one rep) with an even heavier weight – more than you thought you could handle. Try to perform a full rep.
Working down:	Do three sets of three to five reps with the heaviest weight you can handle.
Final set:	Perform one set of eight to ten reps using a moderate weight (but not too light) for a final pump.

After this squat routine, do the barbell deadlift using the very same sequence. Remember that you're working with poundage far greater than the norm. Finally, complete your trilogy of powerlifting exercises with the barbell bench press. Again, train as you did with the other two exercises.

You might have noticed that deadlifts and squats are done together twice in a row, but then on every third workout of this nature the dead-

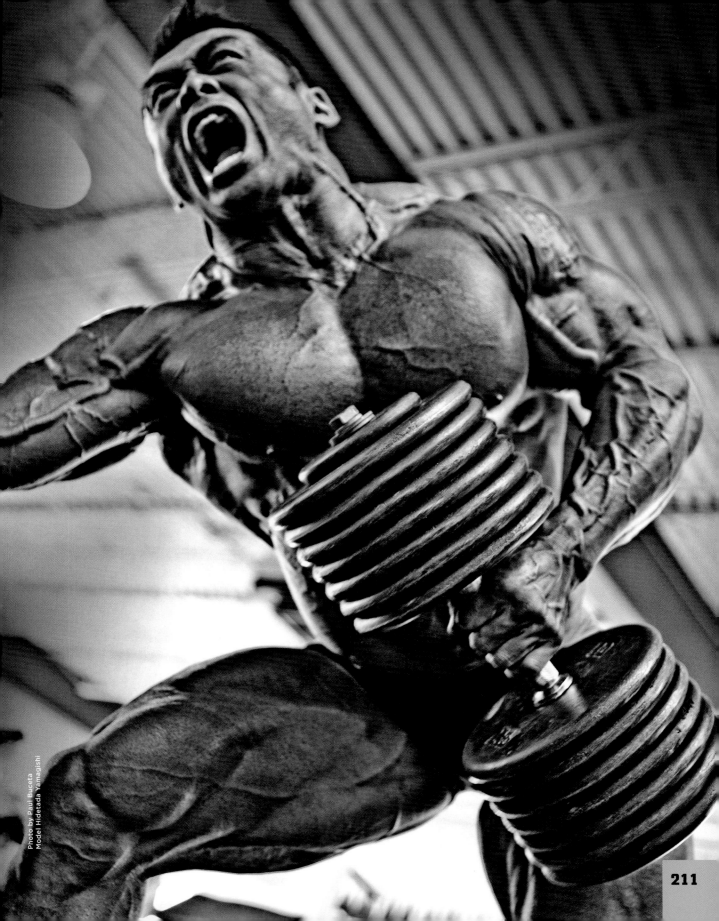

You can adjust this program to suit your needs, depending on which bodyparts you feel need the most work.

lifts are eliminated, for an eight- to nine-day period. Many strength experts feel that your lower back doesn't recover quite as quickly as your legs, and skipping the deadlift every third workout aids your recovery. Adjust the program to meet your needs. You should be using training poundages in excess of 84 to 88 percent of your one-rep maximum. For specific exercises, see the chart below.

3 POWERLIFTS – 12-WEEK CYCLE

WEEK	MONDAY	TUESDAY	WEDNESDAY	THURSDAY	FRIDAY	SATURDAY	SUNDAY
1	Squat & Deadlift	Bench Press			Bench Press	Squat & Deadlift	
2		Bench Press		Squat	Bench Press		
3	Bench Press	Squat & Deadlift				Bench Press	Squat & Deadlift
4			Bench Press		Squat	Bench Press	
5		Bench Press	Squat & Deadlift			Bench Press	
6	Squat & Deadlift	Bench Press			Bench Press	Squat	
7		Bench Press		Squat & Deadlift		Bench Press	
8		Squat & Deadlift	Bench Press			Bench Press	Squat
9	Bench Press				Squat & Deadlift	Bench Press	
10		Bench Press	Squat & Deadlift		Bench Press		
11	Squat	Bench Press			Bench Press	Squat & Deadlift	
12	Bench Press			Squat & Deadlift	Bench Press		

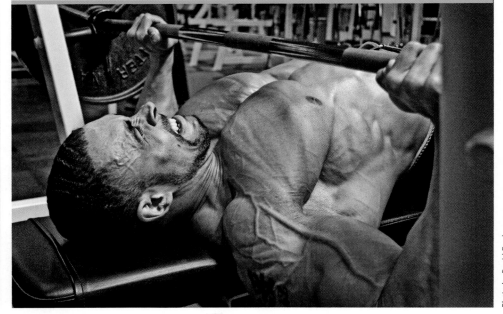

Photo by David Ford
Model Tim Liggins

Once you've completed the high-intensity/ low-volume phase, you can up your working weights to roughly 80 percent of your one-rep max.

GOALS OF PHASE TRAINING

If your bodybuilding gains are leveling off, you must use various methods of training overloads to create a balance between the capacity of your central nervous system and your muscles to respond to the stress of the training method used. You'll have to go partly by instinct – basically, you exercise depending on how you feel, which means you must become an expert in understanding what your body is telling you.

Your brain receives signals from the nerve endings and other receptors in your body. It can indicate to you the response of the various amounts of muscle contraction and stretching and the pressure in the muscle from the sets and reps you're doing. It can also be instrumental in preventing overtraining. When you understand how your body reacts to training stimuli, you'll know exactly when you've done enough reps, sets and exercises in a workout. After six months to a year of consistent training, you'll begin to understand how your body reacts to progressive weight training.

If you want to produce continued gains without worrying about hitting training plateaus or overtraining, then phase training is your answer. Top physique and strength champions have learned that their bodies cannot tolerate peak performance training for too long. As a means to combat this problem, these champions began employing light, medium and heavy training loads in a variety of ways throughout the year.

In general, periods of high-volume / low-intensity and medium-volume / medium-intensity training are effective for a maximum of eight to twelve weeks. Low-volume / high-intensity overloads are generally effective for only five to eight weeks. Before you determine which method of phase training to begin with, you must first establish your goal. If you are coming off a layoff, whether you were just resting your body or recovering from an illness or injury, you should consider the advantages of beginning your training with high-volume/low-intensity workouts. Whatever you do, stay away from attempting to perform high-intensity workouts.

PHASE – A (ENDURANCE)
WEEKS 1 – 4 HIGH-VOLUME / LOW-INTENSITY WORKOUTS

The first four weeks feature endurance training. Begin training with lighter poundages and more sets and reps. Attitude is more important than the number on the plates. The weight must feel light until your enthusiasm for training builds up again. Your workload should be roughly 60 to 78 percent of your one-rep maximum for three sets of 15 to 30 reps.

MAXIMUM REPETITION SET
200 lbs x 20 reps

WEEK 1:

MONDAY (HEAVY DAY)

115 x 20
155 x 20
180 x 20

THURSDAY (LIGHT DAY)

100 x 20
130 x 20
155 x 20

WEEK 2:

MONDAY (HEAVY DAY)

125 x 20
160 x 20
190 x 20

THURSDAY (LIGHT DAY)

105 x 20
135 x 20
160 x 20

WEEK 3:

MONDAY (HEAVY DAY)

130 x 20
170 x 20
200 x 20

THURSDAY (LIGHT DAY)

110 x 20
145 x 20
170 x 20

WEEK 4:

MONDAY (HEAVY DAY)

135 x 20
180 x 20
210 x 20

THURSDAY (LIGHT DAY)

115 x 20
155 x 20
180 x 20

For the final stage of this training method, lower your reps and increase your weight to build max muscle.

To prevent muscle injury and severe soreness, especially after a layoff, never begin training with the intensity of previous workouts. Always start with high volume/low intensity. You can begin medium-volume/medium-intensity workouts after this phase of training is completed to your satisfaction.

PHASE – B (STRENGTH / ENDURANCE)

WEEKS 5 – 8 MEDIUM-VOLUME / MEDIUM-INTENSITY WORKOUTS

Phase B will bring you back to your previously established level of strength and endurance. Your workload should be 80 percent of your one-rep max for three or four sets of eight to twelve reps. Take a look at the chart below for more details.

MAXIMUM REPETITION SET
235 lbs x 12 reps

WEEK 5:

MONDAY (HEAVY DAY)

135 x 12
175 x 12
205 x 12

THURSDAY (LIGHT DAY)

135 x 12
175 x 12

WEEK 6:

MONDAY (HEAVY DAY)

135 x 12
175 x 12
220 x 12

THURSDAY (LIGHT DAY)

135 x 12
175 x 12
190 x 12

WEEK 7:

MONDAY (HEAVY DAY)

135 x 12
185 x 8
205 x 6
235 x 12

THURSDAY (LIGHT DAY)

135 x 12
185 x 12
200 x 12

WEEK 8:

MONDAY (HEAVY DAY)

135 x 12
185 x 8
205 x 6
225 x 4
245 x 14

THURSDAY (LIGHT DAY)

135 x 12
190 x 12
210 x 12

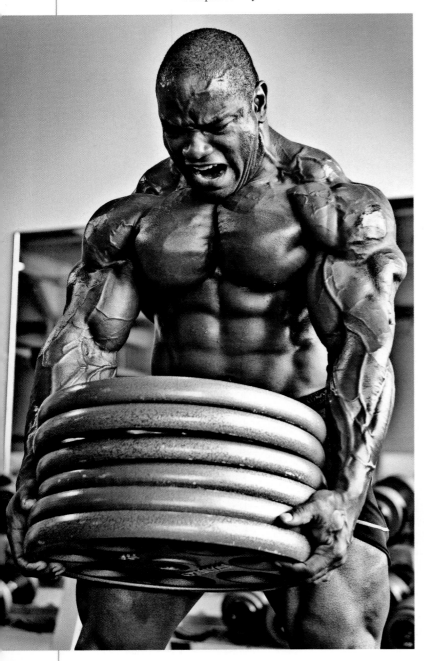

Photo by Rich Baker
Model Johnnie Jackson

Each cycle is four weeks in length, consisting of both a high-intensity growth phase and a low-intensity stabilizing phase.

CYCLE #	NAME	EMPHASIS
1	Body Focus	Standard three-day split emphasizing a strong muscle pump and burn-out in the final sets of each exercise.
2	Megamass	Each muscle group is stimulated with two different movements for a medium volume of sets. Compound exercises are used to focus on developing new muscle mass.
3	Body Blast	A high frequency phase based on traditional full-body training, which hits the major muscle groups in every workout.
4	Preflex	Isolates the target muscle with the first exercise and then stimulates the whole muscle group with a compound movement in the second move.
5	GH Plus	With a focus on heavy lifting and strengthening connective tissues, powerlifting compound movements are used in low volume sets to stimulate a strong growth hormone response.
6	Superflex	Mid-volume superset training combines synergistic muscle groups to flush the target area with maximum blood flow.
7	Powerplay	The compound and isolation exercise mix emphasizes the push-pull system of bodybuilding training. The focus is on power movements.
8	Anabolic Burst	During the bulking phase, do low reps of heavy weights including dynamic stretching. Then do lighter isolation exercises, higher reps and aerobic training during the cutting phase.

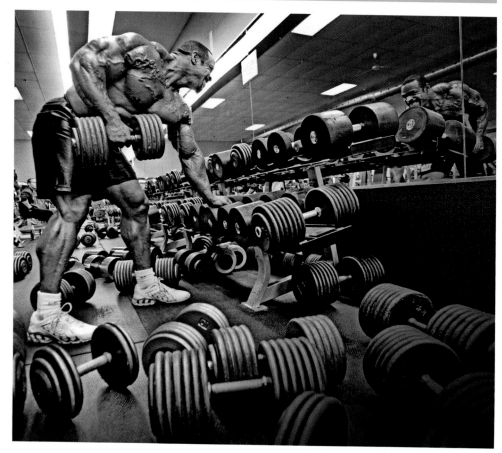

Photo by Paul Buceta
Model Paul Dillet

The leg press is used as part of the growth phase during the Body Focus cycle.

BODY FOCUS CYCLE – GROWTH PHASE WEEK ONE

DAY	MUSCLE GROUP	EXERCISE	SETS/REPS
Monday	Chest	Incline Barbell Press	1 x 10, 1 x 8
	Shoulders	Overhead Barbell Press	1 x 10, 1 x 8
	Triceps	Lying EZ-Bar Triceps Extension	1 x 10, 1 x 8
	Abs	Hanging Leg Raise	1 x 25-50
Wednesday	Back	Lat Pulldown	1 x 10, 1 x 8
	Biceps	Barbell Curl	1 x 10, 1 x 8
	Calves	Standing Calf Raise	1 x 10, 1 x 8
Friday	Thighs	Leg Press	1 x 10, 1 x 8
	Forearms	Barbell (Palms Up) Wrist Curl	1 x 10, 1 x 8
	Abs	Crunch	1 x 25-50

With the exception of the abs exercises, you should do a burn-out set of 12 to 15 reps following each of the other exercises listed.

BODY FOCUS CYCLE – GROWTH PHASE WEEK TWO

DAY	MUSCLE GROUP	EXERCISE	SETS/REPS
Monday	Chest	Incline Barbell Press	1 x 10, 8, 6, 4
	Shoulders	Overhead Barbell Press	1 x 10, 8, 6, 4
	Triceps	EZ-Bar Triceps Extension	1 x 10, 8, 6, 4
	Abs	Hanging Leg Raise	2 x 25-50
Wednesday	Back	Lat Pulldown	1 x 10, 8, 6, 4
	Biceps	Barbell Curl	1 x 10, 8, 6, 4
	Calves	Standing Calf Raise	1 x 10, 8, 6, 4
Friday	Thighs	Leg Press	1 x 10, 8, 6, 4
	Forearms	Barbell (Palms Up) Wrist Curl	1 x 10, 8, 6, 4
	Abs	Crunch	2 x 25-50

With the exception of the abs exercises, you should do a burn-out set of 12 to 15 reps following each of the other exercises listed.

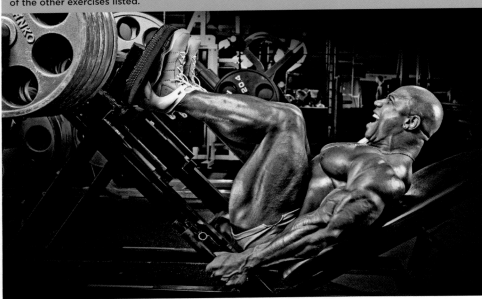

Photo by Robert Reiff
Model Darrell Terrell

You'll do hack machine squats as the stabilizer move for thighs during weeks three and four.

Photo by Robert Reiff
Model Mike Ergas

BODY FOCUS CYCLE – STABILIZE PHASE WEEKS THREE & FOUR

DAY	MUSCLE GROUP	EXERCISE	SETS/REPS
Monday	Chest	Parallel Bar Dip	1 x 10, 1 x 8
	Shoulders	Dumbbell Lateral Raise	1 x 10, 1 x 8
	Triceps	Barbell Close-Grip Bench Press	1 x 10, 1 x 8
	Abs	Incline Sit-up	1 x 25-50
Wednesday	Back	Seated Low Pulley Row	1 x 10, 1 x 8
	Biceps	Dumbbell Curl	1 x 10, 1 x 8
	Calves	Seated Calf Raise	1 x 10, 1 x 8
Friday	Thighs	Hack Squat	1 x 10, 1 x 8
	Forearms	Dumbbell (Palms Up) Wrist Curl	1 x 10, 1 x 8
	Abs	Lying Leg Raise	1 x 25-50

With the exception of the abs exercises, you should do a burn-out set of 12 to 15 reps following each of the other exercises listed.

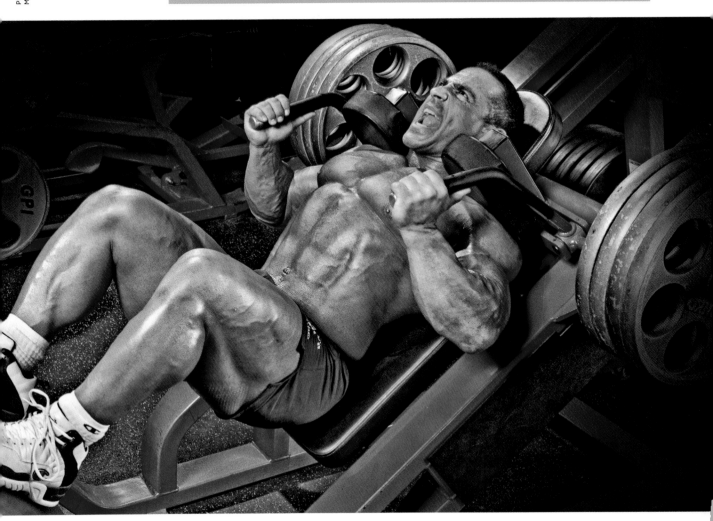

The crunch is paired with the incline sit-up for abs for the first phase of the Mega-mass cycle.

MEGAMASS CYCLE – GROWTH PHASE WEEK ONE

DAY	MUSCLE GROUP	EXERCISE	SETS/REPS
Monday	Back	Seated Row	2 x 10-12
		Lat Pulldown	2 x 10-12
	Chest	Barbell Bench Press	2 x 10-12
		Incline Dumbbell Flye	2 x 10-12
	Abs	Incline Sit-up	2 x 25-50
Wednesday	Thighs	Barbell Back Squat	2 x 10-12
		Leg Extension	2 x 10-12
	Shoulders	Seated Barbell Press Overhead	2 x 10-12
		Dumbbell Lateral Raise	2 x 10-12
	Abs	Hanging Leg Raise	2 x 10-12
Friday	Biceps	Barbell Curl	2 x 10-12
		Incline Dumbbell Curl	2 x 10-12
	Triceps	Close-Grip Barbell Bench Press	2 x 10-12
		Lat Pushdown	2 x 10-12
	Calves	Standing Calf Raise	2 x 12-15
		Seated Calf Raise	2 x 12-15
	Abs	Crunch	2 x 25-50

MEGAMASS CYCLE – GROWTH PHASE WEEK TWO

DAY	MUSCLE GROUP	EXERCISE	SETS/REPS
Monday	Back	Seated Row	3 x 6-8
		One-Arm Dumbbell Row	3 x 6-8
	Chest	Barbell Bench Press	3 x 6-8
		High Pulley Cable Crossover	3 x 6-8
	Abs	Incline Sit-up	2 x 25-50
Wednesday	Thighs	Barbell Back Squat	3 x 6-8
		Barbell Lunge	3 x 6-8
	Shoulders	Overhead Seated Barbell Press	3 x 6-8
		Barbell Shrug	3 x 6-8
	Abs	Hanging Leg Raise	2 x 25-50
Friday	Biceps	Barbell Curl	3 x 6-8
		Chin-up (Palms Facing)	3 x 6-8
	Triceps	Close-Grip Barbell Bench Press	3 x 6-8
		Lying EZ-Bar Triceps Extension	3 x 6-8
	Calves	Standing Calf Raise	3 x 8-10
		Donkey Calf Raise	3 x 8-10
	Abs	Crunch	2 x 25-50

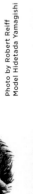

Photo by Robert Reiff
Model Hidetada Yamagishi

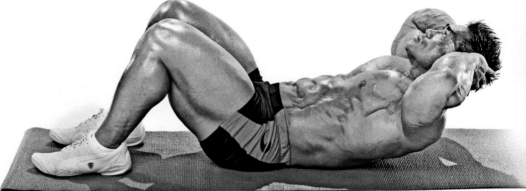

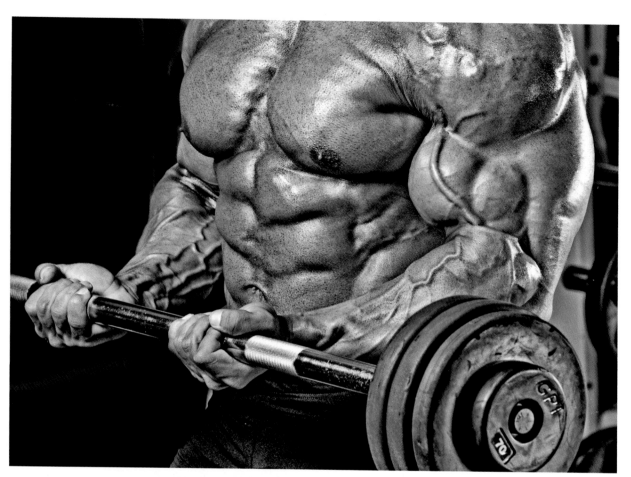

The barbell curl and incline dumbbell curl are the two biceps moves you'll do during weeks three and four on this cycle.

MEGAMASS CYCLE — STABILIZE PHASE WEEKS THREE & FOUR

DAY	MUSCLE GROUP	EXERCISE	SETS/REPS
Monday	Back	Seated Row	2 x 10-12
		Lat Pulldown	2 x 12-15
	Chest	Barbell Bench Press	2 x 10-12
		Incline Dumbbell Flye	2 x 12-15
	Abs	Incline Sit-up	2 x 25-50
Wednesday	Thighs	Barbell Back Squat	2 x 10-12
		Leg Extension	2 x 12-15
	Shoulders	Seated Barbell Press Overhead	2 x 10-12
		Dumbbell Lateral Raise	2 x 12-15
	Abs	Hanging Leg Raise	2 x 25-50
Friday	Biceps	Barbell Curl	2 x 10-12
		Incline Dumbbell Curl	2 x 12-15
	Triceps	Close-Grip Barbell Bench Press	2 x 10-12
		High Pulley Pushdown	2 x 12-15
	Calves	Standing Calf Raise	2 x 12-15
		Seated Calf Raise	2 x 15-20
	Abs	Crunch	2 x 25-50

BODYBLAST CYCLE – GROWTH PHASE WEEK ONE

DAY	MUSCLE GROUP	EXERCISE	SETS/REPS
Monday	Thighs	Barbell Back Squat	1 x 12-15
	Back	Deadlift	1 x 12-15
	Chest	Incline Barbell Press	1 x 12-15
	Shoulders	Overhead Barbell Press	1 x 12-15
	Biceps	Barbell Curl	1 x 12-15
	Triceps	Close-Grip Barbell Bench Press	1 x 12-15
	Calves	Standing Calf Raise	1 x 12-15
	Abs	Hanging Leg Raise	1 x 25-50
Wednesday	Thighs	Leg Press	2 x 10-12
	Back	One-Arm Dumbbell Row	2 x 10-12
	Chest	Dumbbell Bench Press	2 x 10-12
	Shoulders	Dumbbell Lateral Raise	2 x 10-12
Friday	Thighs	Barbell Back Squat	1 x 12-15
	Back	Deadlift	1 x 12-15
	Chest	Incline Barbell Press	1 x 12-15
	Shoulders	Overhead Barbell Press	1 x 12-15
	Biceps	Barbell Curl	1 x 12-15
	Triceps	Close-Grip Barbell Bench Press	1 x 12-15
	Calves	Standing Calf Raise	1 x 12-15
	Abs	Crunch	1 x 12-15

The basis of the Body Blast cycle is traditional full-body training – hitting all the major muscle groups in every workout.

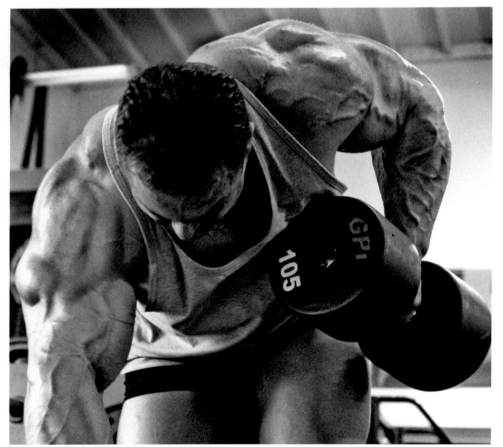

Photo by Irvin Gelb
Model Alexander Fedorov

BODYBLAST CYCLE – GROWTH PHASE WEEK TWO

DAY	MUSCLE GROUP	EXERCISE	SETS/REPS
Monday	Thighs	Barbell Back Squat	2 x 8-10
	Back	Deadlift	2 x 8-10
	Chest	Incline Barbell Press	2 x 8-10
	Shoulders	Overhead Barbell Press	2 x 8-10
	Biceps	Barbell Curl	2 x 8-10
	Triceps	Close-Grip Barbell Bench Press	2 x 8-10
	Calves	Standing Calf Raise	2 x 8-10
	Abs	Hanging Leg Raise	1 x 25-50
Wednesday	Thighs	Leg Press	4 x 6-8
	Back	One-Arm Dumbbell Row	4 x 6-8
	Chest	Dumbbell Bench Press	4 x 6-8
	Shoulders	Dumbbell Lateral Raise	4 x 6-8
Friday	Thighs	Barbell Back Squat	2 x 8-10
	Back	Deadlift	2 x 8-10
	Chest	Incline Barbell Press	2 x 8-10
	Shoulders	Overhead Barbell Press	2 x 8-10
	Biceps	Barbell Curl	2 x 8-10
	Triceps	Close-Grip Barbell Bench Press	2 x 8-10
	Calves	Standing Calf Raise	2 x 10-12
	Abs	Crunch	1 x 25-50

BODYBLAST CYCLE – STABILIZE PHASE WEEKS THREE & FOUR

DAY	MUSCLE GROUP	EXERCISE	SETS/REPS
Monday	Thighs	Hack Squat	2 x 12-15
	Back	Pull-up (Palms Forward)	2 x 12-15
	Chest	Parallel Bar Dip	2 x 12-15
	Shoulders	Overhead Dumbbell Press	2 x 12-15
	Biceps	Incline Dumbbell Curl	1 x 12-15
	Triceps	Standing or Seated EZ-Bar French Press	1 x 12-15
	Calves	Seated Calf Raise	1 x 12-15
	Abs	Lying Leg Raise	1 x 25-50
Thursday	Thighs	Hack Squat	2 x 10-12
	Back	Pull-up (Palms Forward)	2 x 10-12
	Chest	Parallel Bar Dip	2 x 10-12
	Shoulders	Overhead Dumbbell Press	2 x 10-12
	Biceps	Incline Dumbbell Curl	1 x 10-12
	Triceps	Standing or Seated EZ-Bar French Press	1 x 10-12
	Calves	Seated Calf Raise	1 x 12-15
	Abs	Lying Leg Raise	1 x 25-50

Photo by Robert Reiff
Model Troy Tate

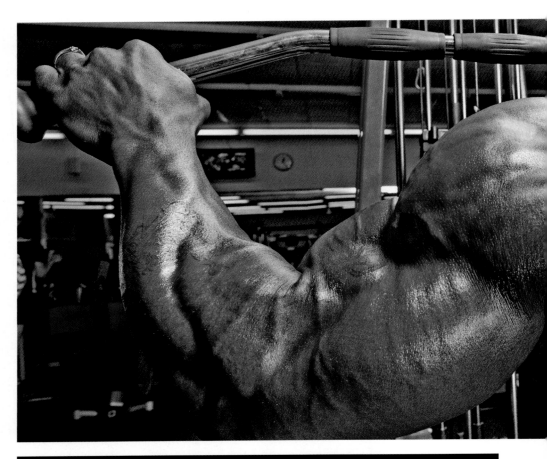

PREFLEX CYCLE – GROWTH PHASE
WEEKS ONE & TWO

DAY	MUSCLE GROUP	EXERCISE	WEEK 1 SETS/REPS	WEEK 2 SETS/REPS
Monday	Thighs	Leg Extension	1 x 10-12	3 x 8-10
		Leg Press	1 x 10-12	3 x 8-10
	Back	One Dumbbell Pullover	1 x 10-12	3 x 8-10
		Bent-over Row	1 x 10-12	3 x 8-10
	Abs	Hanging Leg Raise	2 x 25-50	2 x 25-50
Wednesday	Chest	Incline Dumbbell Flye	1 x 10-12	3 x 8-10
		Barbell Bench Press	1 x 10-12	3 x 8-10
	Shoulders	Dumbbell Lateral Raise	1 x 10-12	3 x 8-10
		Overhead Seated Barbell Press	1 x 10-12	3 x 8-10
	Forearms	Barbell (Palms Up) Wrist Curl	1 x 10-12	2 x 10-12
		Barbell (Palms Down) Wrist Curl	1 x 10-12	2 x 10-12
Friday	Biceps	Dumbbell Concentration Curl	1 x 10-12	3 x 8-10
		Barbell Curl	1 x 10-12	3 x 8-10
	Triceps	High Pulley Pushdown	1 x 10-12	3 x 8-10
		Close Grip Barbell Bench Press	1 x 10-12	3 x 8-10
	Calves	Seated Calf Heel Raise	1 x 10-12	3 x 10-12
		Standing Calf Heel Raise	1 x 10-12	3 x 10-12
	Abs	Leg Raise	2 x 25-50	2 x 25-50

With the exception of the abs exercises, all other bodypart exercises should be done as supersets.

Photo by Kevin Horton
Model Ben White

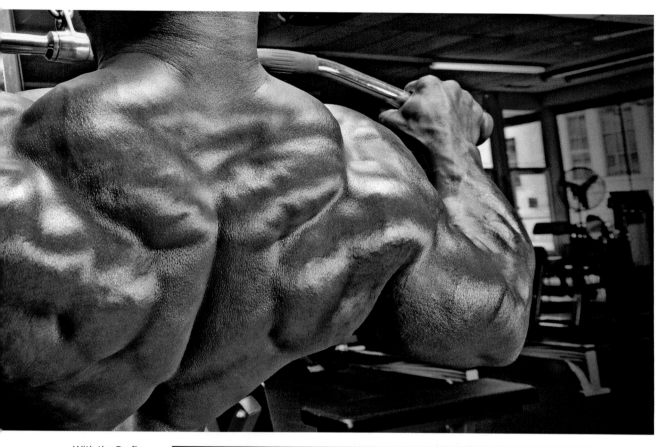

With the Preflex cycle, you isolate the target muscle with the first move for each bodypart and then perform a compound move second to recruit secondary muscles in the group.

PREFLEX CYCLE – GROWTH PHASE WEEKS THREE & FOUR

DAY	MUSCLE GROUP	EXERCISE	SETS/REPS
Monday	Thighs	Sissy Squat	1 x 10-12
		Hack Squat	1 x 10-12
	Back	One-arm Dumbbell Row	1 x 10-12
		Lat Pulldown	1 x 10-12
	Abs	Crunch	2 x25-50
Wednesday	Chest	Pec-Deck Flye	1 x 10-12
		Flat Dumbbell Bench Press	1 x 10-12
	Shoulders	Barbell Upright Row	1 x 10-12
		Overhead Dumbbell Press	1 x 10-12
	Forearms	Dumbbell (Palms Up) Wrist Curl	1 x 10-12
		Dumbbell Hammer Curl	1 x 10-12
Friday	Biceps	Incline Dumbbell Curl	1 x 10-12
		Pull Up (Palms Facing)	1 x 10-12
	Triceps	Dumbbell Kickback	1 x 10-12
		Lying EZ-Bar Triceps Extension	1 x 10-12
	Calves	Leg Press Calf Raise	1 x 10-12
		Donkey Calf Raise	1 x 10-12
	Abs	Hyperextension	2 x 25-50

With the exception of the abs exercises, all other bodypart exercises should be done as supersets.

You'll perform one set of 25–50 reps of the hanging leg raise twice a week during the growth phase of the GH Plus cycle.

GH PLUS CYCLE — GROWTH PHASE WEEKS ONE & TWO

DAY	MUSCLE GROUP	EXERCISE	SETS/REPS	WEEK 2 SETS/REPS
Monday	Thighs	Barbell Back Squat	1 x20	3 x 20
		Leg Extension	1 x 12-15	3 x 12-15
	Calves	Standing Calf Raise	1 x 12-15	1 x 12-15
	Back	Deadlift	1 x 10-12	1 x 8-10
	Chest	Incline Barbell Bench Press	1 x 10-12	1 x 8-10
	Shoulders	Overhead Barbell Press	1 x 10-12	1 x 8-10
	Abs	Hanging Leg Raise	1 x 25-50	1 x 25-50
Wednesday	Biceps	Barbell Curl	2 x 10-12	2 x 8-10
	Triceps	Standing or Seated EZ-Bar French Press	2 x 10-12	2 x 8-10
	Forearms	Barbell (Palms Up) Wrist Curl	2 x 10-12	2 x 10-12
	Abs	Crunch	1 x 25-50	1 x 25-50
Friday	Thighs	Barbell Back Squat	1 x 20	3 x 20
		Leg Extension	1 x 12-15	3 x 12-15
	Calves	Standing Calf Raise	1 x 12-15	1 x 12-15
	Back	Deadlift	1 x 10-12	1 x 8-10
	Chest	Incline Barbell Bench Press	1 x 10-12	1 x 8-10
	Shoulders	Overhead Barbell Press	1 x 10-12	1 x 8-10
	Abs	Hanging Leg Raise	1 x 25-50	1 x 25-50

With the exception of the abs exercises, all other bodypart exercises should be done as supersets.

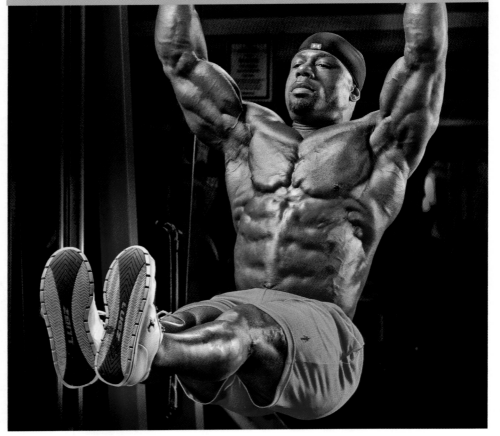

Photo by Michael Butler
Model Tippu Deckard

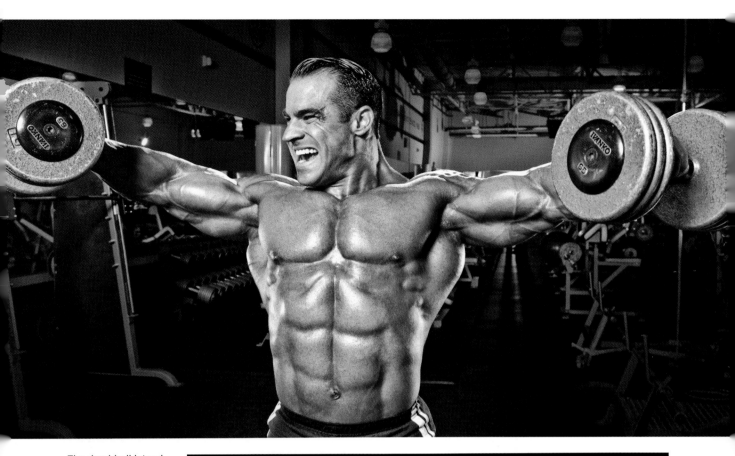

The dumbbell lateral raise is the main shoulder move that you'll perform twice during the weekly split during weeks three and four.

GH PLUS CYCLE — STABILIZE PHASE WEEKS THREE & FOUR

DAY	MUSCLE GROUP	EXERCISE	SETS/REPS
Monday	Thighs	Leg Press	1 x 12-15
		Sissy Squat	1 x 12-15
	Calves	Seated Calf Raise	1 x 12-15
	Back	Lat Pulldown	1 x 10-12
	Chest	Flat Dumbbell Bench Press	1 x 10-12
	Shoulders	Dumbbell Lateral Raise	1 x 10-12
	Abs	Crunch	1 x 25-50
Wednesday	Biceps	Incline Dumbbell Curl	2 x 10-12
	Triceps	High Pulley Pushdown	2 x 10-12
	Forearms	Barbell (Palms Down) Wrist Curl	2 x 10-12
	Abs	Hyperextension	1 x 25-50
Friday	Thighs	Leg Press	1 x 12-15
		Sissy Squat	1 x 12-15
	Calves	Seated Calf Raise	1 x 12-15
	Back	Lat Pulldown	1 x 10-12
	Chest	Dumbbell Bench Press	1 x 10-12
	Shoulders	Dumbbell Lateral Raise	1 x 10-12
	Abs	Crunch	1 x 25-50

With the exception of the abs exercises, all other bodypart exercises should be done as supersets.

Supersets are used in the Superflex cycle to target synergistic muscle groups and promote growth.

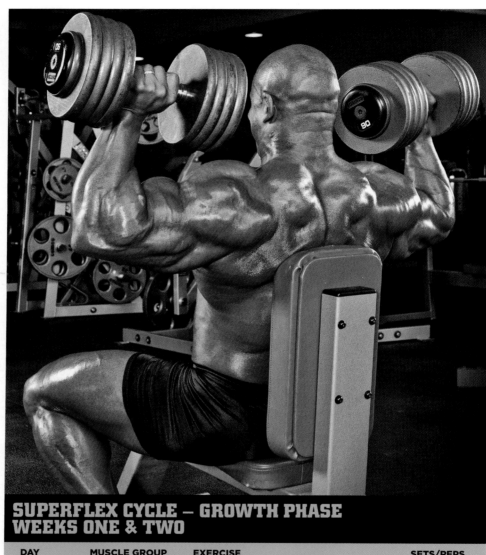

SUPERFLEX CYCLE – GROWTH PHASE WEEKS ONE & TWO

DAY	MUSCLE GROUP	EXERCISE	SETS/REPS
Monday		Superset:	1 x 10-12
	Back/	Seated Low Pulley Row	1 x 10-12
	Chest	Incline Barbell Press	2 x 25-50
	Abs	Hanging Leg Raise	
Wednesday		Superset:	1 x 10-12
	Thighs/	Leg Press	1 x 10-12
	Leg Biceps	Leg Curl	1 x 10-12
		Superset:	1 x 10-12
	Shoulder/	Dumbbell Press Overhead	1 x 10-12
	Calves	Seated Calf Raise	
Friday		Superset:	1 x 10-12
	Biceps/	Barbell Curl	1 x 10-12
	Triceps	Standing or Seated EZ-Bar French Press	1 x 10-12*
	Forearms	Barbell (Palms Down) Wrist Curl	1 x 25-50*
	Abs	Leg Raise	

*In week two, do one additional set.

Photo by Jason Breeze
Model Craig Richardson

The one-arm dumbbell row functions as the main back move during the stabilizing phase.

Photo by Rich Baker
Model Fouad Abiad

SUPERFLEX CYCLE – STABILIZE PHASE
WEEKS THREE & FOUR

DAY	MUSCLE GROUP	EXERCISE	SETS/REPS
Monday		Superset:	1 x 8-10
	Back/	One Arm Dumbbell Row	1 x 8-10
	Chest	Parallel Bar Dip	2 x 25-50
	Abs	Oblique Raise/Side Crunch	
Wednesday		Superset:	1 x 8-10
	Thighs/	Hack Squat	1 x 8-10
	Leg Biceps	Leg Curl	1 x 8-10
		Superset:	1 x 8-10
	Shoulder/	Dumbbell Lateral Raise	1 x 8-10
	Calves	Standing Calf Raise	
Friday		Superset:	1 x 8-10
	Biceps/	Incline Dumbbell Curl	1 x 8-10
	Triceps	High Pulley Pressdown	1 x 8-10
	Forearms	Dumbbell Hammer Curl	1 x 25-50
	Abs	Crunch	

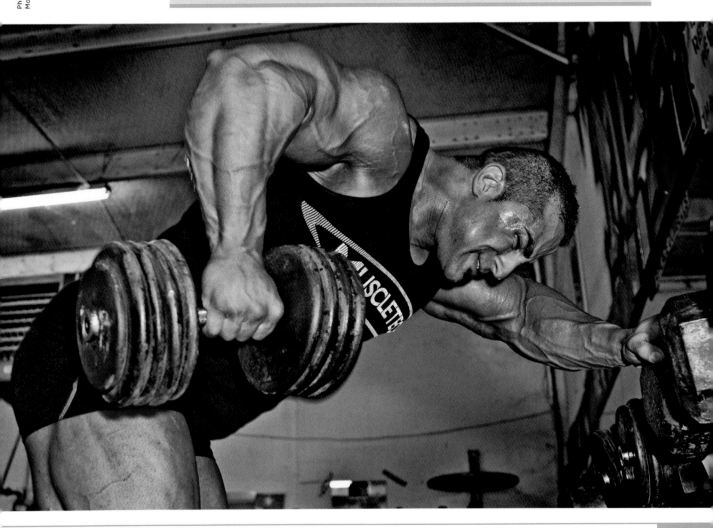

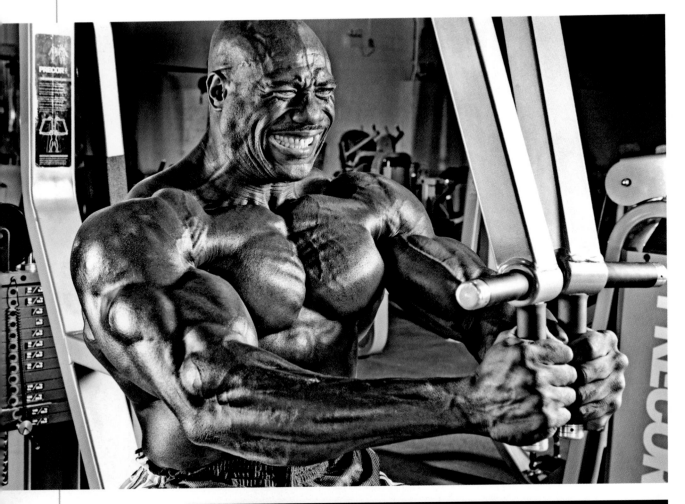

The Powerplay cycle emphasizes the push-pull system with a focus on power movements.

POWERPLAY CYCLE — GROWTH PHASE WEEKS ONE & TWO

DAY	MUSCLE GROUP	EXERCISE	WEEK 1 SETS/REPS	WEEK 2 SETS/REPS
Monday	Thighs	Barbell Back Squat	2 x 10-12	4 x 4-6
		Leg Extension	1 x 12-15	1 x 12-15
	Chest	Incline Barbell Press	2 x 10-12	4 x 4-6
		Pec-Deck Flye	1 x 12-15	1 x 12-15
	Abs	Crunch	2 x 25-50	2 x 25-50
Wednesday	Back	Deadlift	2 x 10-12	4 x 4-6
		Lat Pulldown	1 x 12-15	1 x 12-15
	Biceps	Barbell Curl	1 x 12-15	2 x 12-15
	Calves	Standing Calf Raise	1 x 12-15	2 x 12-15
	Abs	Hyperextension	2 x 25-50	2 x 25-50
Friday	Shoulders	Overhead Barbell Press	2 x 10-12	4 x 4-6
		Dumbbell Lateral Raise	1 x 12-15	1 x 12-15
	Triceps	Close-Grip Barbell Bench Press	1 x 12-15	2 x 12-15
	Forearms	Barbell (Palms Up) Wrist Curl	1 x 12-15	2 x 12-15
	Abs	Hanging Leg Raise	2 x 25-50	2 x 25-50

Photo by Paul Buceta
Model Joel Stubbs

POWERPLAY CYCLE – STABILIZE PHASE WEEKS THREE & FOUR

DAY	MUSCLE GROUP	EXERCISE	SETS/REPS
Monday	Thighs	Leg Press	2 x 10-12
		Sissy Squat	1 x 12-15
	Chest	Dumbbell Bench Press	2 x 10-12
		Incline Dumbbell Flye	1 x 12-15
	Abs	Crunch	2 x 25-50
Wednesday	Back	Bent-Over Row	2 x 10-12
		One Dumbbell Pullover	1 x 12-15
	Biceps	Standing Dumbbell Curl	1 x 12-15
	Calves	Seated Calf Raise	1 x 12-15
	Abs	Hyperextension	2 x 25-50
Friday	Shoulders	Overhead Dumbbell Press	2 x 10-12
		Dumbbell Shrug	1 x 12-15
	Triceps	Pulley Pushdown	1 x 12-15
	Forearms	Barbell (Palms Down) Wrist Curl	1 x 12-15
	Abs	Hanging Leg Raise	2 x 25-50

When doing the close-grip barbell bench press for your triceps, use hand spacing slightly inside of shoulder width.

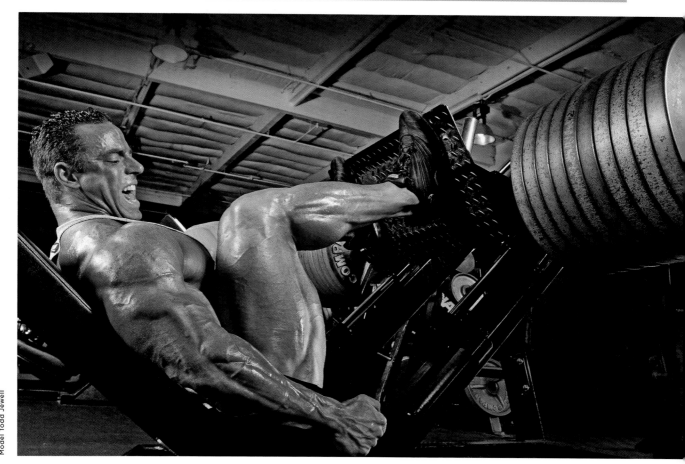

Photo by Irvin Gelb
Model Todd Jewell

CHAPTER 32

TWO POWER BODYBUILDING PROGRAMS

Exercise and set combinations in one 12- to 16-week cycle and another eight-week cycle are designed to create results.

The two Power Bodybuilding Programs consists of two parts. One part lasts 12 to 16 weeks, while the other is an eight-week training cycle.

POWER BODYBUILDING PROGRAM NUMBER 1
12 TO 16 WEEKS

POWER BUILDING CYCLE PART A
MONDAY (DAY 1)
Flat-Bench Barbell Press

Do a warm-up set of 10 reps, followed by a set of six reps using the same weight. Be sure to get a full stretch and use proper form and normal lifting speed when doing the lift. Continue adding weight throughout two sets of five reps. Immediately perform a set of three reps, to set the pattern for the five single attempts that will follow. Select a weight that will allow you to do a solid single attempt with a pause on your chest.

Your next set should be a single rep using additional weight. Follow that up with yet another single rep with additional weight. Be sure you don't bounce; just touch your chest and go. Remember to keep proper form. Next, add weight and do another single rep attempt, again with a touch and go. Your fourth single rep set will be with less weight, but with a pause. The same applies for your fifth and final single. Then, drop weight again and do three reps, all with a pause.

Your last set will be for three reps with blowups. To perform a blowup, you lower the bar to your chest, drive off, but stop the bar about six inches off your chest. Hold it there for a two count and lower the bar back to your chest. Repeat this for your second and third reps, but on your third rep, after holding it six inches off your chest, push the bar up to a completed lift. Take very safe, moderate jumps in weight because you never want to fail in any of your lifting attempts. You should always have a spotter on hand for this exercise.

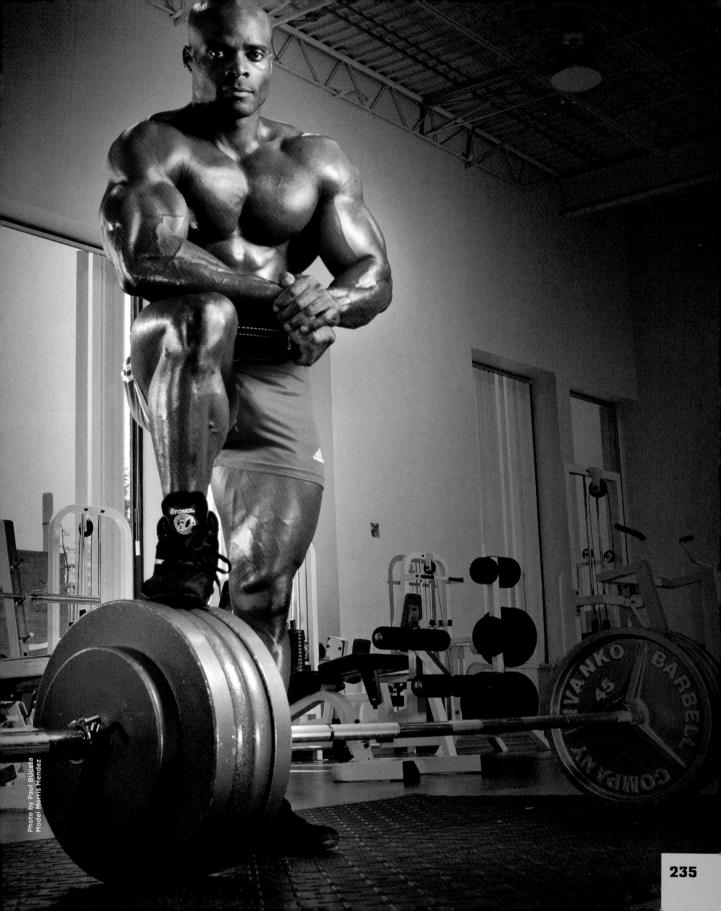

For the barbell deadlift, you'll perform two warm-up sets before doing two working sets. After that, move to a power rack.

BARBELL BACK SQUATS

Your first set will be a warm-up set of 10 reps, followed by a set of six reps with the same weight. Add weight for a follow-up set of five reps. This should be followed by another weight increase and another five reps. Then move on to the power rack. Set the support pins to where your thighs will be two inches above parallel if the bar were racked there. Your first power rack set will have three reps. Add weight and do another set of three reps. Add more weight and do another three-rep set.

Lower the weight and do one set of three reps with blowups. This follows the same pattern as in the bench-press blowup set. Get set with your squat, lower the bar to the support rods, drive up about four inches and hold for a two count. Then lower the bar and repeat the cycle for your next two reps. Do not relax. Never release the tension during the squat blowups. On your third rep, hold for a second and then drive through and complete the squat. The power rack will help you to develop power and style. Remember to squat deep on any of your full attempts.

BARBELL DEADLIFT

Do a set of 10 warm-ups and then another set of six. Add weight for a set of five reps and then add more weight for another set of five. These sets will be your last regular deadlifts. From there, move to the power rack. Set the support rods so the bar will be two inches below your knees. You'll be training the top / lockout part of the deadlift.

Begin with a set of three reps. Add weight and do another set of three. Once again add weight and do your top set of three reps. From there, lower the poundage and complete a closing set of three reps. You cannot perform blowups on the top / lockout part of the barbell deadlift.

Photo by Robert Reiff
Model Brian Yersky

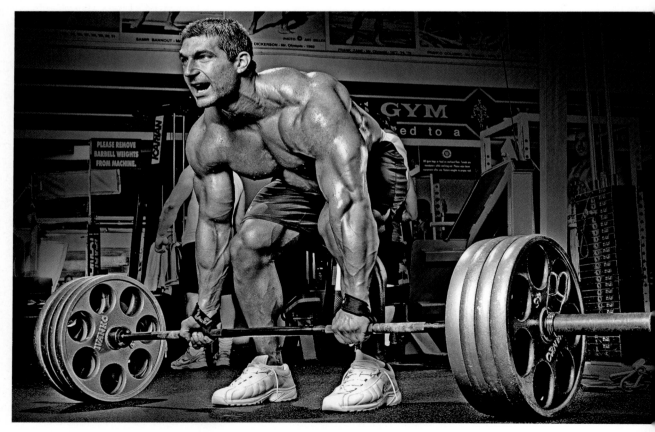

POWER-RACK BARBELL DEADLIFTS

Power-rack training will allow you to conquer and correct any mechanical flaws you may have in your technique. It is meant to assist and build and shouldn't be used as a test of strength or power. While power-rack training, you'll be able to handle weight at least equal to your best.

Here are four important points to consider when it comes to the performance of the power rack barbell deadlift:

1. When doing power-rack barbell deadlifts, always use heavy-duty canvas or cotton lifting straps. These help you complete your reps. They aren't aids to help you cheat. Use them judiciously.

2. Never start the lift from the support rods. Your traps will receive a great workout by removing the weight from the hooks.

3. As you take the weight out, lower it to the rods under control. Use correct form, and keep the bar in its groove (your lifting path). Do not relax. Stay tight. Now start your pull off the pins. Each time you return the bar to the pins, you should remain tight. Don't bounce the weight off the support rods.

4. Concentration is very important. If necessary, upon your direction, have the spotters help you out of the hooks, thereby allowing you to get set in the lockout position. Also have your spotters follow the path of the bar down to the support rods. You should attempt to handle the majority of the poundage. Your spotters are there only to assist you and by using them in this manner, you'll be able to save your strength and apply it to the lift.

WEDNESDAY (DAY 2)

Day two begins with the flat bench barbell press. Start once again with a warm-up set of 10 reps. Follow that up with the same weight for six reps. Increase the weight for a set of five reps. Increase the weight again for another set of five reps. Then comes the first of three sets, which should all be done as a normal touch and go barbell bench press.

Lower the weight on sets four and five. Do all of these reps with a pause. Be sure to pace yourself. You should allow for the same amount of pause time on each rep. Push your chest up and use your lats. Your lats play an important role in the barbell bench press. Strong, thick lats allow you to have a solid base on the bench and they'll assist in the drive off your chest. Remember to get set with a strong, solid base on the bench.

The barbell back squat should be performed as follows: Warm up with a set of 10 reps. Then, perform another set of six reps, followed by two sets of five reps each. Increase the weight between the sets. Follow that up with one set of three reps. Increase the weight again for your top set, which you should perform for two reps. Then, decrease the weight and do another three reps. Your last set of squats will be a set of five reps. During that three-two-three series of squats, it's vital not to miss any reps. Be strong during your set-up and think of each rep as a single lift.

FRIDAY (DAY 3)

On the flat bench barbell press, start with a warm-up set of 10 reps, and then do another six reps. Perform another set of five reps, followed by an additional set of five. Then do another five sets of three reps. The first of these five sets is three reps with a pause. Add weight again, and do a set of three using touch and go. Then, do yet another set of three reps with touch and go. Lower the weight and do a set of three reps with a pause. Your last set of three reps will be blowups.

SATURDAY (DAY 4)

Start with the barbell back squat. The warm-up pattern is the same as before. Perform 10 reps and then six reps. Follow that up with two sets of five reps each. Then do a set of three reps. These reps should set the pace, as your next set is only a single. Add weight again for another single rep. Decrease your poundage for your third and final single-rep attempt. Lower the weight again for three reps. Your close-out set will be five reps. These single attempts are not to be taken as make-it-or-break-

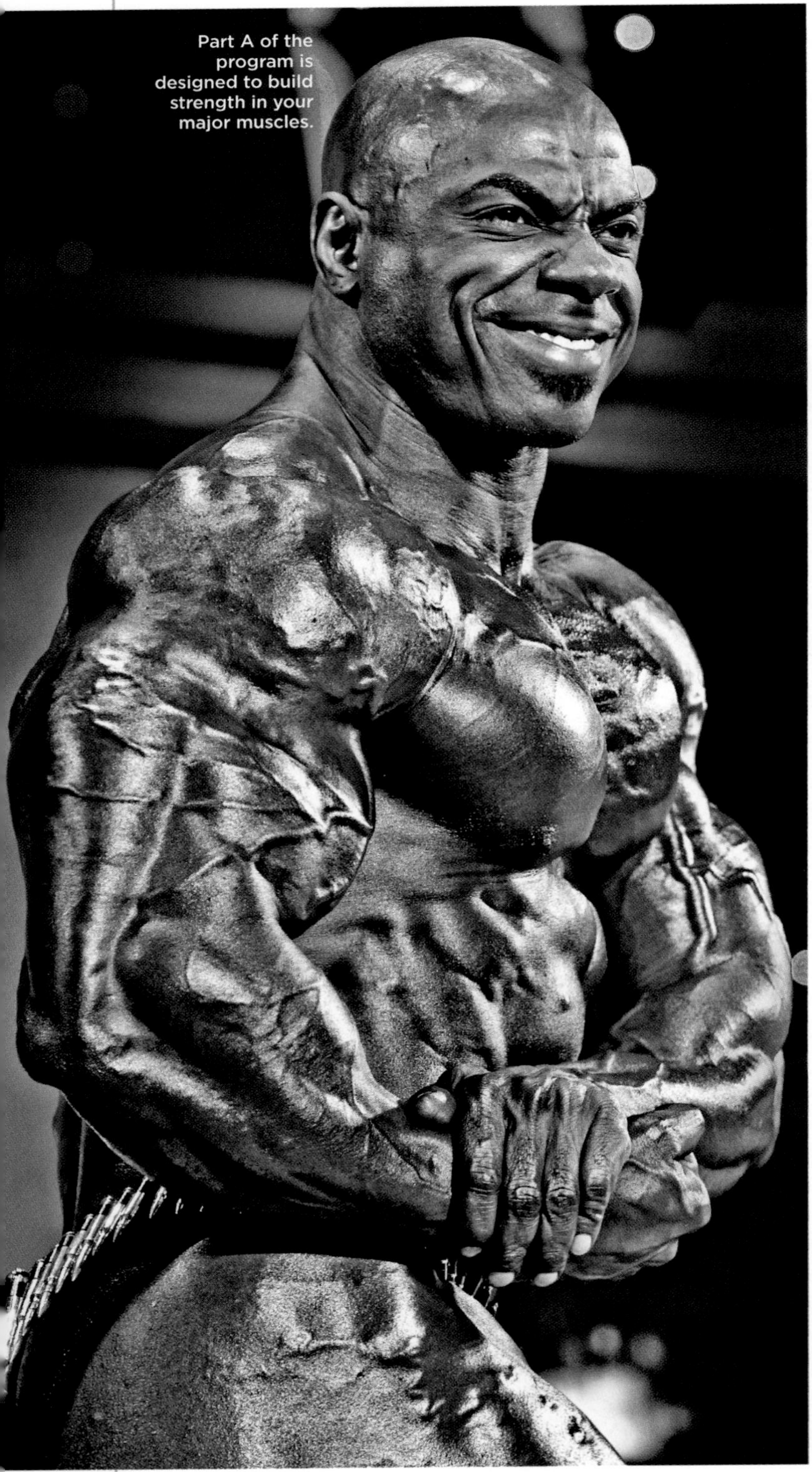

Part A of the program is designed to build strength in your major muscles.

it attempts. Their purpose is to build strength. Put some work into them, but don't try to perform at 110 percent each week.

Move on to regular deadlifts for 10 reps, followed by a set of six reps. Then perform two sets of five reps. Move to the power rack and set the support rods at about six inches below your knees. Start doing four sets of three reps each, and increase your poundage with each set. Your last set is a triple with blowups. Don't deviate from this set and rep structure.

POWER BUILDING — CYCLE PART A OUTLINE

MONDAY (DAY 1)

FLAT-BENCH BENCH PRESS
Warm-up: 2 x 10/6
1 x 5
1 x 5
1 x 3
1 x 1 (plus) Pause
1 x 1 (plus) Pause
1 X 1 (plus) Touch and Go
1 X 1 (plus) Touch and Go
1 x 1 (minus) Pause
1 x 3 (minus) Pause
1 x 3 (minus) Blowups

BARBELL BACK SQUAT
Warm-up 2 x 10/6
1 x 5
1 x 5

POWER-RACK SQUAT
1 x 3 (plus)
1 x 3 (plus)
1 x 3 (plus)
1 x 3 (minus) Blowups

DEADLIFT
Warm-up: 2 x 10/6
1 x 5
1 x 5

POWER-RACK DEADLIFT
Set the support rods to about two or three inches below your knee.
1 x 3 (plus)
1 x 3 (plus)
1 x 3 (plus)
1 x 3 (minus)

In every third week, Monday's program changes from three reps to two reps.

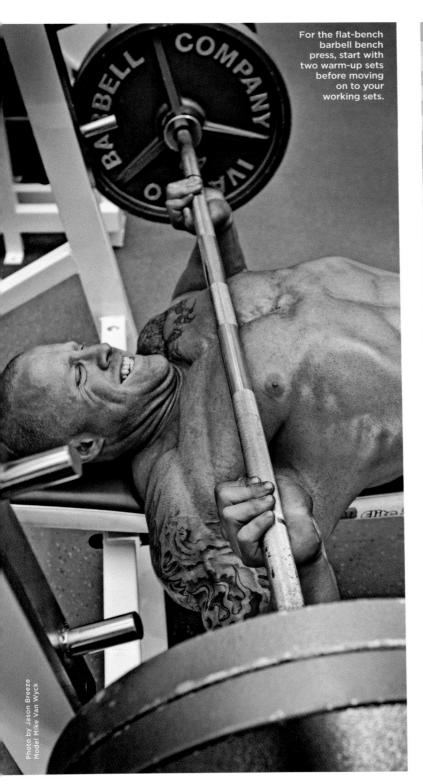

For the flat-bench barbell bench press, start with two warm-up sets before moving on to your working sets.

Photo by Jason Breeze
Model Mike Van Wyck

WEDNESDAY (DAY 2)
FLAT-BENCH BENCH PRESS
Warm-up: 2 x 10/6

1 x 5

1 x 5

1 x 5 (plus)

1 x 5 (plus)

1 x 5 (plus)

The above three sets should be done as touch and go.

1 x 5 (minus) Pause

1 x 5 (minus) Pause

BARBELL BACK SQUAT
Warm-up 2 x 10/6

1 x 5

1 x 5

1 x 3 (plus)

1 x 3 (plus)

1 x 2 (plus)

1 x 3 (minus)

1 x 5 (minus)

FRIDAY (DAY 3)
FLAT-BENCH BENCH PRESS
Warm-up: 2 x 10/6

1 x 5

1 x 5

1 X 3 (plus) Pause

1 X 3 (plus) Touch And Go

1 X 3 (plus) Touch And Go

1 X 3 (minus) Pause

1 X 3 (minus) Blowups

One of the keys to power-rack success is to never relax. Keep your arms locked out and perform as if you were lifting the weight from the floor. Don't jerk into the attempt. Maintain a straight, upright position as long as possible throughout the lift. Try to keep a firm center of gravity and keep the bar close to your legs. If you allow the bar to drift out, you'll be pulled out of your groove. Once the bar is at your knee area, push your hips in, drive the floor away with your feet and pull with your lats. In every third week of the strength program, you should change all reps in the power rack deadlift from triples to doubles.

Use Power-Bodybuilding Program Number 1 for 12 to 16 weeks. After that 12- to 16-week period, follow Power-Bodybuilding Program Number 2 for eight weeks.

SATURDAY (DAY 4)

BARBELL BACK SQUAT

Warm-up: 2 x 10/6

1 x 5

1 x 5

1 x 3

1 x 1 (plus)

1 x 1 (plus)

1 x 1 (minus)

1 x 3 (minus)

1 x 5 (minus)

DEADLIFT

Warm-up: 2 x 10/6

1 x 5

1 x 5

POWER-RACK SQUAT

Set the support rods to six inches below your knee.

1 x 3 (plus)

1 x 3 (plus)

1 x 3 (plus)

1 x 3 (plus)

1 x 3 (minus) Blowups

Every third week, Saturday's program changes from three reps to two reps.

Explanation:
(plus) = Increase Poundage
(minus) = Decrease Poundage

The squat – and all its variations – is the best single move to build lower-body size and strength.

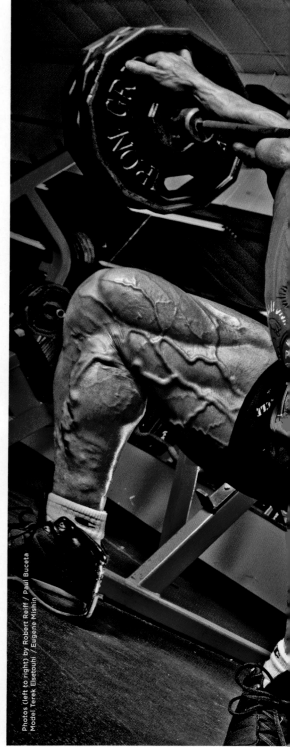

Photos (left to right) by Robert Reiff / Paul Buceta
Model: Terek Elsetouhi / Eugene Mishin

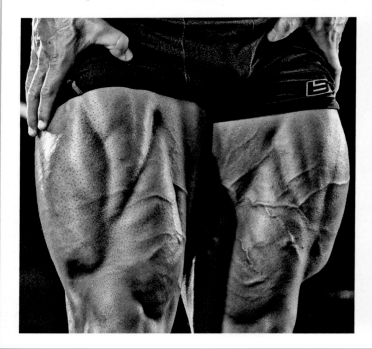

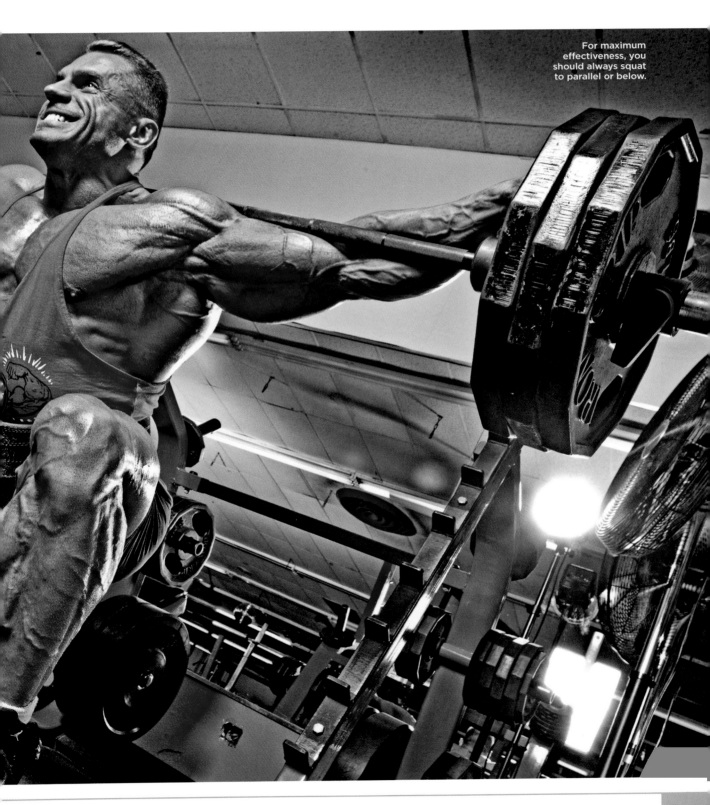

For maximum effectiveness, you should always squat to parallel or below.

HUGE & FREAKY MUSCLE MASS AND STRENGTH SECRETS

On Day 1 of Cycle Part B, you'll do four sets of six to eight reps of all moves, including the wide-grip front lat pulldown.

12-16 WEEK BODYBUILDING – CYCLE PART B

Always try to add weight in your bodybuilding training workouts. Don't do it week to week, but instead do it during the four sets of six to eight reps. You can pyramid your poundage (increase for two sets, then decrease for two sets), or perform your first set with one weight, then increase the weight for the next three sets.

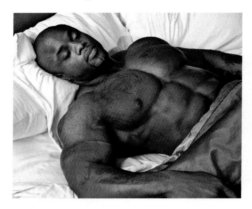

Power Bodybuilding Program Number 1 follows a Monday-Wednesday-Friday-Saturday pattern. However, any combination of four days per week will do, provided that you allow for proper rest and recovery time between your workouts. If your training time is limited, you can add the exercises from the third day to the fourth day and reduce the program to a three-day-per-week program.

BODYBUILDING – CYCLE PART B OUTLINE

MONDAY (DAY 1)

LEG PRESS
4 x 6-8*

LEG EXTENSION
4 x 6-8*

LEG CURL
4 x 6-8

DUMBBELL BENCH PRESS
4 x 6-8*

WIDE-GRIP FRONT LAT PULLDOWN
4 x 6-8

UNDERHAND CLOSE-GRIP FRONT PULLDOWN (PALMS FACING UP)
4 x 6-8*

TWO-DUMBBELL ROW
4 x 6-8*

BEHIND-THE-NECK BARBELL PRESS
4 x 6-8*

EZ-BAR TRICEPS EXTENSION
4 x 6-8 (Lying)

ONE-DUMBBELL TRICEPS EXTENSION
4 x 6-8

EZ-BAR CURL
4 x 6-8*

DUMBBELL CURL
4 x 6-8*

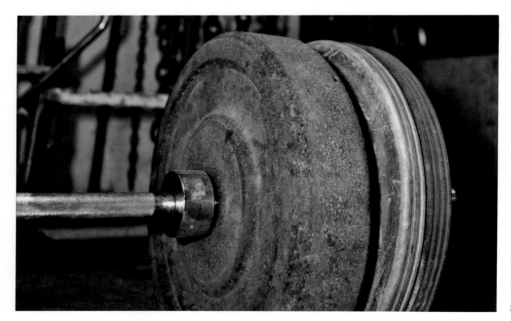

Photo (top to bottom) by Gregory James / Jason Breeze
Model Ben White

WEDNESDAY (DAY 2)

HACK SQUAT

4 x 6-8

LEG EXTENSION

4 x 6-8

LEG CURL

4 x 6-8

EZ-BAR BENCH PRESS

4 x 6-8

DUMBBELL BENCH PRESS

4 x 6-8

ONE-ARM DUMBBELL ROW

4 x 6-8

LONG PULL CABLE ROW

4 x 6-8*

OVERHEAD DUMBBELL PRESS

4 x 6-8*

EZ-BAR TRICEPS EXTENSION

4 x 6-8 (Lying)

TRICEPS PRESSDOWN

4 x 6-8

EZ-BAR CURL

4 x 6-8*

DUMBBELL CURL

4 x 6-8*

FRIDAY (DAY 3)

EZ-BAR BENCH PRESS (WIDER GRIP)

4 x 6-8

DUMBBELL PRESS

4 x 6-8

BEHIND-THE-NECK BARBELL PRESS

4 x 6-8

SATURDAY (DAY 5)

HACK SQUAT

4 x 6-8

LEG PRESS

4 x 6-8*

WIDE-GRIP FRONT LAT PULLDOWN

4 x 6-8*

UNDERHAND CLOSE-GRIP LAT PULLDOWN (PALMS FACING FORWARD)

4 x 6-8

(*) When you're on your last set of six to eight reps, do your reps, stop and count to 10, and then do one more rep. After you do the one rep, rest again, count to 10 and do another rep. Continue this one-rep / rest cycle six times. Your last set would be six reps plus six extra reps. This is based on the rest-pause theory.

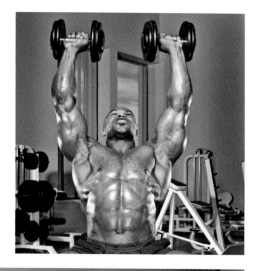

On Day 2, the dumbbell overhead press falls about midway through your workout while the dumbbell curl is the finishing move.

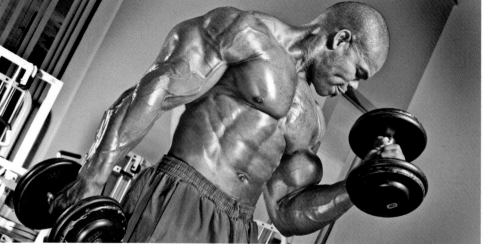

ULTIMATE POWER BODYBUILDING PROGRAM NUMBER 2

8 WEEK POWER BUILDING — CYCLE PART A OUTLINE

MONDAY (DAY 1)

BARBELL BACK SQUAT

Warm-up: 2 x 10/6

1 x 5

1 x 5

1 x 5

1 x 5 (plus)

1 x 5 (plus)

1 x 5 (minus)

1 x 5 (minus)

DEADLIFT

Warm-up: 10 x 6

1 x 5

1 x 5

1 x 5

1 x 5 (plus)

1 x 5 (plus)

1 x 5 (minus)

1 x 5 (minus)

All deadlifts are to be performed from the floor. You shouldn't be doing any rack work.

WEDNESDAY (DAY 2)

FLAT BARBELL BENCH

Warm-up: 2 x 10/6

1 x 5

1 x 5

1 x 5

1 x 5 (plus) touch and go

1 x 5 (plus) touch and go

1 x 5 (minus) touch and go

1 x 5 (minus) touch and go

1 x 8

BARBELL POWER CLEAN

Warm-up: 2 x 6/6

1 x 5

1 x 5

1 x 5

1 x 5 (plus)

1 x 5 (plus)

1 x 5 (minus)

1 x 5 (minus)

1 x 8 Flush Set

FRIDAY (DAY 3)

BARBELL BENCH PRESS: SAME AS WEDNESDAY

BARBELL BACK SQUAT: SAME AS MONDAY

Explanation:
(plus) = Increase Poundage
(minus) = Decrease Poundage

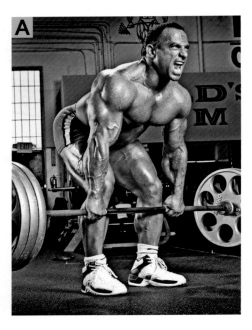

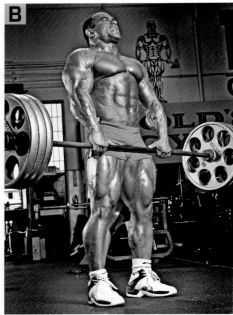

Proper form is crucial throughout the full range of motion on the barbell deadlift.

Photo by Robert Reiff
Model Mike Ergas

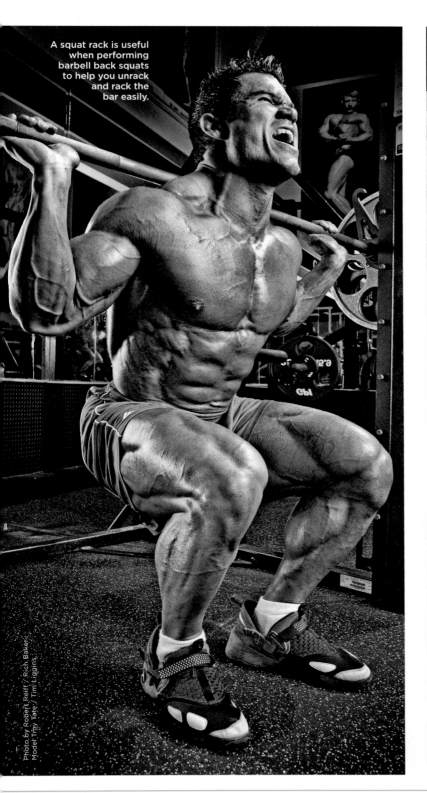

A squat rack is useful when performing barbell back squats to help you unrack and rack the bar easily.

Photo by Robert Reiff / Rich Baker;
Model Troy Tate / Tim Liggins.

8 WEEK POWER BUILDING – CYCLE PART B OUTLINE

MONDAY (DAY 1)

LEG EXTENSION

4 x 6-8*

LEG CURL

4 x 6-8

DUMBBELL BENCH PRESS

4 x 6-8

WIDE-GRIP FRONT LAT PULLDOWN

4 x 6-8*

TWO-DUMBBELL ROW

4 x 6-8

BEHIND-THE-NECK BARBELL PRESS

4 x 6-8

BARBELL FRONT RAISE

4 x 6-8

BARBELL SHRUG

4 x 6-8

EZ-BAR TRICEPS EXTENSION

4 x 6-8

DUMBBELL EXTENSION

4 x 6-8

TRICEPS KICKBACK

4 x 6-8*

EZ-BAR CURL

4 x 6-8*

DUMBBELL CURL

4 x 6-8

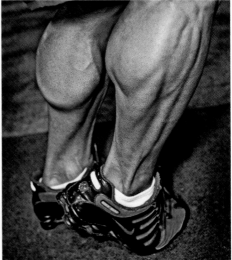

WEDNESDAY (DAY 2)		FRIDAY (DAY 3)
HACK SQUAT		**LEG PRESS**
4 x 6-8		4 x 6-8
LEG EXTENSION		**LEG CURL**
4 x 6-8		4 x 6-8
EZ-BAR CURL BENCH PRESS		**DUMBBELL BENCH PRESS**
4 x 6-8		4 x 6-8
DUMBBELL BENCH PRESS		**DUMBBELL FLYES**
4 x 6-8*		4 x 6-8*
ONE-ARM DUMBBELL ROW		**ONE-ARM DUMBBELL ROW**
4 x 6-8		4 x 6-8
LONG PULL CABLE ROW		**WIDE-GRIP FRONT LAT PULLDOWN**
4 x 6-8		4 x 6-8
UNDERHAND CLOSE-GRIP FRONT PULLDOWN (PALMS FACING UP)		**OVERHEAD DUMBBELL PRESS**
4 x 6-8		4 x 6-8*
BEHIND-THE-NECK BARBELL PRESS		**BARBELL FRONT RAISE**
4 x 6-8		4 x 6-8
OVERHEAD DUMBBELL PRESS		**BARBELL SHRUG**
4 x 6-8		4 x 6-8*
EZ-BAR TRICEPS EXTENSION		**EZ-BAR (LYING) TRICEPS EXTENSION**
4 x 6-8		4 x 6-8
TRICEPS PRESSDOWN ON LAT MACHINE		**ONE-DUMBBELL TRICEPS EXTENSION**
4 x 6-8		4 x 6-8
DUMBBELL TRICEPS KICKBACK		**TWO-DUMBBELL CURL**
4 x 6-8		4 x 6-8*
EZ-BAR CURL		**ONE-DUMBBELL CURL**
4 x 6-8		4 x 6-8
PREACHER BENCH BARBELL CURL		
4 x 6-8		

After your last set, stop for 10 seconds. Then, do one more rep followed by a rest for a total of six times.

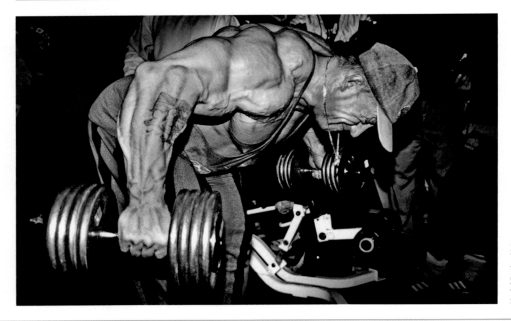

Model Dorian Yates

Photo by Robert Reiff
Model David Hoffman

These two programs combine some of the best exercises along with sets and reps combinations to spark new muscle growth and strength improvements.

5 POINTS ON POWER BUILDING AND BODYBUILDING PROGRAM

1. In power-building cycles, you can use lifting apparel (squat suit, bench press shirt, knee or wrist wraps, a lifting belt, etc.), but use them in moderation. If you find yourself actually needing to use any of these items to complete your sets, then review your training or poundage. It's fine to use any of these items to protect an injured bodypart, however, you should not rely on them to enable you to lift your weights.

2. There is no power-rack training in the Power Building Number 2 cycle. You'll use this phase to build on your full range of movement by performing the deadlift.

3. Depending on which week of the program you're in, your reps will either be five or three. You'll always do four plus and minus gain factor sets, however, the reps will change. You should be doing five reps in each of the eight weeks, with the ex-

ception of the third and sixth weeks. In the third and sixth weeks, you should be doing three reps.

4. The four plus and minus gain factor sets that you do will follow this pattern: Sets one and two increase poundage (plus), while in sets three and four, decrease the poundage (minus).

5. Barbell power cleans have been added to the program and you'll find that these will help with your starting power in the deadlift. When done correctly, barbell power cleans will add muscle mass to your traps and shoulder areas. It's a quick lift, so be extra sure to use proper form.

These two programs provide some of the best exercises as well as set and rep combinations for gaining strength and muscle mass growth. The gains and improvements that you desperately want are waiting for you. If you apply yourself, they'll quickly become a reality.

CHAPTER 33

SOVIET PHASE TRAINING

Overcome a training rut, stagnation or any other barrier to increased muscle mass with this advanced bodybuilding program.

Soviet Phase Training is an 11-week strength and muscle mass improvement program designed by Dr. Yuri Verkhoshansky along with our good friend Rick Brunner. The program is ideal for advanced bodybuilders who have hit a period of stagnation, mass barrier or training plateau.

Soviet Phase Training has a macro-cycle consisting of three blocks. The first block lasts 21 days and has three micro-cycles. The first two micro-cycles are strength oriented and last 14 days. The following chart provides precise details concerning the exercises, sets and reps you should be performing during those first two weeks:

MICRO-CYCLES 1 AND 2

DAY	SETS X REPS
MONDAY	
Barbell Back Squat	1-3 x 3-6
Barbell Bench Press	1 x 10, 3-4 x 3-6
Combination: Lying EZ-Bar Bent-Arm Pullover and Lying Triceps Extension	3-4 x 5-7
Combination: Bent-Arm Dumbbell Flye and Lying EZ-Bar Triceps Extension	4-6 x (2-4) + (2-3)
Work your abs hard.	
TUESDAY	
Deadlift	1 x 10, 2 x 4-8
Wide-Grip Barbell Bent Row	1 x 10, 3 x 4-8
Behind-The-Neck Wide-Grip Barbell Press	1-2 x10, 2 x 5-8
Preacher Bench Barbell Curl	2 x 6-10
Work your abs lightly.	
FRIDAY	
Barbell Back Squat	1 x 10, 3-4 x 4-8
Lying EZ-Bar Triceps Extension	2-3 x 4-6
Triceps Parallel Bar Dip (w/load)	3-4 x 5-7
Work your abs hard.	
SATURDAY	
Barbell Good Mornings	2-3 x 4-8
Wide-Grip Barbell Bent-Over Row	4 x 6
Seated Overhead EZ-Bar Triceps Extension	4-6 x 4-6
Barbell Curl.	3-4 x 4-6 + (1-2 cheat curls)

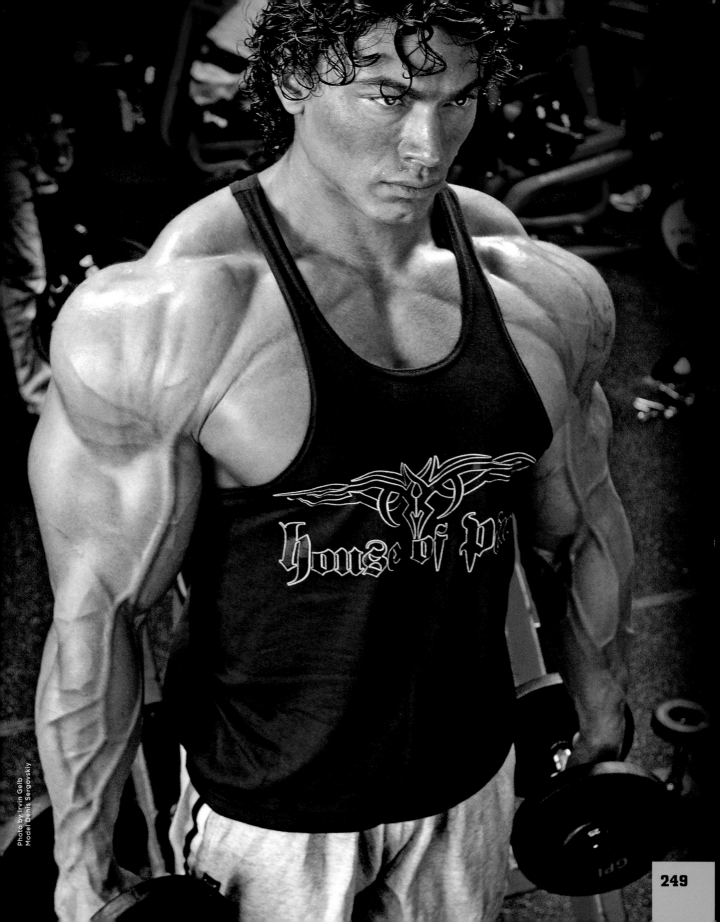

MICRO-CYCLE 3

DAY	SETS X REPS
MONDAY AND THURSDAY	
Barbell Back Squat	3-4 x 6-8
Barbell Bench Press	3-4 x 6-8
Combination: Lying EZ-Bar Bent-Arm Pullover and Triceps Extension	2-3 x 6-8
Parallel Bar Dip	2-3 x 6-8
Work your abs hard.	
TUESDAY	
Deadlift	4 x 6-8
Wide-Grip Barbell Bent-Over Row	4 x 6-8
Behind-The-Neck Barbell Press	4 x 6-8
Barbell Curl	4 x 6-8
Work your abs lightly.	

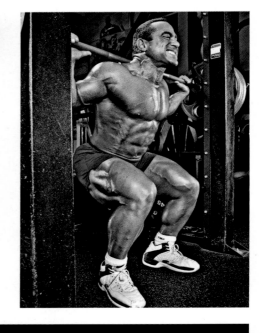

The sets and reps for certain moves will change depending on which micro-cycle you're doing.

MICRO-CYCLE 4

Much like the first block, the second block also consists of three micro-cycles lasting 21 days. We will refer to the first micro-cycle of the second block as the fourth micro-cycle or as a developing stage that is a traditional split system lasting seven days.

DAY	SETS X REPS
MONDAY	
Barbell Back Squat	1-3 x 8-12
Lying Triceps Extension (rest-pause)	3-4 x 6-8
Combination: Lying EZ-Bar Bent-Arm Pullover and Triceps Extension	3-4 x 4-6
Seated Calf Raise	4-5 x 6-10
Work your abs hard.	
TUESDAY AND SATURDAY	
Deadlift	2-3 x 6-8
Wide-Grip Barbell Bent-Over Row	2-3 x 6-8
Behind-The-Neck Barbell Press	3-4 x 8-10
Preacher Bench Barbell Curl	2-3 x 6-8
Work your abs lightly.	
WEDNESDAY	
Wide-Grip Incline Barbell Bench Press	4 x 6-9
Dumbell Flye	4 x 6-8
Parallel Bar Dip	4 x 6-8
Work your abs lightly.	
FRIDAY	
Barbell Back Squat (rest-pause)	3-5 x 6-8
Barbell Bench Press	2-3 x 8-12
Combination: Lying EZ-Bar: Bent-Arm Pullover and Triceps Extension	3-4 x 4-6
Standing Calf Raise	4-6 x 8-10
Work your abs lightly.	

Photo by Robert Reiff
Model Mike Ergas

MICRO-CYCLE 5

Micro-cycle 5 is another seven-day period that will ensure you further develop your muscles. In the following chart you'll find the exact sets, reps and exercises that will stimulate the results you crave.

DAY	SETS X REPS
MONDAY	
Deadlift	1 x 10, 3-4 x 4-6
Wide-Grip Barbell Bent-Over Row	1 x 10, 2-3 x 6-8
One-Arm Dumbbell Row	3-5 x 6-8
Preacher Bench Barbell Curl	2-3 x 6-10
Barbell Curl	1-3 x 6-8 + (1-2 cheat reps)
Work your abs hard.	
TUESDAY AND SATURDAY	
Barbell Back Squat	1 x 10, 3-4 x 8-12
Barbell Bench Press	2-3 x 8-10
Combination: Lying EZ-Bar Bent-Arm Pullover and Triceps Extension	3-4 x 4-6
Parallel Bar Dip	4 x 4-6
Work your abs lightly.	
WEDNESDAY	
Seated or Standing Barbell Good Mornings	2-3 x 4-6
Behind-The-Neck Barbell Press	2-3 x 6-8
Barbell Upright Row	3-4 x 6-8
Dumbbell Lateral Raise	3-4 x 6-8
Bent-Over Dumbbell Lateral Raise	3-4 x 4-6
FRIDAY	
Deadlift	1 x 6-8
Wide-Grip Barbell Bent-Over Row	2-3 x 4-6 + (1-3 cheat reps)
One-Arm Dumbbell Row	3-5 x 6-8
Preacher Bench Barbell Curl	2-3 x 6-8
Barbell Curl	1-2 x 6-8 + (1-2 cheat curls)
Work your abs hard.	

In micro-cycle 5, you'll do a few cheat reps at the end of your regular sets of barbell curls.

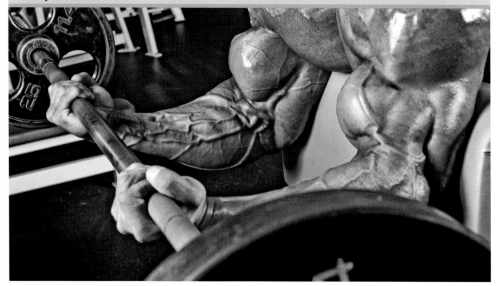

Photo by Paul Buceta
Model Eduardo Correa da Silva

MICRO-CYCLE 6

After two weeks of development, the sixth micro-cycle is a restorative period that lasts seven days. The following chart lists exercises, sets and reps that should be closely followed.

DAY	SETS X REPS
MONDAY AND THURSDAY	
Barbell Back Squat	3-4 x 6-8
Barbell Bench Press	3-4 x 4-8
Combination: Lying EZ-Bar Bent-Arm Pullover and Triceps Extension	2-3 x 6-8
Triceps Parallel Bar Dip	2-3 x 6-8
Work your abs hard.	
TUESDAY AND FRIDAY	
Deadlift	4 x 6-8
Wide-Grip Barbell Bent-Over Row	4 x 6-8
Behind-The-Neck Barbell Press	4 x 6
Barbell Curl	4 x 6
Work your abs lightly.	

You'll target each bodypart with the same exercises twice per week during micro-cycle 6.

Photo by Paul Buceta
Model Bill Wilmore

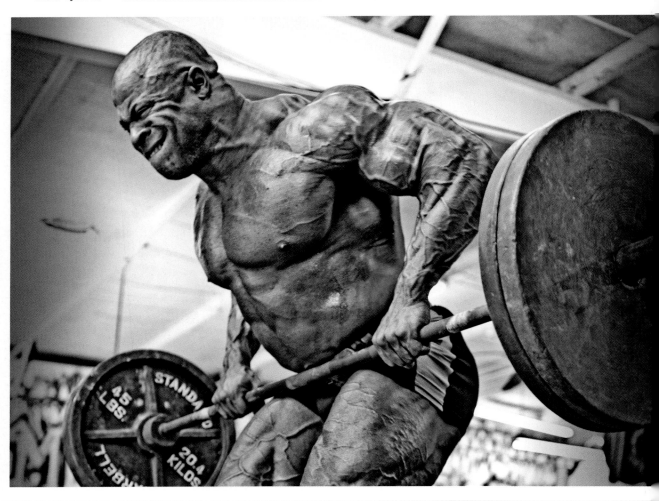

As part of micro-cycle 7 you'll combine EZ-bar bent-arm pullovers with triceps extensions.

MICRO-CYCLE 7

The third and final block has four micro-cycles lasting 32 days. The seventh micro-cycle lasts nine days and is used for developing your legs and chest. Be sure to follow the exercises, sets and reps listed and to use the third, fifth and eighth days to rest.

DAY	SETS X REPS
DAYS 1 AND 6	
Barbell Back Squat (rest pause)	4-5 x 6-10
Barbell Bench Press	3-4 x 8-12
Decline Barbell Bench Press	2-3 x 6-10
Parallel Bar Dip	3-4 x 6-8
Combination: Lying EZ-Bar Bent-Arm Pullover and Triceps Extension	3-4 x 6-8
Work your abs lightly.	
DAYS 2 AND 7	
Leg Press	3-5 x 8-10
Leg Extension	2-3 x 8-12
Leg Curl	2-3 x 6-10
Dumbbell Bench Press	3-5 x 6-8
Incline Dumbbell Flye	3-4 x 6-8
Triceps Pressdown	3-5 x 6-8
DAYS 4 AND 9	
Deadlift	1 x 10, 4-5 x 3-5
Wide-Grip Barbell Bent-Over Row	1 x 10, 2-3 x 3-5
Behind-The-Neck Wide-Grip Barbell Press	1-2 x 8-10
Preacher Bench Barbell Curl	3-4 x 6-10
Work your abs hard.	

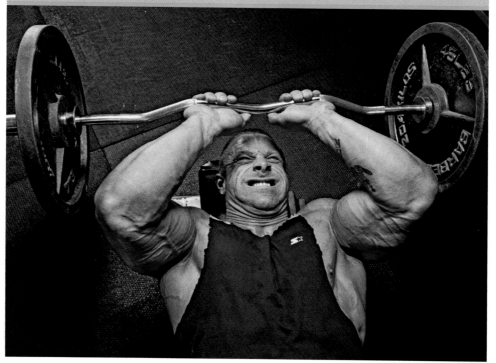

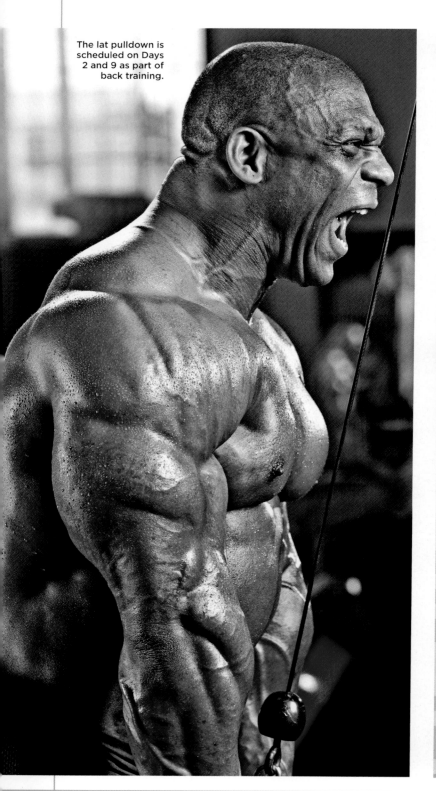

The lat pulldown is scheduled on Days 2 and 9 as part of back training.

MICRO-CYCLE 8

The eighth cycle is a seven day restorative period. Follow the exercises listed and be sure to use the first, fourth and seventh days for rest.

DAY	SETS X REPS
DAYS 2 AND 5	
Barbell Back Squat	3-4 x 6-10
Barbell Bench Press	3-4 x 4-6
Combination: Lying EZ-Bar Bent-Arm Pullover and Triceps Extension	2-3 x 6-8
Parallel Bar Dip	2-3 x 6-8
Work your abs hard.	
DAYS 3 AND 6	
Deadlift	4 x 6-8
Wide-Grip Barbell Bent-Over Row	4 x 6-8
Behind-The-Neck Barbell Press	4 x 6-10
Barbell Curl	4 x 6-8
Work your abs lightly.	

MICRO-CYCLE 9

The ninth micro-cycle lasts nine days and is for developing your back and shoulders. Use the third, fifth and eighth days for rest.

DAY	SETS X REPS
DAYS 1 AND 6	
Deadlift	1 x 10, 4 x 3-6
Wide-Grip Barbell Bent-Over Row	1 x 10, 3-4 x 4-6
Behind-The-Neck Wide-Grip Barbell Press	3-4 x 8-10
Preacher Bench Barbell Curl	4-5 x 6-10
Work your abs hard.	1-3 x 4-6 + (1-2 cheat reps)
DAYS 2 AND 7	
Seated or Standing Barbell Good Morning	4 x 6-8
Lat Pulldown	3-4 x 6-10
Low-Pulley Seated Row	4-5 x 6-10
Barbell Upright Row	4-5 x 6-8
Bent-Over Dumbbell Lateral Raise	3-5 x 6-8
Preacher Bench Barbell Curl	4-5 x 6-10
DAYS 4 AND 9	
Barbell Back Squat (rest pause)	2-3 x 8-12
Barbell Bench Press	2-3 x 8-12
Parallel Bar Dip	3-4 x 6-8
Combination: Lying EZ-Bar Bent-Arm Pullover and Triceps Extension	3-4 x 4-6
Work your abs lightly.	

Photo by Robert Reiff
Model Quincy Taylor

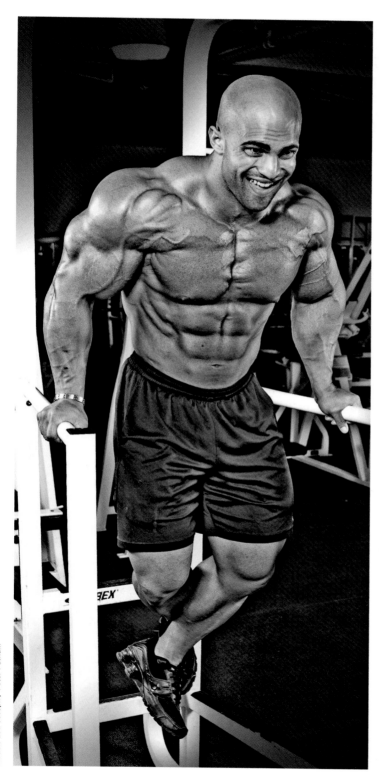

Photo (left to right) by Jason Breeze / Robert Reiff
Models Lou Joseph / Peter Putnam

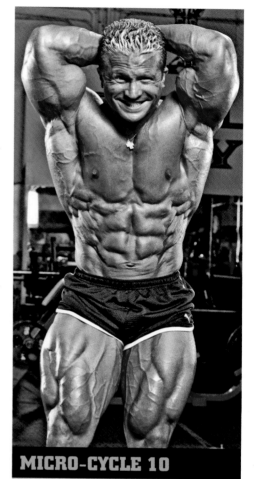

MICRO-CYCLE 10

The tenth cycle is a seven-day restorative period similar to the eighth micro-cycle. Use the first, fourth and seventh days for rest.

DAY	SETS X REPS
DAYS 2 AND 5	
Barbell Back Squat	3-4 x 6-10
Barbell Bench Press	3-4 x 4-6
Combination: Lying EZ-Bar Bent-Arm Pullover and Triceps Extension	2-3 x 6-8
Parallel Bar Dip	2-3 x 6-8
Work your abs hard.	
DAYS 3 AND 6	
Deadlift	4 x 6-8
Wide-Grip Barbell Bent-Over Row	4 x 6-8
Behind-The-Neck Barbell Press	4 x 6
Barbell Curl	4 x 6-10
Work your abs lightly.	

CHAPTER 34

CONTEST PREPARATION

Mike Sable's four-phase approach – including a workout cycle, program prescription, aerobic training and pre-contest dieting – is intricately designed so bodybuilders can peak eight times over a six-month period.

We've always approached our training with the goals of getting into the best shape possible and staying in peak condition. Fortunately, we've been able to learn from some of the greatest bodybuilders in history. From Frank Zane and his 10 Phases of Training to Steve Davis and his Seven Progression Levels of Training, the greats all follow a plan that ensures optimum condition.

Former Mr. America and Mr. World, Mike "The Zipper" Sable also followed a plan. However, Mike's plan was quite different. Mike used a four-phase approach that miraculously had him in peak form eight times over the course of a six-month period. The four phases in this unique approach include a workout cycle, program prescription, aerobic training and pre-contest dieting. The approach led to great successes, including a significant Overall Professional Bodybuilding Association championship.

Mike's workout consisted of eight-day and 10-day training splits. The 10-day training split featured four consecutive workout days followed by a day of rest. On the first day, he trained his legs. The second day featured chest, triceps and traps workouts. On day three, Mike exercised his biceps and back. The deltoids were then worked on day four. The fifth day was reserved for rest. This pattern was then repeated once again in days six through ten.

The eight-day training split followed a similar pattern. Mike worked out for three consecutive days and then rested on the fourth. On the first day he trained his legs and shoulders. His back and biceps were trained on the second day. In the third day, the traps, triceps and chest were trained. Mike rested on day four and repeated this cycle on the fifth through eighth days.

On his road to winning the Overall Professional Bodybuilding Association championship, Mike divided his time into quarters. Depending on the amount of time between contests, the length of time in the quarters would vary. For discussion's sake, let's assume each quarter was 30 days. Mike used the ten-day and eight-day split methods throughout the period. If you're seeking his type of success try following his example.

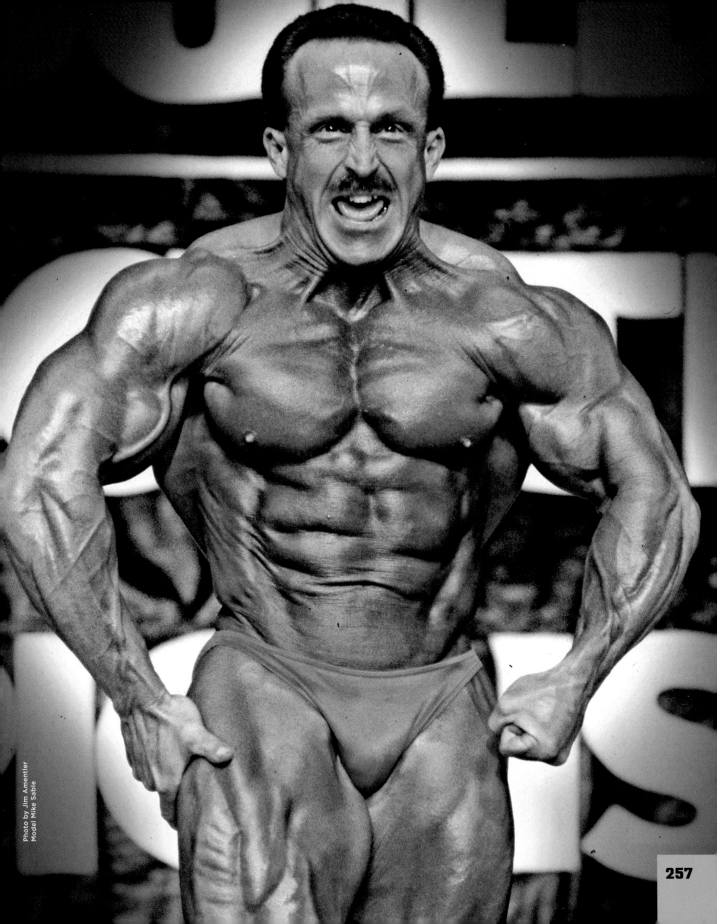

257

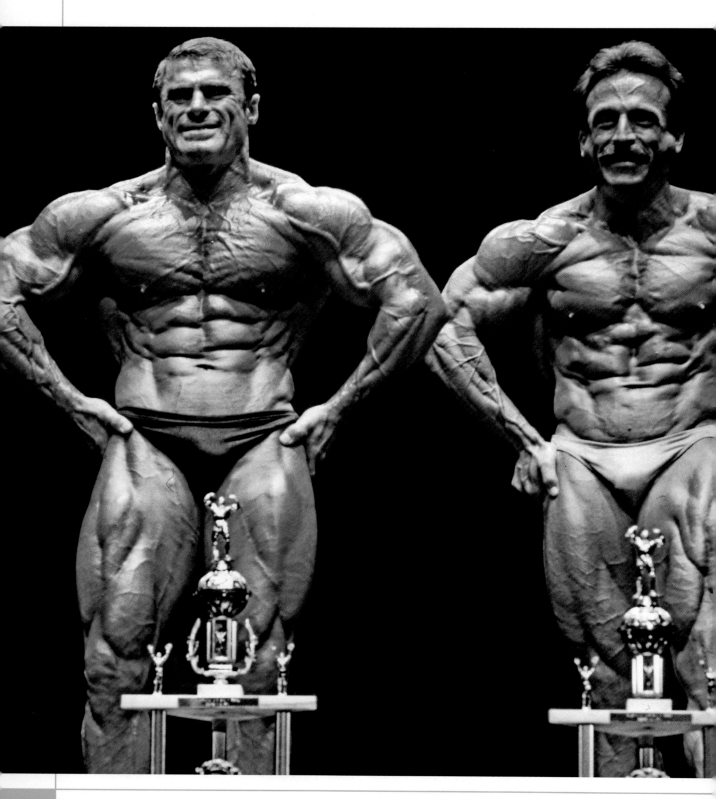

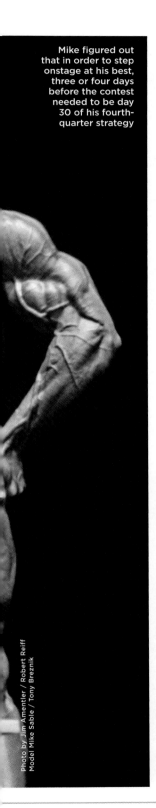

Mike figured out that in order to step onstage at his best, three or four days before the contest needed to be day 30 of his fourth-quarter strategy

Photo by Jim Amentler / Robert Reiff
Model Mike Sable / Tony Breznik

FOUR QUARTERS

If you're planning on using Mike's championship method, in the first quarter you should use two core-growth free-weight-only movements for each muscle group you'll be training. It's important to use the pyramid principle of steadily increasing the poundage while decreasing the corresponding rep scheme (12, 10, 8, 6, 4) for five sets each. You should finish by performing one muscle-specific exercise for three sets of eight reps.

In the second quarter, you should once again perform two core-growth free-weight-only movements. However, instead of decreasing reps while increasing your poundage, you should alter your rep scheme (12, 10, 8, 10, 12). Upon completing this, finish off with two isolation exercises for three sets of eight reps.

The third quarter should consist of the same pyramiding principles and free-weight-only movements. You should also include some variable resistance and cable machine work performed in a tri-set fashion.

Finally, the fourth quarter should feature the use of cable equipment and variable-resistance machines for muscle isolation. Use no free weights or any of the pyramiding principles that were used in the previous three quarters. You could also use supersetting techniques. Mike ensured that day 30 of the fourth quarter would arrive three or four days before a contest.

Mike spent the first two-and-a-half quarters, or 65 percent of his pre-contest training, using the 10-day-split method. The remaining one-and-a-half quarters, or 35 percent of his training, he used the eight-day-split method. Mike's aerobic sessions began at 30 minutes and gradually increased to 60 minutes during the four quarters. Unfortunately, the frequency of his aerobic training is unknown.

PRE-CONTEST DIET

To say that Mike's pre-contest diet is surprising is an understatement. While most bodybuilders cut calories, Mike actually continually increased his daily caloric intake by 100 calories throughout the four quarters. Mike feasted on six hearty meals each day. The meals consisted of such things as oatmeal, chicken breast, tuna, halibut, shark, baked potatoes, steamed vegetables, tomatoes, raw onions, egg whites and assorted fruits. The results speak for themselves. Mike was able to gain 18 pounds of rock-hard muscle and thereby create a championship physique following such a diet and training program.

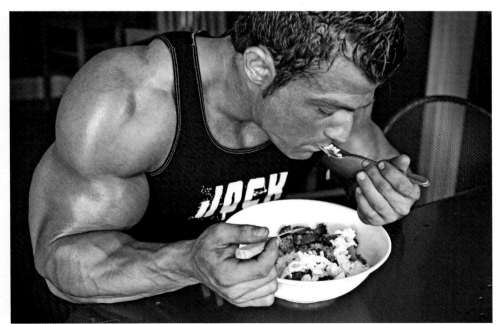

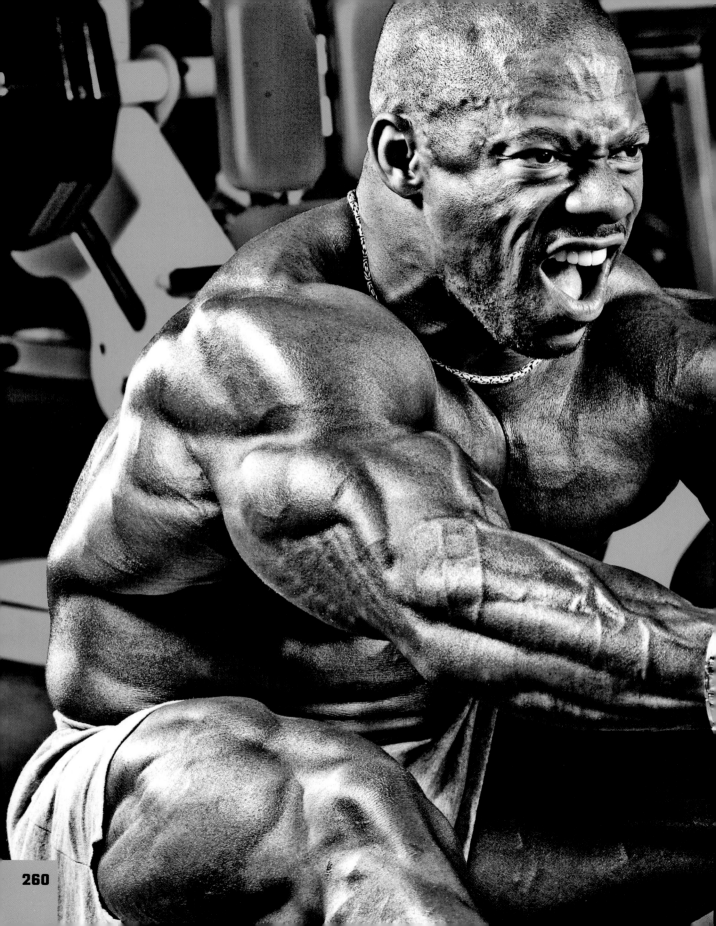

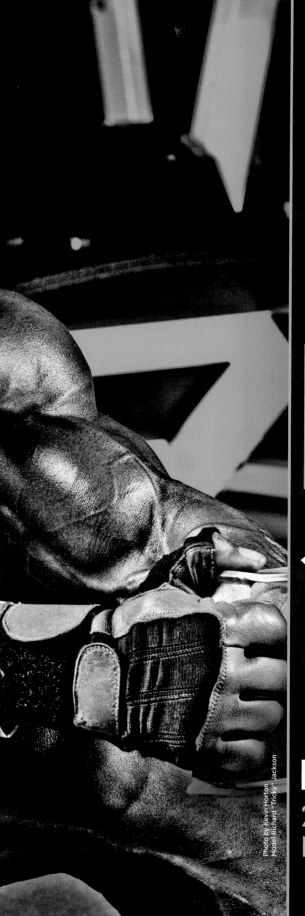

BOOK
10

29 Red-Line Intensity
Manipulation Techniques

CHAPTER 35

TECHNIQUES 1 TO 29

Keep your training fresh and your muscles constantly facing new demands with endless combinations of 29 effective techniques.

To increase your muscle size and strength, you must carefully place new demands on your muscles. Here are some unique and easy strategies that are sure to provide you with optimum muscle blasting. Don't use all of these techniques at one time, as this would increase your risk of overtraining. At most, use two or three of them so your central nervous system remains activated, fresh and in a constant state of adaptation.

BURNS

Burns are a type of partial cramping movement that can be used during and at the end of a set. For example, at the top of your barbell curl, lower the barbell back about three inches from the top position and immediately curl the barbell back to full tension at your neck. Hold the tension about one-quarter of a second, then lower the barbell back and contract to full tension. Each burn should accumulate more tension than the last.

One way to work burns into your plan is to perform two complete full-range reps of an exercise, then two burns, and so on, until you've completed your set. Another way to introduce burns into your rep pattern is to do six to ten at the end of a set when you can't do any more full-range reps.

BURNOUT CHALLENGE

With a training partner of equal strength, select an exercise (we'll use barbell curls) and a poundage that will allow you 12 reps. Do 12 reps, then immediately have your partner do a set of 12. When your partner's set is complete, grab the barbell and do a maximum repetition set. (Vary the hand spacing on the bar from set to set.) You should perform all sets to momentary positive failure. The first person who fails to correctly execute a maximum triple set loses the challenge.

CUMULATIVE REPETITIONS CLARIFIED

This technique can be utilized in bodyweight-only exercises (incline sit-up, parallel bar dip, pull-up, push-up, seated-position dip, sissy squat, one-leg squat, squat jumps and others) and in free-weight exercises. As an example of bodyweight-only exercises, let's consider the parallel bar dip. Do one rep and then rest for two seconds. Then do two reps and rest again for two seconds. Continue this way by doing three reps and

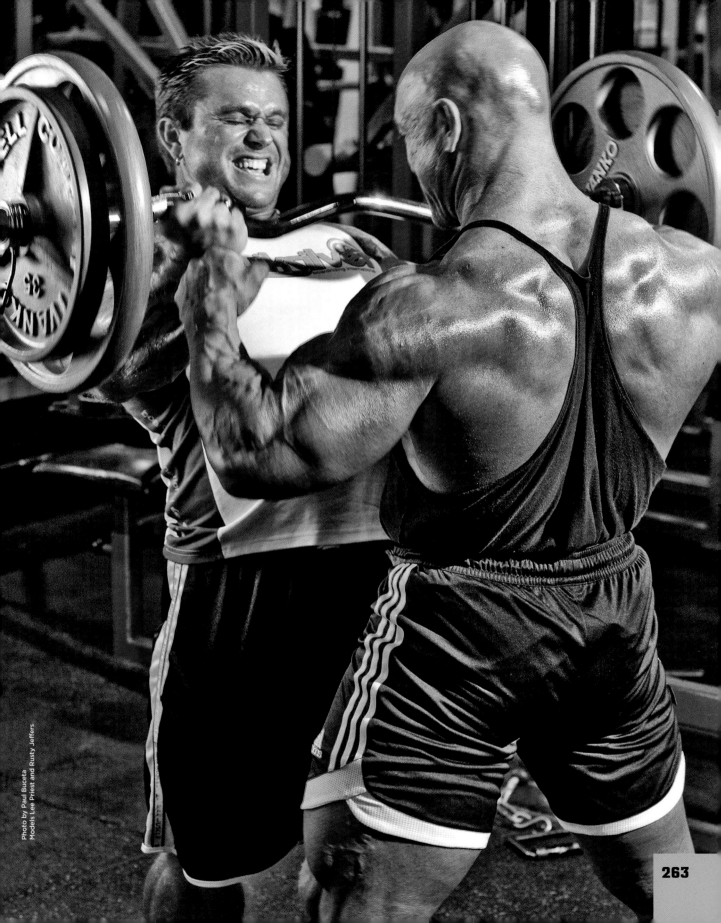

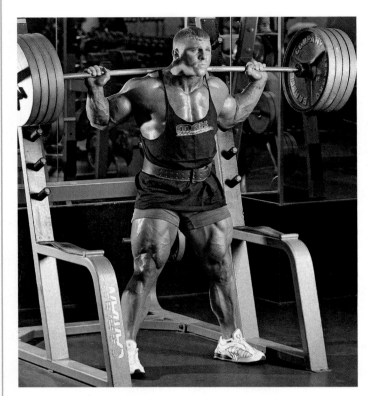

The squat rack can be a very useful tool for quickly racking and unracking the bar between sets.

three to five reps in proper form. Perform one rep of the high-bar Olympic-style barbell squat and then put the barbell back into the squat rack and rest for 10 seconds. Perform two reps and then take a 10-second rest. Then do three reps and take a 10-second rest. Continue increasing your rep count until you simply can't do anymore. For example, let's say you worked up to four reps and find that after the 10-second rest you can't do another five reps. At this point, stop performing the high-bar Olympic-style barbell squat for this workout. Continue from workout to workout using the same poundage until you are able to complete eight reps successfully. After you've reached this goal, a poundage increase is in order. Add only enough poundage to drop your repetition scheme back down to a base of three to five reps and begin this cycle over again.

The base repetition of three to five should be used only with general or anabolic core growth exercises, as well as some tendon-strengthening movements. The best way to apply the cumulative rep plan to a specific exercise is to begin with a rep base of 10 and gradually work up to a goal of 15 reps. When you reach 15 reps, you'll essentially be entering into a dimension of endurance training with a poundage you previously used for building strength.

DEMON TRAINING TECHNIQUE

The Demon Training technique (or Past Failure training technique) was popularized by the late Trevor Smith. Performing this technique, you'll be faced with at least one of four demons: The pre-exhaust principle, regular reps to positive failure, forced reps or drop sets. Demon Training provides an intense shock to the central nervous system and muscles that even the most experienced trainers will feel. This training technique suggests that sets performed for muscle-specific and anabolic core growth exercises be carried to momentary muscle failure (where you can't complete a full range of motion on your own). Once that happens, your training partner or spotter must assist you in completing an additional number of forced reps (six to eight) before you stop.

resting again for two seconds. Maintain this pattern until you simply cannot exceed your previous rep count. For example, if you get up to 10 reps and find that after a two-second rest you can't do 11 reps, consider this set complete. We recommend a maximum of 25 reps. Remember: Your objective is to get your muscles accustomed to doing more reps with each workout.

We realize that your success or failure in performing a bodyweight-only exercise is directly related to your weight. If you weigh 175 pounds, chances are you'll have an easier time completing more reps than if you weigh over 200 pounds. If your weight proves prohibitive, then use this technique instead: Work up to 10 repetitions and then back down to one.

The instruction for free-weight exercises is somewhat different from that of a bodyweight-only exercise. The exciting part about training with cumulative repetitions as it applies to free weights is the progressive levels you can place on your muscles. Let's assume that you decide to do the high-bar Olympic-style barbell squat. Use a poundage that will allow you to blast out

Photo by Jason Mathas
Model Ty Young

You'll feel as though you're in terrible agony and your muscles will be pumped beyond belief, but you're not finished yet! Your training partner must immediately decrease the poundage by 30 to 40 percent. Continue the set until you can't perform another rep. Once again your training partner must help you get additional reps.

Your training partner will now decrease the poundage so you can continue your journey into the growth zone. Whenever you begin to fail, your partner must assist you. It may make you feel nauseated and give you tremendous pain, but that's the only way to complete the exercise.

DEMON TRAINING QUADS EXERCISE
Pre-Exhaust 1
Leg Extension

Set 1: Select a poundage you can do on your own for 10 to 12 solid reps. Perform the leg extensions in a rhythmic manner (for example, three seconds up and then three seconds down). Once you hit positive failure, have your partner assist you in completing an additional eight reps past positive failure.

Set 2: Have your partner immediately decrease the poundage by 30 to 40 percent and then continue performing reps until you achieve positive failure without help. Have your partner assist you in completing an additional six to eight reps.

Set 3: Decrease the resistance by an additional 30 to 40 percent and continue performing reps until failure. Once you reach failure, have your partner assist you in completing an additional eight reps.

The first series is always the easiest. You'll find your anxiety levels building as you prepare to start the following:

Pre-Exhaust 2
Leg Extension

Repeat the exact same procedure as described in Pre-Exhaust 1. Upon completion of Pre-Exhaust 2 leg extensions, you'll likely be ready to call it a day. But it's not over yet!

ANABOLIC CORE-GROWTH EXERCISE
Barbell Back Squat, Leg Press or Hack Squat, One Set Only (Regular and Forced Reps)

Choose one of the three squatting exercises listed and load up the bar or machine with enough

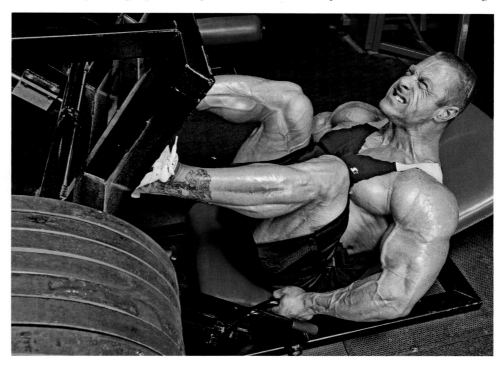

Photo by Kevin Horton
Model Ed van Amsterdam

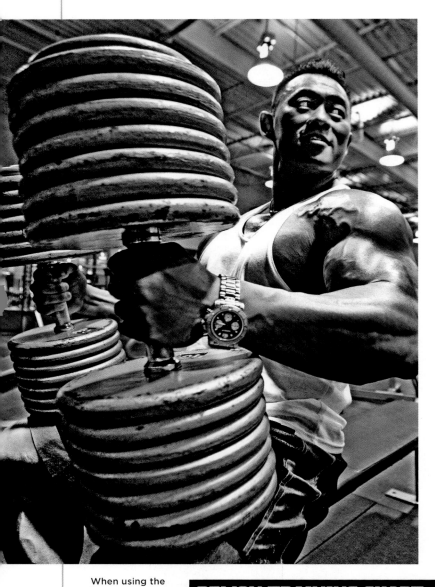

poundage to successfully perform eight to ten reps. Remember to have your partner nearby as you perform your set. When you reach positive failure, have your spotter assist you in getting a few reps (five or six) beyond failure and then call it a day. On to hamstrings!

HAMSTRINGS
Pre-Exhaust 1
(Sets 1 & 2)
Leg Curl

Follow the same principles you used during the leg extensions, but do two sets. Pay attention to your instincts. After the first set you may have nothing left in the tank. You may have so much blood in your quads that it'll be very painful to perform a curling motion. Suffer through if you can. After following these Demon Training principles, you will jumpstart your body to new levels of muscle growth.

ANABOLIC CORE-GROWTH EXERCISE
Stiff-Leg Barbell Deadlift (3/5 range movement) One Set Only (Regular and Forced Reps)

Follow the instructions given for the anabolic "core growth" exercise squat movement.

CALVES
Pre-Exhaust 1 & 2
(Sets 1, 2 and 3)
Seated Calf Raise

ANABOLIC CORE-GROWTH EXERCISE
Standing Calf Raise One Set Only (Regular and Forced Reps)

When using the Demon Training System, make sure your time in the gym is no more than 45 minutes per session – this program is painful.

DEMON TRAINING CHART
This chart illustrates Demon Training for other muscle groups.

	PRE-EXHAUST 1 & 2 (SETS 1, 2, 3)	ONE SET ONLY (REGULAR & FORCED REPS)
MUSCLE GROUP	MUSCLE SPECIFIC EXERCISES	ANABOLIC "CORE GROWTH" EXERCISES
Back	Pullover Machine or One Dumbbell Pullover	Bent-Over Row and Lat Pulldown
Chest	Pec Deck or Dumbbell Flye	Incline Barbell Press or Smith-Machine Incline Bench Press
Delts	Single-Arm Low-Pulley Cable Lateral or Dumbbell Lateral Raise	Overhead Barbell Press of Smith-Machine Incline Bench Press
Triceps	Triceps Pressdown	Close-Grip Barbell Bench Press
Biceps	Concentration Curl	Narrow-Grip Chin-Up

Photo by Paul Buceta
Model Jea Jung

6 DEMON TRAINING
BASIC REQUIREMENTS

1. Take an hour after your workout to recover before resuming your daily activities.
2. You can't train in this manner for more than five or six weeks at a time.
3. Train only once a day for a maximum of four times per week, and take rest days. Here's a typical schedule you might want to follow:

    Day 1: Chest and calves
    Day 2: Delts and triceps
    Day 3: Off
    Day 4: Back and biceps
    Day 5: Quads and hams
    Day 6: Off
    Day 7: Off

4. Spend a maximum of 45 minutes in the gym per workout session.
5. Demon Training is extremely painful. You may experience anxiety before a workout.
6. You must keep all other physical activities to a bare minimum during your five- or six-week training cycle. Doing so will ensure that you reach maximum recovery and have energy available for workouts.

It's imperative that you get plenty of sleep and have adequate nutrients in your body at all times. We want to make it perfectly clear: As opposed to Mike Mentzer's stance on Heavy Duty Training, we don't think of Demon Training as the only way a bodybuilder should train. There are many paths to the mountaintop. Some are more painful but can yield greater results. In the end, it's your choice. Perhaps the greatest challenges you'll face using Demon Training will be fighting the urge to train more than four days per week, and generating sufficient intensity to make certain you go beyond failure.

DOGGCRAPP TRAINING

Doggcrapp Training is a weight-training method created by Dante Trudel, a southern California power bodybuilder. Dante promoted it heavily back in the mid-nineties in his bimonthly journal called *Hardcore Muscle*. At the time, it was simply known as a multi-rep rest / pause theory, which employed the use of very heavy weights on compound exercises.

Recently we began to hear stories about IFBB pro bodybuilder David Henry and the sensational muscle gains he was making with a

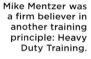

Mike Mentzer was a firm believer in another training principle: Heavy Duty Training.

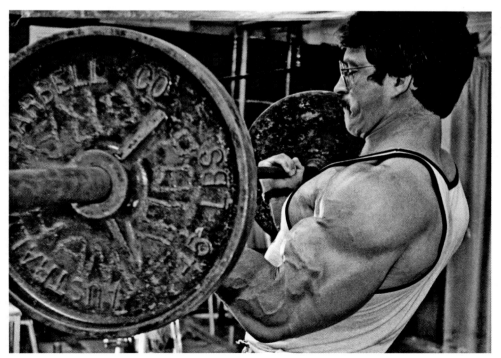

Model Mike Mentzer

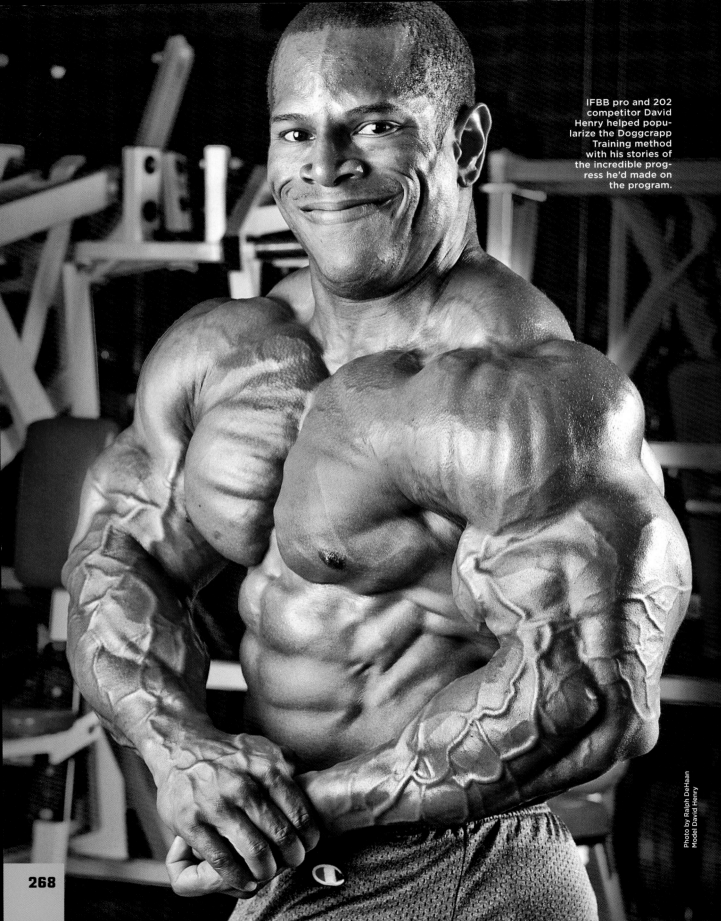

IFBB pro and 202 competitor David Henry helped popularize the Doggcrapp Training method with his stories of the incredible progress he'd made on the program.

program called Doggcrapp Training. When we found out he was training under the guidance of Dante, suddenly it all made sense. What we had known earlier as the multi-rep rest / pause theory had been re-dubbed Doggcrapp Training. (Doggcrapp was the screen name Dante used around a decade ago when he wrote posts discussing his training protocol.)

WWE Hall of Famer Ricky "The Dragon" Steamboat once said that to become a successful main event wrestler it was necessary to have some sort of hook that would spark interest and generate worldwide publicity. With that theory in mind, the unusual name of Doggcrapp Training certainly makes sense. Once you add in the association of popular IFBB pro bodybuilder David Henry, the newfound success of the weight-training method is unsurprising. It's sad to say, but without a big name on board many worthwhile training concepts never reach the level of prominence they might deserve.

DOGGCRAPP FLAT-BENCH BARBELL PRESS

As a hypothetical example assume you can do 200 pounds for eight to ten hard-fought reps. Do three specific warm-up sets in a moderate to fast, controlled cadence. The first will be 60 pounds (30 percent of the eight- to ten-rep maximum) x 10 reps, then 100 pounds (50 percent) x 8 and finally 160 pounds (80 percent) x 4. With these out of the way, perform the main pec-bursting set with 200 pounds and do it in Doggcrapp style for three all-out sets, as follows:

Set 1: 8-10 reps to positive failure (10-15 deep breaths)

Set 2: 3-4 reps to positive failure (10-15 deep breaths)

Set 3: 1-3 reps to positive failure

On the final rep of the third set, do a 20-second static hold (iso-tension) three or four inches from a peak contraction lockout position. Then, immediately upon finishing the static hold, do 60 to 90 seconds of fascia stretching.

Push the barriers and explode in the positive phase of the flat-bench barbell press (two seconds or less). On the negative return (down phase) of the main set (200 pounds), it's very important to take eight seconds lowering the bar down to your chest. Remember, this applies only to the main set and not the three warm-up sets. All of the muscle fibers in your pecs will feel as though they've been pounded into oblivion the next morning because the flat-bench barbell press is a brutal exercise when done Doggcrapp style.

Three anabolic core-growth exercises (never muscle-specific or shape-training exercises) are recommended for each muscle group when training Doggcrapp style. However, all three are not to be performed in the same workout. For instance, in the first training session of the week for your pecs, perform only one exercise. Let's assume you're going to do the flat-bench barbell press. On the second non-consecutive training session for your pecs, you might consider doing the incline barbell press. When a third training session is scheduled, use yet another exercise, such as the Smith-machine decline press.

Every three pec workouts, rotate through the three individual exercises and then start the rotation over again. Always try to increase the resistance at least two-and-a-half to five pounds in each exercise when doing a new rotation. You should train each major or minor muscle group only twice on non-consecutive training days (an eight-day period). If you have above normal (localized muscle and central nervous system) recovery abilities, you can train the same muscle group twice in a seven-day period. Check out some of the split routines in this book – you'll find them especially helpful when putting together a Doggcrapp training program. As with any intense training of this nature, Doggcrapp training will remain effective for about 10 to 12 weeks. At that point you will require a 10- to 21-day layoff.

EXTENDED SETS

This dual-purpose training principle was developed by Joe Weider for targeting muscle power, size and definition within a certain bodypart. The conventional set-rest-set training stimulated either more muscle power and size or definition, but usually not both. With this training principle Joe covered both aspects of development. Here are a few examples of Extended Sets:

LATS

Part 1: Wide-grip front lat pulldown (to upper chest) – five sets of six reps
Part 2: Close reverse-grip front lat pulldown (to upper chest) – five sets of 10 to 12 reps

CHEST

Part 1: Wide-grip barbell bench press – five sets of six reps
Part 2: Narrow-grip barbell bench press – five sets of eight to twelve reps

DELTS

Part 1: 60- to 70-degree incline dumbbell laterals (supine) – five sets of six reps
Part 2: 60- to 70-degree incline dumbbell laterals (prostate) – five sets of eight to ten reps

TRICEPS

Part 1: Lying (flat bench) barbell kickback – five sets of six reps
Part 2: Lying (flat bench) half-movement barbell kickback – five sets of 10 to 12 reps

BICEPS

Part 1: Incline dumbbell curl – five sets of six reps
Part 2: Incline dumbbell curl with hands at side near parallel to body (half crucifix) – five sets of eight to ten reps

To further clarify the extended set principle, let's use the lat exercises as an example. Begin by performing wide-grip front lat pulldowns (to upper chest) for one set of six heavy reps, and then immediately do the close reverse-grip lat pulldowns (to upper chest) for one ruthless set of 10 to 12 reps. Once you've completed those reps, take a 60- to 90-second rest. Immediately after this period, perform another set of both exercises. Repeat this procedure until you've completed five sets of each exercise.

The transition from Part 1 to Part 2 of an exercise is usually nothing more than a simple change in positioning as well as an increase in the repetition factor. With a little ingenuity, chances are you'll be able to come up with some

other exercises to do in extended-set fashion. You might even want to try doing six reps in part one and then a ruthless 20 reps for part two.

UNORTHODOX EXTENDED SETS

When performing unorthodox extended sets it's important not to waste any time between the first and second exercises. For the lats and biceps exercises, do not let go of the bar; simply lean back and begin performing the upper pulley cable curl exercise.

QUADS/CALVES

Part 1: Leg press
Part 2: Leg press calf raise

LATS/ABS

Part 1: Pull-up
Part 2: Hanging knee raise

LATS/BICEPS

Part 1: Reverse-grip lat pulldown to chest
Part 2: High-pully cable curl to forehead

MODIFIED REPS

"The Golden Eagle" Tom Platz was known to use this set-extender technique when training for his impressive showings at the IFBB Mr. Olympia contests. Once you've completed your absolute maximum, full range-of-motion reps to positive and negative failure, continue to move the bar through a partial range of motion. This may be a three-quarter, half or quarter-rep (such partial reps are scarcely visible to the untrained eye when training the calves and forearms). As long as you can still move the barbell, your muscles are firing and contracting against the resistance. The set ends when you are squeezing and contracting the muscles but there's absolutely no movement.

WHAT IS FST-7?

FST-7 is a training system Hany Rambod devised after years of research and a great deal of trial and error with many of his pro bodybuilding clients. FST-7 stands for Fascia Stretch Training, and the seven refers to the seven sets of 8 to 12 reps (rest 30 to 45 seconds between sets) performed for the final exercise of a target muscle group. Here's an example of FST-7:

EXERCISE	REP RANGE
Dumbbell Curls	3-4 x 8-12
Preacher Bench Curls	3 x 8-12
FST-7: EZ-Bar Curls	7 x 8-12*
*Rest 30-45 seconds between sets.	

Hany has had many of his client's use this system for overall growth and especially to improve stubborn muscle groups that were seemingly resistant to just about anything else the person had tried. For more detailed training information on FST-7 go to www.fst-7.com.

FORCED REPS (ASSISTED REPS)

A forced rep is an extension of a particular set of reps where your strength level has been reduced to a point of positive failure (where you can no longer move the weight under your own power). To clarify, let's assume that you have chosen to perform a set of barbell presses for eight to twelve reps. A quick look at the Holistic Training Guide (p. 485) indicates that you should use 80 percent of your one-rep max in order to accomplish this set. Taking into account the high and low reps (eight to as many as twelve), you might hit the point of positive failure on the 11th rep. You're simply not strong enough to accomplish reps 11 and 12 because your strength has been reduced to less than your one-rep max.

At this point, a training partner should immediately help you push or pull the weight through the point of positive failure for two or three additional reps. In order to achieve maximum intensity, your training partner must give you only enough assistance to make up the difference between your existing strength level and your original one-rep max poundage. One way to be sure just enough assistance is being applied in a forced rep is for your training partner to count off the seconds required to push the weight up. If the weight is being pushed up to lockout in less than two seconds, the spotter might be assisting you more than he should. Likewise, if it takes longer than 10 seconds, he might not be helping you enough.

Forced reps success is dictated by the recovery rate of a particular muscle group, diet, attitude and physical environment. This type of training is not for beginners, those who are coming off a training layoff or bodybuilders who are plagued with a training injury, because it can lead to overtraining or a worsened injury in these individuals.

Advanced bodybuilders generally approach their forced-rep style of training in one of three different ways. They might do one forced-rep workout per week for each bodypart, or they

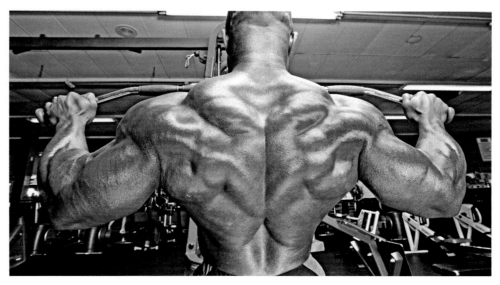

With the Extended Sets System you transition from part one to part two of a move (e.g., wide-grip to front reverse grip of the front lat pulldown), doing one set of each, before resting.

may do forced reps at every other workout. Some bodybuilders will do two forced-rep workouts in succession followed by three regular workouts without forced reps. Of the three training situations, the most sensible is the first, especially if you want to avoid overtraining and tendon and ligament injury.

GIANT SETS

Giant sets are an extension of supersets and tri-sets, where you perform anywhere from four to six exercises for either one particular muscle group or two opposite muscle groups. It's very important that you do your exercises in sequence, one right after the other, without the rest you would normally take between exercises. Take only one to two minutes of rest after you've completed the last exercise in the sequence before beginning a second or third giant set sequence.

You can vary your approach to performing giant sets in any number of ways. One sugges-

tion is using a general exercise followed by a specific exercise. In other words, your first, third, and fifth exercises are the heavier size- and power-building movements, while your second, fourth and sixth exercises are the lighter muscle-specific isolation or shaping movements. You could also reverse the order and do a combined pre-exhaustion giant set. Here's how:

CHEST GIANT SET

1. Dumbbell flye
2. Barbell bench press
3. Incline dumbbell flye
4. Incline barbell bench press
5. Decline dumbbell flye
6. Decline barbell bench press

Exercises one and two work the mid-pecs, three and four hit your clavicular or high-pec region, while the the fifth and sixth exercises finish off your lower pecs.

If you're considering a pre-exhaust giant set for your back, try the following:

BACK GIANT SET

1. Bent-over lateral raise
2. Bent-over row
3. Decline pullover
4. Lat pulldown
5. Hyperextension
6. Stiff-leg deadlift

The first and second exercises work your middle lat and rhomboids, the third and fourth work your upper/outer lats, and exercises five and six work your erectors spinae. To work your trapezius rather than your middle lats you could replace the first two exercises with barbell shrugs and power cleans.

Remember the double pre-exhaustion sequence (one specific exercise followed by a general and finished up with a specific) mentioned in the information on tri-sets? Instead of working one particular bodypart, why not work opposing parts? Using the chest and back examples, simply arrange the sequence so that chest exercises one, two and three are followed by back exercises one, two and three. You could work the biceps and triceps, erectors spinae

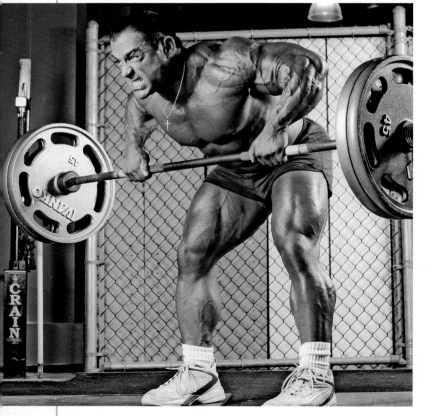

The bent-over row works well in a giant set for back to target your middle lats and rhomboids.

Photo by Ralph DeHaan
Model Mike Ergas

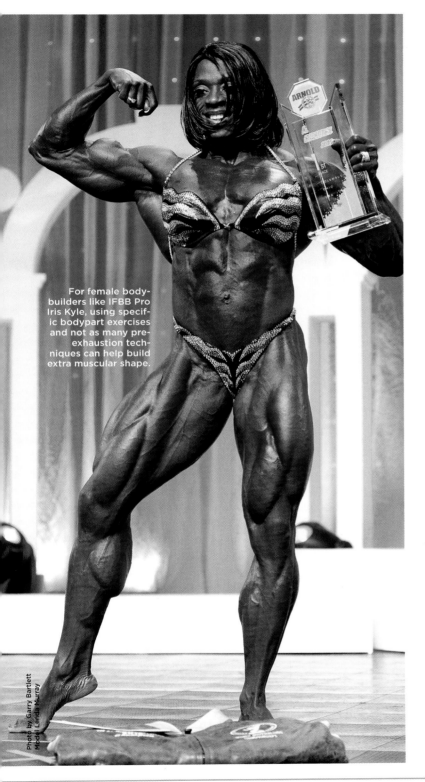

For female body-builders like IFBB Pro Iris Kyle, using specific bodypart exercises and not as many pre-exhaustion techniques can help build extra muscular shape.

Photo by Garry Bartlett
Model Lenda Murray

and abs, delts and traps or quads and hamstrings using the same method.

Another way to vary your giant sets is through the use of specific exercises and fewer pre-exhaustion techniques. This method is appropriate for female bodybuilders who wish to add extra shape to their muscles. You can perform four to six specific exercises for one particular bodypart, or two or three specific exercises each for two opposing bodyparts. If you're an intermediate or advanced bodybuilder, use the minimum number of exercises and perform only two cycles of the giant set for one particular muscle group or four cycles for a giant set consisting of two bodyparts. If you're an intermediate bodybuilder looking at specialization, it's a good idea to do three cycles with five exercises per giant set. For those of you who are advanced bodybuilders, you'll find you may want to perform six exercises and four cycles.

Here are a couple more examples of some intriguing giant sets:

JOHN PARILLO'S MENTAL ACUITY GIANT SET (QUADS & HAMSTRINGS)

Leg Curl 20 reps	
Leg Extensions 20 reps	
Leg Press 20 reps	
Safety Squat Bar or Barbell Back Squat 20 reps	
EZ-Bar Squat (hold bar overhead) 20 reps	

*Do one giant set, rest two minutes and repeat.

SUPER GIANT SET SHOULDER BLITZ

Overhead Barbell Press	1 x 8–12
Barbell Upright Row	1 x 8–12
Lateral Raise	1 x 8–12
Barbell Shrug	1 x 8–12
Overhead Barbell Press	1 x 8–12
Barbell Upright Row	1 x 8–12
Bent-Over Dumbbell Lateral Raise	1 x 8–12
Barbell Shrug	1 x 8–12

HEAVY-LIGHT SYSTEM

If you follow the Heavy-Light system exactly the way it was originally intended, you will develop maximum size, power and shape. The deltoids are a great example. Flip to the back of the book and consult with the Holistic Exercise Selection Chart (on p. 480-484). Choose one core-growth or general exercise from Group 1 and one muscle-specific exercise from Group 2. Let's say your selections are the seated behind-the-neck barbell press from Group 1 and the seated lateral raise from Group 2. Begin by performing two sets of six to eight reps (with 84 to 88 percent of your one-rep maximum) in the press. Be sure to rest about three minutes between sets. Immediately after you've completed the second set, perform one set of 10 to 12 reps (with approximately 80 percent of your current single-rep maximum) of the lateral raise. Rest one or two minutes and repeat the process.

After you've completed the entire process a second time, take a five-minute rest. This rest period will give you time to select a new core-growth and muscle-specific exercise from the Holistic Exercise Selection Chart. Now go through another series of the Heavy-Light system. Upon completion of this series, you'll have done 12 sets in total (four sets each of two anabolic core-growth exercises and two sets each of two muscle-specific exercises). An intermediate bodybuilder will find this is an excellent method to specialize on a muscle group. An advanced bodybuilder could adapt this method of training for a specialization program simply by performing four sets for each of three general exercises and two sets for each of the selected three muscle-specific exercises (performing a total of 18 sets).

MUSCLE ROUNDS

The foundation of the Titan Training system, Muscle Rounds is one of the most ingenious and simple intensity techniques for increasing muscle gains. Select a poundage that allows you a maximum of eight to ten reps in a muscle-specific or core-growth exercise. Perform four full reps with a 10-second rest. The four full reps plus 10-second rest is one round. Fol-

For the Heavy-Light System, the behind-the-neck barbell press is a good core growth exercise option for the heavy portion.

low those directions again for five more rounds. Six Muscle Rounds equals one series. For each particular exercise, perform four series, resting for roughly one minute after each.

If you've chosen the correct poundage for Muscle Rounds, you will find the first three reps fairly easy to complete. However, beginning with reps four through six, your muscles will almost immediately go into lactic-acid paralysis. You'll have to be extremely tenacious to make your muscles contract during the final three reps. It may seem hopeless to complete, but don't give up. By persisting, you'll be training your muscles to obey your will.

MYO-GENETIC SET

Dr. G. Kerry Knowlton, a former pro wrestler and chiropractor, came up with the idea of the Myo-Genetic Set. The Myo-Genetic Set is generally known as a strip set, but is more structured. The basic six-step premise is:

1. Always warm up with a muscle-specific (isolation) exercise before beginning steps two and three.
2. Load up a barbell with an amount near your one-rep max.
3. Do your first rep. If the weight is not quite heavy enough, then use very strict form and do a super-slow rep (10 seconds up and 10 seconds down). If the weight is too heavy, then you may use some controlled cheating. After a few workouts, you'll be able to gauge your starting poundage more accurately.
4. After each single rep, quickly remove enough poundage that you can get another. Don't stop or rest.
5. Perform eight to ten consecutive single reps (with a subsequent decrease in poundage) per set. Do only one or two sets per muscle group. Do only four to six sets per workout and only on compound or core-growth exercises (barbell squat, bench press, deadlift, curl, etc) and not on muscle-specific, or isolation exercises (dumbbell flye, lateral raise, etc)
6. Work each muscle group only once per week and continue this program for a maximum of four to six weeks.

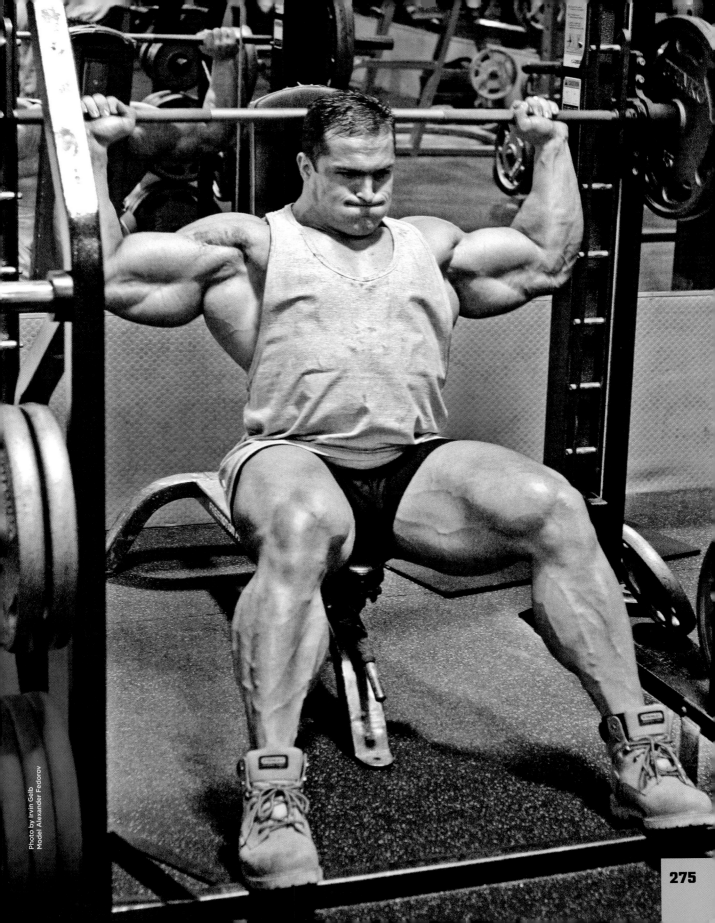

275

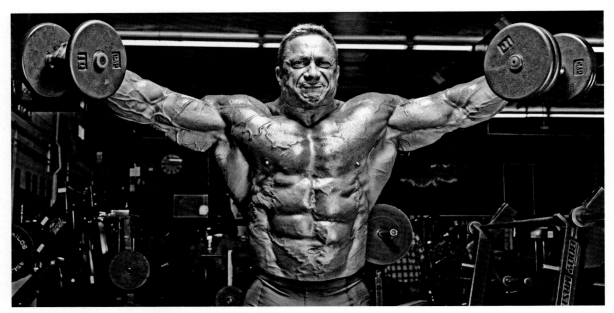

To perform negatives correctly, the negative portion of one rep (lowering the dumbbells back to the start position shown here) should take four to five seconds.

NEGATIVE TRAINING

Negatives (eccentric contractions) are basically the contractions of a muscle belly while it's being lengthened. The negative phase of the bench press would be the process of lowering the weight from the extended-arms position (where the pecs are contracted) to chest level (where the pecs are stretched). Generally you can do a negative with 20 to 40 percent more poundage than you can lift in the positive phase.

This method of training offers the physiological benefit of increased strength by conditioning the body to overload stress. It can also be used in a dual capacity with forced reps. After you've completed the forced-rep portion of a conventional set of bench presses, for example, have a training partner of comparable strength carefully pull the barbell back to arms' length. He will then release the bar and you can bring the barbell to the lowest position of the movement without his aid. At that point, he helps you lift the barbell again.

A properly performed negative rep in a conventional set should take approximately four to five seconds. As a general rule, when the descent takes less than four seconds per rep, it's time to end the set. For the greatest stimulation while performing negatives you should do roughly three reps (never more than six per set).

The purest form of Negative Only (N-O) training is to do one set of eight or nine consecutive reps with a poundage 20 to 30 percent over your one-rep max. Perform the negative phase of each rep (five to eight seconds each) under your own power and be sure that your spotter is available to provide all the necessary assistance through the positive phase of each rep. If you really want to experience the ultimate in N-O training, take a poundage that is 20 to 30 percent over a positive or negative six-rep maximum and perform four sets of six reps. The first three negative reps in each set should take approximately six seconds each, and the final one should take four seconds. This style of training will require the use of at least one spotter. This strategy can be used for any pre-exhaust sequence.

Some bodybuilders carry N-O training to another intensity level. Instead of doing multiple reps, they do a Single-Rep Negative (SRN). Essentially, they take a poundage that is 20 to 30 percent over their one-rep max and attempt to hold it for as long as possible (for example, lockout on a barbell bench press). As their strength depletes, the barbell begins to lower. This means you slowly and deliberately fight the lowering process (never allowing your muscles to relax), taking as long as 40 seconds to

Photo by Kevin Horton
Model Markus Ruhl

complete the negative phase of the rep in good form. It's extremely important to have at least one spotter during this process. For added safety, use a power rack or Smith machine.

Most negative training requires the presence of a spotter. However, you can perform Negative Accentuated (N-A) training by cheating the weight (using your own body momentum) through the positive range of the exercise and then performing the negative rep (usually with 70 percent of the maximum poundage involved that can be lifted with either both of your arms or legs). This would be applicable to most barbell, dumbbell and pulley cable exercises. If you wanted to do unilateral exercises that would solicit the use of an arm (one-arm dumbbell curls) or leg (one-leg squats), you would use the opposite arm or leg to assist you through the positive portion of the exercise.

You need at least 72 hours of recovery time before you can perform another similar work-

out. With that in mind, you might want to try doing negatives no more than twice a week per muscle group. Unless otherwise indicated, you shouldn't perform negatives on more than two sets per exercise, and those two sets should be in the conventional range of six to twelve reps. You might consider doing a brief 15- to 25-minute total-body workout with 10 to 12 reps per muscle group and using a combination of the three negative training styles.

MUSCLE MASS NEGATIVES

Perform four reps to positive failure with the most poundage involved (for example, 200 pounds in the flat barbell bench press). Quickly add 20 percent more to the bar (200 x .20 = 240 pounds) and with the help of a competent spotter do two or three negatives. Each negative should take no less than five seconds to perform. Upon completion of the negatives, rest about a minute and then repeat for two or

Negative Accentuated training can be applied to cable moves like the cable reverse flye by cheating on the positive portion and then performing the negative rep.

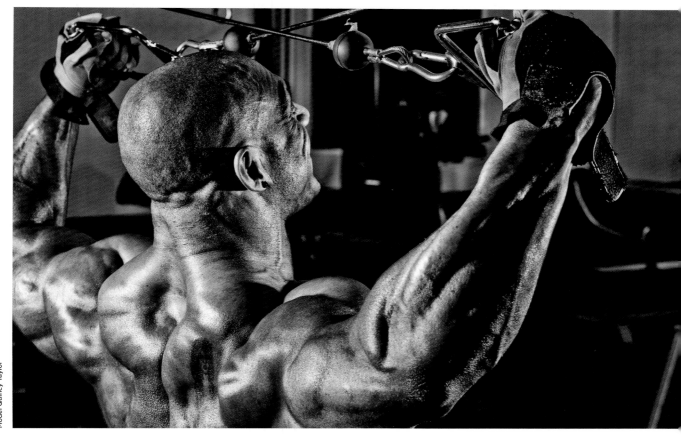

Photo by Paul Buceta
Model Quincy Taylor

three more cycles. To avoid overtraining, muscle mass negatives are best performed once every 10 days.

MUSCLE MASS NEGATIVES AND POSITIVES

Select a poundage for the Smith machine incline bench press or back squat that's approximately 75 percent of your four-rep max. If you're able to perform with a maximum poundage of 200 pounds, this means you should initially load the bar to total 150 pounds.

Perform the Smith machine incline bench press or back squat using a slow, smooth and precise movement for four complete reps to positive failure. Begin the fifth repetition by descending through the negative phase of your rep. When the bar touches your chest or you're in the bottom position of the barbell squat, have a spotter remove 25 pounds off each side of the

Just before stepping onstage, these two pros, Dexter Jackson and Kai Geene, are hoping their training techniques and strategies are enough to earn the title.

bar, leaving it with only 150 pounds (or 75 percent of your four-rep max). Power through the positive phase to the lockout position without any assistance from your spotter. Pause just long enough in the lockout position so your spotter can quickly add 25 pounds to each side of the bar (bringing it back up to 200 pounds) for your negative, at which point your spotter will remove the 25 pounds from each side again. Do a seventh and eighth rep exactly the same way. This completes one set. Rest for five minutes, perform a second set, and rest for another five minutes before completing your third and final set. Remember, you'll be using more weight on the negative phase of the exercises and 25 percent less weight on the positive phase for the fifth through eighth add-on reps in each of the three sets.

Note: Prior to the performance of a heavy or moderate workout for either of the two ex-

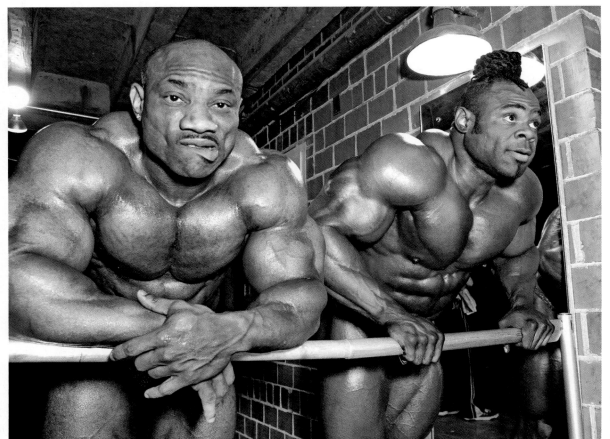

Photo by Rich Baker
Models Dexter Jackson and Kai Greene

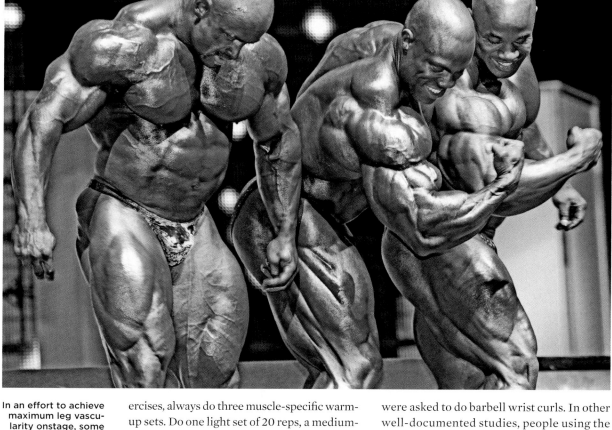

In an effort to achieve maximum leg vascularity onstage, some competitors elevate their legs backstage so when they step out in front of the judges, the blood vessels are popping.

ercises, always do three muscle-specific warm-up sets. Do one light set of 20 reps, a medium-weight set for 15 reps and then a medium-heavy set for 15 reps. After that point you're ready for your work sets.

OCCLUSION TRAINING

Occlusion training originated at the University of Tokyo. To train this way, you cut off the blood supply to your worked muscles by pumping up a blood-pressure cuff or velcro straps on the upper arms or thighs for two minutes. During the two-minute period, exercise with slightly less than 50 percent of your maximum for roughly 20 seconds. After the two-minute period elapses, quickly remove the cuff or straps. A rush of blood will reach your muscles. It's our understanding that a 20-percent strength gain can be achieved using this technique as was evident in some test studies where subjects were asked to do barbell wrist curls. In other well-documented studies, people using the technique for a 14-day period made an eight percent gain in quad muscle size using leg extensions. These results are especially remarkable considering that those same subjects made only a seven percent gain in the previous four months of conventional training.

A variant of the occlusion technique has been used backstage at bodybuilding contests. Bodybuilders keep their legs elevated (with no pressure cuffs or velcro straps attached) for a period of time and then step onto the stage to pose with the blood vessels in their legs popping, thereby creating a rather dramatic vascular look. You can achieve a similar effect with timed breath control during posing.

We must caution you that if the pressure cuff is too tight or it it's on for too long, it could cause thrombosis. We feel two minutes is short

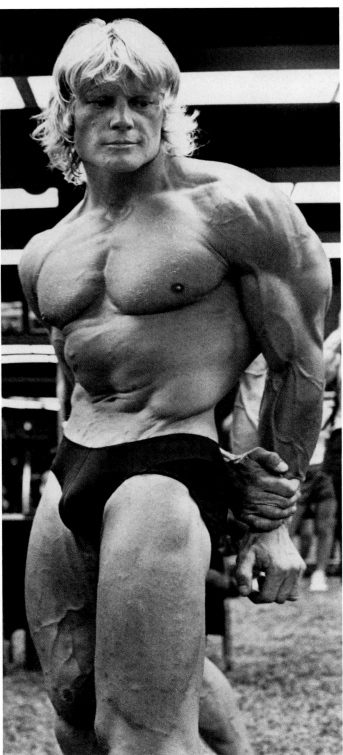

Model Dave Draper

enough that this should not happen. Body-builders who are on anabolic steroids should be especially careful because they may be candidates for hemorrhages – they're already over-hydrated and have their blood vessels expanded to the max.

Steve Holman and Jonathan Lawson address a modified version of occlusion training in their *Ultimate Mass Workout.* We believe that occlusion training is probably a waste if you're dedicated to building strength simply because nerve stimulation of muscle fibers is more important than the blood supply (at least in the early stages of heavy training).

PRE-EXHAUST PRINCIPLE

The Pre-Exhaust Principle was invented by one of the authors of this book, Robert Kennedy, back in the late 1960s, and it continues to be used by bodybuilding champions looking to shock their muscles into new growth. Essentially, it takes out the weakest link in a compound movement, allowing you to work your target muscle more effectively. For example, let's say you want to work your pecs but you find when you perform a bench press that your triceps give out before your pecs are fully fatigued. If you start with an exercise that works your chest but takes your triceps out of the equation (isolation) and then fully blast your pecs with a compound exercise, you have successfully used the pre-exhaust method.

If you're an intermediate bodybuilder, do about 10 to 12 reps of your isolation exercise and then immediately do you six to eight reps of the compound exercise. Do not rest between these exercises. If you allow even three seconds of rest before beginning your compound exercise, your muscles will have recovered at least 50 percent of their ability to contract and you'll lose some of the effectiveness of the routine. Rest after your compound exercise, and then do two or three more pre-exhaust / compound combination sets.

If you're an advanced bodybuilder looking for the ultimate experience in pre-exhaust training, begin with the isolation exercise for 10 to 12 reps. After you've finished these, immediately do another set with a lighter weight. Do

Dave Draper had his own strategy for the pre-exhaust technique – he'd do sets of his core-growth, compound moves before performing pre-exhaust cycles.

a third set with a lighter weight still. Move on to the compound exercise for six to eight reps until positive failure. Next, strip 20 percent of the poundage off the barbell and do as many extra positive reps as you can. When these are done, drop another 20 percent off the barbell and finish off with reps to positive failure. Rest three to five minutes and complete this cycle again. A training partner is very helpful in this case.

PRE-EXHAUST PRINCIPLE PLUS MUSCLE MASS AND STRENGTH BUILDING

"The Blonde Bomber" Dave Draper, bodybuilding champion of the late 1960s, has a rather unique way of incorporating the pre-exhaust technique into his strength training. He realized early in his bodybuilding career that the real mass and strength-building exercises are core growth or compound (multi-joint) exercises, and these are the ones he initially attacks. For instance, he might begin with the seated behind-the-neck press done in straight sets pyramid style for four sets of 10-8-6-6 and adding five to ten pounds per set. Only after he completes these size- and strength-building sets does he use the pre-exhaust technique.

To sufficiently isolate the lateral deltoids, he attacks them with dumbbell lateral raises (10 to 12 reps) and then immediately goes to seated high incline (80 to 90 degree) dumbbell presses (six to eight reps) for four to six pre-exhaust cycles. You don't want to fatigue a muscle that will assist in a core growth or compound exercise, especially if that exercise is with poundages that pose the risk of injury or expose the muscle to such stress that it fails to perform.

Some bodybuilders do their strength-building sets in the same manner as Dave Draper, but their approach to pre-exhaust adaptation is slightly different. They do an isolation exercise and immediately follow it with a core growth or compound exercise performed in a negative-only fashion. The secret to the success of this method is that the negative exercise requires only 15 percent as much oxygen as a compound exercise done in the negative and positive phase.

If you've weighed the pros and cons of the pre-exhaust technique and wish to try it out for yourself, see the following chart and you'll find techniques that are guaranteed to accelerate muscle size and vascularity:

PRE-EXHAUST CHART

MUSCLE GROUPS	MUSCLE-SPECIFIC (ISOLATION) EXERCISES	CORE GROUP (COMPOUND) EXERCISES
Quads	Leg Extension Hack Squat	High Bar Squat Barbell Front Squat
Hamstrings	Leg Curl	Stiff-Leg Barbell Deadlift (3/5 range movement)
Trapezius	Barbell or Dumbbell Shrug	Barbell Power Clean or Wide-Grip Up-Right Row
Latissimus Dorsi	Barbell Decline Pullover Stiff-Arm Lat Pulldown	Lat Pulldown (to sternum) or Pull-Up (palms forward) Bent-Over Row or Pull-Up
Middle Back	Bent-Over Lateral Raise	Wide-Grip Bent-Over Row
Spinal Erectors	Prone (Hyper) Extension	Conventional Deadlift
Upper Pectorals	Incline Dumbbell Flye Cable Crossover	Incline Barbell Press
Mid Pectorals	Dumbbell Flye	Bench Press
Low Pectorals	Decline Dumbbell Flye	Decline Bench Press
Deltoids	Dumbbell Lateral Raise Cable Lateral Raise	Press Behind Neck Overhead Barbell Press
Biceps	Barbell Preacher Curl Barbell Curl (Gironda style)	Regular-Grip Chin-Up (palms facing) Lat Pulldown (palms facing sternum / torso upright)
Triceps	Triceps Pressdown	Parallel Bar Dip or Close-Grip Bench Press
Forearms	Barbell Wrist Curl (palms down)	Barbell Reverse Curl
Calves	Seated Calf Raise	Standing Calf Raise

MORE PRE-EXHAUST OPTIONS
Deltoids Sequence
1. Bent-over dumbbell lateral raise
2. Dumbbell front raise
3. Barbell overhead press (followed by a 60-second rest)
4. Lateral raise
5. Barbell press behind neck

Biceps Sequence
1. Biceps curl with barbell and standing
2. Lat pulldown behind head
3. Preacher curl
4. Chin-up (palms facing) to a negative only
5. Lying dumbbell curl
6. Lat pulldown to chest (palms facing)

Triceps Sequence
1. One-dumbbell triceps extension (holding dumbbell with both hands)
2. Parallel bar dip
3. Lying EZ-bar triceps extension
4. Close-grip barbell bench press
5. Triceps pressdown
6. Barbell press behind neck
7. Parallel bar dip, negative only

MODIFIED PRE-EXHAUST
This technique involves performing three sets of a specific exercise (resting 60 to 90 seconds between sets) for a predetermined number of reps. Once you have completed the third set, rest for 60 to 90 seconds. Then advance to the Pre-Exhaust Cycles (refer to chart). Remember, you should not rest between the muscle-specific and anabolic core-growth exercises. Upon completion, you may rest for two to three minutes between each individual cycle.

Quads
The quadriceps modified pre-exhaust cycle is one of the most demanding routines ever devised. It consists of leg extensions with three sets of 15 reps. Do this exercise in straight-set fashion, resting 72 seconds between sets. Finish the third set and rest for 60 seconds. Then, begin the pre-exhaust technique with four sets of 12 reps for each of the following exercises: Leg extensions, leg presses and parallel barbell squats (which you can perform for 10 to 12 reps). At this point, you can rest for three to four minutes between cycles.

For those of you who train at home and don't have a leg-press apparatus, perform barbell hack squats (heels on a two-and-a-half inch block) for three sets of 10 reps. Do this exercise in straight-set fashion, resting 72 seconds between the first two sets. Upon completion of the third set, you may rest for 60 seconds. Then, perform barbell hack squats followed by barbell front squats (three sets of 10 reps for each). Don't rest between the hack squats and front squats! Make sure to use a squat rack for safety.

The tension superset technique is similar to the pre-exhaust technique, but it has two main differences: A compound, or multi-joint, exercise can precede an isolation exercise, and supersets can be performed for opposing muscle groups. A basic example of the tension superset designed to maximize the exercise effect is the sissy squat superset with barbell front lunges for your quads.

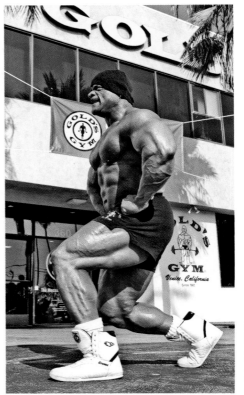

Front lunges, shown here without the barbell, can be paired with sissy squats for a tension superset.

Photo by Robert Reiff
Model Will Harris

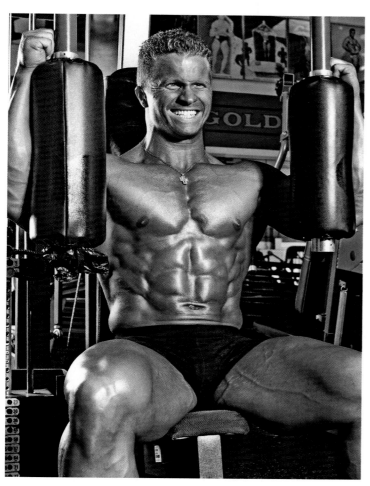

A good double pre-exhaust option for chest is the incline dumbbell press and pec-deck, plus the decline dumbbell press.

Biceps

Perform low-incline (20 degrees) dumbbell curls for three sets with 12 reps. Do this exercise in straight-set fashion, resting no more than 72 seconds between sets. When you finish your third set, rest for 60 seconds and begin the following pre-exhaust technique: Low-incline (20 degrees) dumbbell curls for four sets of 10 to 12 reps. At this point, you may take a 90-second rest. Following that rest, perform narrow reverse-grip chin-ups for four sets to failure.

DOUBLE PRE-EXHAUST
Chest

1. Perform the barbell bench press to neck, immediately followed by the dumbbell flye. Follow that up with a parallel bar dip (negative only).

2. Perform the incline dumbbell press, immediately followed by the pec-deck machine. Then, follow that up immediately with the decline dumbbell press.

Triceps

1. Perform the triceps pressdown, immediately followed by the one-dumbbell triceps extension. Follow that immediately with a parallel bar dip (negative only).

2. Perform the lying EZ-bar triceps extension, immediately followed by the lat machine pushdown. Follow that up with a flat barbell bench press.

3. Do a one-repetition negative parallel bar dip (30 seconds up and 30 seconds down), immediately followed by one dumbbell triceps extension (holding the dumbbell in both of your hands). Instantly follow that up with a parallel bar dip (negative only).

Biceps

1. Do preacher bench dumbbell curls and immediately follow that up with standing barbell curls. Then, perform chin-ups (negative portion only).

2. First do the standing barbell curl, and then immediately follow that with seated incline dumbbell curls. After that, you should immediately perform the barbell bent-over rowing exercise with an underhand grip.

3. Perform one super-slow chin-up (30 seconds up and 30 seconds down), immediately followed by a preacher curl with a barbell. Then, perform one chin-up (negative only).

4. Do the lat pulldown. Immediately follow that exercise with a lying dumbbell curl. Then, without wasting any time, perform the barbell bent-over rowing with a wide grip. This completes your biceps routine.

THE PRE-EX POST-PUMP METHOD
Thighs

Leg extension
Front squat
Sissy squat

Photo by Irvin Gelb
Model Peter Putnam

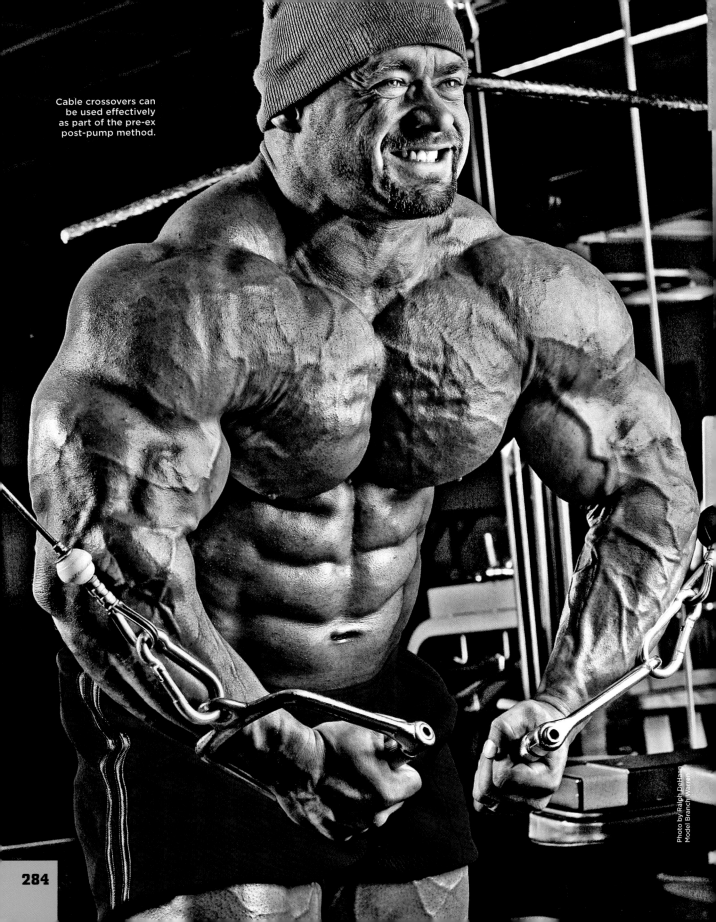

Cable crossovers can be used effectively as part of the pre-ex post-pump method.

Back

Straight-arm pulldown
Chin-up
Straight-arm barbell pullover

Chest

Dumbbell flye
Bench press
Cable crossover

Shoulders

Lateral raise
Barbell press behind neck
Barbell upright row

Biceps

Incline dumbbell curl
Reverse-grip lat pulldown to chest
Standing barbell concentration curl

Triceps

Triceps pressdown
Parallel bar dip
Lying dumbbell kickback

You wouldn't use this form of training for your calves. Of course, if you're like most people, you'll be performing higher repetitions for your calves anyway.

You can vary the combinations, as well as the number of sets and reps. The ideal number of reps is eight to ten. You should perform between two and four sets. Even if you're performing only two sets, you'll still give yourself a tremendous pump. If you can manage three or four sets, you can assure yourself of fast growth.

It's best to work only one muscle group per session. If you try and cover all of your body, it'll only be counterproductive. Give it all you've got, and you'll find that any lagging muscle group will quickly catch up with the rest of your body.

Pro Tip Pre-Exhaust: Do a muscle-specific (isolation) exercise movement for 30–50 reps then immediately do an anabolic core growth (compound) exercise movement for 4–6 partial reps.

PSYCHO-BLAST SET CONCEPT

Denie Walter popularized the Psycho-Blast Set Concept. The concept was actually just one element of the total system of training Denie wrote about in his book entitled *Psycho*

Blast: The Ultimate Pumpout. Psycho-blast sets consist of only four sets per exercise. The first set is performed for 10 to 12 maxi-pump reps followed by a 45-second rest. Then perform a second set using the same poundage or you can even increase it by 10 pounds. Your reps on this second set may decrease, but never let it fall below six power reps. Take another 45-second rest and then perform a third set, followed by yet another 45-second rest and a final fourth set. Every rep should take roughly three to five seconds to complete the full range of movement. According to Denie, you should perform every third rep of a set doing what he calls total stop-pauses, where you might stop the movement completely during any phase of the movement, however, only momentarily. In addition to that, Denie feels that if you're unable to accomplish this the weight is simply too heavy. If you're looking for another way to increase the intensity of the psycho-blast concept, you should perform double, half and full reps (21s) in the final set. Now that's intense!

PSYCHO-BURST TRAINING

Psycho-Burst training is a one super-slow rep-per-set concept that was popularized by former NABBA Mr. U.S.A. Rob Colacino. In this style of training, you will accomplish the most amount of work involving the highest number of possible muscle fibers in the least amount of time.

Rob explains that it's important to warm up by performing two sets of eight to ten reps using a light weight. He adds that you initially need to do some experimenting and he stresses the importance of having two spotters you trust on either side of the bar. To perform one slow-motion rep per set for the bench press, Rob says to grab the weight and bring it down very slowly on the negative part of the exercise. Just touch your chest. Three quarters of the way up, hold the bar there. At this point Rob quickly counts to 50 in his head. He may hold it for a little less time or even a little longer, depending how he feels. Rob says to bring it up the rest of the way very slowly. Hold the bar locked out for as long as you can, then lower it back for the negative. Stop one-quarter of the way down and hold it there. Again count to 50 in your head (more or less). Bring it down very slowly to about halfway. Stop there. Now it really gets tough. You hold it there for as long as you can, then lower it very slowly down to touch your chest. Once you've accomplished this, you must then bring the bar back up. Tell your spotters to let you do it on your own and push the weight off your chest. "I don't care if it doesn't even go off your chest – just contract, contract, contract," says Rob. "You don't stop until you feel you are dead. And then you

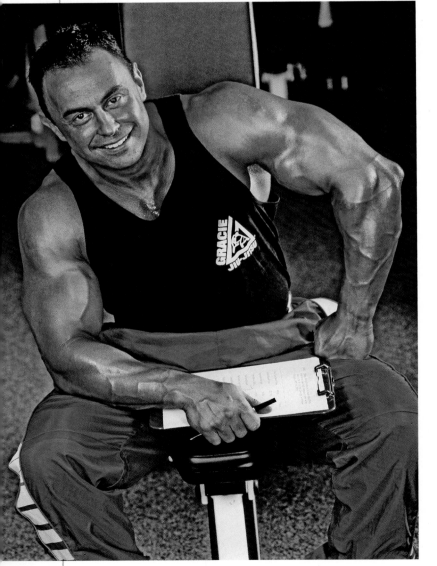

Charles Poliquin, one of the two creators of reciprocity training.

say 'Take that damn weight away from me.'" At that point, you can take a much-deserved two- to five-minute rest before moving on to incline bench presses, which you should perform in the exact same way.

PYRAMID TRAINING

In Pyramid training, you simply add poundage and decrease the repetition scheme in each succeeding set. Assuming you were doing barbell curls, a typical pyramid for your biceps and delts would start with you doing two sets of 12 reps using a weight that's 80 percent of your one-rep maximum (1RM). In your next two sets, you should decrease your total reps to only six and increase your poundage to 84 percent of your 1RM. If you were doing the standing dumbbell lateral raise exercise for your delts in pyramid style, you'd start out doing two sets of 14 reps with a weight that's 68 percent of your 1RM. In the next two sets, you would decrease your reps to 12, and increase your lifting to 72 percent of your 1RM. For your third round of two sets, you should increase your poundage to 76 percent of your 1RM, but decrease your rep count to only 10. In your fourth attempt at two sets, you should decrease your reps to only eight, but increase your weight to 80 percent of your 1RM. Simply stated, as you decrease your rep count, you slightly increase the poundage.

Unless otherwise indicated, when performing core growth and specific exercises, you should always meet the requirements in the Holistic Training Guide. If you want to know more about the strategies of pyramiding, information can be found in our book entitled *Anabolic Muscle Mass*.

RECIPROCITY TRAINING

The basic idea behind reciprocity training, as designed by Charles Poliquin and Paul Gagne, revolves around the use of agonist and antagonist exercise movements. Essentially, you use the whole spectrum of the strength curve in the involved muscles. By doing so, you're able to lift as much as two percent more weight.

If you're using your biceps and triceps, with one arm you'll do a one-arm triceps pressdown and with the other arm you'll perform the one-

Photo by Alex Ardenti
Model Charles Poliquin

dumbbell curl for a predetermined number of repetitions. When this dual set is finished, switch sides. These movements are done simultaneously, which means you cut your workout time in half. Another way of looking at it is that you'll be able to do twice as much work without increasing the amount of time you put in.

Some other examples of exercises you might do for these muscles include lying on a bench and simultaneously performing a one-dumbbell curl and one-dumbbell triceps extension and, using the cable crossover unit, performing low-pulley cable one-arm triceps extensions overhead and one-arm biceps curls using the high pulley cable.

REST-PAUSE TRAINING

Rest-pause training and its variations is an intense form of training that combines brief amounts of rest with selected poundage and repetition schemes in a particular set.

METHOD 1

Use 75 to 80 percent of the maximum poundage you currently use when you do a normal set of an exercise. For example, if you can perform the press behind the neck with 200 pounds for 10 reps, reduce the weight to 150 to 160 pounds and begin your program. Perform 10 reps and then rest for 10 seconds. Then perform nine reps and rest for 10 seconds. Continue in this manner until you are down to only one rep. Depending on your stamina, you may be able to do more than one rep. Go to failure in this final set until you can't even budge the barbell.

METHOD 2

Begin by warming up with 60 percent of your current six-rep maximum and perform eight to ten reps. Increase the poundage, making certain you are able to perform six solid reps. Perform these six reps and then rest for 60 seconds. Continue in this manner for a total of 10 sets per individual exercise. If at any point during the 10 sets your rep count drops to five, decrease the poundage only enough to ensure you're able to perform the basic six-rep pattern.

METHOD 3

Using a 10-set pattern, warm up with 60 percent of your current maximum for the number of reps you plan to perform. Let's assume that you want to acquire some power in your 35-degree incline bench press. Currently, your best incline bench press might be 300 pounds for five reps. Begin your first set of 35-degree incline bench presses with 80 percent of your five-rep poundage (240 pounds). Rest for one minute between succeeding sets. During each of these rest periods you'll add five percent to the barbell until you are using 100 percent or your five-rep maximum for the fifth set. Use the same weight for your sixth set. Starting with the seventh set you will decrease the poundage by five percent on each of the final four sets. See the chart for clarity.

35-DEGREE INCLINE BARBELL BENCH PRESS (300 POUNDS X 5 REPS)

SETS	REPS	POUNDAGE	PERCENTAGE
1	5	240	80
2	5	255	85
3	5	270	90
4	5	285	95
5	5	300	100
6	5	300	100
7	5	285	95
8	5	270	90
9	5	255	85
10	5	240	80

In the fifth and sixth sets you may not be able to perform the suggested five reps per set because of the minimal rest of one minute between sets as compared to the conventional requirement of resting three to eight minutes. Do whatever you can until you're able to perform five reps each set, and then upgrade your poundage-percentage (based on a new five-rep maximum) scale and begin a new cycle of the 10-set rest pause.

You might also try utilizing the one-minute rest period for a superset pattern on an opposing bodypart. You can employ different rep patterns based on your particular goals. In general exercises, you can use reps of three to six for power, seven to eleven for size and strength and 12 to 15 for endurance.

METHOD 4: SIX SETS OF TEN REPS

Find a poundage you can perform for 10 reps. Add 10 percent more weight to the barbell. You'll do 10 reps in each set, but the secret to accomplishing this task is the length of your rest periods. When the first set ends, take a 30-second rest. Add 15 seconds to each subsequent rest period. After the second set rest for 45 seconds and so on. When you get to the point where you can do all six sets rather easily for 10 reps, add more poundage.

METHOD 5

The fifth method is similar to the six-set/ten-rep method, but with slightly less weight and a shorter rest. Select a poundage you can perform for 10 reps. Decrease this poundage by five percent. Your rest intervals between sets should each be exactly 30 seconds. Your first set should be 10 reps, but in subsequent sets that number will likely decrease. When you get to the point where you're doing 10 reps rather easily for all six sets, it's time to add more poundage to the barbell.

RIOT BOMBING

As far as we can tell, the only published mention of riot bombing appeared in one of the Weider magazines back in the mid-1960s. It was the brainchild of the late Irvin "Zabo" Koszewski, a champion bodybuilder known for his dia-mond-cut abdominals. Many west coast Muscle Beach bodybuilders used this method with tremendous results. It basically consists of a mega-volume number of sets and rotating rep scheme.

Riot bombing involves only two exercises – one for each opposing muscle group. Some exercise combinations for riot bombing include alternating barbell front squats with leg curls, bench presses with bent-arm pullovers, seated alternating dumbbell presses with lat pulldowns, bent-over rows with bench dips and incline dumbbell curls with triceps pressdowns.

THE 10-STEP APPROACH TO RIOT BOMBING THE QUADS AND HAMS

1. Do 20 sets for each muscle group. For example, perform 20 sets of barbell front squats and 20 sets of leg curls.
2. Performing 20 sets for one muscle group before going on to the next exercise could make the workout very long. Perform the sets in superset fashion.
3. Start with a poundage that you can easily handle for 10 reps in a compound (anabolic core growth) exercise or 14 reps in an isolation (muscle-specific) exercise.
4. After the second set, add poundage and do eight reps (compound exercise) or 12 reps (isolation exercise).
5. Add weight on your eighth set and do sets of six reps (compound exercise) or 10 reps (isolation exercise).
6. On your 14th set, increase to a poundage that will accommodate a rep scheme of four reps (compound exercise) or eight reps (isolation exercise).
7. On the 16th set, reduce the poundage so you can complete the same rep pattern listed in step 5.
8. On the eighteenth set, reduce the poundage to allow the same rep count detailed in step 4.
9. In the 20th set, reduce the poundage so you can complete 15 reps whether the exercise is compound or isolation.
10. The intensity level in riot bombing is extremely high because of the limited rest intervals between the supersets. If your goal is to increase your muscle

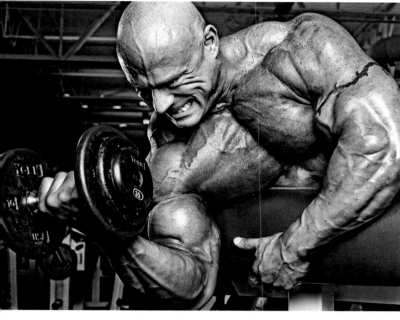

If you're superset-ting biceps and tri-ceps, try preacher curls and EZ-bar French presses.

Photo by Kevin Horton
Model Mark Antonek

EZ-bar French press for the triceps, which is a pushing muscle, and the preacher curl for the biceps, which is a pulling muscle. Another example is doing the bench press for the chest and the lat pulldown for the back.

When you perform the exercises in superset fashion for opposing muscle groups, one exercise generally uses a pushing muscle while the other is pulling. You can come up with many superset exercise combinations of your own in the push/pull style that involve two opposing muscle groups. You can also superset exercises by performing either two pulling or two pushing exercises in succession, such as heavy barbell curls with preacher bench dumbbell curls. Since you'll be working the same muscle group with two exercises (this is called a true superset), you'll need to rest for 15 to 30 seconds between supersets as opposed to taking no rest at all when working opposing bodyparts in superset fashion. Because of the intensity involved in working two exercises for the same muscle group, we recommend that you do not superset two compound exercises.

The most commonly accepted mode of training superset style is to begin with a compound exercise and follow up with an isolation exercise. Most advanced trainers are well aware of the various popular and published superset combinations, but there are some unorthodox supersets you should consider. For your delts and biceps, you could perform the overhead barbell press and then immediately do body-weight-only curl-grip chin-ups. If you want to work your delts and triceps, you could perform upright barbell rows, followed immediately by bodyweight-only parallel bar dips.

If you're a steroid-free bodybuilder, you can gain muscle mass through moderate or even light weights using supersets, especially if you pay attention to your nutrition and have sufficient glycogen for that super pump. A lot of advanced power bodybuilders fear using lighter weights. You must overcome this because of the legitimate potential that supersets offer in the form of growth and a great pump. You may encounter a metabolic adjustment period going from the slow, heavy-training tempo to the brisk training pace of supersets. Some bulked-up

mass, you should rest for 30 to 45 seconds between supersets. You should rest for only 15 seconds if you are aiming at sharper muscularity.

Be creative – mix and match different exercises. You can do compound exercises for both muscle groups, isolation exercises for both, or compound for one and isolation for the other. Refer to the Exercise Selection Chart when choosing exercises.

Riot bombing is recommended only for advanced bodybuilders. Perform riot bombing no more than twice a week. If you decide to do riot bombing twice per week then make sure to work a different set of opposing muscles on the second day, and don't do riot bombing on consecutive days. Use this advanced strategy for a maximum of 30 to 45 days at a stretch.

SUPERSETS

Also known as alternates, supersets are one of the most popular training principles amongst advanced bodybuilders – sure to enhance your pump. You can alternate between two exercises for opposing muscle groups (called antagonistic supersets) in a nonstop fashion, i.e. no rest between sets. For example, you can do the bodybuilders' cardiovascular systems have a hard time adjusting. If this describes you, try easing into this training to give your system time to adjust.

TRISETS

Performing a triset is very similar to performing a superset in that it requires you to do back-to-back exercises for the same muscle. The difference is that you'll perform three exercises together rather than two. For example, if you're working on your deltoids, you might begin with behind-the-neck seated presses for six to eight reps, go to standing dumbbell lateral raises for 10 to 12 reps, and finish off with roughly 10 reps of bent-over lateral raises. Rest approximately one to two minutes and begin the cycle a second time. The deltoid exercises represent one generalized movement that works the overall delt followed by two specific movements that attack the medial and posterior segments of the deltoid respectively. If you want to blitz the posterior segment of the delt only in a triset, you would pick three specific exercises for this area and do them in the manner described.

TWENTY-ONES

Twenty-ones were very popular with West Coast bodybuilding champions many years ago. Essentially, you choose a poundage you can perform for eight to twelve reps. Using the standing barbell curl as an example, begin by doing seven half curls from the starting position (thighs) to the navel region. After you've completed these reps, immediately perform seven half curls from your navel to your neck. Remember to contract your biceps hard at the top. You might also want to do a couple of burns every other rep. Without any rest, finish off with seven complete curls.

There are other variations of the 21 movements, such as 18s (6x6x6), 15s (5x5x5) and the fraction method which can be adapted to any muscle group.

UP-AND-DOWN-THE-RACK SYSTEM

Larry Scott, the first and two-time Mr. Olympia, used a shoulder-blasting routine incorporating the up-and-down-the-rack system to build his incredible deltoids. He would perform overhead dumbbell presses followed by bent-over dumbbell lateral raises, and finally end with standing dumbbell lateral raises. He would do six to ten sets per series and about six reps on the press, as well as eight to ten reps on the lateral raises per set. He would work his way up and down the rack with no rest between sets and very little rest between exercise series. Most of the time, Larry used dumbbells rather than barbells because he feels that barbells aggravate the shoulder region as a result of the improper torque that's applied to the shoulder joint.

Up and down the rack refers to where the dumbbells sit (when they've been properly returned to the rack, that is). With each set you move further up the rack by choosing a heavier weight until you reach the peak weight, at which point you decrease the weight with each set, moving down the rack. You can do both the "up" and "down" segments together in one set (a pyramid set) or you can perform two or three sets going up the rack and then two or three going down.

For our example we'll use the dumbbell overhead press. Begin with a pair of dumbbells that you can press overhead for six solid reps. After you've finished those reps, you should immediately pick up a heavier set of dumbbells and press those overhead. Continue in this manner until you've reached a poundage that will allow you to complete only three reps. That's your last set going up the rack, or increasing your weight. Going down the rack usually takes place after you've gone up the rack. It's simply the reverse of the previous procedure and it's usually done for two or three sets. You should minimize your rest time between sets. The only way you can do that is to have your dumbbells set up ahead of time so that you can move rapidly from one set to another.

When moving down the rack you must keep in mind both moderation and speed. You will not be able to use this method to your benefit if you're struggling with limit loads. Speed is required both in the actual performance of the movements and in the pace you follow as you go through the program. For example, if you wanted to perform dumbbell curls, you should begin with a pair of 60s and perform a set of six reps. Then, without resting, pick up 55s and perform six more reps. Immediately following that, do six more with 50s. Continue in this manner until you've completed six reps with 35s. You should complete these six sets in less than five minutes. After a three-minute rest, begin a second combination of six sets, using the same weights and repetitions as the first time.

In addition to performing a high number of sets at whirlwind speed, you can get the best results by using a wide variety of exercises that will help you reach every fiber in your muscles. Keep in mind that on compound exercises you shouldn't go below three reps, and with isolation exercises you shouldn't go below eight reps in a final set of the up-the-rack system. The up-and-down-the-rack system does work and there are countless bodybuilders around the world that can vouch for it.

When moving down the rack with dumbbell curls, remember to focus on the speed of the movement and your pace as you decrease weight.

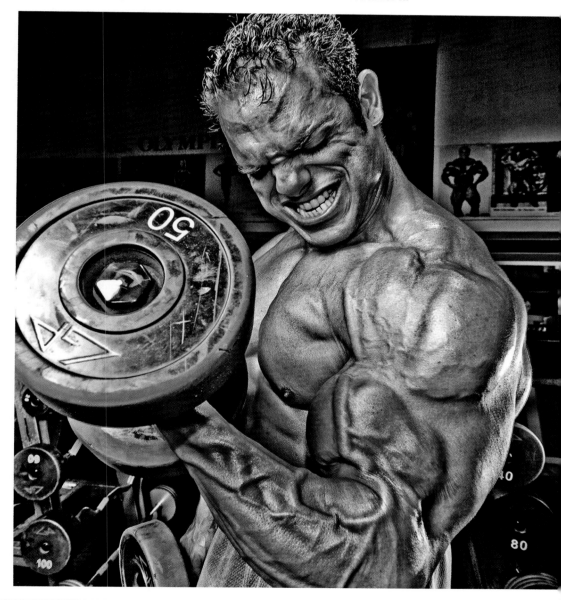

Photo by Michael Butler
Model David Hughes

X-SIZE TRAINING PLAN

This system is the brainchild of Germany's Oliver Wolter. To prepare the muscle fibers of a select muscle group for maximum growth, a workout begins with a preparatory one rep only of a compound exercise. For this one rep, use a weight that's 50 percent of your 1RM.

The preparatory one-rep-only set is performed in super-slow fashion using a cadence of 60 seconds from beginning to end in the positive phase and then another 60 seconds immediately thereafter to complete the negative phase. Directly after the preparatory set, do a set of six to eight reps maximum using either a compound or isolation exercise. Without resting, decrease your poundage by 30 percent and rep out to positive failure. For example, if you're using 200 pounds for the maximum set in the lat pulldown, you should drop that amount to 140 pounds for the sub-maximum set and go till you can't go anymore. During the last rep, perform a static contraction by holding the poundage at the fully contracted (positive phase) position for 15 to 20 seconds.

Training frequency is an important consideration and X-Size Training can be structured into a modified every-other-day split whereby you perform back, chest and delts in the first day, biceps, triceps and forearms on the third day and on the fifth day you work on your quads and hamstrings. You can also use the push/pull split variation. On the first day, work on your quads and hamstrings. Rest on the second day.

On the third day, work on your back and biceps and rest on the following day. Work on your chest, delts and triceps on day five and then take the next two days to rest and recuperate.

When doing exercises such as the barbell squats, bench presses or leg presses, begin your one-rep set in the positive phase of the movement. Train safely by doing the rep in a power rack, if possible. Follow the X-Size program for three weeks. The X-Size program is such a unique, high-intensity program even advanced bodybuilders cannot use it for a long time. This program may be short, but it will ignite a tremendous gain of five to ten pounds of pure muscle mass.

ZERO-EFFORT TECHNIQUE

The most important factor in stimulating muscle growth is the intensity at which a particular muscle or muscle group is worked. In stimulating the maximum muscle gain factor, the effectiveness is dependent upon how close you come to the point of momentary muscular failure or a specific point during an exercise when the muscles can no longer lift (positive phase) or lower (negative phase) the weight.

In 1982, the late Scott Chinery and his team at Cybergenics sought to develop a training protocol that would bring muscles close to complete failure, increase strength capacity and stimulate muscular growth as quickly and efficiently as possible. After extensive research, they developed the Zero-Effort technique.

X-SIZE TRAINING CHART

MUSCLE GROUP	PREPARATORY SUPER-SLOW ONE REP	MAXIMUM SET 6-8 REPS POSITIVE FAILURE	SUB-MAXIMUM SET 30% LESS POUNDAGE REP TO POSITIVE FAILURE HOLD FOR 15-20 SECONDS
Quads	Leg Press	Leg Extension	Leg Extension
Hamstrings	Stiff-Leg Barbell Deadlift	Leg Curl	Leg Curl
Chest	Bench Press	Flye Pec Deck or Cable Crossover	Flye Pec Deck or Cable Crossover
Delts	Overhead Dumbbell Press	Lateral Raise and Bent-Over Lateral Raise	Lateral Raise and Bent-Over Lateral Raise
Triceps	Lying Barbell Triceps Extension	One-Dumbbell Triceps Extension or Triceps Pressdown	One-Dumbbell Triceps Extension or Triceps Pressdown
Biceps	Standing Barbell Curl	Concentration Curl	Concentration Curl
Forearms	Barbell Reverse Curl	Barbell Wrist Curl (palms up)	Barbell Wrist Curl (palms up)

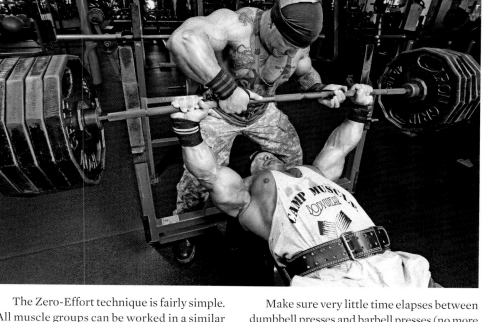

Stimulating max muscle growth depends how close you come to a point of absolute muscle failure – a spotter can help you get just past that point.

Photo by Kevin Horton
Models Rodney Roller and Brian May

The Zero-Effort technique is fairly simple. All muscle groups can be worked in a similar manner. If you want to train your pecs, a thorough warm-up at the beginning of this type of exercise is imperative, as it'll minimize the potential for injury. Perform two sets of slow, high-repetition barbell bench presses (35 percent maximum for 15 to 18 reps). Emphasize a slow, controlled movement in the warm-up and concentrate on your pectoral muscles. After completing the two warm-up sets, stretch the muscles by lying on a bench and holding two light dumbbells in a bent-arm flye position at the bottom of the movement. Hold this for 45 to 60 seconds and then contract your pectorals a few times and swing your arms back and forth. Psych yourself up for an intense experience.

Start with bent-arm flat dumbbell flyes using 80 to 90 percent 1RM. Complete as many repetitions as possible until you can no longer lift the dumbbells, and then bring your arms in and do as many dumbbell bench presses as possible using the same weight. Upon completion of this set, launch into a set of flat barbell bench presses using 50 percent of your 1RM. Your muscles will already be in a pre-exhausted state and 50 percent of your 1RM in the bench press will now be closer to 90 percent of your maximum.

Make sure very little time elapses between dumbbell presses and barbell presses (no more than three seconds) and do as many barbell bench presses to positive failure as possible. When you hit your sticking point, have a spotter or training partner assist you in lifting the barbell and then lower (five seconds minimum) it on your own. Continue until you can no longer lift or lower the barbell. At this point, set the barbell on the upright support rack and, before three seconds elapse, grab yet another set of dumbbells and begin a final set of dumbbell flyes. These dumbbells should be 40 percent of your maximum. Repeat the flye movement until you hit a sticking point and proceed into dumbbell presses with these same weights. When you've reached a point of momentary positive failure, you have completed the set.

In essence, you've done five sets of chest exercises beginning at near-maximum poundage and ending at 40 percent of your maximum poundage. You should not be able to lift the weight at the end of this set. In order for the set to be effective, you must hit a point of positive failure four times and a point of both positive and negative failure one time. The following chart outlines exactly how to perform a chest zero-effort cycle:

CHEST ZERO-EFFORT CYCLE

2 SETS WARM-UPS	BARBELL BENCH PRESS	35 PERCENT 1RM 15–18 REPS
CYCLE #1		
(+) failure	Dumbbell Flye	80 percent 1RM
(+) failure	Dumbbell Bench Press	Same wt. as Dumbbell Flye
(+) and (-) failure	Barbell Bench Press	50 percent max
(+) failure	Dumbbell Flye	40 percent 1RM
(+) failure	Dumbbell Bench Press	Same wt. as Dumbbell Flye
REPEAT CYCLE 2–3X		
CYCLE #2		
(+) failure	Parallel Bar Dip	Bodyweight only
(+) and (-) failure	Incline Barbell Press	70 percent 1RM
REPEAT CYCLE 2X		

The key to Zero-Effort training is to exert all-out muscle effort! A point of momentary muscular failure can be achieved only when you summon 100 percent of your strength reserves, yet cannot complete the rep. Make sure to take little to no rest between the three exercise sequences. If your muscles rest more than three seconds, they will partially recover and much of the benefit will be voided. After three to six months of Zero-Effort training, you should see dramatic improvements in muscular growth and strength capacity.

Experiment with alternative moves in the first Zero-Effort cycle. Be sure to have variety and alternate the exercises within the weekly cycle. Keep your poundage at the recommended percentage of max capability. When a specific weight starts to feel light, go heavier. You'll benefit from utilizing all-out effort, markedly improving strength capacity.

It's extremely important that you do not attempt this method without the aid of a competent training partner. Your training partner or spotter should give you only enough assistance to help lift the weight and nothing more. Don't train any muscle group more than two times a week. Remember to warm up thoroughly before each training session and put your full concentration into every workout.

Bodyweight parallel bar dips can be used in a zero-effort cycle for chest.

POINTS TO REMEMBER

1. Don't rest between sets in a cycle. Rest for one minute between cycles if you're training solo, or just as long as it takes for your training partner to complete a cycle.
2. The time allotted for a Cybergenics exercise set is the calculated number of seconds it takes to move the weight in the positive and negative phase of a full-range-of-motion rep. Since your desire is to build maximum muscle size coupled with huge reserves of power, accelerated high-speed positive phase reps is a good option. Here is how it works: Each rep in the positive phase should be completed as quickly as possible (two seconds or less), not using momentum, but with perfect motion and precise form (never jerky). The negative

Photo by Michael Butler
Model David Hughes

The Cybergenics rep speed tempos aren't a factor for abs, as the muscles have a limited range of motion.

phase of each rep should take five to eight seconds to complete. Because of the limited range of motion for muscle groups such as the calves, abs and traps, the rep speed tempos mentioned don't apply.

3. Upon completion of a cycle, stretch the working muscle group for 30 seconds. After stretching, rest the muscle for another 30 seconds. With conscientious practice and all-out 100-percent effort, the Cybergenics technique will yield phenomenal results. As with any other endeavor, your success will be mainly determined by the effort you put forth.

A helpful chart detailing the Zero-Effort Cycle for all the muscle groups listed in the following training summaries can be found at www.dennisbweis.com.

CYBERGENICS
4-DAY SPLIT TRAINING SUMMARY

Monday – Thursday
Chest / quads-hams-calves / triceps / lower back

Tuesday – Friday
Lats / traps / shoulders / biceps / abs

Wednesday – Saturday – Sunday
Rest and recuperation

6-DAY SPLIT TRAINING SUMMARY

Monday – Thursday
Quads-hams-calves / traps / abs

Tuesday – Friday
Chest / back

Wednesday – Saturday
Shoulders / biceps / triceps

Sunday
Rest and recuperation

Here is a Split Training summary, where you train for five consecutive days in the first week and then three non-consecutive days in the second week.

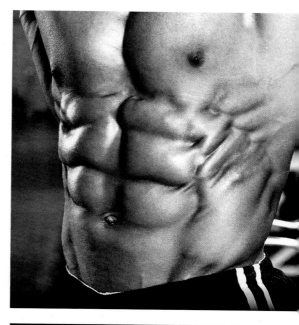

WEEK ONE	
DAY	**BODYPART(S) WORKED**
Monday	Quads, hamstrings, calves
Tuesday	Chest
Wednesday	Traps, lats, lower back
Thursday	Shoulders, biceps, triceps
Friday	Quads, hamstrings, calves
Saturday	Rest
Sunday	Rest

WEEK TWO	
DAY	**BODYPART(S) WORKED**
Monday	Chest
Tuesday	Rest
Wednesday	Traps, lats, lower back
Thursday	Rest
Friday	Shoulders, biceps, triceps
Saturday	Rest
Sunday	Rest

*Repeat Two Week Cycle. Don't go bonkers and incorporate many different Red-Line Intensity Manipulation Techniques into your workout programs all at once. You're better off doing only one or two. After giving your body a chance to recover, you can then try another intensity technique.

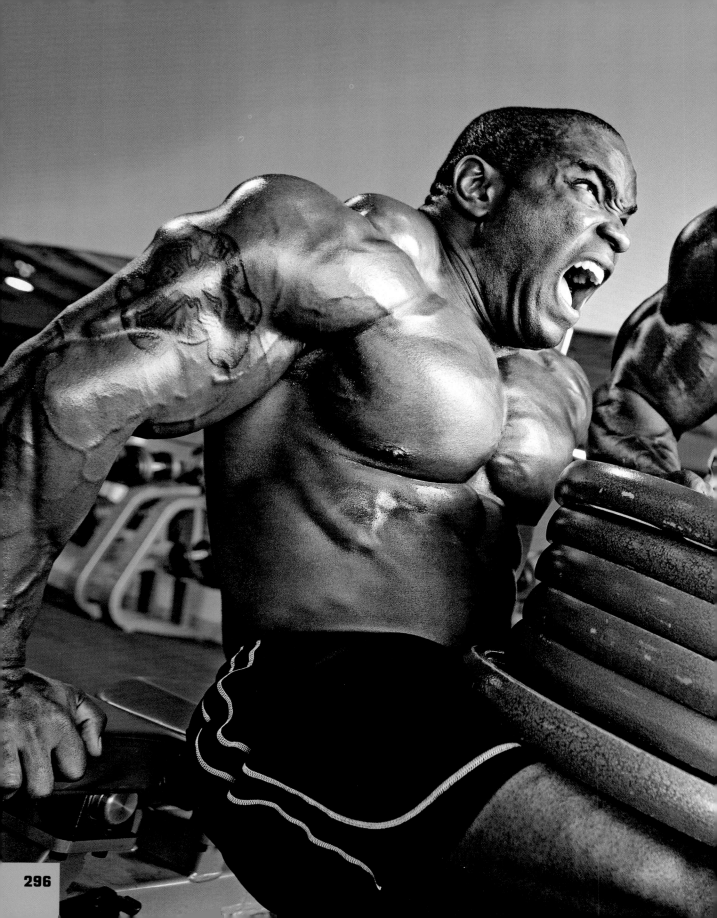

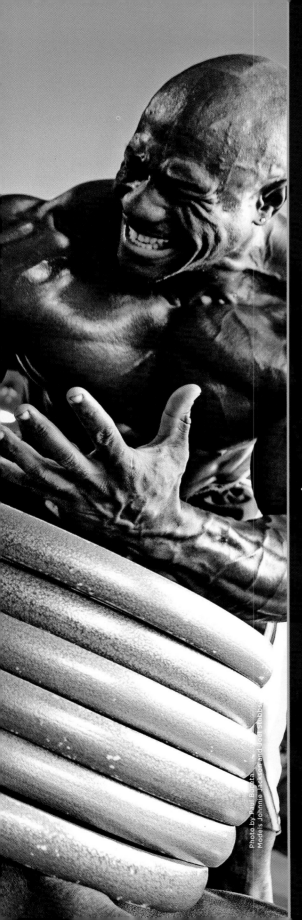

BOOK
11

Super Muscle And
Strength Specialization

CHAPTER 36

TEN GUIDELINES FOR SPECIALIZATION

Not all your muscles will respond the same to training, and this is where specialization techniques come into play.

Every bodybuilder who trains with heavy iron eventually discovers a lack of growth in certain muscle groups. Sometimes this is because of training – the bodybuilder may not enjoy working that muscle, for example, or he may work it too much. A few reasons for this lack of response include the habit of ending sets too soon, overtraining either the muscles of nervous system, lack of training consistency, poor mind-to-muscle link, and bad technique or form.

In theory, if you were to exercise all of your muscle groups equally hard, everything would balance out in time. However, while every muscle group should develop equally in proportion to its potential, you'll soon discover that some muscle groups are more responsive to training than others. When you notice that a particular muscle area isn't responding as it should, you should use specialization for bringing that lagging muscle group up to par. In general (though this is not the case for each individual) the most to least responsive muscles are: Lats, pecs, biceps, triceps, quads, hamstrings, abs, delts, calves and forearms.

Before we make any specific recommendations regarding proper specialization techniques, you should be aware of and consider four aesthetic qualities when building muscle: Separation, definition, shape and symmetry. Separation is where you see a visible division between one segment of a muscle and another. The different heads of the quads are a great example. Definition, often referred to as being cut or ripped, means the muscles are highly visible through the skin, due in large part to the reduction of bodyfat and water under the skin's surface. Shape is the actual shape of the muscle itself, from origin to insertion. This is partly determined by genetics – some people have short muscle bodies and some have long; some muscles "peak" naturally and some don't; some are round and full while some look stretched out. Symmetry is the even development of a muscle on a vertical axis. This term is often used also to refer to overall proportional development. This means your development on the left and right sides of your body should look identical,

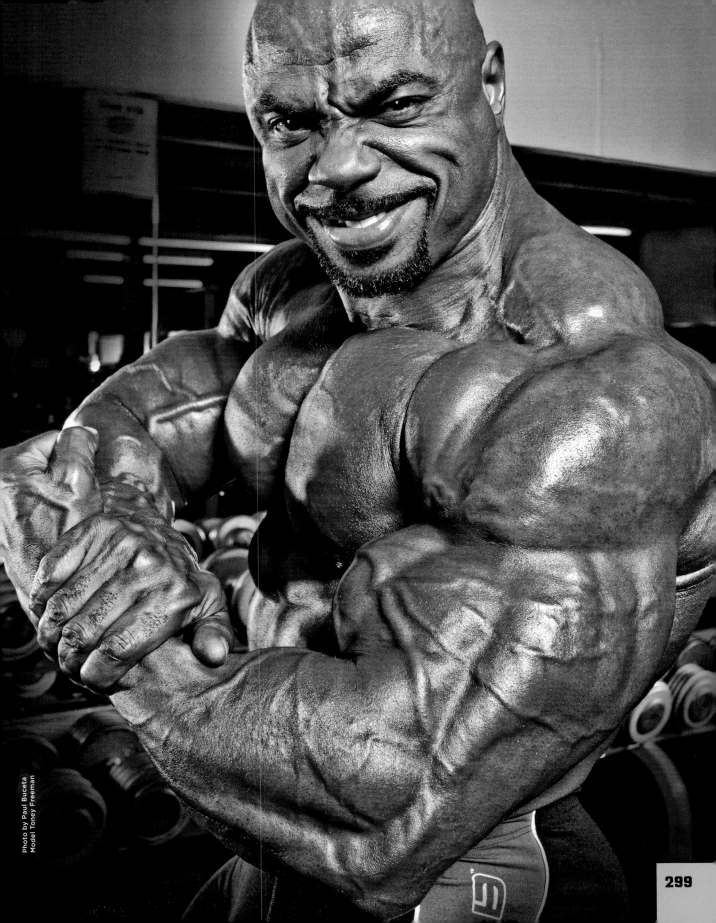

299

and you should have an equivalent level of development from your upper to lower half and again from front to back.

The major muscle groups of the body all contain more than one head or muscle segment. For example, the triceps consists of three heads: The long head, lateral head and medial head. While your triceps may seem to be of equal proportional development with the other muscles of your body, it may not be because most pressing exercises for your chest and shoulders tend to activate the long head of your triceps. As a result, the lateral and medial heads may be disproportionately smaller than the long head, and this throws off the proportion of your triceps. You must take the necessary steps to correct this by focusing some quality priority training on your lateral and medial heads while decreasing the workload

on the long head of your triceps. For a breakdown of the muscle groups and the exercises that work a specific segment of a muscle group, refer to the Holistic Exercise Selection Chart at the end of this book.

Old-school bodybuilders used to train four or five days a week, with two non-consecutive days being devoted entirely to upper-body training and another two non-consecutive days dedicated exclusively to lower-body training. The fifth day was devoted to specializing on any muscle group that needed extra work. Specialization training is a little more evolved. First, you must evaluate the muscle needing priority training. Does it need more strength, size, better shape or a combination of these qualities? Once you've truthfully answered and evaluated your physique, it's time to begin planning your specialization program.

Competitive bodybuilders spend a great deal of time working on any lagging bodyparts they may have in order to bring their best package to the stage.

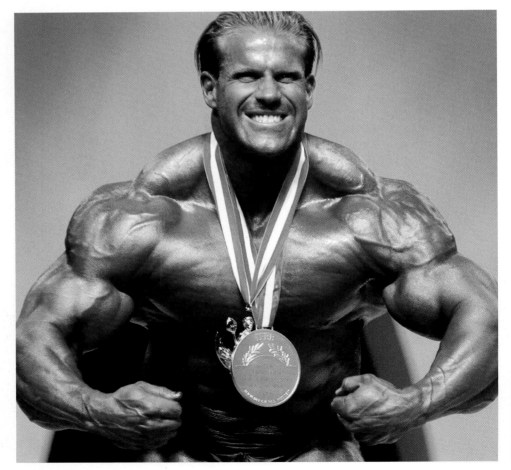

Photo by Garry Bartlett
Model Jay Cutler

Some argue that no other bodybuilder has ever matched the leg development of Tom Platz.

TEN SPECIALIZATION GUIDELINES

1 Choose exercises (refer to the Anabolic Core Growth Exercise Selection Chart) that enhance the most stimulation of size and strength of the muscle group needing specialization. If you want a subpar muscle group to exhibit a combination of size, strength and more fullness or muscularity, refer to the huge Holistic Exercise Selection Chart for more options.

2 To see positive results from a specialization program, you'll generally need a minimum of four to eight weeks of diligent, hard training. Don't follow such a plan for more than 12 to 14 weeks. There have been cases where bodybuilders have been able to shock a stubborn muscle group into a new dimension of growth with as little as one day to two weeks of specialization training.

Former three-time Mr. Olympia Frank Zane has been known to bring up a lagging bodypart in as little as two weeks of concentrated priority training. On the other hand, Arnold Schwarzenegger would specialize on a muscle group for as much as nine months. It took the legendary Lou Ferrigno (former Mr. Olympia contender and TV's The Hulk) even longer. Lou found that one of the biggest challenges in his bodybuilding career wasn't winning titles, but trying to bring his leg development up to par with his upper torso. Interestingly, the "Golden Eagle" Tom Platz had the opposite problem.

3 Specialization training will be most beneficial before mental burnout (exhaustion or overtraining, which is the third and final phase of the general adaptation syndrome) is experienced. When you become aware of this condition, you should take a three-week layoff from specialization training before embarking on another priority program for any other muscle group. This will give you the opportunity to fully recover, and your attitude toward your training will become more focused for the next phase of specialization. Unless otherwise advised, weekly specialization procedures shouldn't be performed more often than ev-

ery other day. The exceptions to this are your abs and calves, which can be worked five or six days per week if necessary.

Research from the former USSR reveals a slight modification to this rule. This research indicates that highly advanced bodybuilders should perform shock training specialization in the following manner: Using your quads as the target muscle for specialization purposes, minimally train your back, chest, shoulders and arms on Monday and Thursday. Do one or two sets per muscle group using muscle specific or isolation exercises. You should only do muscle specific exercises because they take less energy to perform and the energy conserved will be better used in the forthcoming core growth

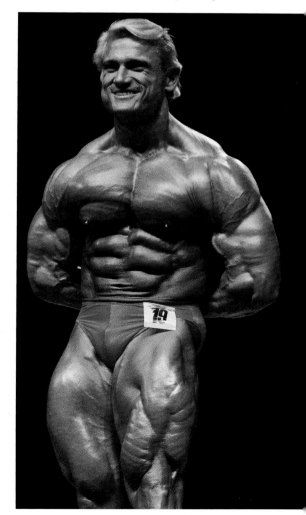

Model Tom Platz

exercise (or compound exercise) shock training program. Specialization training for your quads should be performed once on Wednesday and shock trained twice on Saturday in morning and evening workouts. The morning workout should be intense but not as extensive as the evening workout (perform one less set per exercise during the morning workout).

If you're using Soviet Quad Shock Train Specialization for your quads, you should do a superset of leg extensions followed by 45 degree leg presses. Perform three sets of 12 to 15 reps for each of those exercises. Remember to rest for 60 to 90 seconds between supersets and then perform four or five sets of 10 to 15 reps of the barbell back squats exercises. You should rest for two or three minutes between each set. Go to positive failure on the final two sets of each of the three exercises. Rest on Tuesday, Friday and Sunday. Use extensive physical and mechanical restorative modalities every day to derail overtraining or injury, and to accelerate the recovery time between workout sessions.

4 Usually it's a good idea to do a variety of exercises from many different angles to stimulate maximum gains for a lagging muscle group. The late Don Ross, co-author of the bestseller *MuscleBlasting!*, called this uni-angular bombing (also known as diversified training). He advised bodybuilders to target the same lagging muscle group by using different exercises every two weeks. The late Peary Rader, original owner and publisher of *Iron Man* magazine, first introduced this method of specialization back in the 1960s, calling it The Ten Set Variable System. The idea is to choose 10 different exercises for a muscle group. Begin with a compound exercise, followed by an isolation exercise sequence using a variety of training equipment such as barbells, dumbbells and cables. Complete seven or eight reps for each set. Rest for one minute between each set.

Peary felt that the Ten Set Variable System was not limited to specializing on one muscle group, but could be used very successfully to specialize on the entire upper body. For ex-

ample, a bodybuilder could train up to five different upper-body muscle groups (lats, pecs, delts, biceps and triceps). If doing this, you should rest for five to ten minutes between training each muscle group. This is a tough system, recommended only for advanced bodybuilders if they've reached a sticking point, have the capacity for very hard training and can fully recuperate between workouts.

5 Aside from specialization techniques, the remainder of your training program for moderate and superior muscle groups should follow this rule: Perform two exercises of two sets on each of your moderate muscle groups and one exercise of two sets on your superior muscle groups. If you're a hardgainer, decrease the number of sets by an additional 25 percent.

6 Specialize on only one muscle group (with the exception of Methods Of Specialization: 5 and 6) at a given time. For example, you shouldn't attempt to do priority training for two major muscle groups such as the chest and back at the same time. However, you can work two minor muscle groups such as biceps and triceps or a combination of one major and minor muscle group, if need be.

7 Maintain a positive attitude and the willpower to make the specialization program work. Use visualization techniques frequently. Imagine yourself achieving an improvement in muscle density.

8 Put your specialization (muscle-priority) program at the very beginning of a scheduled morning or evening daily workout. Generally, blood testosterone, glucose, muscle glycogen and the psychosomatic cycle (mental and physical feeling) toward training are at heightened levels during the first 20 to 45 minutes of a workout. As a result, you'll be able to apply maximum training effort.

Upon completion of the specialization program, rest for 20 minutes prior to training other muscle groups. This allows for the proper adaptive biochemical responses at the cellular level and the muscle group receiving the

Vary your exercises, using different angles, to stimulate maximum gains for a lagging bodypart.

priority training. You should probably have a small amount of food or a protein shake to give yourself some energy for the rest of your workout at this point. Interestingly enough, Soviet bodybuilders and lifters plan the volume and intensity of their training sessions around such measurable indexes as diastolic blood pressure, early-morning heart rates, venous blood acidity and white blood cell counts.

9 Another way to structure your specialization training is to perform it in the morning and then come back later in the day and complete the remaining workout for the number of other muscle groups you planned on working that particular day. This incorporates the principle of double-split training.

10 Perform an easy-to-implement effective specialization routine on days that don't have a workout scheduled. For example, do a specialization program on Tuesday, Thursday and Saturday. Train the rest of your other muscle groups once or at most twice per week on non-consecutive days (perhaps on Monday and Friday) and reduce the number of sets you normally do by approximately 25 to 75 percent. For the extreme hardgainer, we suggest only doing one set per muscle group of an isolation exercise.

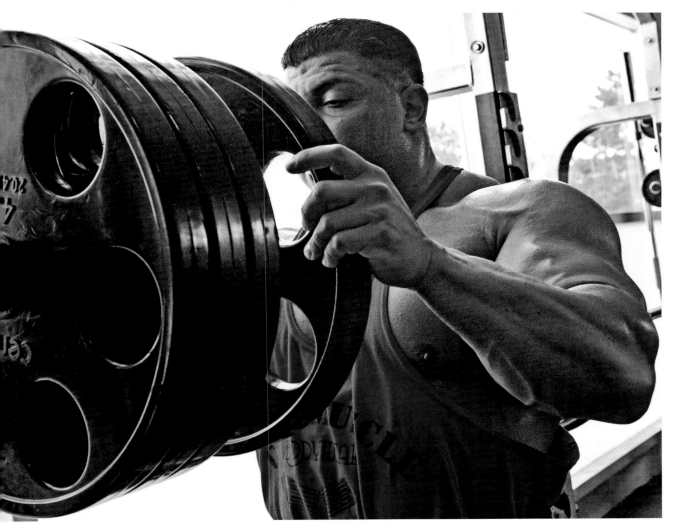

CHAPTER 37

METHODS FOR SPECIALIZATION: METHODS ONE TO FIVE

When it comes to the "how," there are many ways to incorporate specialization into your training routine.

METHOD #1 – STRENGTH ADVANTAGE STRATEGY: ONE-EXERCISE-ONLY SPECIALIZATION

Specialization isn't always about just adding size, shape and muscularity to a subpar muscle group. Sometimes it's advantageous to specialize on one exercise only to the exclusion of doing a group of exercises, especially if it's your mission to gain the most amount of strength in the shortest possible time. Generally the acquisition of strength is reserved for core growth exercises such as barbell squats, deadlifts, bench presses, overhead presses and curls.

Collectively, we've been involved in the iron game for over 100 years and have yet to hear a person ask how much weight another can lift in the lateral raise, incline flye, leg extension or cable crossover. They want to know about big weights on the big lifts.

With that thought in mind, we're going to reveal a couple of easy strategies for improving strength. Through the years, bodybuilders, Olympic lifters and strongmen have made outstanding gains using the strategies we're about to reveal, and these gains are lasting.

The four strength-advantage strategies we are going to detail are the One-Rep Gain Factor, Five x Five Methodic, Six-Week Flashpoint Strength Technique and 12 Workouts to Superior Strength Gains Program. You should choose one of these in conjunction with your One-Exercise-Only Specialization.

ONE–REP GAIN FACTOR

The One-Rep Gain Factor was created by the late Doug Hepburn in the 1950s to acquire a giant reserve of strength and power necessary for the many

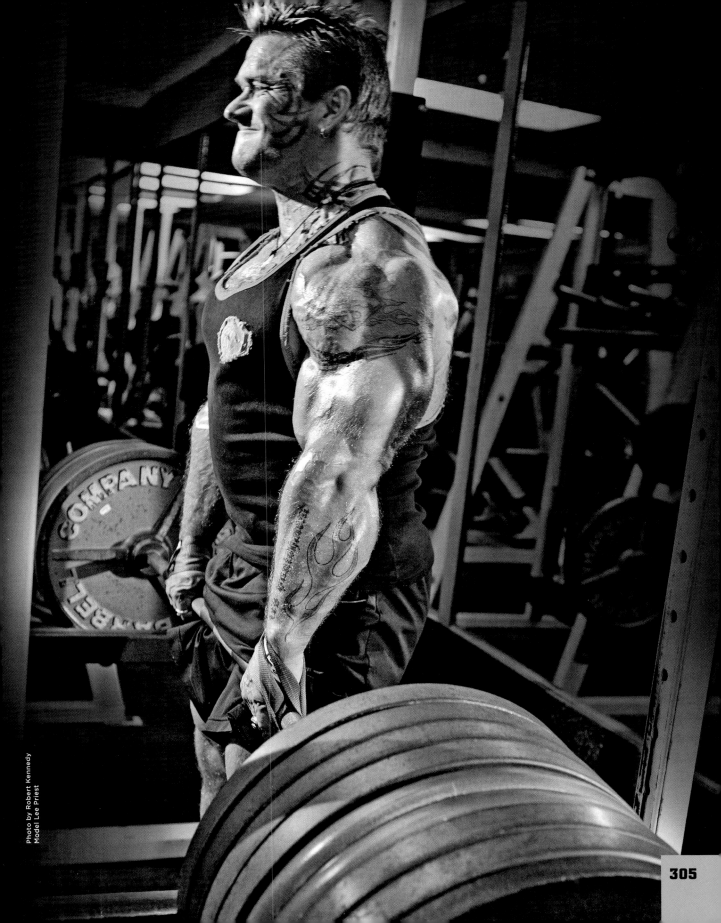

lifts he performed at a world-class level. The workout consists of two parts.

PART 1 – ONE–REP PER WORKOUT

Select a core growth exercise you want to specialize on. Load a bar to a starting weight you can lift for five consecutive reps for a specific warm-up (use a weight you can use comfortably without straining). When you have completed the fifth consecutive repetition, rest for three to five minutes. From there, you advance to single reps. Perform three sub-maximum single reps (rest three to five minutes after each single repetition) while increasing the weight of each proceeding sub-single so that a near-limit weight can be performed for the third and final sub-maximum single. This will generally be about 30 pounds less than you can do in the selected exercise for a one-rep maximum. Now do one rep at your 1RM. Build up the numbers by striving to add one additional rep

at your 1RM each workout until you are doing four maximum single repetitions.

When you're able to perform four maximum single reps, increase your specific warm-up, sub-maximum and maximum single repetition weights by five to ten pounds. It's very important that you don't increase the poundage until the four maximum single reps can be performed. Otherwise, you may create an environment of overtraining of both the localized skeletal muscle and central nervous systems.

PART 2 – MAXI-REP SETS

Upon completion of part one, decrease the weight until you're able to perform four sets of three consecutive reps with the most weight involved. Rest for three to five minutes between each set. With each scheduled workout, add one additional rep until you can manage four sets of five consecutive reps.

When you're able to perform the ninth workout, you should increase the weights on

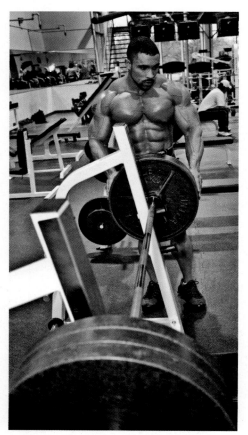

One specialization technique involves building up your rep numbers by trying to add one extra rep each workout at your 1RM until you reach four reps.

WORKOUT #1
4 sets / 3 reps
WORKOUT #2
1 set / 4 reps
3 sets / 3 reps
WORKOUT #3
1 set / 5 reps
3 sets / 3 reps
WORKOUT #4
1 set / 5 reps
1 set / 4 reps
2 sets / 3 reps
WORKOUT #5
2 sets / 5 reps
2 sets / 3 reps
WORKOUT #6
2 sets / 5 reps
1 set / 4 reps
1 set / 3 reps
WORKOUT #7
3 sets / 5 reps
1 set / 3 reps
WORKOUT #8
3 sets / 5 reps
1 set / 4 reps
WORKOUT #9
4 sets / 5 reps

Photo by Rich Baker
Model Tim Liggins

all four sets by five pounds and begin a new series of four sets of three consecutive repetitions, following Workouts #1 through #9. If at any time you can't seem to make the required one-rep gain for two consecutive workouts (this usually happens within the grid of the single-rep sets), you may be experiencing a mild onset of overtraining. In that case, you should temporarily eliminate part one (single-rep sets) from your next three or four workouts, but continue part two (maxi-rep sets), and perform six sets instead of four. When you reinstate part one (single-rep sets) into your program (beginning at where you left off previously), you must reduce the number of maxi-rep sets back to only four. You'll have to recalculate parts one and two so the progressive one-rep gain factor, in both, once again increases somewhat proportionately.

The One-Rep Gain Factor workout seems to garner the most productive cumulative results in strength advantage when it's performed every third or fourth specialized training day. In some severe cases of overtraining, we would suggest decreasing the frequency to once every seventh day.

FIVE X FIVE METHODIC

One of the most effective systems devised for strength gains is the Five x Five Methodic. The exact genesis of this system is unclear, but it appears to have been developed in the U.K. and then brought to the U.S. shortly thereafter. Its major proponent in the U.S. is *Iron Man* Magazine contributor Bill Starr, who deserves credit for disseminating information of this excellent system through his writings and coaching.

The Five x Five Methodic should be used only on core growth exercises (squats, benches, deadlifts, etc.) and shouldn't be applied to muscle-specific or isolation movements (lateral raises, leg extensions, heel raises, etc). Here's a typical 5 x 5 system:

Set 1 65% Max. for 5 reps
Set 2 80% Max. for 5 reps
Set 3 88% Max. for 5 reps
Set 4 89% Max. for 5 reps
Set 5 90% Max. for 5 reps

When you're able to consistently perform each of these last three sets, increase the weight used for each set by about five pounds to ensure you'll be operating at that 88 to 90 percent maximum load as your strength increases.

The Five x Five system is meant for core growth exercises, not isolation moves.

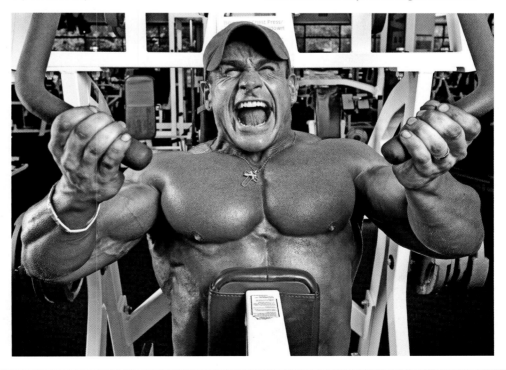

Photo by Kevin Horton
Model Lee Powell

In this method of training it's extremely important to rest between sets, especially in the last three sets, as the stress loads and concurrent rep demands are quite high. You should rest for two to four minutes between sets whenever performing multiple sets at stress loads exceeding 85 percent of maximum. When building strength it makes little sense to battle fatigue.

The Five x Five Methodic system is effective for many reasons, including that it demands you don't fatigue a muscle on your initial warm-up. Another key reason for its effectiveness is that most of the work and maximal output is demanded in the latter three strength sets where you're expected to lift 88 to 90 percent of maximum. As a result, fatigue becomes a factor only toward the last set, which means that you've performed a good degree of high-quality work in an unfatigued state. Of course, everyone has a specific limit as to how quickly they respond to high stress loads, so progress is as much a factor of genetic predispositions as it is of stress loads.

Over time, progress will slow or become non-existent. To help prevent this, the pure 5 x 5 methodic can be modified with a light-training day. If you want to perform a twice-weekly One Exercise Only Specialization procedure using a modified 5 x 5 methodic, follow the chart below:

Most of the demand on your muscles will come in the third, fourth and fifth sets when you're using a higher percentage of your 1RM.

SET NUMBER	DAY 1	DAY 2
1	65% 1RM – 5 reps	65% 1RM – 6-8 reps
2	80% 1RM – 5 reps	80% 1RM – 6-8 reps
3	88% 1RM – 5 reps	84% 1RM – 6-7 reps
4	88% 1RM – 5 reps	84% 1RM – 6-7 reps
5	88% 1RM – 5 reps	84% 1RM – 6-7 reps

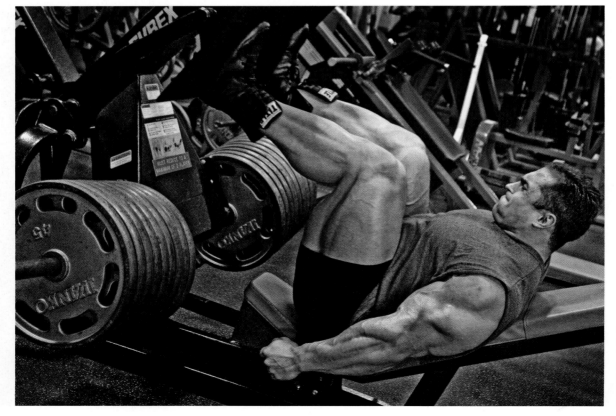

Photo by Alex Ardenti
Model Alexander Fedorov

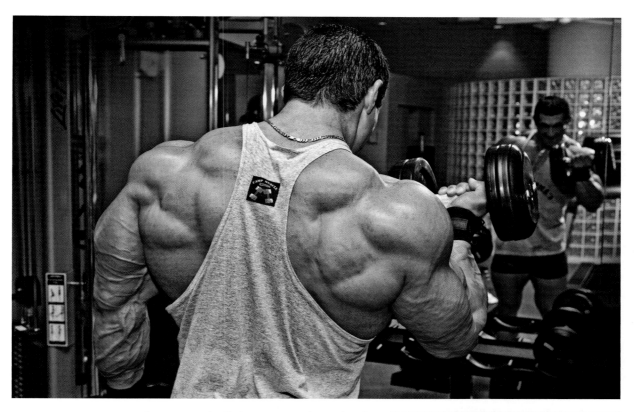

Photo by Rich Baker
Model Brian Yersky

With the flashpoint strength technique, you'll get the greatest strength gain in the least amount of time.

The 5 x 5 methodic is an extremely good tool to develop strength, but remember to use this system only when specializing on core growth exercises. The stress loads are far too high for isolation movements and you may injure yourself badly if you don't follow the system properly.

SIX-WEEK FLASHPOINT STRENGTH TECHNIQUE

We've researched every strength advantage strategy, so we know what works and what doesn't. The Flashpoint Strength technique is a six-week strength advantage strategy that will give you the greatest strength gain in the least amount of time. It uses a fixed poundage percentage of a one-rep max (1RM). Increase the percentages of maximum and corresponding poundages no more than once every seven days, over a six-week period. On the right you'll find an outline of the six progressive training levels. Be sure to perform a couple of light exercise-specific warm-up sets at each level of your training.

MONDAY AND FRIDAY OR TUESDAY AND SATURDAY

LEVEL ONE (WEEK #1)

After a couple of light exercise-specific warm-up sets, perform five sets of 10 maxi-pump reps using 65 percent of your unfatigued 1RM.

LEVEL TWO (WEEK #2)

5 sets x 8 maxi-pump reps with 72 percent of your 1RM

LEVEL THREE (WEEK #3)

5 sets x 6 power reps with 79 percent of your 1RM

LEVEL FOUR (WEEK #4)

5 sets x 4 power reps with 86 percent of your 1RM

LEVEL FIVE (WEEK #5)

4 sets x 3 power reps with 93 percent of your 1RM

LEVEL SIX (WEEK #6)

1 set x 2 power reps with 100 percent of your 1RM

The Superior Strength Gains system requires only two workouts per week and involves three different workouts.

12 WORKOUTS TO SUPERIOR STRENGTH GAINS PROGRAM

During the course of our exhaustive research, we've discovered at least a dozen excellent strength programs that would help the bodybuilding community increase their strength in core exercises such as the barbell bench press, curl, deadlift, overhead press, bent-over row, back squat, etc.

One of the most productive strength programs is the 12 Workouts to Superior Strength Gains program that a bodybuilder named John Robbins used to blast his own and others' strength into the stratosphere. The intensity threshold of his program requires only two workouts per week, usually on Mondays and Thursdays, to avoid the overtraining syndrome.

Workout A takes place on the first training day of the week. Your training stress loads for your barometer one-rep sets will consist of working with 95 percent of your current 1RM. If you were a natural, steroid-free bodybuilder with a 300-pound max in the barbell bench press, your workout would be performed as follows: 135 (45%) / 10 reps, 185 (62%) / 5 reps, 225 (75%) / 3 reps, 255 (85%) / 2 reps and 285 (95%) / 4 single-rep sets.

On the second training day (workout B), you'll use 85 percent of maximum (300 pounds) for three triple-rep strength-building sets. This second workout is performed as follows: 135 (45%) / 10 reps, 185 (62%) / 5 reps, 225 (75%) / 3 reps and 255 (85%) / 4 single-rep sets.

The third training sequence (workout C) requires you to use 75 percent of your critical threshold 300-pound maximum for two or three five-rep sets. Lift 135 (45%) / 10 reps, 185 (62%) / reps and 225 (75%) for three sets of five reps.

A brief overview of this program would show that in the first week you're doing workout A on Monday, workout B on Thursday, and then workout C on Monday at the beginning of the second week. On Thursday of the second week, you perform workout A, and so on. If you prefer a visual aid, please see the following chart:

WEEK NUMBER	MONDAY OR TUESDAY WORKOUT	THURSDAY OR FRIDAY WORKOUT
1	A	B
2	C	A
3	B	C
4	A	B
5	C	A
6	B	C

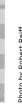

Photo by Robert Reiff
Model Monty Rogers

To maintain a systematic strength progression in this three-program training approach, it's vital that you strive to add five pounds over your previous training barometer one rep (workout A) or multiple-rep strength-building sets (workouts B and C) every workout, if possible. At the conclusion of the six-week cycle, you'll have accomplished approximately a six- to eight percent strength gain in the barometer sets of programs A, B and C. At that point, you can test for a new 1RM and, after taking a one-week layoff of active rest, begin a new six-week cycle.

Choose one of the four strength-advantage strategies for a One-Exercise-Only specialization procedure, and follow Guidelines of Specialization one to ten.

The floor barbell press lockout training system is a single-exercise bench-press building program that can help you make great increases in poundage on the standard bench press.

ONE-EXERCISE-ONLY SPECIALIZATION CONCLUSION

Just to illustrate the thought and creativity that can go into planning a One-Exercise-Only Specialization program, we thought you might enjoy reading about the measured movement floor bench press and deadlift. Here's some interesting instruction on each one.

FLOOR BARBELL PRESS LOCKOUT TRAINING SYSTEM (WOODEN-PLANK CONCEPT)

How would you like a One-Exercise-Only super bench press-building program that will guarantee an increase to your limit in the barbell bench press by 30 to 50 pounds in just 45 to 60 days? If you want to blast your regular bench press into the stratosphere, try this failsafe system for building tremendous tendon and ligament mass and strength faster than you ever thought possible!

TENDON AND LIGAMENT MASS AND STRENGTH THEORY

If you want to build huge reserves of great muscle strength, you must train for greater tendon and ligament mass and strength. This isn't as difficult as it seems and can be accomplished with the use of heavy poundage on the floor barbell press with measured movement lockouts.

One of the most simplistic ways of accomplishing this task is to secure approximately four dozen 1" x 12" wooden planks which measure 18 inches long.

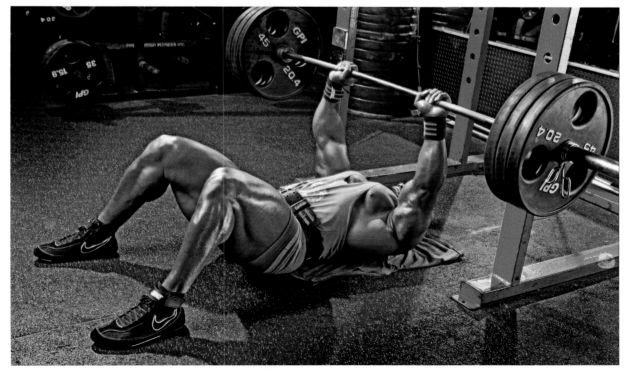

Photo by Robert Reiff
Model Johnnie Jackson

Place two stacks of wooden planks evenly a correct distance apart so you can initiate the Barbell Floor Press. The number of wooden planks used in each stack will be dependent on the diameter of the plates (i.e. use 25 pound plates, more planks, 45 pound plates, less planks etc.) of a previously positioned and loaded barbell. All in all the wooden plank and barbell plate diameter considerations should definitely allow for a 2–3 inch measured movement in the lockout position of the Barbell Floor Press.

Begin by doing the regular Barbell Bench Press for two warm up sets of 15 and 10 reps each. (See the proceeding set and rep schedule.) When you have finished the warm-up sets lie down on the floor between the two wooden planks and begin doing the first of 8 sets of the Barbell Floor Press.

On the sixth set you shouldn't have any problems locking out 40 percent (125 pounds) over your best maximum single effort in the barbell bench press.

Follow the program as prescribed on two non-consecutive workout days. One of the best strategies is to perform the barbell floor press on one day and then rest for a total of three days. In this case your workouts for the barbell floor press will be structured around an eight-day cycle as opposed to the common seven-day cycle. Don't worry, this will allow for maximum recovery of your muscles and systemic recovery of your central nervous system. You should remove a plank from each side of the stack on every fourth barbell floor press workout. The cool thing is you will continue to move the same top poundage (set number 6) through an increased range of movement to where the back of the upper arms almost touch the floor.

Concentration is extremely important. You have to work up your adrenaline for an explosive push. Imagine how thrilled you'll be when you're able to do the floor barbell press measured movement lockouts off just a very few planks and at 40 percent over your 1RM in a regular barbell bench press! Your new 1RM in the regular barbell bench press will have increased by at least 30 to 50 pounds.

FLOOR BARBELL PRESS MEASURED MOVEMENT LOCKOUT SYSTEM

Floor barbell press lockouts are a very rigorous form of exercise, and you must take special care to avoid injuries. When handling a poundage considerably greater than you're accustomed to, it's very important to warm up properly. Here is a sample workout schedule based on a flat barbell bench press 1RM of 300 pounds:

EXERCISE WARM-UP	POUNDAGE	REPS	1RM %
Flat Barbell Bench Press	135	15	45
	185	10	60
Floor Barbell Press Lockout	225	8	75
	305	6	120
	355	3	120
	385	2	130
	405	1	135
	425	1	140
	355	3	120
	305	6	102

After six to eight weeks of performing this measured movement lockout routine, go back to a regular barbell bench press program for at least one month before going back to floor presses.

We caution you to take it easy the first couple of days back. While you've improved your tendons, ligaments, mass and strength and your old poundage limit feels light, your pectoral muscles have not been accustomed to full-range movements with maximum poundage for the last few weeks. Take at least a week to get your pecs and delts ready for hoisting the heavy iron. You'll find that this will greatly reduce the possibility of an injury.

If you're going to use planks, you may want to drill a hole in the front and back of each plank so the holes line up with all the other planks in the stack. This will allow you to drop a long 1/2″ steel rod into the front and back hole to act as a pin to stop the planks from shifting off center when they're hit.

MEASURED MOVEMENT BARBELL DEADLIFT (WOODEN-PLANK CONCEPT)

How would you like to add as much as 10 percent onto your power deadlift 1RM within a few short workouts? Here's how:

BARBELL DEADLIFT WORKOUT

Load a bar to your best 10-rep maximum poundage and then perform two sets of six reps (rest for three minutes between the sets). This exercise should be performed like the regular conventional deadlift except for two important differences. First, as you reach the vertical lockout position, motion your shoulders up and back as far as possible while slightly bending your arms to activate your biceps. Hold this position for two seconds and then lower the barbell until the plates are about two inches off the floor. Stop any further movement and hold in place for about two or three seconds. Then, begin the upward pull again and repeat the whole process once more for two sets of about six reps. Once you've completed this, rest for eight to ten minutes.

Specialization techniques like the Barbell Deadlift Workout and the Measured Movement Power Deadlift will effectively target your back to promote increased gains.

MEASURED MOVEMENT POWER DEADLIFT (WOODEN-PLANK CONCEPT)

The measured movement power deadlift is the secret exercise that will give you the fantastic boost of power you've always wanted when performing the conventional barbell deadlift. Prior to beginning this exercise, use the wooden planks from the previous barbell floor press and arrange them in even stacks so that when a barbell is placed on them, the bar will be positioned at your knees.

Place the barbell on the planks and load it up to a poundage that's 10 percent over your 1RM. For example, if your 1RM in the barbell deadlift is 400 pounds, you should add 40 pounds more to the bar. Begin performing this lift in a conventional deadlift style, but for only one single effort in a slow, deliberate manner

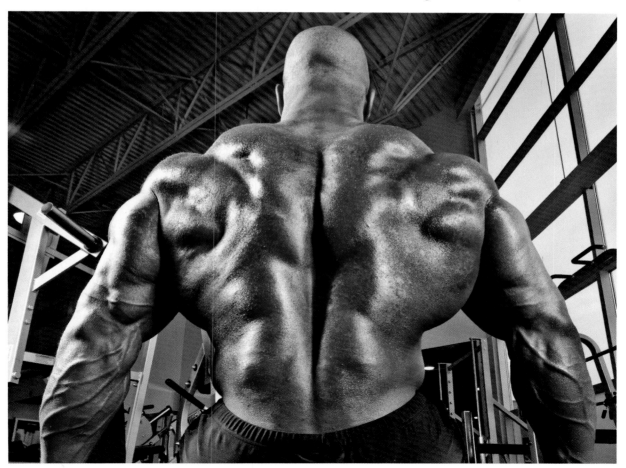

Photo by CW Photography
Model David Fenty

Giant Cycles, with a specific order of isolation and compound moves for a muscle group, will increase muscle hypertrophy.

and with a firm lock-out. Perform six to ten single attempts (depending upon your existing energy level), resting three to five minutes between attempts. Even though you are deadlifting 10 percent more poundage than you normally lift, the pull will seem less difficult since the lifting motion is only a few inches (from knees to lockout).

The key to improving in this exercise is to remove two 1" wooden planks from each stack each workout. Continue with the plank removal until you're finally doing the single-rep deadlifts from the floor. You may discover that removing one plank each workout isn't always possible. You might only remove a plank from each stack every fourth workout. Regardless, the wooden plank removal exercise is still a fast way to gain strength in the deadlift.

Always begin the first single effort of the measured movement power deadlift from knee level to lockout even if you have removed many planks by that point. Work your way down the planks to your present level of strength. Once you've worked your way down to pulling the deadlifts off the floor, add 10 percent more to the barbell and begin the procedure all over again. After two cycles of the measured movement barbell deadlift, you should eliminate them from your deadlift program for two or three months. Following this period, you can implement them back into your workout again.

METHOD #2 – SIZE, SHAPE AND MUSCULARITY – GIANT CYCLE SPECIALIZATION

Using a group of exercises in a specific way can be a great way to add size while improving shape and muscularity. One of the most efficient training principles to use is the Giant Cycle (not to be confused with giant set).

The Giant Cycle principle is a tested and proven brutally intense program for maximizing metabolic and cosmetic muscular hypertrophy. By employing the Giant Cycle principle, you'll increase cellular energy production and strength by increasing the number of mitochondria within the muscle cells themselves. As a result, you may find that you suddenly have the ability to perform an increased number of

reps, and your muscles will grow more quickly.

Giant Cycle is a term used to describe the performance of a series of exercises for a muscle group. The exercises will consist of a muscle specific (single joint) movement and a compound (multiple joint) movement. The exercises are normally set up for most standard giant cycles and reverse giant cycles as seen below.

STANDARD GIANT CYCLE
Isolation Move
Isolation Move
Compound Move
Isolation Move
REVERSE GIANT CYCLE
Compound Move
Compound Move
Isolation Move
Compound Move

On the right are some examples of standard giant cycles for quads, hamstrings and upper pecs. You must first select a weight that can be performed for the desired number of repetitions. Keep the rep number the same for all four components in any given giant cycle. Don't rest between any of the four sets.

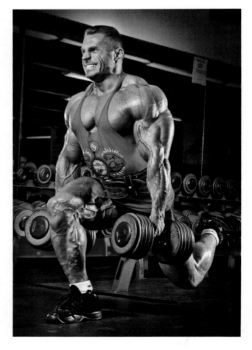

Photo by Paul Buceta
Model Evgeny Mishin

QUADS

Leg extensions for 10 reps using 100 pounds.

Leg extensions for 10 reps using 75 pounds. (Drop weight by 25 percent.)

Wide stance hack squat for 10 reps using 210 pounds.

Leg extensions for 10 reps using 50 pounds. (Always use 50 percent of weight used in step 1.)

HAMS

Leg curl for 12 reps using 80 pounds.

Leg curl for 12 reps using 60 pounds.

Stiff-leg deadlift for 12 reps using 135 pounds.

Leg curl for 12 reps using 40 pounds.

CHEST (UPPER PECS)

Incline flye for 12 reps using 60 pounds.

Incline flye for 12 reps using 45 pounds.

Flat bench press for 12 using 135 pounds.

Incline flye for 12 reps using 30 pounds.

**EXAMPLE OF A REVERSE GIANT
CYCLE FOR BACK THICKNESS**

T-bar or angled leverage row for 10 reps using 150 pounds.

T-bar or angled leverage row for 10 reps using 110 pounds.

Straight-arm pulldown or one-dumbbell pullovers for 10 reps using 100 pounds.

T-bar or angled leverage row for 10 reps using 75 pounds.

If the initial poundage drop of 25 percent results in uneven or unusable poundage, you should select the next lower poundage available. For example, if you to take 25 percent from 50 pounds, the result is 37.5 pounds. In that case, use 35 pounds. If you cannot perform 10 reps with the weight you selected for the compound movement in set 3 but you can perform at least five reps, you may continue to use that weight. However, if your selection allows you to perform fewer than five reps, you must lower the weight. Rest only two minutes between each standard or reverse giant cycle series, or as long as it takes for your training partner to complete his giant cycle. You should perform three to five series of a standard or reverse giant cycle for any subpar muscle group needing specialization.

The leg extension can be used as the isolation move for a standard Giant Cycle for legs.

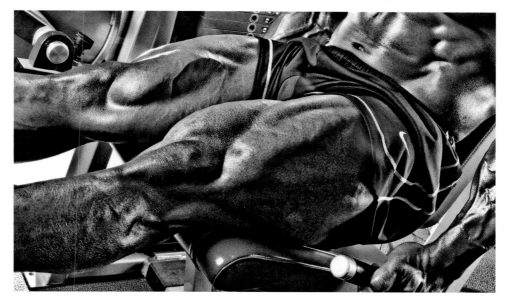

STANDARD AND REVERSE GIANT CYCLES

QUADS – STANDARD GIANT CYCLE

Leg Extension

Leg Extension

Barbell Back Squat or Hack Squat

Leg Extension

HAMS – REVERSE GIANT CYCLE

Leg Curl

Leg Curl

Stiff-Leg Deadlift

Leg Curl

BACK – REVERSE GIANT CYCLE

T-Bar Row

T-Bar Row

Straight Arm Lat Pulldown or One-Dumbbell Bench Pullover

T-Bar Row

PECS – STANDARD GIANT CYCLE

Flat Dumbbell Flye

Flat Dumbbell Flye

Flat Barbell Bench Press

Flat Dumbbell Flye

DELTS – STANDARD GIANT CYCLE

Standing Dumbbell Lateral Raise

Standing Dumbbell Lateral Raise

Barbell Upright Row

Standing Dumbbell Lateral Raise

TRICEPS – STANDARD GIANT CYCLE

Two-Arm Dumbbell French Press

Two-Arm Dumbbell French Press

Close-Grip Barbell Bench Press

Two-Arm Dumbbell French Press

BICEPS – STANDARD GIANT CYCLE

Concentration Curl

Concentration Curl

Cheat Barbell Curl

Concentration Curl

METHOD #3 – POWER-BODY-BUILDING SPECIALIZATION

"A power bodybuilder, regardless of the exercise, forces toward the heaviest weight in that exercise because he has two goals: One, to gain muscle mass, the other, to max out the weights he measures his life and performance by. If he's not making gains on the one level, he looks to the other level for satisfaction. Therefore, he does not feel he is wasting himself because in every exercise he must be making a gain in poundage or reps." Bodybuilding expert and photojournalist Denie Walter once said this and it's still true today.

Power-building specialization is physiologically constructed to provide a high level of concentrated training intensity for ultimate gains in strength while simultaneously providing high volume (pump training) to add size and improve shape and muscularity to a subpar muscle group.

To add strength, you should perform one of the strength-advantage strategies (One-Rep Gain Factor, Five x Five Methodic, Six-Week Flashpoint Strength Technique or the 12 Workouts to Superior Strength Gains Program) from the one-exercise-only specialization method. If you're looking to add size as well as improve your shape and muscularity for a subpar muscle group, you should select a standard or reverse giant cycle and perform three or four series.

HOLISTIC 6-12-40 REPS

Bodybuilders are always looking for different ways to shock a lagging muscle group into new strength, size and muscularity, and the Holistic 6-12-40 Reps technique delivers. The ideal number of sets and reps will allow you to establish an excellent mind-to-muscle link without fatigue derailing it. Once the link is in full force, the ideal number of sets and reps will allow you to use the most poundage involved for the stimulation of the strength gain factor, as well as the much desired muscle pump and muscular endurance.

One exercise protocol that's excellent in this regard is the heavy poundage / low reps, medium poundage / moderate reps and light poundage / high-reps principle, or the Holistic 6-12-40 Reps technique. It has proven to be very effective in bringing up a lagging muscle group such as the biceps, and it's equally effective as a growth stimulator for just about any muscle group.

To use a nine-set program design for your biceps, load a barbell with just enough poundage to do one light warm-up set for 20 full-range-of-motion reps of the barbell curl. Take a 30-

If you want to bring up your biceps, combine concentration curls with cheat barbell curls using the standard Giant Cycle.

to 45-second rest, load additional poundage and perform six full reps to positive failure. Immediately begin performing the preacher bench barbell curl for 12 reps to positive failure. Right after completing of the 12th rep, do seated alternating dumbbell curls for 40 maxi-pump reps to positive failure. The biceps' time under tension will go beyond 60 seconds for this series. Repeat the series at least two more times.

Remember you shouldn't rest within the 6-12-40 series other than the time it takes to move from one piece of equipment to the other. Upon completion of the first series of three exercises, you may have to reduce the poundage as a result of tension and fatigue. If so, remove five to ten pounds for the second and third series. Be sure you take four or five days of rest between each Holistic 6-12-40 Reps workout scheme.

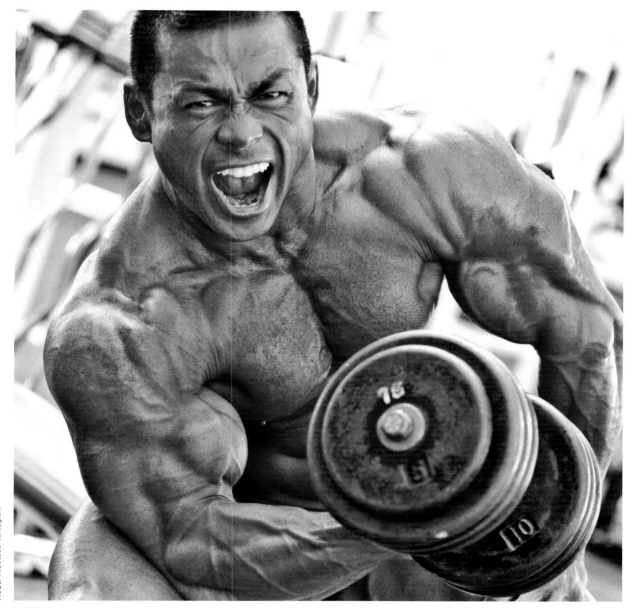

Photo by Paul Buceta
Model Hidetada Yamagishi

Some bodybuilding pros will do the 6-12 rep scheme on the standing calf machine (works the 60 percent fast-twitch fibers of the gastrocnemius) and immediately finish off with 40 reps on the seated calf machine (works the 88 percent slow-twitch fibers of the soleus).

that if a person trains both sides equally but concentrates more on the weaker side, muscle development and strength will eventually become balanced. We disagree and would like to offer you a rather easy solution to solve a bilateral deficit in symmetry or strength output.

HOLISTIC 6-12-40 REPS SPECIALIZATION

EXERCISE	SETS	REPS	%OF 1RM	METHOD
Barbell Curl	3	4-6	85	Explosive – Pause between each repetition.
Preacher Bench Barbell Curl	3	12-15	75	Rhythmic Cadence – Moderate speed, with a relaxation pause of a second or less between each repetition.
Seated Dumbbell Curl	3	40	40	Slow Tension – Perform each rep in a slow, sustained fashion (i.e., keep continuous tension on the muscle throughout the concentric and eccentric phases of the movement). No rest pauses through the entire set.

Prior to performing the nine sets, do one or two warm-up sets for each exercise. Perform one exercise after another and take no rest.

Stretch after specialization training to avoid delayed-onset muscle soreness. By following the above sets and reps guidelines, you'll achieve an increase in strength and size and improve your shape and muscularity.

METHOD #4 – BILATERAL DEFICIT SPECIALIZATION FOR BALANCE, SIZE, STRENGTH AND SYMMETRY

Bilateral deficits (asymmetrical deficits) are very common. A bilateral deficit is where the symmetry and strength of the muscles on one side of the body is better than those on the other side.

When measuring your biceps, forearms, thighs and calves, there can be as much as an inch of difference from one side to the other. Bilateral deficits are not exclusive to symmetry and muscle group measurements. There have been extensive studies where the strength outputs of two arms or two legs were tested against the strength outputs for the same exercise using just one arm or one leg. Guess what? You tend to generate about 20 percent more strength output with the dominant arm or leg.

Some experts say that no extra reps or sets are needed for your weaker side. They argue

Simply add one limb (arm or leg) exercise to your current exercise program. Better yet, you could do a four- to six-week specialization program to derail bilateral deficits.

Virtually any exercise that you can perform with both arms and legs using a barbell can be done with one arm or leg using a dumbbell. The same applies for any exercise machine or cable where you would normally use both arms or legs. Machine exercises can be effectively adapted to one arm or leg without having to worry about balance or stabilization issues.

To give you an idea of how bilateral deficit training can be accomplished, here's a brief peak at the one-limb strategy IFBB legend and Hall of Famer Flex Wheeler used when he was training for a pro bodybuilding contest: For quads, Flex performed hack squats using both legs and then did leg extensions one leg at a time. For his back, he did bent-over rows using both arms. Then, using one arm at a time, he used the seated cable row. Flex then went to work on his triceps. He used both arms on triceps pressdowns (V-bar) before using only one arm at a time for reverse-grip pressdowns.

Some of the top pros use the alternate-rep method. With a dumbbell in each hand, they perform exercises such as curls, flyes, lateral raises, overhead presses, bent-over rowing and triceps kickbacks with each hand simultaneously. As the muscles begin to fatigue, they

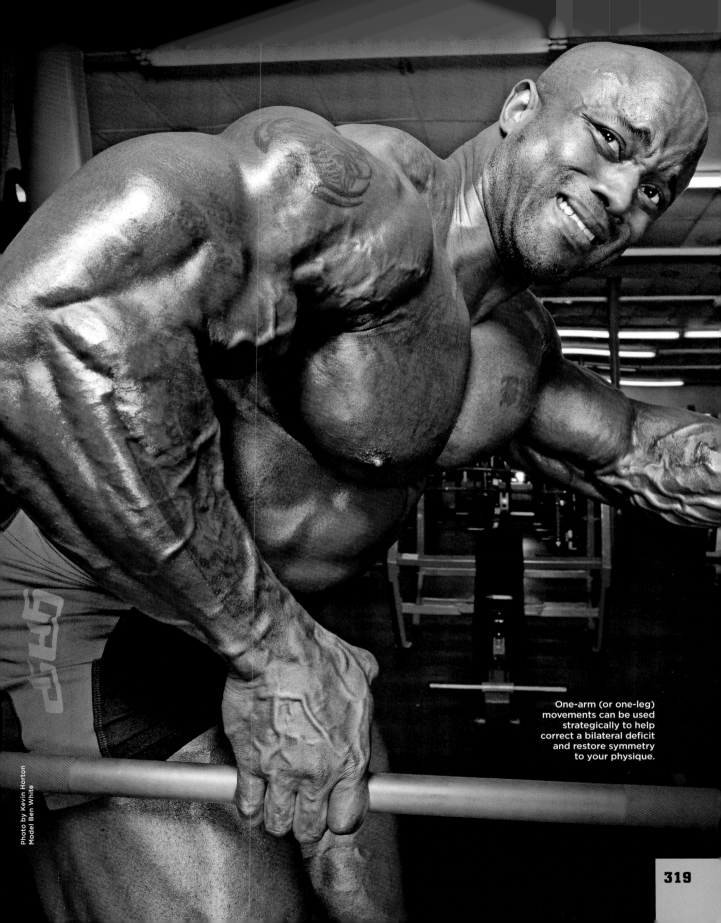

One-arm (or one-leg) movements can be used strategically to help correct a bilateral deficit and restore symmetry to your physique.

Photo by Kevin Horton
Model Ben White

If you're going to modify a standard two-leg movement to a one-leg version, it's imperative that you maintain the standard body posture as much as possible.

switch to doing the reps in alternating style (left, right, left while maintaining maximum concentration etc.). This gives the non-working limb a very brief rest, which results in a few more reps.

It's extremely important when training one limb at a time to make sure your body is aligned in nearly the same posture as it would be when doing the movement with both limbs. For instance, if you decide to do one-leg barbell back squats for the left leg in a power rack or Smith machine, don't thrust the non-working right leg out in front of you. This will change the adaptive response of your nervous system to your thigh muscles in a way that will prevent the best improvement of bilateral deficit. Take the normal squat stance with both of your legs and then do as much of the lift in the positive (under two seconds) and negative (five to eight seconds) phase of each rep as you possibly can with your left leg. Use the right leg only to assist in stabilization and balance.

A good way to accomplish this is to pretend a bone in your right leg is broken and you can't exert any pressure on it. As a result, the quads in your right leg will not contribute or generate any type of significant strength or force output to complete the assigned reps. Here's a four-set combo (considered one cycle) that you can gradually incorporate into your workout program for the one-leg barbell back squat:

Set #1 – Squat two inches above parallel for 6 to 10 reps

Set #2 – Squat to parallel for 6 to 10 reps

Set #3 – Squat two inches below parallel for 6 to 10 reps

Set #4 – Squat four inches below parallel for 6 to 10 reps

Stay with the four-set combo and assigned reps until you feel completely comfortable doing the one-leg barbell back squat. Then gradually decrease the number of reps down to eight, followed by three and then two, using as heavy

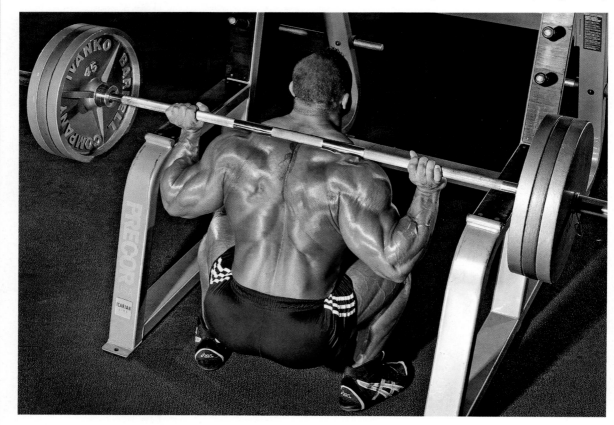

Photo by Paul Buceta
Model Fouad Abiad

poundage as possible for each unique squat position (above or below parallel, etc.). Stay at a particular rep range for two or three weeks before moving down to the next rep scheme. Work up to doing two cycles of the four-set combo. Do the four-set combo cycle no more than twice per week (on non-consecutive training days) when doing rep ranges of six to ten, eights and threes. When you get down to two reps or fewer, do them only once every couple of weeks. Always do three sets on the non-dominant side to every one set you do on the dominant side.

When doing an exercise for one limb, hold a dumbbell in the non-working hand (unless otherwise instructed) at the customary start position as a means of balance and bilateral posture. Don't grab any part of the vertical upright support rack with the non-working hand, as this will change the adaptive response of your mind-to-muscle link and to your chest muscles. Instead, hold a dumbbell in the non-working hand at chest level.

Another bilateral deficit strategy is to do one-limb movements in negative-only style. For example, on machines such as the hack squat, leg extension or leg press, use both legs when doing the positive phase of each rep, but then lower through the negative using only one leg. Use about 30 percent less poundage than normal. Each negative-only rep should take between five and eight seconds. Even negative-only pull-ups can be done by pulling up through the positive phase with both arms and lowering with one arm. Use the hand of your non-working arm to hold onto the wrist of your working arm as a control mechanism.

Though Vince Gironda didn't believe in unilateral movements, he did emphasize the need to develop the neural connections in the non-dominant limb. To do this, he would try to concentrate on slow, bilateral reps while counting to six and mentally directing the nerve force to feel it more on his weaker side. Vince also believed in using the non-dominant side for ordinary tasks such as combing your hair or picking up an object, viewing it as a way to develop your neural pathways for that side. Theoretically, the non-dominant side could

then catch up to the dominant side as he continued to do bilateral movements.

Vince Gironda trained the non-dominant side of his body for one year using specific exercises, yet reported no change in strength or size. Mike Mentzer, on the other hand, tried extra one-armed exercises for the non-dominant bicep that was lagging and it helped. Despite Vince's unsuccessful experience training the non-dominant side, according to anecdotal evidence there's at least the physiological possibility of developing the non-dominant side muscle group, through specific unilateral movements or exercises.

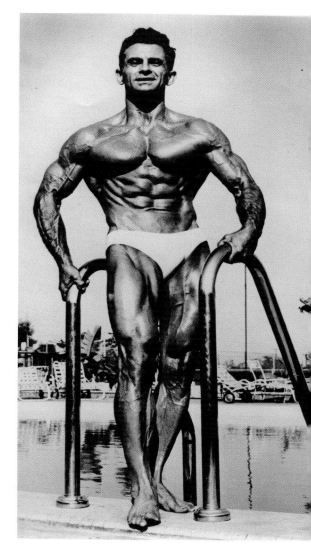

Model Vince Gironda

METHOD #5 – TENDON AND LIGAMENT MASS SPECIALIZATION

All bodybuilders are searching for training methods to increase their muscle mass and power in order to attain that Herculean look. We were no different. We'd gobble up stories about some of the strongest men in the world, and in time, we discovered one of their most important secrets: They all believed in developing tendon and ligament strength through the use of power assistance exercises.

For those of you who are not familiar with the differences of tendon and ligament connective sinews, we'll briefly describe each of them. Tendons are a sort of tough cord or strap-like connective tissue that connect the ends of the muscle to bone tissue. They are typically quite strong and somewhat elastic and transmit the tensile load produced by the muscles to the bone, causing all motion of the body. Tendon strength may be twice that of the muscle belly itself. Ligaments, on the other hand, connect one bone to another at the joints. They help keep bones and joints firmly in place while allowing movement. In other words, they prevent joints from dislocating or otherwise moving in ways they were not meant to. We should also mention cartilage. Cartilage is a simple semi-transparent, firm elastic material found on the surfaces of bones where they form joints. Cartilage prevents bones from rubbing against each other.

Tendons and ligaments are composed primarily of collagen fibers. These fibers give strength and allow the tendons and ligaments to respond mechanically to the forces (stress or strain) applied through power-building movements. Compared to the skeletal muscles, tendons and ligaments have a poor blood supply.

The collagen fibers in tendons and ligaments give strength and enable mechanical responses to the forces applied through various exercises.

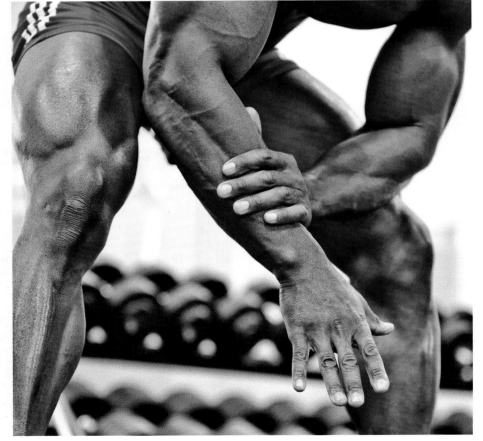

Photo by Paul Buceta
Model Morris Mendez

Some experts suggest doing high-volume training consisting of two or three exercises per muscle group with five to ten sets of around 10 to 20 reps. They theorize that the constant repetitive action of huge volume training stimulates tendon and ligament strength and growth because of the larger workload and increased blood flow to the muscle group. Some of these armchair trainers carry this philosophy to the ultimate extreme by suggesting that tendon and ligament strength is actually increased by doing 50 to 70 reps with a weight only 30 percent of your one-rep max. Nonsense! About the only thing this type of training will do is develop what we call a "suck pump," and it only lasts a few hours. Sure the muscles might swell relatively quickly to a seemingly huge size from the two systems of training, but they will usually do so without a corresponding rise in strength. Big muscles are not always an indicator of great strength. Remember, it is through tendon strength that the potential power of a muscle is transmitted to the joints where movement and pressure is directly applied. Aside from improving your appearance, this type of seemingly massive muscle is largely ineffective.

The late Chuck Sipes, IFBB bodybuilder, often told us that tendon and ligament strength is developed in three phases: Stretching movements, isometric concentrated sustained drives and heavy supports. To obtain real power, bodybuilders need to specialize on exercises that build greater tendon and ligament strength. The way to build this fortress is to use exercises that give your larger muscle groups such as your thighs, glutes, pecs and back plenty of action. Work these muscles over a short range of movement doing half- and quarter-squats and deadlifts, lockout presses and heavy negative curls from the finish position. It's this type of training, which Joe Weider coined short-range and limited-motion principles, that will give you rugged and powerful tendon and ligament strength.

The human body cannot fail to respond to the stimulus of the short-range and limited-motion principles. Your biggest challenge might be finding the heavier poundages for your tendon and ligament strengthening exercises. If you're training in a hardcore gym alongside competitive bodybuilders and powerlifters, this may not be a huge obstacle, but what about the power bodybuilder who trains at home? There's no possible way to perform quarter- or half-squats, overhead supporting and lockout exercises at home unless you pick up a heavy-duty power rack. With this apparatus, any of the short-range and limited-motion power exercises can be performed safely even if you are forced to train on your own. The exercises that were previously out of the question can become part of your repertoire.

TENDON AND LIGAMENT STRENGTHENING PROGRAM

The exercises, sets and reps constitute a workout schedule of their own but it's possible for you to instinctively devise your own program by improvising on the regular exercises you do.

MONDAY

LIGHT BARBELL FLAT BENCH PRESS
Perform four sets of five reps. Use a poundage that allows you nine reps, but do only five.

PARTIAL-MOVEMENT BARBELL BENCH PRESS
Perform three sets of six reps. You'll want to use a heavy-duty power rack for this exercise. To determine how many inches you should lower the bar during the partial bench presses, measure from the highest point of your chest to your wrists while you are lying on the bench with your arms completely extended. Roughly every two weeks, lower the starting point for the partial bench press movement by one-sixth of your total arm length. During the first two weeks, lower the bar four inches from lockout. In the next two weeks, lower it another four inches.

BARBELL TRICEPS EXTENSIONS (LYING ON A FLAT BENCH)
Perform four sets of six reps. Holding an EZ-bar, lower it to your nose and extend. You might want to use elbow ACE supporters for this exercise (maybe even two on each elbow, as there's a lot of stress on the elbow joint).

As part of the Tendon and Ligament Strengthening Program, perform alternating reps of lat pulldowns to the front and behind the neck.

PARTIAL BARBELL TRICEPS EXTENSIONS (LYING ON A FLAT BENCH)

Perform three sets of six reps. Working within the confines of the power rack, adjust the flanged steel rod's safety catches so you have only two or three inches to extend, or press the bar, to lockout. Add variety to the movement by turning the palms of your hands either up or down, and by alternating the width of your hand spacing each set so that all three heads of the triceps are worked.

BARBELL OVERHEAD PRESS

Perform four sets of six reps. Work up to two good sets of high weight.

BARBELL CURLS

Perform three sets of six reps. Use an EZ-bar and maximum weight.

LAT PULLDOWNS

Perform four sets of ten reps. Alternate one rep in front of the neck and one rep behind the neck.

TUESDAY
REST AND RECUPERATION

THURSDAY
HEAVY FLAT BENCH PRESS

(USE THIS CYCLE SEQUENCE)

Weeks 1 to 3 perform four sets with six reps using maximum poundage.
Weeks 4 and 5 perform four sets of five reps.
Weeks 6 to 8 perform three sets of three reps.
Week 9 perform two sets of 3 reps.
Week 10 go for an 1RM attempt.

HEAVY BARBELL FLAT BENCH SUPPORTS

Perform four one-rep sets of 20 seconds. Begin with about 20 to 40 percent over your best 1RM in the bench press and press just off the supports. The idea is to do this with a very slight elbow bend at most to support the massive poundage at arm's length for five to twenty seconds. When you're able to hold the weight for four sets of 20 seconds, it's time to add more weight.

BARBELL PRESS OVERHEAD

3 sets of 7 reps use a poundage that you can do for 11 solid reps but only do 7.

PARTIAL BARBELL PRESS OVERHEAD

Three sets of six partial reps. This exercise is a fine tendon and ligament movement for the triceps and shoulder girdle. Use a poundage 10 to 20 pounds lower than your best (un-

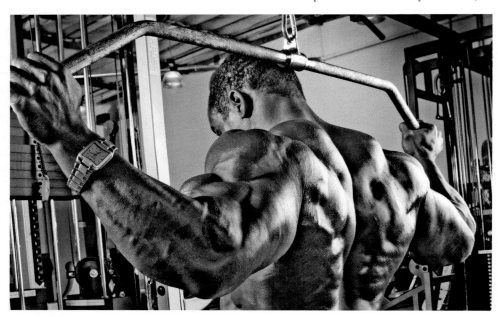

Photo Ralph DeHaan
Model Omar Deckard

psyched, non-adrenalin fueled) full-range one-rep max (1RM) in the overhead barbell press. Adjust the height of the bar within the power rack so it just clears the top of your head. Remember to do all overhead presses while standing and not seated.

For the first set, take a grip with normal hand spacing, press the weight up to arms' length overhead, then lower and repeat for the required partial reps. For the second set take a grip two inches wider than the first. For the final third set use a grip an inch or so closer than that of the first set. If you find it difficult to get the required reps with the hand spacing suggested, take some weight off the bar rather than changing the width of hand spacing.

BARBELL CURLS

Perform three sets of six reps. Use 20 pounds less than on the previous curl day.

PARTIAL POWER CURLS

Perform two sets of six to ten reps. Adjust the height of the bar in the power rack to a fixed position just an inch or so above the horizontal position of your forearms. Do the partial power curls from this area. Vary the exercise by using various widths of grips. Hold the partial contraction at the top of the movement for two seconds or more. Within a few workouts, you should see no less than five to ten pounds of improvement on your regular full-range-of-movement curl. Use a straight bar on this exercise.

FRIDAY
COMPLETE REST AND RECUPERATION

SATURDAY
BARBELL BACK SQUATS

Perform three sets of 10 reps. Increase the weight by 40 pounds and go for three sets of six reps. Given the stress that the squats will put on your knee joints, you might want to put on some knee wraps for these sets. Knee wraps can be purchased at any sporting goods store.

BARBELL QUARTER SQUATS

Perform three sets of six reps. Use about 50 pounds more than your parallel squat to begin with and go only a quarter of the way down. Don't lock your knees.

HEAVY BARBELL SQUAT SUPPORTS

Perform four sets of 20 seconds. Don't do this exercise after quarter squats, but alternate them from week to week. Keep your legs straight and locked.

DEADLIFTS
Perform two sets of five reps.

The key to fantastic power in the tendons and ligaments is the rep scheme and the use of partial and support movements in the day-to-day workouts. We advise you to keep the reps to around six.

In a 1986 interview, Ted Arcidi explained, "Sixes are great. You get good endurance and strength. I feel that sixes are the greatest thing that man ever came across for repetition, especially in the bench press. With sixes you're away from heavy, heavy weight but you still have to throw some weight around because it's not exactly light weight. Imagine going for your best six reps. That means for me I've got to get 560-570 pounds in the bench press. This gives me (and you) a lot of tendon and ligament strength. This is a very important factor when getting into weeks six through nine on the heavy bench press day cycle."

Add weight to the barbell whenever possible, while still performing the specified reps. Perform using maximum effort for every set. Never hold back for a future exercise.

With this program, you're going to find that your muscles will develop to a huge size, but with a corresponding high development of all the tendon connections at the intersection of each muscle. You won't get this type of two-power development from high-volume training systems. Low reps and heavy poundages are the keys to a foolproof system of building greater tendon and ligament strength. Following these points will ensure you get more out of your training efforts.

SUNDAY
COMPLETE REST AND RECUPERATION

CHAPTER 38

METHODS FOR SPECIALIZATION: METHODS SIX TO ELEVEN

The list of methods continues for incorporating specialization techniques into your regimen.

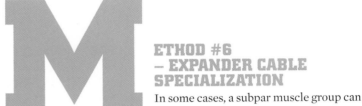

METHOD #6 – EXPANDER CABLE SPECIALIZATION

In some cases, a subpar muscle group can be the result of not exposing those muscles to enough continuous tension. One way to combat this problem is to do super-slow reps or, even better, specialization training. Using expander cables in addition to weights is a good idea. There is very little danger of overtraining when using expander cables. When using weights (barbells, dumbbells), your whole body is forced to exert a tremendous amount of energy just supporting your bodyweight and the barbell or dumbbell. As a result, whatever bodypart you're exercising will be in a constant state of exertion for the entire set and fatigue will occur much faster. Expander cables are so light that energy is not being wasted. Only the muscle being exercised is using energy.

Expander cables are quiet and very easy to store or transport, which means they're also great for travel. The three distinct types of expander cables are steel spring, flat rubber and elastic rubber cord. The steel spring seems to offer more uniform or consistent strength per spring. The main disadvantage is that they have a tendency to pinch your skin with any movements close to your body. The flat rubber and elastic rubber cord will not behave in this manner, but neither will provide as much tension. Some very general expectations from expander training include: Increased chest expansion, better breathing capacity and a more grainy muscularity in the upper torso. If your goal is to achieve greater upper-body muscularity, it's best to perform a specialized cable-training program of 30 minutes to one hour, three days per week. This type of program requires rest between days for your body to repair.

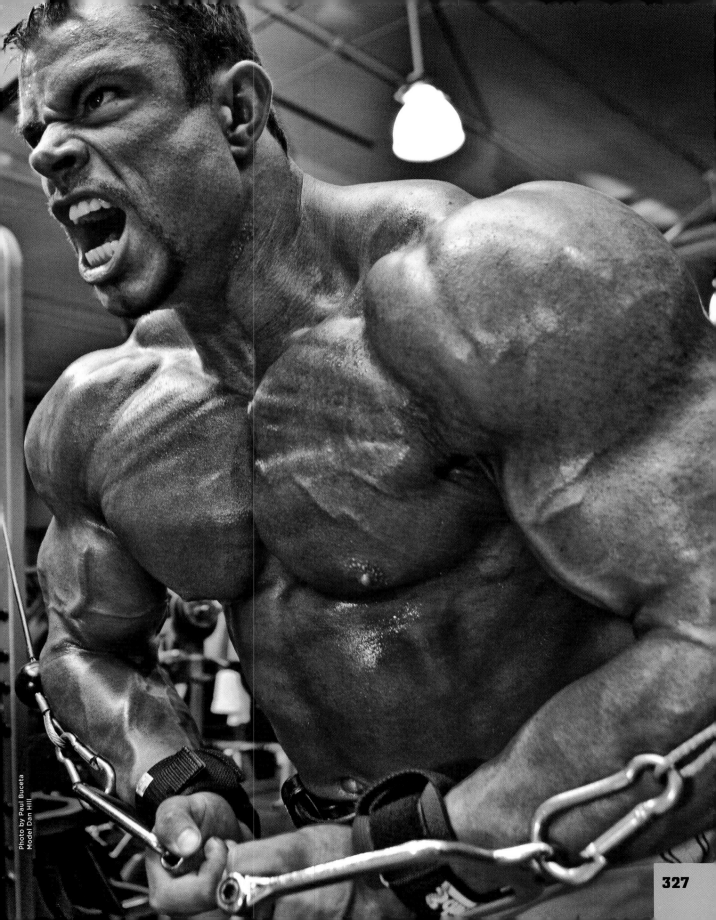

327

FOUR SPECIALIZED EXPANDER CABLE TRAINING TIPS

1. Use speed with smooth movement in each of your exercises.
2. Strive for shorter rest periods between each set. By accomplishing this, you'll be able to add more sets in the 30- to 60-minute program.
3. One of the most important points to remember is that expander cables have the power of stimulating growth faster because of the increased resistance and stretching that occurs through the full range of the movement. In the high range or completed areas of the exercise movement, concentrate on a deeper, wider stretch.
4. For added muscularity, hold the maximum stretched position for a second before beginning the next rep.

If you don't want to do expander cable training three days a week as suggested, then we encourage you to use cables in a heavy barbell program. You should do that by planning your total barbell and expander cable training program at least six months ahead of a contest. During the first two months of contest training, perform two sets (per bodypart) of expander cable work after all of your sets. For example, after you have completed all of your biceps work, finish off with two sets of expander cable curls. In the third and fourth months of training, perform three sets of expander cable work per bodypart. Finally, during the fifth and sixth months, perform four sets of expander cable work per bodypart.

YOUR SIX-MONTH TRAINING SHOULD LOOK AS FOLLOWS:
MONTHS 1-2

You should perform two sets of cable movements following your weight-related work on your deltoids, biceps, triceps, chest, lats, traps and forearms.

MONTHS 3-4

At this point, you may add one additional cable set for each bodypart. Remember to keep track of this in your training journal for your reference.

MONTHS 5-6

During this final two months, you will perform a total of four expander cable movement sets per bodypart. Some of the very best movements in expander cable training are:

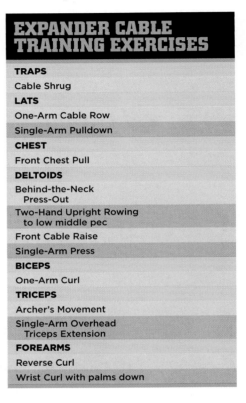

EXPANDER CABLE TRAINING EXERCISES
TRAPS
Cable Shrug
LATS
One-Arm Cable Row
Single-Arm Pulldown
CHEST
Front Chest Pull
DELTOIDS
Behind-the-Neck Press-Out
Two-Hand Upright Rowing to low middle pec
Front Cable Raise
Single-Arm Press
BICEPS
One-Arm Curl
TRICEPS
Archer's Movement
Single-Arm Overhead Triceps Extension
FOREARMS
Reverse Curl
Wrist Curl with palms down

The best repetition schedule to follow when using cables is 10 to 12 reps. When you feel as though you're able to perform the 10 to 12 reps easily and that you aren't getting a deep burn or ache in the muscle being worked, it's time to add another progressive strand or band to your cable apparatus. The arrangement of movements in cable training is overwhelming. For instance, if you're into a specialized expander cable program, you might consider supersetting muscle groups with your cables as you do with barbells.

We suggest that you have two cable sets available to accomplish this because not all bodyparts are strong enough to use the same cable strand. By having them ready before you begin, you'll also save time in making cable strand strength changes. Here's a sample program:

FOUR- TO SIX-WEEK BARBELL / EXPANDER CABLE SYSTEM

TWO TIMES PER WEEK

The following workout could be adjusted very well to the Soviet Quad Shock Training Specialization program.

SUPERSET:

Bench Press 2 X 10-12

Expander Front Chest pulls 2 X 10-12

Rest three minutes, then

SUPERSET:

Wide-Grip Barbell Bent-Over Row 2 X 10-12

Expander Cable Overhead Pulldown 2 x 10-12

Rest three minutes, then

SUPERSET:

Standing Barbell Press Overhead 2 X 10-12

Expander Cable Front Raise 2 X 10-12

Rest three minutes, then

SUPERSET:

Standing Barbell Curl 2 X 10-12

Expander Cable Biceps Curl

Rest three minutes, then

SUPERSET:

Standing Barbell French Press 2 X 10-12

Expander Cable Archer Movement 2 X 10-12

You can also reverse the order of your supersets. For example, do the expander cable flyes first, followed by the bench press. This makes the bench press more difficult to perform and is another way to increase the intensity of your workout. Spend a month with the cables alone. See how many cables you can use per exercise, how many reps you can manage and how long you can hold the exerciser at full extension.

Another type of expander cable training system you might want to try is the 21 Movement. You begin by stretching, curling or pulling – depending on the exercise you're performing at the time – to the halfway point for seven reps. Then, you pull from the locked out or high position to halfway for seven reps and finally finish off with seven complete reps. This constitutes one complete set.

Combining barbell and expander cable exercises or specialized cable work should result in better muscle shape, definition and muscular power. Expander cables will also bring out muscle density, but only after you've built them with weights.

Expander cable training puts increasingly more tension on your tendons, ligaments and

Cables provide continuous tension for the muscles and therefore function as an ideal piece of equipment for specialization techniques such as super-slow reps.

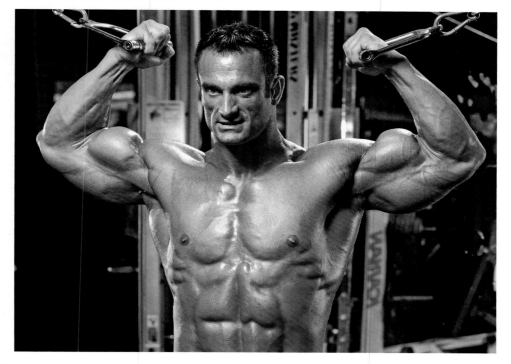

Photo by Robert Reiff
Model Dan Decker

Preacher curls are an effective biceps move to shape train for muscle separation and hardness.

muscle areas, meaning that these areas are strengthened in a different way than when you use weights. With this in mind, if you're a powerlifter, you would be wise to consider including expander cables as a part of your schedule because of the tremendous strength factors involved from the added tendon and ligament work. Expander cables are great for pumping up at a physique contest and a vitally important conditioning tool for a powerlifter. They build tendon and ligament strength and give added muscle tone and sharpness, which cannot be obtained by weights alone. For more information on expander cables, visit: www.ironmind.com.

METHOD #7 – 50/50 COUNTER-SPLIT

One of the most radical methods of specialization we have come across is the old-school 30-Day 50/50 Counter-Split Specialization. It's a little-known training secret that many top bodybuilders have used for years as a means of forcing rapid gains and naturally stimulating improved muscle shape. Basically, it's a counter-split that consists of priority training a lagging muscle group six days per week. You train the muscle group needing specialization for muscle size and strength on Monday, Wednesday and Friday. Countering (hence the term

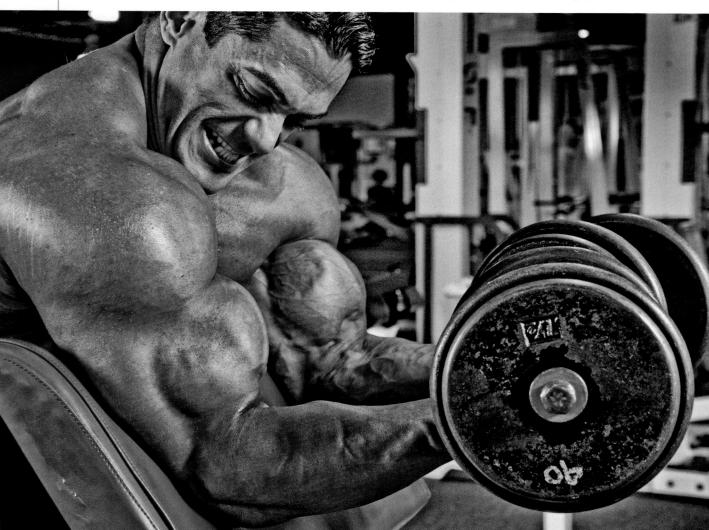

Photo by Jason Breeze
Model Gustavo Badell

counter-split) those training days, you train that same muscle group for shape on Tuesday, Thursday and Saturday.

MUSCLE BULK AND STRENGTH MONDAY-WEDNESDAY-FRIDAY

Choose one compound exercise from the Exercise Selection Chart / Group No. 1 that will work the belly of the muscle. Here's how it works for biceps:

Week 1 – Begin the program by doing the standing barbell curl for four sets of nine reps on each training day.

Week 2 – On each training day, do a total of five sets of seven reps of the seated or kneeling barbell curl.

Week 3 – Do six sets of five reps of standing alternating dumbbell curls on each training day

Week 4 – During this final week, perform seven sets of three reps of the standing barbell curl on each training day.

This four-week progression is adaptable for the intermediate bodybuilder. If you're an advanced bodybuilder, you can begin with five sets per major or minor muscle group needing specialization in each workout day during the first week of priority training. You should do seven sets in the second week of training and nine sets in the third and fourth weeks. Very few advanced bodybuilders will ever need to do more than nine sets of one exercise per muscle group in each workout session. You should rest between sets for two to five minutes.

SHAPE TRAIN TUESDAY-THURSDAY-SATURDAY

In the remaining 50 percent of specialization training, you'll shape train for the development of sharp separation and granite-like hardness. Choose one muscle-specific, or isolation, exercise from the Exercise Selection Chart / Group No. 2 that will target the muscle group needing specialization. Do four to nine sets of each with high reps (nine to twelve), using light to moderate weights.

Week 1 – Begin the program by doing the preacher bench barbell curl for four sets of

nine reps on each training day.

Week 2 – Do dumbbell hammer curls for a total of five sets of 10 reps on each training day.

Week 3 – Perform one-dumbbell concentration curls for six sets of 11 reps on each training day.

Week 4 – Do the Gironda body-drag curl for seven sets of 12 reps on each training day during this final week of training.

You should rest between each set for 45 to 90 seconds.

In order for the 30-Day 50/50 counter-split specialization program to be successful, you must use impeccable form. It's only through impeccable form that you're able to accelerate the muscle gain and strength factors and derail the onset of training injuries. Make sure to always perform exercises correctly for the specified number of reps. Never do your exercises in an uncontrolled (jerking or bouncing) manner.

By following our advice, you'll be able to use impeccable exercise form and increase your exercise poundage in a logical manner. The speed of the negative (eccentric) and positive (concentric) phase of consecutive reps is important to your progress. It's a good idea to do the first half of your reps of a set in an extremely slow manner. Take 10 seconds in the positive phase and five seconds per rep in the negative phase. In the last half of your reps, you should take two seconds in the positive phase, one second in the iso-tension (peak contraction) phase and four seconds in the negative phase. Do this speed system for only one or two sets on a scheduled training day.

POUNDAGE INCREASE

Use the Kaizen (Japanese for constant and never-ending improvement) method for a particular set scheme at the beginning of each training week. You should add $1\frac{1}{4}$ to $2\frac{1}{2}$ pounds to each side of a barbell and as little as $\frac{1}{4}$ to $\frac{1}{2}$ pounds per dumbbell used. (Tip: Add 1 $\frac{1}{8}$th inside diameter cast iron flat washers or magnetic PlateMates to the barbell or dumbbells to accomplish these small weight jumps.) While the increases are almost insignificantly small, you will constantly improve. The weight increases may be imperceptible to you but over time you will get stronger, as opposed to adding substantial weight to a bar and almost instantly hitting a plateau.

The 30-Day 50/50 counter-split specialization technique is somewhat similar to the Zane and Schwarzenegger methods of specialization (consecutive training days etc.). The main difference is that it lasts twice as long. As with any regular or specialization training program, you'll experience periods when your results just aren't what you expect. Also, you will use the system only so long before gains stop. Therefore, after this intense 30-day specialization program is completed, you should stop and take a seven-day layoff from all training and then go back into a regular training schedule of sets and reps for the previously lagging muscle group.

FOUR-DAY MODIFIED TRAINING APPROACH

Training six days per week is a bit much for the full recovery of your muscles and nervous system. We think a modified training approach, where you perform the muscle bulk and strength program on Monday and Friday and the muscle-shape program on Tuesday and Saturday, is far more muscle friendly. Another option would be to train on Monday and Tuesday, rest on Wednesday, and then train again on Thursday and Friday and rest on Saturday and Sunday.

If the weekly four-day modified training frequency still doesn't allow enough time for proper rest and recovery, then you should do the muscle bulk and strength program on Monday, Wednesday and Friday and the muscle-shape program on Saturday only, assuming that your priority training is geared more

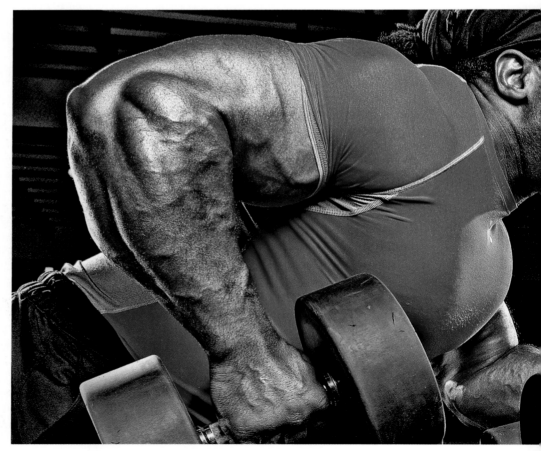

Photo by Robert Reiff
Model Jerome Ferguson

One of the most intense specialization methods is designed to stimulate a new burst of muscle growth in the shortest time possible – the nine-hour, one-day muscle blitz.

towards the increase of muscle bulk and strength. If muscle shape is your priority, then you should do the muscle bulk and strength training on Monday only and the muscle shape training on Tuesday, Thursday and Saturday.

METHOD #8 – NINE-HOUR ONE-DAY MUSCLE BLITZ

Want to add a half-inch of muscle in one day? If so, try the radical muscle blitz system. Bodybuilders are always on the lookout for new and innovative high-intensity training techniques that will stimulate new muscle growth in the shortest time possible. When muscle growth and development stop beyond the norm, certain specialization methods should be implemented to stimulate a new burst of the muscle growth curve. One of the most distinctive methods is the nine-hour, one-day muscle blitz. It employs a blood volume approach

that will see you performing maxi-pump reps (where four or more repetitions are executed in all sets). It's done through a dispersal of very brief, brutal, and extremely intense micro-training sessions (often called time-compression workouts) on the hour and half-hour during a nine-hour period. If you're like most people, work will get in the way of performing the one-day muscle blitz, so it's best to do it on a weekend or when you're on vacation. Whatever the case, you should devote a whole day to uninterrupted training. Go to the gym in the morning and don't leave until the evening.

Although radical, this method of training has been battle-tested in some of the most hardcore gyms around the world. The one-day muscle blitz system consists of 16 stepping stones that help give you an extra edge in your fight for more muscle size. Here's a detailed look at each one.

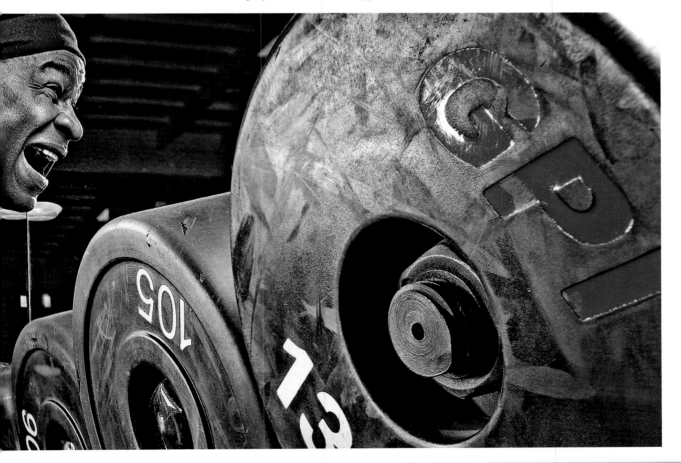

16 STEPPING STONES

#1 THE WEEK PRIOR

Your last training session should be two days prior to performing the one-day muscle blitz system. Your training sessions during this week should be of medium-intensity loads (72 to 84 percent of your current un-fatigued one-rep maximums) and high to very high volume. German volume training (GVT) is an excellent workout choice.

Pick 10 exercises to work your total body and do 10 reps per set. Choose either a compound or isolation exercise, depending on your wants or needs. Rest for 20 to 60 seconds (maximum) between each growth set of a selected exercise. If possible, use a fixed poundage (no pyramids) for all 10 sets. If it's not possible, reduce the poundage to no more than five to ten pounds every two to five sets. Other options include eight sets of eight reps or six sets of six reps. You should rest for 15 seconds (for increased muscularity) or 30 to 45 seconds (for muscle mass increase) between each training set of a selected exercise.

Don't begin your first regular training session feeder workouts until Tuesday and Wednesday of the following week and be sure to use medium-intensity loads and high volume for one week only. Then go back to your previous training protocol, whatever that may be.

#2 REST AND RECOVERY

Don't perform any workouts two days before or after the one-day muscle blitz.

#3 USE A TAPE MEASURE

An excellent system of feedback for monitoring muscle growth is using a non-shrinkable / stretchable nylon tape measure. On Friday, have a training partner place a tape measure snugly around the largest circumference point of your contracted muscle. Don't pump up your muscles ahead of time.

#4 12 HOURS PRIOR

Sleep and recovery before your muscle-blitz day is of vital importance.

#5 THREE HOURS PRIOR

It's 6:00 AM on a Saturday morning. It's time for you to get out of bed. Don't suffer from 3-D! If you delay/defer/dawdle, you're weakening your willpower.

#6 BODY CORE TEMPERATURE

By waiting for three hours to pass from the time you wake up (6:00 AM) to the beginning of your first micro-blitz training session (at 9:00 AM), you'll allow your body core temperature to reach a level that's high enough to speed up the chemical reactions involved in

Protein shakes are a great option to continuously shuttle amino acids into your bloodstream.

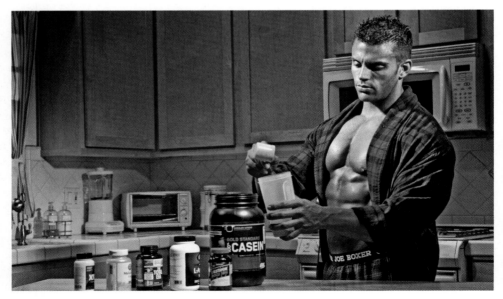

Photo by Robert Reiff
Model Chris Jalali

muscular contraction. Body core temperatures have a profound effect on your strength and stamina during the blitz-training sessions. We suggest that before your first micro-training session at 9:00 AM you do no more than some light aerobic work, PNF stretching and specific warm-up sets.

Atmospheric temperature and humidity are important as well. Make sure the room temperature doesn't go below 68 degrees. Make your body core and room temperatures work for you, not against you. Use internal and external temperatures to help you build bigger, better and stronger muscles faster.

#7 CORE GROWTH EXERCISES

Choose two mass-building compound barbell exercises for a lagging muscle group. The nine-hour one-day muscle blitz works most effectively when training your calves and upper arms. Some of the best upper-arm exercises are the classic standing two-handed barbell curl (for biceps), the seated EZ-bar French press (for triceps) and two dumbbell exercises. Any of those should be quite effective.

#8 SUPER-INTENSE TIME-COMPRESSION WORKOUTS

Take your first workout at 9:00 AM and perform three supersets with barbells. At 9:30 AM, perform two supersets with dumbbells. At the top of every hour, you should continue to do three supersets (methodic *) of barbell movements. At the half-hour mark of every hour, you should exercise with the dumbbells for two supersets (methodic **). Your last workout should be at 5:30 PM. Each even and odd hour and half-hour workout will take an average of only five to seven minutes to complete. (Please see the following day's itinerary.)

9:00 AM Superset:

Perform three sets of four to six reps of the classic standing two-handed barbell curl. Do three sets of four to six reps of the seated EZ-bar French press.

Methodic*

Positive phase speed reps / slow negative return

supersets. Rest for 90 seconds between each of the three supersets.

On every hour (until 5:00 PM), you should perform the arm exercises you did at 9:00 AM, making sure to keep the set / rep schemes identical.

9:30 AM Superset:

Do two sets of 10 to 12 reps of alternating dumbbell curls. Perform two sets of 10 to 12 reps of the one-dumbbell triceps extensions.

*Positive Phase Speed Reps / Slow Negative Returns

You should complete the positive phase of every rep of the barbell biceps and triceps exercises as quickly as possible. Don't use momentum. Use perfect motion and precise form (never jerky). Each positive phase speed rep should take approximately one-and-a-half seconds or less to complete. Slow negative returns should take more than two times longer (around four to five seconds). Control the weight, don't let it control you!

Methodic **

Tension super-sets. You should take no rest-pauses between the two supersets.

At the half-hour mark of each hour (until 5:30 PM), you should perform the arm exercises you did at 9:30 AM, making sure to keep the set / rep schemes identical.

**Tension Supersets

The rep-contraction tempo for dumbbell(s) biceps and triceps exercises should be of a medium or moderate speed. Also, when performing a shaping exercise for your biceps or triceps, use a non-pausing rhythm of performance. This deliberate, rhythmic performance allows your muscles to re-engage themselves at every point in the rep. It could be said that the muscles coax themselves to work. Never perform in a haphazard or jerky fashion and don't allow for the assistance of any other muscles in your body. Take no pauses at any point during the reps or after a rep – go smoothly from one rep to the next.

• Be sure to always stretch after each set of 9:00 AM superset exercises. Hold each stretch

You should aim to consume three moderate whole-food meals during this blitz program and obtain the rest of your daily calories from scheduled protein shakes.

for 10 to 20 seconds. Never force a stretch and never hold it if you begin to feel pain or cramping.

• Rest as much as possible between each workout throughout the day.

#9 PHYSICAL AND MECHANICAL RESTORATIVE MODALITIES

It's important to employ physical and mechanical restorative modalities during and after (post-workout) the one-day muscle blitz system or any other exercise protocol.

#10 EAT FOR STRENGTH AND EXPLOSIVE PERFORMANCE!

You should eat three moderate meals, but don't overstuff yourself. Eat your first major meal (breakfast) at home before leaving for the gym. Eat your second major meal (lunch) after 1:00 PM, and the third major meal (supper) at around 6:00 PM. You will also need to ingest protein every hour.

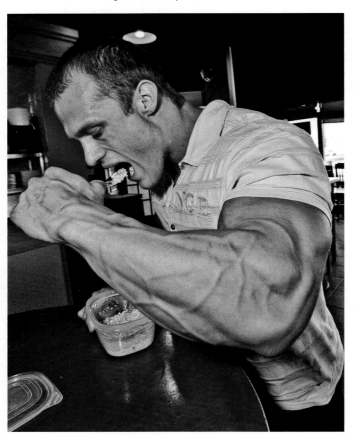

You should eat your lunch and have your hourly protein feedings at the gym. Prepare your foods (bananas, cheese slices, oatmeal, papaya spears, whole wheat pasta, egg whites, sweet potatoes/yams, steamed brown rice, low-sodium water-packed tuna, skinless chicken and turkey breasts, watermelon, flank steak, lean ground and roast beef, etc.) ahead of time. Poached egg whites topped with a cup of unsweetened frozen or fresh strawberries (when in season) make for an excellent high-protein dessert. You can add a teaspoon of fructose. Pack your food and plenty of low-sodium distilled water in a cooler and lug it to the gym. Drink plenty of water during this specialization program.

#11 HOURLY PROTEIN PUMP (FEEDING)

Beginning at 7:00 AM, and after every on-the-hour training session, take 15 grams of complete protein if your lean bodyweight is under 198 pounds. If you're over 198 pounds, consume 23 grams of complete protein.

#12 MIND-MUSCLE VISUALIZATION

Refer to chapter 19 for advice on this topic.

#13 EXAGGERATED MEASUREMENTS

At the conclusion of the nine-hour one-day muscle blitz, measure your arms. Your arms will be pumped beyond belief and they may show an exaggerated measurement of as much as three-quarters of an inch. The initial burst of peak muscle growth pump will usually result in a half-inch permanent gain, and a half-inch pump gain will usually result in a permanent gain of a quarter-inch or so the next morning.

#14 TWO DAYS AFTER

Don't work out on Sunday or Monday. Aggressively utilize the appropriate physical and mechanical restorative modalities to accelerate the complete recovery process of your localized muscles, biceps, triceps and central nervous system.

#15 RESUMING TOTAL-BODY WORKOUTS

Refer to #1, The Week Prior.

Photo by Ricg Baker
Model Matthew Roberts

#16 FREQUENCY OF THE ONE-DAY BLITZ SYSTEM

The one-day muscle blitz system is just that, a 24-hour system. After one day, the muscle gains generally stop. Some pro bodybuilders have modified the blitz system, training two days in a row rather than just one, for example. In this case they would use two different core growth exercises such as the supinated dumbbell incline curl for biceps and the EZ-bar close-grip bench press or the parallel bar (vertical) dips for triceps.

Summary

The one-day muscle blitz system seems to encourage upper-arm growth for a number of reasons. One reason is that each methodic training session takes approximately five to seven minutes to complete. This accumulated work time will allow you to demonstrate a very acute level of the mind-to-muscle link during each set of the selected exercise. Another advantage of these brief, brutal and intense micro-training sessions is that the body gets almost an equal ratio of accumulated rest to work. Another reason the one-day muscle blitz system works so efficiently is that you're performing as much as 80+ sets for your arms, and that's three or four (perhaps even 10) times the number of sets they are used to. They have no other option but to grow.

You can come up with some terrific exercise combinations of your own for other muscle groups such as quads/hamstrings, mid-chest/mid-back, upper chest/lats and delts/mid-back etc., especially if you review the Holistic Exercise Selection Chart. And it will be well worth the effort! Lasting gains of one-half inch or more can be realized in one day on this program when followed exactly as outlined.

METHOD #9 – RHEO H. BLAIR'S FOUR-WEEK SPECIALIZATION TRAINING SYSTEM

In the 1960s, *Iron Man* magazine brought to the attention of the bodybuilding world the unmatched success of a nutritionist named Rheo H. Blair, aka Irvin Johnson. He was supervising the nutritional programs of top physique champions. Many Southern California-area physique champions such as Gable Paul Boudreaux, Dave Draper, Vince Gironda, Don Richard Howorth, Larry Scott and Frank Zane would go to Rheo's house in Los Angeles and load up on his wildly popular and result-generating milk and egg protein powder, as well as other Blair supplement formulas.

A fact not so well known about Rheo H. Blair was his vast knowledge of lifting heavy iron. He actually promoted a system of training that would up the size and strength gain factor of anyone willing to use it diligently. The Rheo H. Blair four-week specialization training system begins with a 30-day preparatory phase.

PREPARATORY PHASE: WEEKS 1 TO 4

Suggested Exercises: Back squat, bench press, bent-over row, barbell overhead press, barbell curl and overhead barbell triceps extension. Perform the exercises in the precise order listed.

Sets and reps: During the first month using the Blair System of training, perform three sets of 10 to 15 reps of each exercise with light to moderate weights.

Training Frequency: Train three times per week (Monday, Wednesday and Friday or Tuesday, Thursday and Saturday).

After performing this preparatory program for one month, add a specialization technique.

SPECIALIZATION PHASE: WEEKS 5 AND 6

At the beginning of each training session, you'll specialize on one of the six exercises. For example on Monday, begin with the back squat by doing one or two light warm-up sets and then load weight on the bar to about 10 to 15 pounds less than your best three-rep maximum. Then, it's just a matter of performing 10 sets of three reps and resting for two to three minutes between sets. This part of the workout will take approximately 30 to 40 minutes to complete.

Once you've completed the 10 sets of three reps, continue the workout by doing the remaining five exercises for three sets of 10 of 15 reps. During the next workout, begin by specializing on the bench press for 10 sets of three reps, and then do the remaining four exercises for three sets of 10 to 15 reps and so on. It will take you five workouts / two weeks to complete the specialization technique, one time, on each of the five exercises.

SPECIALIZATION PHASE: WEEKS 7 AND 8

This two-week session is almost identical to the last, except instead of doing 10 sets of three reps on your specialization exercise, you'll do 12 sets of three reps. Blair advised his bodybuilding clientele to use this program.

While we like the 10 sets of three reps concept because it really enhances contractile power and strength within the selected muscles being worked, we feel training for 30 to 40 minutes (10 sets times three with a total of two to three minutes of rest between each set) on just one exercise is a bit long. As an alternative you could use a best 10-rep maximum weight and perform 10 sets of three reps, but resting only 10 seconds or so between sets.

METHOD #10 – ARNOLD'S FORGOTTEN MUSCLE GROUP PRIORITY TRAINING

MONDAY-WEDNESDAY-FRIDAY

Arnold's training philosophy was to train what he considered the forgotten muscle groups (traps, forearms, lower back and calves) with as much intensity as the upper arms. Here's an example of how Arnold would initiate forgotten muscle group priority training for the forearms: He would perform barbell wrist curls (with the palms up) for five sets of 10 reps and superset them with a calf exercise. After completing these supersets, he would then begin his next forearm exercise which was the one-dumbbell wrist curl (again with the palms up) performed for five sets of 10 reps and again superset with another calf exercise.

TUESDAY-THURSDAY-SATURDAY

Arnold would superset standing barbell (EZ-curl bar) reverse curls for five sets of 10 to 12 reps with a triceps exercise such as feet-elevated triceps pushups. After these supersets were completed, Arnold would do reverse preacher curls with an EZ-curl bar for five sets of 10 to 12 reps, again superset with a triceps exercise. Arnold was known to specialize on a lagging muscle for as long as nine months!

METHOD #11 – FRANK ZANE'S TWO-WEEK SPECIALIZATION STRATEGY

On Monday, do a heavy workout performing 25 sets (five exercises for five sets of eight to ten reps per exercise). Some of the exercises Zane used for his back were bent-over rows, T-bar rows, one-arm dumbbell rows, V-bar pulldowns to front and hanging upside-down barbell rows. Frank once said, "Another thing I find that helps my lower back is hanging by my feet. I got a special pair of [inversion or gravity] boots in Pasadena, California. This chiropractor makes them there and you just clamp them on and hang upside down by your feet. What I started doing was rowing while hanging upside down by my feet. You know, just like a bent-over row. But I would hang by my feet and do rowing with 100 pounds for sets of 10 repetitions and it not only helped my back development, but it really brought the lower lats out and cured my lower back."

Using different exercises on Tuesday (to attack the muscles from different angles), drop from five sets to three sets per exercise. On Wednesday, do 10 to 15 overall sets for your back using the same exercises as the Tuesday routine. Take Thursday off for rest and relaxation. On Friday, hit the back in the same way as for Monday's routine. Do only a minimal amount of back work on Saturday (maybe three or four sets of some lat stretches).

Training the back in this manner for two continuous weeks will bring startling improvement. On a short-term blitz program of this nature, two weeks is about the maximum amount of time that you can expect to obtain decent results. Since you'll be working the back hard five times per week, you may find it to your advantage to do it a different time from the rest of your daily exercise routine (perhaps utilizing the daily double-split principle).

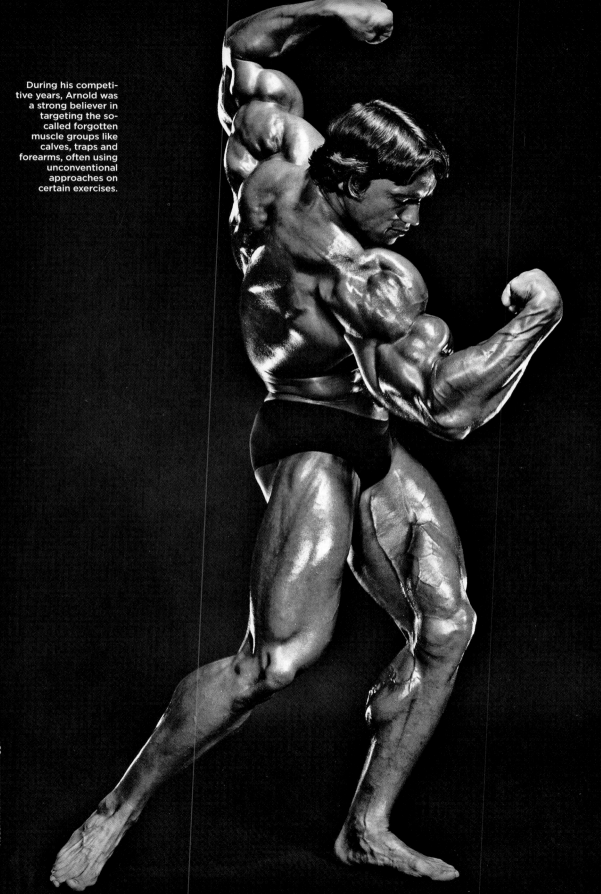

During his competitive years, Arnold was a strong believer in targeting the so-called forgotten muscle groups like calves, traps and forearms, often using unconventional approaches on certain exercises.

Model Arnold Schwarzenegger

CHAPTER 39

SIXTY-PLUS BODYBUILDING SPECIALIZATION PROGRAMS

Target your quads, hamstrings, calves, pecs and delts like never before with over 60 specialization techniques

In this chapter, we'll explore over 60 bodybuilding specialization programs. We'll begin by looking at overall leg and quads exercises, followed by hams, calves, pecs and delts. You should follow these programs every other day for four to six weeks, with the exception of the exercises for abs and calves, which can be performed five or six days per week.

LEGS
1. (OVERALL LEG SIZE)

Parallel Barbell Squat	2 x 8, 6, 4, 2
Power-Rack Quarter Squat	4 x 10
Non-Lock Leg Press	6 x 6

2. (QUADRICEPS)
No-Barbell Squat Workout

We learned about the no-barbell squat workout back in the '70s from a top California bodybuilder named Dan Howard. Your thighs will be pumped to the max and you should experience very little fatigue in your lower back. To safeguard against future knee injuries, we suggest that you warm up your knees with five minutes on the stationary bike before this leg workout, and then do some quad stretches.

Begin with leg extensions in a two-part movement. Bring the legs up and do the top quarter of the movement only for 20 reps, making sure to maximally tense your quads upon lockout of each rep. Upon completion of the 20th and final quarter-rep, bring your lower legs all the way

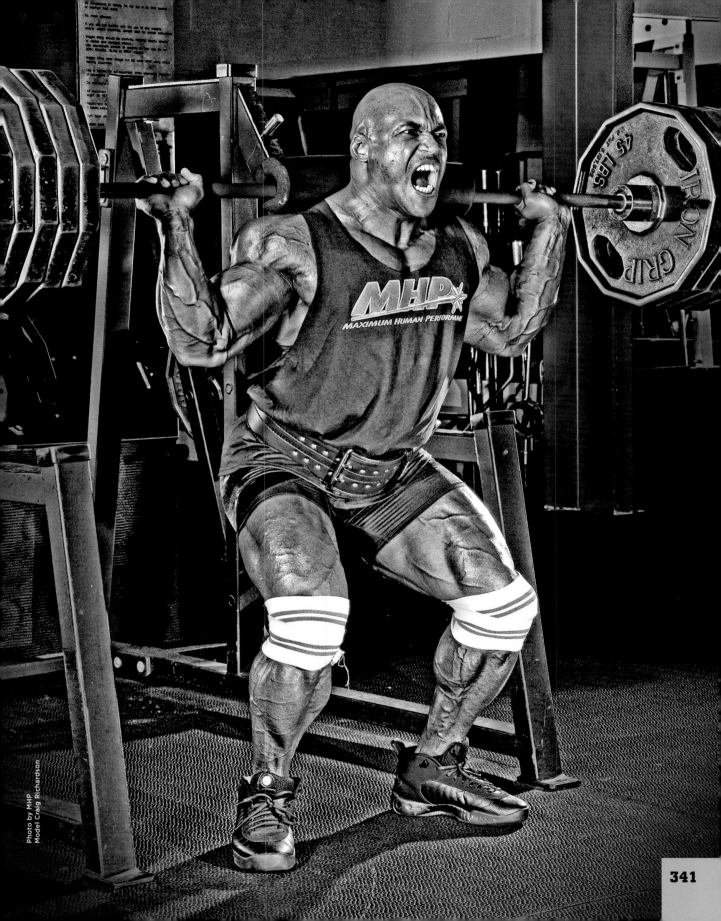

back and then immediately do 20 full-range-of-motion reps. The lactic acid burn you experience should be almost unbearable.

Without taking any rest, walk over to the leg press and do at least 20 (up to 50) non-locked reps: Lower your legs until the front of your thighs touch your chest and then push your legs up just shy of lockout (for maximum muscle tension). Some bodybuilders go as high as 50 to 75 reps in this exercise, which of course involves maximum effort from the quads, hamstrings and glutes. Upon completion of the leg presses, immediately perform 20 full reps of bodyweight-only sissy squats (or if you're feeling up to it, you could do barbell front squats). Do three tri-sets in the manner described. Your cardiovascular system will demand a three- to five-minute rest upon the completion of each tri-set.

As with any exercise program, it's important to not only train hard, but also smart. Some bodybuilders can overwhelm their ACL (anterior cruciate ligament, which crosses over the front of the knee) when doing leg extensions, so proceed with caution. Perform all your reps in a smooth, continuous-tension manner. When you perform the leg press, be sure that your back is flat against the seat and that your glutes also stay against the seat, especially in the bottom position of the rep. Whatever you do, don't devate from this method or try to cheat. In the end, you'll only be cheating yourself.

3. (QUADRICEPS)

Superset:	
Barbell Front Squat	5 X 8-10
Leg Extension	5 X 12
Non-Lock Leg Press	2 X 8-10
Leg Curl	5 X 10-12

4. (QUADRICEPS)

Leg Extension (Strict)	2 X 6
	4 X 4
Superset:	
Leg Extension (Strict)	2 X 8
Bodyweight Jumping Squat	2 X Failure
Rest Two Minutes Between Supersets	
Leg Extension (Semi-Cheat)	3 X 12
Leg Curl (Strict)	3 X 12
Bodyweight Jumping Squat	1 X Failure

5. (QUADRICEPS)
Leg Press Mad Sets

IFBB pro bodybuilder "Marvelous" Melvin Anthony uses a basic and brutal approach consisting of three exercises when working his quads, including the torturous leg press mad sets. He calls them mad sets because they will drive you insane.

Melvin begins and ends his quad workout with leg extensions. He warms up with four light sets of 12 to 15 reps. Next, Melvin does four sets of eight to ten reps of barbell front squats, using an ascending weight progression (example, 135, 225, 315 and 415). From there, he moves on to the leg press mad sets. Melvin does just two master sets (consisting of nine sub-sets each) one to two times a week to build his quads. On paper this may look easy, but it's an adrenaline-depleting process. Melvin uses 75 percent of his best 10-rep maximum weight.

He begins his first master set of nine sub-sets performing them with just six seconds of rest between each, using a decreasing rep scheme of 15, 12, 10, 8, 6, 5, 4, 3 and 2. This completes a total of 65 reps. He then rests for around a minute and does a second master set.

To end his quad workout, Melvin uses two or three times the poundage on leg extensions that he used on the warm-up sets. He does four sets of 12 to 15 reps. He also does a body shift by moving his butt and back away from the seatback support of the leg extension unit. This changes the emphasis of the exercise to high hip flexors and mid quads.

6. (QUADS / HAMS)
Shape Train the Quads and Hams

Here's a blood volume quad and hamstring routine that will gratify your ego by changing your rate of progress from ordinary to spectacular. Do a set of 30 fast, strict reps of leg extensions and then take a brief rest. Follow that up with a set of 20 and rest again. Next, do five growth-zone sets of 15 reps each, and then a pump set of 20 and then another 30 followed by a 10-minute rest. Then do leg curls, which affect the soleus muscle of the calf. Do the exact same sets and reps as above. Finally do hack squats, again using the same sets and

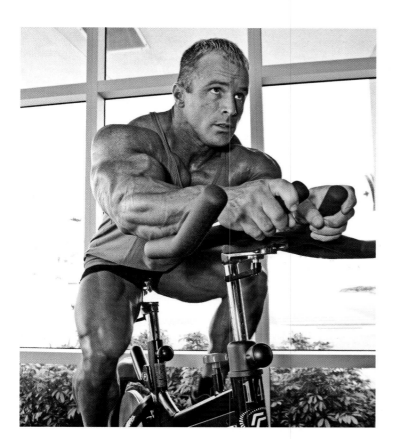

Before doing the high-rep leg program, start with a five- to ten-minute ride on the stationary bike as a warm-up.

reps. For additional definition, you could do lunges using a very light weight across your shoulders for four sets of 15 reps for each leg.

If you wish to shape your legs even further, you won't find a more effective or enjoyable method than riding a racing bicycle. Rent, borrow or buy one and ride it in sprints for five to ten minutes at a time, as if you were doing sets. It will considerably improve the contour, shape and definition of your entire leg.

7. (QUADS / HAMS)
High-Rep Leg Program

Warm up using the stationary bike for five to ten minutes.	
Barbell Back Squat	4-5 x 15-20
Jump rope for 30 seconds between each set.	
Leg Press	3 x 15 2 x 50
Leg Curl	4 x 15-20
Stiff-Leg Deadlift	4 x 15-20
Always stretch between sets.	

8 (QUADS / HAMS)
Barbell Front Squat

Barbell Front Squat	4 x 8-10
Superset:	
Leg Press	5 x 10
Leg Curl	5 x 10

9 (QUADS / HAMS / CALVES)
Mike Dadigan's Mr. Western America's Favorite Leg Routine

3X PER WEEK	
(Mon-Wed-Fri)	
Leg Extension	3 x 20
Non-Lock Barbell Back Squat+	6 x10
Leg Curl	3 x 20
Seated Calf Raise	9 x 20
One-Dumbbell Calf Raise	3 x 12-15
Tibilias Contraction	3 x 50

+On the non-lock barbell back squats, instead of always doing six sets of 10 reps, try doing six sets of six reps but with a little twist: Take six seconds to do the negative and six seconds to do the positive phase of each rep. Also, don't forget to pause for two seconds at the bottom of each rep.

4X PER WEEK	
(Tues-Thur-Sat-Sun)	
Standing Calf Heel Raise	5 x 20-30
(light weight and go for a pump)	

3X PER WEEK	
(Tues-Thur-Sat)	

Jog one to two miles and then do five wind sprints of 50 to 75 yards.

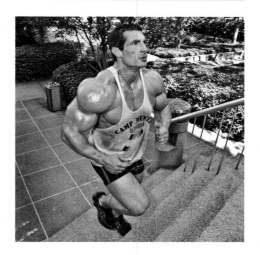

Photos by Rich Baker
Model Con Demitriou / Brian Yersky

10 (QUADS / HAMS / CALVES)
Super Circuit Leg Shaper

Six-time Ms. Olympia, Cory Everson, revealed this leg-shaping workout on her ESPN "Body-Shaping" TV show viewers many years ago. The following eight progressive-resistance exercises should be performed in the order listed as a nonstop circuit for 20 repetitions each. Rest for one to two minutes, after completing the circuit. Do three circuits.

Alternating Front Lunge
Dynamic Lunge
Bodyweight Only Single-Leg Heel Raise
Barbell Front Squat
Leg Extension
Leg Curl
Barbell Back Squat
Step-Up

Step-ups should be performed on a sturdy exercise bench or wooden box. The vertical measurement of these items should correspond to your height. If you're:

5' or under	(Use a box 12 inches in height)
5'1"-5'3"	(Use a box 14 inches in height)
5'4"-5'9"	(Use a box 16 inches in height)
5'10"-6'	(Use a box 18 inches in height)
Over 6'	(Use a box 20 inches in height)

The program may look simple, but it's very demanding. It's also an excellent specialization program for both male and female bodybuilders who are interested in shape-training their legs without acquiring additional muscle bulk and power. Many bodybuilders make the mistake of neglecting to shape-train their legs and walk on stage looking very awkward.

11. (QUADS / HAMS / CALVES)
Volume Training Specialization

1X PER WEEK	
(Monday Or Tuesday)	
Workout 1 – Power Phase	
Olympic Barbell Back Squat	5 x 5
Hack Squat	4 x 8-10
Leg Curl	6 x 6-12
Stiff-Leg Barbell Deadlift	4 x 8-12
1X PER WEEK	
(Wed Or Thur)	
Workout 2 – Building Phase	
Olympic Barbell Back Squat	5 x 8-10
Hack Squat	4 x 8
Leg Extension	4 x 8
Leg Press	4 x 8
Leg Curl	4 x 6-12
Stiff-Leg Barbell Deadlift	4 x 8-12
1X PER WEEK	
(Fri Or Sat)	
Workout 3 – Muscle-Sculpting Phase	
Barbell Front Squat	5 x 6-12
Leg Press	3 x 8-12
Leg Extension	4 x 8-12
Leg Curl	4 x 6-12
Stiff-Leg Barbell Deadlift	4 x 8-12
CALF MUSCLE	
Seated Calf Raise	2 x 12
Standing Calf Raise	3 x 12

After you do the sets for calves, do three cycles of the triple-drop method. Work at getting a rep pattern of 12, 12 and 8 on each cycle. Finish off your calf work with two sets of 20 reps of donkey calf raises.

The Super Circuit Leg Shaper includes the leg curl as one of eight moves performed in the circuit.

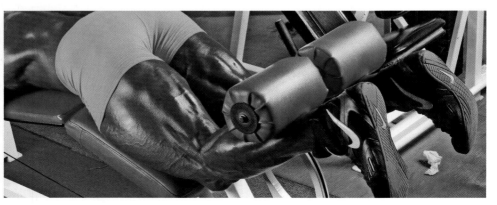

Photo Ralph DeHaan
Model Omar Deckard

CALVES

1.

Standing Calf Calf Raise	5 x 20
One-Leg Heel Raise (Hold Heavy Dumbbell In One Hand)	4 x 20

Following these two exercises, you should lean against a wall and rise up on your toes (with just your own bodyweight) while flexing your calves very hard in the top contracted position for a 10- to 20-second count. Do this four times, pausing to rest slightly between sets.

2.

Standing Calf Raise	4 x 25
One-Leg Heel Raise (Bodyweight Only)	4 x 60

In the first 30 reps, concentrate on the downward stretch. Bounce through the final 30 reps, concentrating on the high flex position.

TIBIA CONTRACTIONS

Sit on a high bench so your legs are free to hang. Then work your feet back and forth and add poundage to the exercise when the reps become easy. However, don't sacrifice form just for the sake of adding poundage.

3.
STAGGERED-SETS CALF TRAINING

When consecutive sets of an exercise prove too great a demand on your muscles – especially when going to momentary positive failure – you should use staggered sets (or interspersing exercises) as an alternative to minimize the effects of mental and localized muscle fatigue. For example, assume that your calves fatigue dramatically when doing consecutive sets. The solution to this is to do one set of a calf exercise after every two sets of exercises for other bodyparts.

The following calf program will incorporate Staggered Sets Training (SST). Select one calf exercise and perform one set immediately after every two sets of exercise for another muscle group until you've completed eight sets of the calf exercise. Here's an example using Stan McQuay's post competition push / pull superset (compound sets) combos workout.

PUSH / PULL SUPERSET COMBOS
(MODERATE POUNDAGE – STRICT FORM – HIGH REP VOLUME)

Do a superset consisting of wide-grip lat pulldowns and triceps pressdowns. For each exercise, you should perform two sets of 15 to 20 reps and then another superset. This second superset should consist of seated rows, as well as one-arm reverse-grip triceps pushdowns. Perform two sets of 15 to 20 reps of each of these exercises. Your third superset should follow the same rep and set scheme and consist of 45-degree incline barbell presses and standing barbell curls. Finally, finish off with a superset consisting of high pulley cable crossovers, as well as standing alternating dumbbell curls. For these exercises, you should perform two sets of 20 to 30 reps each.

Stan used these push / pull superset combos a couple of days after winning the 2006 NPC Nationals, as a means to merely maintain his upper torso muscle size and density.

Let's assume you're using Stan's program and want to apply Staggered Sets Training (SST) into it. In that case, immediately after concluding each of the 16 superset combos, you should perform one set of a calf exercise, such as the standing and/or seated calf machine heel raises, for a total of eight sets.

Here's a couple of nifty strategies to choose from when implementing Staggered Sets Training (SST) for the calves into Stan McQuay's push/pull superset combos or any workout for that matter.

Standing and/or Seated Calf Raise

1. Heavy poundage: Begin with 20 reps per set and progressively add poundage to each remaining set until you can perform only three reps in the eighth and final set.
2. High reps: Simply add reps and not poundage. Start with 20 reps and work to the highest reps possible by the eighth and final set of the selected calf exercise.

Remember, these are Staggered Set Training guidelines and not rules. While we suggested doing a ratio of one staggered set to every two sets of another exercise, you may feel it's best to go with a ratio of one to five. That decision is entirely up to you.

Staggered Sets Training (SST) for your calves and abs seems to work quite well when worked in with most major and minor muscle groups. However, you must use common sense. It isn't a good idea to do an ab exercise in between sets of lower back exercises (deadlifts, bent-over rowing) because weakening your ab muscles through exercise may compromise the integrity of your lower back area. Likewise, you shouldn't work your biceps in between sets of back work (bent-over rowing, lat pulldown and pull-up etc.), since you rely on your biceps to assist you in your back work.

4.
LEO COSTA JR. FAST BLAST CALF SECRET

Here's an ultimate Fast Blast secret from Leo Costa, Jr., co-author of *Titan Training*. When Leo was training for some of the top bodybuilding shows he did not neglect the development of his calves. One of his favorite calf exercises was the standing calf raise. For this exercise he would select a poundage he could do for 10 reps for full range of motion. He would mount the machine and before he even began the first rep he would stretch his calves in the very low stretch contraction position. His heels would be quite a bit lower than the top of the calf block he was standing on. He would hold his static stretch for 20 seconds. Then, in a slow-medium tempo he would do three full heel raises. Upon completion of the third rep, he'd go into a deep stretch in the bottom position, holding it for 15 seconds. He would then do four more full reps (seven so far) and upon completing this rep, he'd stretch at the bottom for 10 seconds.

Leo would then reposition his feet on the calf block to achieve a different stress angle and blast out three final full reps. This completed one set. He would do a total of five sets of 10 reps, each rep performed in a slow-medium cadence. Upon completion of the five sets of the standing calf raise, Leo's calves were pumped beyond belief, but he wasn't finished working them yet. He would then change the emphasis of his calf training to the soleus. For this he would do the seated calf raises for a total of four sets of 10 reps, using the same training method as described for the standing calf raises.

Leo performed the entire fast blast calf program, consisting of nine tough sets, three times per week on non-training days for a maximum of three weeks. After the three weeks, Leo would go back to his regular calf workouts for a few months or until he felt his calves needed another jolt. Give Leo's routine a go the next time you need to specialize on the calves.

5.
MCLELLAN CALF PROGRAM

This specialization program is almost the opposite of Leo Costa's program You will be perform a few sets of a calf exercise. The secret is the utilization of certain training principles such as rest-pause, burns and supersets. When these three training principles are combined in the unique manner about to be described, you can literally shock your calves into greater dimensions of size and shape.

We learned about this calf program back in the '60s after reading an *Iron Man* magazine article, "BLAST Those Calves To Greater Size," by Jim McLellan. What intrigued us most about this calf program was the guarantee of a 1½- to 2-inch gain of new muscle growth in just three months. Using the standing calf raise as our example, here is a description of the McLellan calf-jarring technique.

TECHNIQUE-EMPHASIS

Load the calf machine with a weight that will allow you to maximally complete 15 slow, burning, full-range-of-motion repetitions. You can use one of two foot positions: The first possible position is with your big toes wide apart and your heels only three or four inches apart. This places a great deal of muscle tension on the inner aspect of your calf when performing the movement. The second position is with your big toes eight to twelve inches apart and your heels spaced further apart than that. Keep your bodyweight on the edge of your feet in this pigeon-toed position and you can't help but create stimulus to the outer aspect of your calf.

By angling your toes outward with your heels only three to four inches apart, you transfer the emphasis to your inner calf during the movement.

Lock your legs straight at the knee joint, muscles tensed and your upper torso aligned with your pelvis throughout the movement as opposed to leaning forward or backward. Begin the actual calf movement (using one of the two described foot positions) by allowing your heels to slowly descend as far below the plane or level of your toes as possible. If the balls of your feet are correctly positioned on the near edge of the foot block, you'll feel as if you're teetering (but not slipping off the block). This foot placement will give you the maximum range of motion.

Without cheating, thrust your heels upward forcefully by the quick, powerful pull of your calves until the balls and the heels of your feet are as near to vertical alignment as possible. Look up at the ceiling while doing this and try to raise your heels even higher. You should feel the instep shift forward at the apex of the movement (support pressure is over the ball of your foot and big toe).

Lock your knees so your legs are straight and slowly lower your heels as far beneath toe level as possible. Change directions and repeat for the number of reps indicated in the workout plan. Note: Breathe out as your heels rise and breathe in as they lower.

Upon completion of the 15th rep, and while in the deep stretch position, lift one foot off the calf block, and with your muscles relaxed, shake your leg twice for about four seconds. Repeat with your other leg. Immediately do eight unhurried, slow-burning full repetitions, then take four seconds shaking each leg twice. Then do eight more full reps and the leg shakes. Do a final eight full reps, but this time omitting the leg shakes.

Immediately upon completion of the third set of eight full reps, do quick partial-rep heel raises (burns) in the 3/5 range of the movement until failure (the calves will feel like they have been firebombed). You aren't done yet. With your calves already feeling the lactic acid burn, then, with both of your feet, do a full rep to the high contracted position. While there, take your right foot off the block and lower it. In short, go up on two feet and come down on one. Then, go back up on two feet and down on your right foot, continuing in the alternating manner described for 10 to 20 more times (depending on your willingness to tolerate the pain).

Rest for five minutes (massaging your calf muscles slightly and shaking your legs to get the blood circulating once again). Then begin the whole sequence once again. Do this every other day for two weeks. In the third to twelfth weeks, immediately upon completing the two-up and one-down, begin doing another dose of 3/5-range burns followed by 10 to 20 more reps in the two-up and one-down. A 1½-inch permanent gain is average for those giving the McLellan calf routine a three-month ride.

Photo by Jason Breeze
Model Craig Richardson

6.

NINE-WEEK GIANT SET CALF ROUTINE (FOUR SUBSETS IN ONE)

This principle was designed in 1992 by Gustavo Barni (co-author of *The Muscle Augmentation System*) and is one of the most effective ways to add considerable muscle mass to your calves. Frequency and duration of the week-by-week training will be addressed in the training frequency table.

GIANT SET ONE

Subset 1: Select a poundage that allows you 12 slow, full reps in a calf exercise such as the standing calf raise, toe press or donkey calf raise (keep your legs straight and your feet spaced six inches apart and parallel to each other).

Rest for 20 seconds and quickly shake or massage your calves. This will assist you in the removal of lactic acid accumulation.

Subset 2: Continuing with the same poundage, do as many slow reps to positive muscular failure as possible. Within a couple of seconds of completion, bend your knees very slightly and use one of the toe / heel positions detailed in the McLellan Calf Program.

Subset 3: Do as many rapid bouncy reps as possible, keeping your legs slightly bent when your heels descend through the negative phase of each rep. Then, slightly extend (semi-straighten) your legs as your heels rise through to the top contracted positive phase of the movement. Rest for 10 seconds and quickly shake or massage your calves

NINE-WEEK GIANT SET CALF ROUTINE (FOUR SUBSETS IN ONE)

WORKOUT WEEK NO.	MON OR TUE A) STANDING CALF RAISE	WED OR THUR B) LEG PRESS CALF RAISE	FRI OR SAT C) DONKEY CALF RAISE
1-3	4 Giant sets	4 Giant sets	4 Giant sets
4	4 Giant sets + *Seated Calf Raise 2 sets to positive failure	4 Giant sets + *Seated Calf Raise 2 sets to positive failure	4 Giant sets + *Seated Calf Raise 2 sets to positive failure
5	Train Mon – Exercise "A" Tue – Exercise "B" Use week 4 exercise protocol *Note: When doing the add a 5th sub-set within each giant set on Tuesday*	Rest	Rest day: Friday Exercise "C" Train Saturday Use week 4 exercise protocol
6	5 Giants sets + *Seated Calf Raise 3 sets to positive failure	5 Giant sets + *Seated Calf Raise 3 sets to positive failure	5 Giant sets + *Seated Calf Raise 3 sets to positive failure
7	" "	" "	" "
8	*Train Mon – Exercise "A" Tue – Exercise "B" Use week 6-7 exercise protocol* Note: When doing the 5 giant sets and on Tuesday add a fifth subset within each	Train Wed – Exercise "C" Use week 6-7 exercise protocol Note: When doing the 5 giant sets and on Tuesday add a fifth subset within each Rest day Thursday	Rest days Fri – Sat
9	6 Giant sets (5 subsets)	6 Giant sets (5 subsets)	6 Giant sets (5 subsets)

Notes:
1. *Seated calf raise – Upon completion of each set of reps to positive failure, do bouncy heel raises (burns) in the top peak contraction range of each heel raise until failure.
2. Unless otherwise noted in the table, every giant set consists of four subsets.
3. Upon the completion of a calf-training session, consider using massage.
4. Sunday is always reserved for rest.

Shrugs (shown here with dumbbells) can be used as one exercise in a giant set for shoulders.

Subset 4: Repeat Subset 3. This completes Giant Set One. Rest for 60 to 90 seconds while shaking or massaging the calves. Perform three more in the following manner:

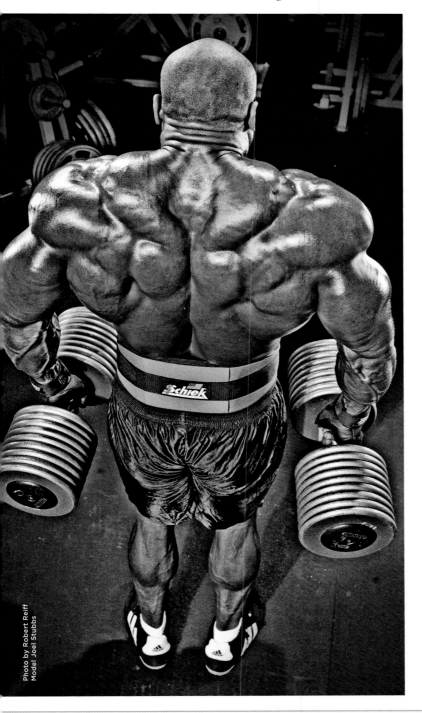

7.

25-15-10 CALF BLAST

Here's a short and sweet calf routine called the 25-15-10 extended-set technique. While doing the standing calf raise, do 25 full reps (from the bottom stretch to the top peak contraction). Perform each one in a slow and deliberate manner, stretching at the bottom and squeezing and contracting at the top.

Upon completion of the 25th rep, and without taking any rest, do 15 super-fast speed reps in the top one-quarter to one-third range of the movement. Once you have completed the 15 reps without rest, finish off with a final 10 full reps in super-slow fashion. This completes one cycle. Do three cycles. In the 25- and 15-rep phase of the cycle, stretch your calves for approximately 10 to 15 seconds every fifth rep. The three cycles of this calf blast should be performed three non-consecutive training days per week.

TRAPS

1.

Barbell Shrug	4 x 20–25
Kneeling Barbell Power Clean	6 x 6
Dumbbell Upright Row	4 x 15
Bent-Over Laterals	4 x 15–20

2.

Barbell Shrug	4 x 8
Standing Barbell Hang Clean	4 x 12
Narrow-Grip Upright Row	4 x 12
Barbell High Pull	4 x 16
Please note that when performing the upright rows and barbell hang cleans, you should breathe twice between reps.	

3.

SUPERSET	
Haney Barbell Shrug/Row	3 x 8-10
Upright Cable Row	3 x 8-10
SUPERSET	
Seated Dumbbell Shrug	2 x 10-12
Barbell High Pull	2 x 6-8
Rest for one minute between supersets.	

4.

TRI-SET	
Bent-Over Rear Dumbbell Lateral	3 x 10
Haney Barbell Shrug/Row	3 x 10
Barbell or Dumbbell Shrug	3 x 10

BACK

1.

(SPINAE ERECTORS, LATS)	
Hyperextension	3-4 x 15-25
Deadlift	3-4 x 3-5
Power Clean	3-4 x 3-5
Bent-Over Row	3-4 x 8-12
Bent-Over Laterals	3-4 x 10-15

2.

BACK SUPREMACY WORKOUT	
Deadlift	3-4 x 10-12
Barbell Shrug	4-5 x 8-12
Curl-Grip Lat Pulldowns to Front	4-5 x 6-10
Curl-Grip EZ-Barbell Bent-over Row	4-5 x 6-10
One-Arm Dumbbell Row	3-4 x 6-10

The bent-over dumbbell row is a classic back move to increase density, size and strength in your upper back.

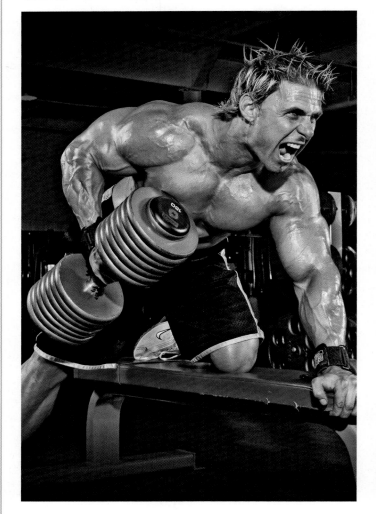

3.

THREE-WAY BACK ATTACK RICH GASPARI STYLE	
MONDAY (THICKNESS)	
Deadlift	5 x 10, 8, 6, 6, 10

– Add poundage on each of the first four sets and decrease in the fifth set.

Medium-Grip Barbell Bent-Over row	4 x 8-10

– Increase poundage each set.

Seated Row	4 x 10-12

– Increase poundage each set.

Hyperextension	4 x 10-12

– Hold a weight behind head.

WEDNESDAY (WIDTH)	
Wide-Grip Pull-up to Front	4 x Failure
Lat Pulldown Behind Neck	4 x 10-12

– Increase poundage each set.

Superset

Close-Grip Pulldown to Chest	4 x 10-12

– Do this while lying on a flat exercise bench.

One-Dumbbell Bench Pullover	4 x 10-12

– Don't do this movement lying across a flat exercise bench because doing so creates over tearing and stretching of your medius rectus (abs) and lower back (lumbar region) hyperextension.

FRIDAY (WIDTH AND THICKNESS)	
Superset	
Wide-Grip Lat Pulldown to Front	4 x 8-10
T-Bar Row	4 x 8-10

– Increase poundage each set.

Superset	
Close-Grip Lat Pulldown to Chest	4 x 8-10
Low-pulley cable row	4 x 8-10

– Increase poundage each set.

Superset	
Lat pulldown Behind the Neck	4 x 6-8
Low Incline Bench Prone Dumbbell Row	4 x 6-8
Hyperextension Or Stiff-Leg Barbell Deadlift	4 x 8-10 4 x 8-10

4.

TRI-SET
Wide-grip Pullup to Chest
Lat Pulldown to Chest
Seated Row

Do these three exercises in tri-set fashion for eight reps and five burns in each set. Don't rest between sets and take only minimal rest between each tri-set series. Do four to six tri-sets.

Photo by Jason Breeze
Model Andre Rzazewski

5.

Wide-Grip Pull-up to Chest	6 x 6-8
– Arch your back and use a weight belt.	
Heavy Bent-Over Row	4 x 6-8
– Use a curl grip and pull the bar into your stomach area.	
Seated Row (medium grip)	4 x 8-10
One-Arm Dumbbell Row	4 x 8-10
Straight-Arm Lat Pulldown (to thighs)	4 x 10-12

6.

MID-BACK / ERECTOR THICKNESS	
Bent-Over Row	4 x 6-8
– Use a curl grip and pull bar into your stomach area.	
Seated Row	4 x 10-12
– Use a V-bar	
Bent-Over Lateral	3 x 10
T-Bar Row	4 x 6-8
Bent-O ver EZ-bar Row	3 x 8-10
– close grip	

CHEST

1.

18X NON-BENCH PRESS BLASTER

The 18x Non-Bench Press Blaster is a little-known program that can add muscle or at least keep you from losing strength. You perform four fundamental exercises, none of which involves the mechanics of the bench press. You may find the movements difficult, depending on your weight, because they are bodyweight-only exercises.

The four exercises we're going to reveal are for your upper torso. Don't perform any other upper-body exercise during this session, but you can do some leg training. The four exercises you'll be performing are: Pull-up, parallel bar dip, chin-up and vertical hangs from the pull-up bar. The workout program frequency is three non-consecutive days per week for a total of six weeks.

Stretch	(5 to 10 minutes)
Pull-up:	5 sets x 8 reps

With your palms away from you, knees bent and legs crossed, pull to your upper chest.

Parallel bar dip:	5 sets x 10 reps

Do this exercise with your hands in the nor-mal dipping hold position (knuckles facing outward) and your elbows close to your up-right torso with your knees bent and legs crossed. Be sure to go deeper with each set until your upper arms are parallel or below. Deliberately lock out your elbows at the top, as this will help you develop triceps strength. If you have an adjustable set of dipping bars, you should occasionally vary your grip width. A grip width of 26 inches or less will activate more triceps. With a wider grip, you can expect more shoulder and pec stimulation.

Chin-ups:	3 sets x 8 reps

With your palms facing you, your knees bent and legs crossed, pull up till your upper chest touches the bar.

Parallel Bar Dip (again):	4 sets x failure

Do tandem triceps double dips. With your knuckles pointed inward towards your body, do a set to failure. Then, without pause, read-just your grip to the normal dipping hold (knuckles pointed outward) and rep out until failure. This constitutes two sets. Take a rest and begin once again.

Stretch	(2-3 minutes)
Vertical Hang From Pull-up Bar:	3 sets x 15-20 seconds each

With the pull-ups and chin-ups, there should be no swinging or any other unnecessary body motions such as bouncing. If you can't perform the desired reps, try to find someone to assist you. Whatever the case, it's very important that you use proper form throughout.

2.

Barbell Bench Press	2 x 8, 4, 2, 1
Superset	
Incline Dumbbell Flye	4 x 12
Incline Barbell Press	4 x 8
Straight-Arm Pullover	2 x 20
Notes: On the regular bench press, use the heavy-light system. Add weight and decrease your reps. Perform the incline barbell press with a wide grip and high on your chest (to work the shoulder-girdle / pec region). You should take two deep breaths between reps. Use a light weight for the straight-arm pullover. Work toward a deep stretch.	

3.

Wide-Grip Barbell Bench Press to Neck	6 x 6-8
Superset:	
35-Degree Incline Dumbbell Press	3 x 8-10
Parallel Bar Dip (with weight)	3 x 8-10
Decline Dumbbell Flye	3 x 12

4.

Flat Barbell Press	6 x 8,6,4,2,2,1
– Do one set of each rep count on one chest-training day per week, adding weight in each set.	
Incline Barbell Press	6 x 6
– Add weight for each set.	
Superset:	
Decline Dumbbell Flye	5 x 10-12
Incline Dumbbell Press	5 x 6-8
Wide-Grip Pec Dip	3 x 8-10
– Use a weight belt.	

5.

COUNTER-SPLIT FOR CHEST	
MONDAY-WEDNESDAY-FRIDAY (MUSCLE MASS)	
Decline Bench Press	5 x 10
Incline Bench Press	5 x 8
Incline Dumbbell Press	5 x10
TUESDAY-THURSDAY-SATURDAY (SHAPE TRAIN)	
Decline Dumbbell Flye	5 x 12
Decline Dumbbell Press	5 x 6
– Rapid-pump, non-lock reps	
Decline One-Dumbbell Pullover	5 x 15

6.

PEC-DELT TIE-IN	
Flat Barbell Bench Press	6-8 x 6
– Add poundage for each set.	
35-Degree Dumbbell Incline Press	4 x 6-8
Decline Dumbbell flye	3 x 8-12
Behind-the-Neck Barbell Press	5-6 x 6
Standing Dumbbell lateral Raise	3 x 8-12
One-Dumbbell Lateral Raise on Incline Bench	3 x 8-12
– Sit or lie sideways on an incline bench.	
Incline-Bench Reverse Dumbbell Lateral Raise	3 x 8-12
Bent-Over Dumbbell Lateral Raise	3 x 8-12
– Sit on the end of a flat exercise bench.	

This specialization routine is one of the rare ones where two muscle groups are worked together in a high volume number of sets. In other words, using the specialization routine will get you a solid return on your investment.

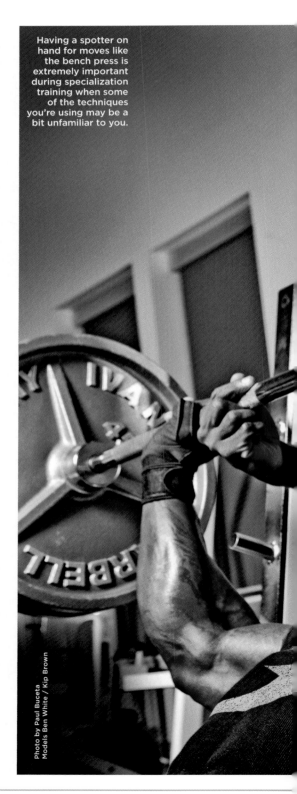

Having a spotter on hand for moves like the bench press is extremely important during specialization training when some of the techniques you're using may be a bit unfamiliar to you.

Photo by Paul Buceta
Models Ben White / Kip Brown

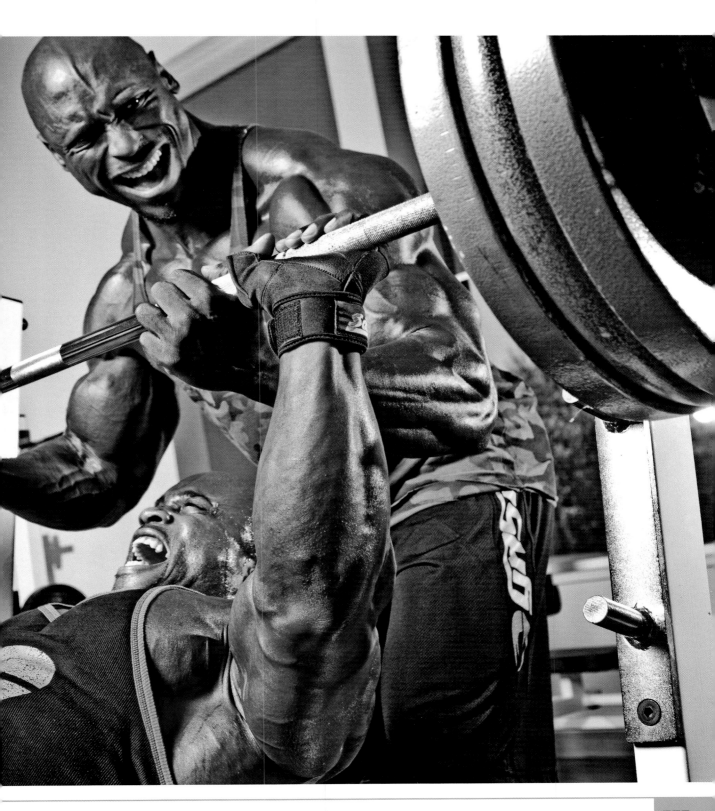

HUGE & FREAKY MUSCLE MASS AND STRENGTH SECRETS

DELTOIDS

1.

Barbell Front Press	4 x 8
Barbell Front Raise	2 x 12
Behind-The-Neck Barbell Press	4 x 8
Lateral Raise	2 x 12
Bent-Over Rear Lateral Raise	2 x 10

Do the first and third exercises while seated and the second, fourth and fifth while in a standing position.

2.

Superset	
Behind-The-Neck Barbell press	6 x 6
80-Degree Incline Dumbbell Press	5 x 6-8
– Perform while seated.	
Superset	
Low-Incline One-dumbbell Lateral Raise	5 x 10
– Sit or lie sideways on a bench.	
Bent-Over Lateral Raise	5 x 10-12

3.

DOWN-THE-RACK DUMBBELL PRESS
–Warm up first and then start heavy. Make five- to ten-pound jumps with no rest between sets. Do eight sets of six reps.
Lateral Raise (standing)
–Perform these in down-the-rack fashion for six sets of 10 reps. Take no rest between sets.
Bent-Over Lateral Raise
–Perform these in down-the-rack fashion for six to eight sets of eight to ten reps. Take no rest between sets.
NOTES: Use a shoulder-width grip on the seated front press and a fairly wide grip on the behind-the-neck press in routine 1. On the seated dumbbell press listed in routine 2, your repetitions should be performed very slowly and with heavy concentration. On the standing lateral raise in routines 1 and 3, be sure to tilt the front end of the bells down as you lift them out to the side. Use a slight elbow bend on the lateral movements.

4.

Behind-The-Neck seated Barbell Press	6 x 6
– Use medium to wide grip and add poundage as you go.	
Superset:	
Incline (80 degrees) Dumbbell Press	5 x 6-8
Low-incline One-dumbbell Lateral Raise	5 x 10
– Sit or lie sideways on a bench.	
Bent-Over Lateral Raise	3 x 10-12

5.

SHOULDER WIDTH IN 90 DAYS	
Standing Lateral Raise	2 x 12
Seated Barbell Press Overhead	2 x 10
45-Degree Incline Prone Rear Lateral Raise	2 x 12
Behind-The-Neck Seated Barbell Press	2 x 10
One-Arm Cable Lateral Raise	2 x 15-20
– Stand sideways to pulley and pull cable from behind your back.	
Barbell Upright Row	2 x 12
Bent-Over Lateral Raise	2 x 15
– This exercise can also be done in low pulley cable crossover style.	

6.

RUSSIAN DELT ROUTINE

The Russian seated alternating dumbbell press is a dumbbell workout that will firebomb your deltoids into new growth. Strategically position four pairs of dumbbells in 10-pound increments from the lightest to the heaviest.

After a warm-up set of 20 reps using 10 pounds, do three series using three different rep schemes. Within each series, perform one set after another with absolutely no rest. You should rest only between series. For our example we'll say your maximum eight-rep set is with 60-pound dumbbells.

SERIES ONE
30 pounds x 8
40 pounds x 8
50 pounds x 8
60 pounds x 8
Rest for three minutes.

SERIES TWO
60 pounds x 6
50 pounds x 6
40 pounds x 6
30 pounds x 6
Rest for three minutes.

SERIES THREE
30 pounds x 4
40 pounds x 4
50 pounds x 4
60 pounds x 4

Anything left in the tank finish off this workout with the 5 x 10 x 15 Standing dumbell lateral raise. (Refer to page 423)

7.

MASSIVE DELTS POWER RACK ATTACK

Massive deltoids are the mark of a man. Unfortunately, the deltoids are slow growing and sometimes frustrating to train, since that training often produces meager observable development. Nothing will stimulate the whole deltoid complex as completely as compound, or anabolic core growth, exercises. If you have a power cage (rack) where you train the following workout will strengthen and thicken your deltoids: To work your deltoids brutally hard, begin your first exercise with the overhead standing barbell press. This should be performed in a power rack using isometric style and doing isometric stops at three different stages or positions of limited movement. The three stages or positions are:

- Pressing the barbell from shoulder level to eye level
- Pressing the barbell from eye level to six inches from lockout
- Pressing the barbell from six inches from lockout to lockout

Do the most difficult stage of the isometric stop first, then the next hardest before finally performing the least difficult.

Let's assume that the most difficult position is stage 2 of the standing overhead barbell press. Place a barbell on the set of starting pins (where the movement will begin) at eye level, beginning with a poundage that's approximately 70 percent of your current full-range one-rep maximum for this exercise. As your workouts progress, you'll want to use training loads of 80 to 90 percent of your one-rep maximum.

A second set of power rack pins (called holding pins) should be placed approximately six inches from the actual lockout position of the standing military press. These are the pins that you will be pressing the barbell against. Begin the exercise by pressing the barbell off the starting pins. As the barbell makes contact with the holding pins, apply a measured resistance of three seconds to reach a peak contraction. Then hold this sustained contraction for nine to twelve seconds. At the completion of the measured sustained contraction, take two additional seconds to release the tension as you lower the barbell back to the starting pins. This completes the second stage.

Set up for the next hardest position (this could be either the top third or bottom third of the movement) and go through the same procedure. Finally do the same with the least difficult position. After you've completed the standing military press (in isometric style, performed only once for each stage), you can do seated overhead dumbbell presses for three sets of six reps each.

We favor the use of dumbbells for a couple of reasons. First, they develop a greater stabilization of the muscular structure of your deltoid region than the use of a barbell. Second, the deltoids are best exercised from a range of 45 degrees below shoulder level to 45 degrees above shoulder level (after which the synergist muscles of the scapula, trapezius and the triceps muscles do the rest of the work). Performing in this range with a set of dumbbells is easier than with a barbell. Press the dumbbells from 45 degrees below shoulder level to the top of your head in non-lock style. Remember to concentrate on contracting your thighs and abdominals. Doing so will help you press more weight overhead.

Perfect execution on the bent-over lateral raise.

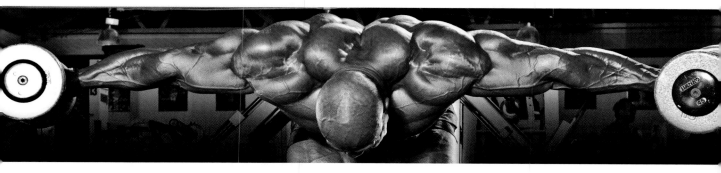

BICEPS
BICEPS MASS POTENTIAL

Figuring out your potential for building biceps mass is not rocket science. Simply measure the distance from the inside of your elbow joint to the edge of your contracted biceps. A half an inch or less means that you have a long biceps length and your potential for building muscle mass in this area is great. If the measurement is a half an inch to a full inch, you're still above average and the potential is good while one to one and a half inches is average in length and potential. You can kiss your pro bodybuilding career goodbye if the measurements fall to one-and-a-half to two or more inches, because that length is below average and the growth potential is poor to minimal.

If you find that you're on the lower end of the potential for building muscle mass on the upper arms, don't worry too much. Remember, there's always the concept of shape training or cosmetic illusion that Bob Kennedy and the late Vince Gironda endorsed for years.

1.

Heavy Barbell Curl	4 x 12, 6, 4, 2
Concentration Curl (seated)	2 x 12
Preacher Bench Barbell Curl	2 x 12

2.

Superset	
Preacher Bench Barbell Curl	4 x 6
Incline Dumbbell Curl	4 x 6-8
Superset	
Preacher Bench Dumbbell Curl	4 x 6
Concentration Curl	4 x 12

3.

Preacher Bench Dumbbell Curl	
–Use maximum weight for six reps and then do four burns at the top-contracted position of the movement.	
Preacher Bench Barbell Curl	
–Use a wide grip for six reps and then do four burns at the contracted position.	
Preacher Bench Reverse Curl	
–Do six reps and four burns at the top of the EZ-curl bar (each rep).	

A series is only complete once you've performed one exercise after another with absolutely no rest between sets. Do four to six series. Work hard and you'll be pleased with the results.

4.

Barbell Curls	5 x 21s (7x7x7)
Cheat Barbell Curl	15 x 4

Alternate one set of the 21 curls to each three sets of the barbell cheat curl. Notes: On the heavy barbell curls in 1, use the heavy-light system. Add weight and decrease your reps.

5.

Superset	
Preacher Bench Barbell Curl	3 x 6
Incline Dumbbell Curl	3 x 6-8
Superset	
Preacher Bench Dumbbell Curl	3 x 8
Concentration Curl (slow)	3 x 12
Note: At the end of the sixth rep in the two variations of the preacher bench curl, do partial movements from the bottom position (burns) for six reps per set. This will total 12 movements in each set. Perform all preacher curls slowly.	

6.

Superset	
Heavy Barbell Cheat Curl	3 x 6
Heavy Dumbbell Seated Alternating Curl	3 x 8
Preacher Bench Dumbbell Curl	4 x 8-10

7.

SUPER-PEAK BICEPS PUMP ROUTINE

Preacher Bench Spider Curl	5 x 8
– Use the vertical side of the bench (spider curl) and be sure to get four burns at the top of each rep. Rest for 60 seconds or less between sets.	
Standing Barbell Curl	3 x 8-10
– Rest for 30 seconds or less between sets.	
Squatting/Barbell Curl	3 x 10-12
– Use narrow hand spacing (six inches apart).	
Standing Concentration Curl	3 x 12-15
– Perform this exercise while standing and do the reps for one arm immediately followed by the other.	

8.

ALL ANGLE BICEPS SPECIAL

High-Incline Dumbbell Curl	5 x 8
45 Degree Incline Dumbbell half-Curl	5 x 8
– With your forearms parallel to the floor, curl five sets of 12 to 15 reps or you could do five sets of 12 to 15 reps when you're at the top of the movement.	
Lying Dumbbell Curl	4 x 10
– Lie supine (face up)	
Preacher Bench Barbell Curl	5 x 15s (5x5x5)
– These follow the same concept of 21s but you do only five reps per one-third rep.	

Supersets are an effective intensity technique to bring up the triceps.

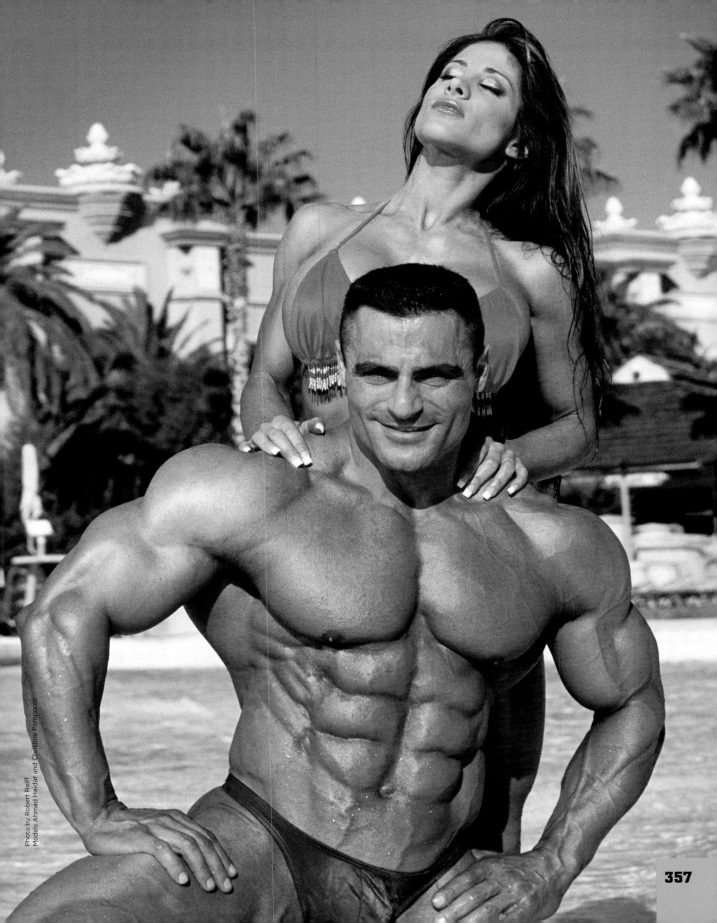

TRICEPS
TRICEPS MASS POTENTIAL

If you want to determine your potential for building triceps muscle mass, simply take a steel measuring tape and measure the distance between the elbow tip and the top of the inside of the horseshoe shape of the triceps. If your triceps length is three inches or less, that means you have a long triceps head and your

The triceps press-down is a good finishing move for this bodypart.

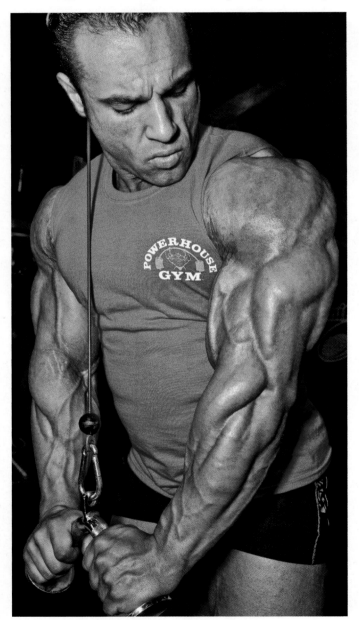

potential is great. If it measures three to four inches, your triceps are above average with good potential while a four- to six-inch measurement means your potential is average. Measurements start reading in the six to seven inch range. A measurement over seven inches indicates your potential is poor to very minimal.

1.

Lying Barbell French Press	2 x 12, 8, 6, 4
Superset	
Triceps Pressdown	2 x 10
One-Arm Dumbbell Triceps Extension	2 x 10

2.

Superset	
Lying Triceps Pullover and Press (EZ-curl bar)	6 x 6
High-Incline French Press	6 x 8-10
Kneeling Cable Extension	5 x 10-12
– Perform these while kneeling, your elbows flat on a bench.	
Triceps Pressdown	3 x 6

3.

Superset	
Lying Triceps Pullover/Press	5 x 6-8
Kneeling Cable Extension	5 x 10
Superset	
Standing Barbell (EZ-curl bar) French Press	3 x 8-10
Triceps Pressdown	3 x 10-12

4

The following triceps routine is a favorite of two-time Mr. Olympia Larry Scott. The routine is extremely difficult, but it does an incredible job of blowing up your horseshoes.

- Supine triceps press using EZ-curl bar – eight reps and four burns at the top
- Kneeling cable extension – eight reps and five burns at the top

Superset these two exercises for five sets of eight reps each. Don't forget the burns because they're important. After you've completed this phase of the program, move on to the kneeling cable extension. Do about eight to ten sets of those, decreasing the poundage every two to three sets. Try to reduce your rest periods down to the point where you're only taking 10 deep breaths between sets.

Photos by Rich Baker
Model Steve Nama

5.

Heavy Barbell Curl	4 x 12, 6, 4, 2
Concentration Curl (seated)	2 x 12
Preacher Bench Barbell Curl	2 x 12

In the French press and supine triceps press movements, keep your elbows pointed up toward the ceiling, making your triceps do all of the work. The triceps pressdown exercise listed in routine 2 should be performed as follows: Begin each set with poundage that will allow you to complete six reps. Then, drop some poundage (20 percent) and do as many reps as possible. Finally, drop another 20 percent and pump to a point of momentary positive failure. This constitutes one set.

6.

Lying Triceps Pullover and Press (EZ-curl Bar)	6 x 6
Superset	
Incline Barbell French Press (EZ-curl Bar)	5 x 8-10
Kneeling Cable Extension	5 x 10-12
– Use the high pulley cable and rest your elbows on a bench.	
Triceps Pressdown	3 x 6

Finish off your triceps with pressdowns in the following manner: Use a weight that allows you to perform six complete perfect reps. Upon completing the sixth rep, drop some weight and do as many reps as possible to failure. Once again drop some poundage and do as many reps as possible. You have completed one set. Do two more sets in the same manner and you'll see growth!

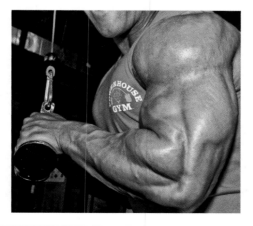

BICEPS-TRICEPS

1.

FRACTION METHOD (JREPS)
Total Upper Arm Specialization

This research-based fraction method is a total upper-arm specialization first used in 1991. It consists of three biceps and three triceps exercises. These exercises are chosen for the direct stress they place on a muscle group. The method of execution is devised to concentrate a continuous tension on particular sections of a muscle group.

The following exercises should be performed on three non-consecutive specialized training days each week. The days you choose to train are up to you, as long as you use an every-other-day pattern. Don't take more than two consecutive days off during this specialization period, which can last from 45 to 90 days for most effectiveness.

EXERCISES

1. Standing barbell curl and/or close-grip barbell curl
2. Triceps pressdown
3. Seated dumbbell curl
4. Lying barbell triceps extension
5. Concentration curl
6. One-arm overhead triceps extension

Do four sets of each exercise, with the reps performed in full or partial range of motion.

To begin, load or select the poundage for the exercise you'll be doing. Place yourself in a position where it's easy to see the clock because it's important to keep your muscles experiencing tension for the correct amount of time. If a clock isn't handy, then have someone time each of your sets.

Set 1: Full range-of-motion reps – Perform these reps in the full positive and negative range of the movement. Do consecutive reps for 30-45-60 seconds and then rest for 30 to 60 seconds.

Set 2: Fraction reps – Imagine the reps of a biceps or triceps exercise divided into three parts, each beginning from the top contracted (finish) position (one-third of the way down, two-thirds of the way down, etc.). Move to each position and return each time. For example, lower the weight one-third of the way down and then raise it. Then, lower it two-thirds of the way down and raise it. Finally, lower the weight to full extension and lift it all the way back up to a full contraction. Do nonstop reps for 30-45-60 seconds and then rest for 30 to 60 seconds.

Set 3: Middle cramp – Do measured movement constant-tension reps from the one-third to two-third range for 30-45-60 seconds and then rest for 30 to 60 seconds.

Set 4: Upper cramp – Perform these as half-reps. From the top contracted range of the exercise, lower the weight halfway down (forearms parallel to the floor) and back up. Work only the upper half of the target reps range and squeeze and contract your biceps or triceps hard. Repeat for 30-45-60 seconds.

For the first two weeks do only exercises one through four in the exact order specified. Beginning in the third week, you should add the fifth and sixth exercises.

The biceps and triceps moves in the total upper-arm specialization program are chosen for the direct stress they place on the muscles.

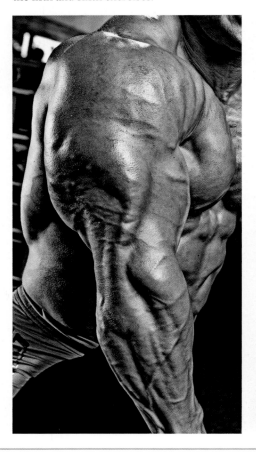

2.

NON-ANABOLIC STEROID BIG ARMS WORKOUT	
Russian Low-Pulley Cable Curl	4 x 8-12
Modified Half-Crucifix Incline Dumbbell Curl	4 x 6-8
Preacher Bench Half Barbell Curl (top half of rep)	2-4 x 6-8
Two-part Pulley Cable Extension	4-6 x 8-12
Two-hand One-Dumbbell Incline Triceps Extension	4-6 x 8-10
– Unorthodox grip	

The standard way is to hold a dumbbell vertically, hands overlapping each other, and your upper palm flat against the inside dumbbell plate. The unorthodox way is with your hands overlapped around the bar with your little fingers against the inside plate. Do one set with your right hand over top of your left. Do the next set with your left hand over top of your right.

3.

Cheat barbell Curl	4 x 4
Concentration Curl	4 x 8-10
Preacher Bench Barbell Curl	3 x 10
Lying Barbell French Press	4 x 6
Triceps Pressdown	3 x 20
Parallel Bar Dip	4 x 8

4.

Superset:	
Cheat Barbell Curl	4 x 6
Preacher Bench Barbell Curl	4 x 15
Barbell French Press	4 x 12
Parallel Bar Dip	3 x 10

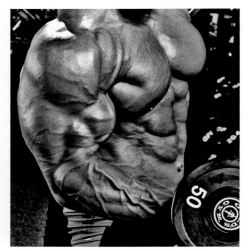

Photos by Robert Reiff
Model Hidetada Yamagishi

5.

MATRIX MASS BICEPS / TRICEPS SPECIALIZATION

UPPER-ARM SPECIALIZATION WEEK 1

DAY	EXERCISES	SETS / REPS
Monday	Barbell Curl Triceps Pressdown (use revolving 20" cambered bar)	4 x 25 4 x 25
Tuesday	Dumbbell Curl Standing EZ-Bar Triceps Extension	4 x 25 4 x 25
Wednesday	Barbell Curl Close-Grip Bench Press (inside shoulder-width hand spacing)	6 x 5 6 x 5
Thursday	Preacher Bench Barbell Curl Lying EZ-Bar Triceps Extension	5 x 7 5 x 7
Friday	Concentration Curl Triceps Pressdown (use rope)	3 x 20 3 x 20
Sat / Sun	Rest and Recuperation	
Rest times	1 minute between sets 3 minutes between exercises Perform each set to positive failure.	

UPPER-ARM SPECIALIZATION WEEK 2

DAY	EXERCISES	SETS / REPS
Monday	Barbell Curl Triceps Pressdown (Use revolving 20" cambered bar)	5 x 25 5 x 25
Tuesday	Dumbbell Curl Standing EZ-Bar triceps extension	5 x 25 5 x 25
Wednesday	Barbell Curl Close-grip Bench Press	7 x 5 7 x 5
Thursday	Preacher Bench Barbell Curl Lying EZ-Bar Triceps Extension	6 x 7 6 x 7
Friday	Concentration Curl Triceps Pressdown (Use rope)	4 x 20 4 x 20
Sat / Sun	Rest and Recuperation	
Rest times	45 seconds between sets 3 minutes between exercises Perform each set to positive failure.	

UPPER-ARM SPECIALIZATION WEEK 3

DAY	EXERCISES	SETS / REPS
Monday	Barbell Curl **Tri-Set:** Close-grip Bench Press Standing EZ-Bar Triceps Extension Lying Dumbbell Triceps Extension	5 x 10 2 x 20 2 x 20 2 x 20
Wednesday	Close Grip Barbell Bench Press **Tri-set:** Barbell Curl Incline Dumbbell Curl Concentration Curl	5 x 8 2 x 20 2 x 20 2 x 20
Friday	Preacher Bench Barbell Curl Standing EZ-Bar Triceps Extension	5 x 8-10 5 x 8-10
Sat / Sun	Rest and Recuperation	
Rest times	1 minute between sets On tri-sets, move from one exercise to another. Perform each set to positive failure.	
Sat / Sun	Rest and Recuperation	
Rest times	45 seconds between sets 3 minutes between exercises Perform each set to positive failure.	

BICEPS-TRICEPS-FOREARMS
ASCENDING-DESCENDING SETS ARM-BLAST ROUTINE

Many bodybuilding champions use Ascending-Descending sets in their arm-blasting routines. As the weight increases with each set, the repetitions decrease. Here's a sample routine:

BICEPS WORKOUT
STANDING BARBELL CURL

Do five sets using the following rep scheme: 15, 12, 10, 8 and 6. Be sure to keep your knees slightly unlocked to ensure strict movements. It's also important to curl the bar up to your chin and then lower it slowly.

    40-Degree Incline Dumbbell Curl
    Do four sets using the following rep scheme: 12, 10, 8 and 6.

PREACHER BENCH BARBELL CURL

Do three sets using the following rep scheme: 12, 10 and 8. Use a false grip and medium hand spacing on the bar. Try to keep your elbows in and curl the bar up to your neck. Extend your arm fully at the bottom of the movement.

ONE-DUMBBELL CONCENTRATION CURL

Do three sets using the following rep scheme: 12, 10 and 8. Keep your arm at a right angle to your body, do slow reps and concentrate!

TRICEPS WORKOUT

Do a light set of 20 reps in the first exercise to facilitate the lubrication of your elbow joints and to warm up the outer head of your triceps. Begin with the lying barbell triceps extension. Do five sets using the following rep scheme: 20, 15, 12, 10 and 9. Use an EZ-bar and be sure to employ a false or thumbless grip.

Follow that up with four sets of the close-grip behind-the-neck barbell presses using the following rep scheme: 12, 10, 8 and 6. Do a press rather than the French curl to prevent elbow injuries. Use a false grip with your hands four inches apart. Lower the barbell to your neck and press it to lockout.

You should then do four sets of triceps pressdowns – 12, 10, 8 and 6 reps. Remember to use a false grip with your wrists locked. You should also fully extend your forearms until lockout.

On to one-dumbbell two-hand triceps extensions. Again, do four sets for 12, 10, 8 and 6 reps. Keep your upper arm against your head and lower the dumbbell below the back of your neck. Raise the dumbbell slowly to lock position.

At this point, you're finally ready to finish off your arm-blasting routine. You can do either preacher bench barbell reverse curls or standing barbell reverse curls with the EZ-curl bar. Whichever exercise you choose, you should perform four sets and do 12, 10, 8 and 6 reps.

Do your movements slowly and use the negative action of each repetition. Remember, contraction is the key.

FOREARMS

1.

Exercise	Sets x Reps
Preacher Bench Reverse Barbell Curl (EZ-curl bar)	4 x 8
One-dumbbell Wrist Curl	4 x 15
– Perform these with your palm up and your upper arm parallel to the floor.	
Rubber Expander Cable Curl	4 x 12
Squeeze Rubber Ball	4 x 40

2.

Exercise	Sets x Reps
Superset	
Barbell Wrist Curl (palm up)	6 x 15
Reverse Barbell Curl	6 x 8
Forearm Gripper Machine	3 x failure
Wrist Roller	3 x failure

3.

Exercise	Sets x Reps
Superset	
Reverse Barbell Curl	4 x 8-10
One-dumbbell Wrist Curl (palm up)	4 x 15-20
Hammer Curl (alternating)	2 x Failure

4.

Exercise	Sets x Reps
Superset	
Barbell Wrist Curl (palms up)	2 x 12-15
Reverse Barbell Curl	2 x 12-15
Superset	
Hammer Curl	3 x 10-12
Two-dumbbell Wrist Curl (palms up)	3 x 10-12
Superset	
Barbell Wrist Curl (palms down)	2 x 25
Barbell Wrist Curl (palms up)	2 x 25
Note: Forearm size and gripping power rely on intense mental concentration.	

ABS

1.

Crunches	2 x 50
45-degree Incline Sit-Up (30 degree bent knee and weight behind head)	2 x 20
Hanging Leg Raise	4 x 15
Kneeling Cable Twist	4 x 15
Jog for half a mile	

2.

Hanging Leg Raise	4 x 15
Crunch	4 x 20
Knee-Ins off Bench	4 x 25
Hanging Leg Raise with Twist	4 x 15

Note: You can use either of the programs every other day. However, for a more intense ab workout, you should alternate programs every other day for six days per week

Hanging leg raises primarily target the lower abs, but you can bring the obliques into the movement by adding a twist.

3.

ANDREAS CAHLING AB GIANT SET

When getting ready for a competition, Swedish-born, 1980 IFBB Mr. International Andreas Cahling used to do a giant set using the following six ab exercises.

1. Roman Chair (or hyper bench) Sit-up – Be sure your torso never goes below a horizontal plane to the floor.	1 x 80-100
2. Incline Sit-Up (with weight)	1 x 15-20
3. Crunch	1 x 60-70
4. Flat Bench Reverse Crunch	1 x 60-70
5. Flat Bench Reverse Crunch (with weight on your feet)	1 x 15-20
6. Hanging Leg Raise (from a pull-up bar)	1 x 30-50

Note: To maximize the effect of this program, you might try doing the exercises in the following sequence: 4, 5, 6, 2, 3 and then 1.

4.

TRI-SETS	
Hanging Knee Pull-In	4-5 x 15-20
Crunch	4-5 x 15-20
Reverse Crunch	4-5 x 15-20

5.

TRI-SETS	
Hanging Bent-Knee Leg Raise	3-4 x 10-12
Crunch with Twist	3-4 x 15-20
Reverse Crunch	3-4 x 20-25

6.

GIANT SET	
Hanging Leg Raise (knees bent)	3 x 15
Crunch	3 x 10
Reverse Crunch	3 x 25
Crunch with Twist	3 x 20
Reverse Crunch	3 x 25
Crunch with Twist	3 x 20

NECK

Refer to book 13, page 448

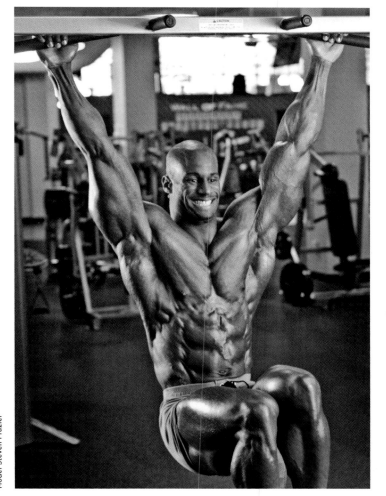

Photos by Ralph DeHaan
Model Steven Frazier

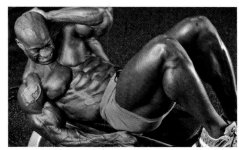

CHAPTER 40

SPECIALIZATION TRAINING WISDOM & QUOTES

There's no better advice than the training insights from some of the greats in this sport.

Dale Adrian, the 1975 AAU Mr. America, was known for his superior physique. One of the key reasons for his success was his off-season approach. "I always try and work my weak points very hard during this time," relates Dale. "It can take a lifetime sometimes to correct a weakness. My back was my weakness, but I'm glad to say this is no longer so. My back is as muscular as all of my other bodyparts. During the specialization period, whether done in the off-season or the competitive season, I would work my back four or five days per week." Dale's results speak for themselves.

Former IFBB bodybuilder **Steve Davis** also specializes on lagging bodyparts. During the off-season, Steve structures his routine so the bodypart being specialized on is worked Mondays, Wednesdays and Fridays. He does minimal work for the rest of the body, once or at most twice per week. For Steve, performing minimal work using a set system means he will only perform a maximum of eight sets per muscle group. If after two months following the specialization routine he hasn't gained the desired results, he makes additional adjustments in his minimal training by reducing the number of sets he performs per bodypart in half. He does as many as 35 to 40 sets for the bodypart he is concentrating on.

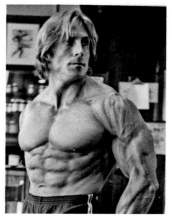

Model Steve Davis

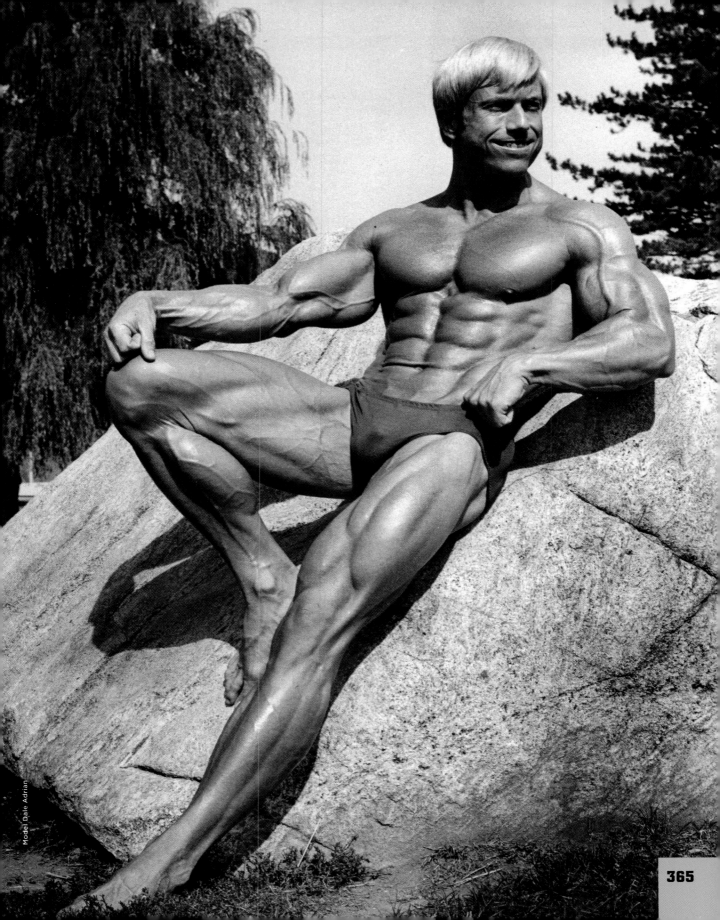

MONDAY-WEDNESDAY-FRIDAY
SPECIAL DELTOID PROGRAM: CYCLE AND CONVENTIONAL SET SYSTEM

A specialization routine for Steve's deltoids would see him performing two cycles of each of the four following movements using eight-rep patterns: Press behind the neck, high-incline-bench rear laterals, low-incline-bench rear laterals and close-grip upright rows.

Steve finishes off his delt specialization routine with cable laterals. He does eight to ten reps per conventional set. Minimal training is done for the rest of his bodyparts twice per week using four to eight sets.

Steve says that whether the bodybuilder is amateur, intermediate or advanced, if he has a weak point in symmetry, proportion or muscle size for any of his muscle groups, then he should work the muscle group or segment by performing an additional two or three sets and increasing the reps by 10 to 25 percent.

Here's one of Steve's favorite forearm programs: Do five sets of eight reps of barbell reverse curls, five sets of 15 reps of barbell wrist curls (palms up) and five sets of 15 reps of reverse wrist curls (palms down). Perform these in tri-set fashion without any rest. You should rest for only 45 seconds between each tri-set.

Jeff King, the 1983 AAU Mr. America and NABBA amateur Mr. Universe, feels it's best to work a lagging bodypart using the same number of exercises as you would for any other area. "I separate the (lagging) bodypart from the rest of my workout [different time of the day] or I just concentrate more on that bodypart. I increase my awareness and intensity level of the workout, how much work I do in a specific period of time when training the [lagging] bodypart with forced reps and negative type work. I don't train any bodypart more than once per day."

As far as bringing a lagging bodypart up to par, Jeff says: "Just allow as long as it takes. You can't rush your body to gain. It's gonna do what it's gonna do, assuming you are working it the right way." Jeff tends to stick with the same routine, but makes sure to increase his intensity. He explains that with some bodyparts he does specialized movements, adding: "it might

just be one movement that specializes on my particular weakness." For example, he does prone barbell shrugs. Jeff relates that you perform this by "lying on a [flat] rowing bench and instead of shrugging the shoulders up to the ears, as you would in the standing upright (barbell) shrugs, here you are lying down on the rowing bench, your body is parallel to the floor and you're pulling your shoulder blades back and actually concentrating on the center of the back, which I consider my weakness." For his abdominals, Jeff performs leg raises (lying on a flat exercise bench) while curling his body (reverse crunches). He explains the curling action as trying "to lift the lower end of the body (the legs) up." He adds that, as his legs "reach just shy of perpendicular to the floor, I then curl my hips up off the bench."

Shelton Leger, 1970s Mr. USA and Junior Mr. America contender, says his system is simple but effective. Shelton explains that he simply uses "four or five exercises on the bodypart." He adds that he begins his priority training at the beginning of his workout session,

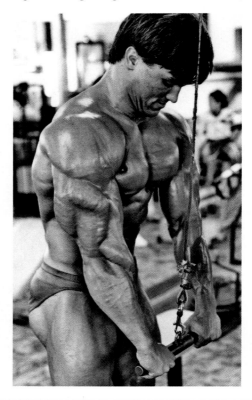

Jeff King believes that the utmost patience is needed when trying to bring up a lagging bodypart.

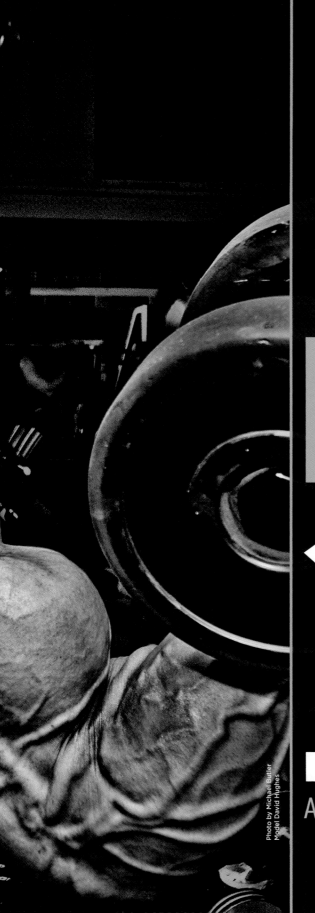

BOOK
12

Aerobics: The Secret Weapon

CHAPTER 41

YOUR PULSE & HEART RATE

If you can find the balance between too much and too little aerobic activity – at the best intensity level – you can do wonders for your health and physique.

After years of research, exercise scientists have determined that one of the best ways to improve your heart, lungs and circulatory system is through the use of aerobics. Another advantage to aerobic activities is their ability to burn fat. In fact, the effects of an aerobic training session will continue to burn fat calories for as long as 12 to 14 hours after the end of your workout. Therefore, aerobics has become the secret weapon of bodybuilders looking to get ripped and cut.

Aerobic training is any mild (low-stress) exercise that's performed nonstop for anywhere from 12 minutes to one hour. For health and fat-loss benefits you should perform aerobics at least three times and as often as six times per week. Aerobics will sustain your pulse at 60 to 80 percent of an age-adjusted maximum heart rate. Three factors determine your optimal heart rate during aerobics (which translates into how hard you are working).

Age – At birth you're capable of 220 beats per minute. Generally speaking, your maximum heart rate will decrease by one stroke for each year of life.

Maximum heart rate – Two hundred beats per minute is the maximum a 20-year-old can sustain under the most active conditions. While technically there are variations in maximum heart rates within any given population, your max heart rate will decrease as you age and the numbers we spout here are good estimates.

Resting heart rate – Your resting heart rate is the number of times your heart beats per minute while you're in a state of rest. The normal resting heart rate for a healthy man is 63 to 72 beats per minute while for women it is 69 to 80 beats per minute. In extremely fit athletes, the resting heart rate can be as low as 30 beats per minute, since their hearts are so strong one beat pushes blood very far. On the other end of the spectrum, a resting pulse that exceeds 88 for

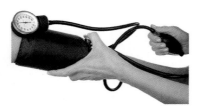

a man or 94 for a woman is considered extremely poor and you should consider taking an EKG test to determine the condition of your heart. Take every step possible to ensure you maintain a healthy heart.

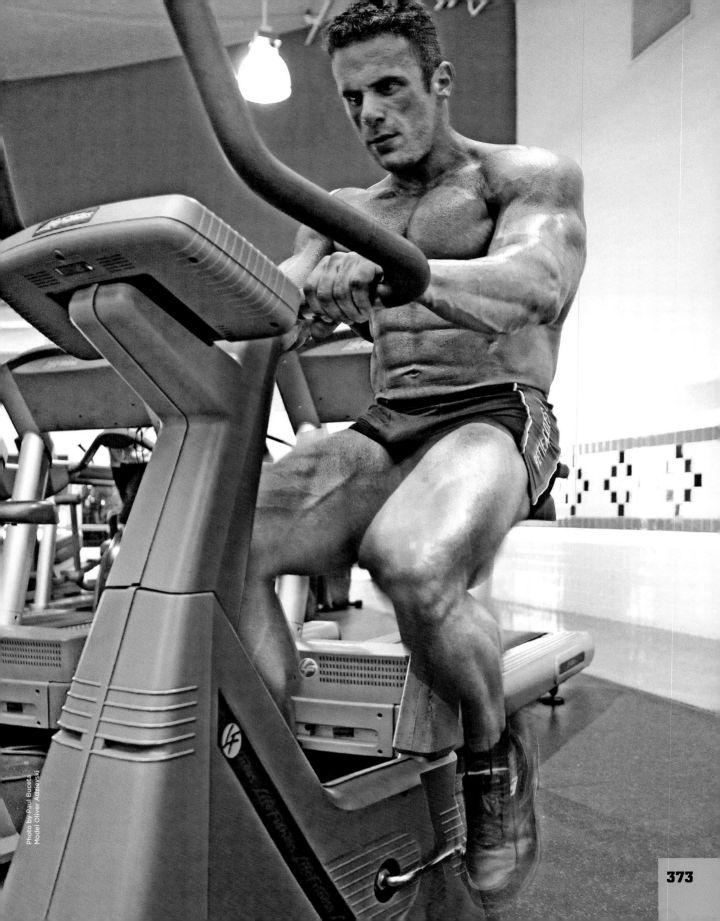

373

MEASURING YOUR RESTING HEART RATE

The most accurate way to determine your resting heart rate is through the use of a pulse-monitoring device. You could also perform a couple of self tests in the following manner:

1. Place your index finger on the carotid artery (located alongside your Adam's apple on the side of your neck). If it's hard to find, you might try tilting your head back and to the left.
2. With your hand in a palm-up position, lightly touch the vein that runs along the surface of your wrist.

PULSE ACCURACY

Be sure that any pulse readings are taken while you're in a healthy state – illness often increases your heart rate. Your resting pulse should be taken as soon as you wake up, before getting out of bed. The most accurate reading would be taken over 60 minutes, but you can take a reading for as little as six seconds. Fig-

ure out how many times the number of seconds you choose goes into 60, and then multiply your beats counted by that number. So if you count for six seconds, multiply the beats counted by 10; if you count for 15 seconds, multiply by four, etc.

A TRAINING TIP

If you're into heavy athletic training and want to know if you're approaching a state of overtraining, then you should monitor your resting heart rate each morning. If you find that your resting pulse is 10 or more beats per minute (BPM) greater than normal, it's possible that you're overtraining and need to decrease your training.

ACHIEVING THE PROPER TRAINING HEART RATE

To achieve the proper training heart rate, begin your aerobic sessions at a minimum of 60 percent of your age-adjusted maximum heart rate and gradually, over a period of weeks, work

The normal resting heart rate for a healthy male is 63 to 72 beats per minute; for a very fit athlete it could be as low as 30.

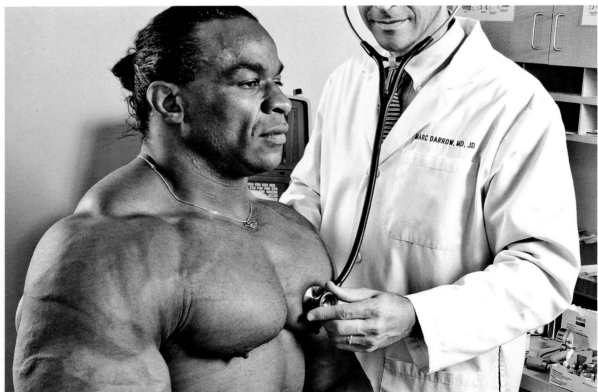

Photo by Robert Reiff
Model Jerome Ferguson and Dr. Darrow

up to 80 percent of the age-adjusted heart rate. Don't stray from these amounts for two very good reasons:

1. An age-adjusted heart rate of less than 60 percent will not be enough to cause the necessary adaptive responses in aerobic efficiency. In many cases, even heart attack victims will aerobically train at slightly more than 60 percent in their very first session.

2. Exercise that's strenuous and performed at more than 80 percent of an age-adjusted maximum puts you in an anaerobic state (which depends upon glucose/glycogen as energy substrate). In addition, this hard work requires you to take prolonged periods of rest between exercises, which lowers your pulse and level of breathing well below the aerobic requirements.

TWO TRAINING HEART RATE FORMULAS

One way to determine your ideal training heart rate is to subtract your age from 220. Then, take that answer and multiply it by the training heart rate percentage you're striving for, whether it be the base requirement of 60 to 70 percent (recovery zone), 70 to 80 percent (aerobic zone) or any percentage up to the 80 to 90 percent (anaerobic zone) maximum. Once you have that figure, you should divide it by 100. For example, let's say you are 40 years old and want to train at 60% of your maximum heart rate. You would subtract your age from 220, and then multiply that number by .60 to find your target heart rate. In this case:

- **(220 – 40) x .60 = 108**

A second formula for determining your ideal training heart rate is called the Karvonen method, named after Finnish physician, Dr. Martti Karvonen. Let's say you are the 40-year-old man from the example above, and your resting heart rate is 55 bpm. Using the Karvonen formula, you would again first subtract your age from 220, but you would then also subtract your resting heart rate from that number, multiply by .60 and add your resting heart rate (see below).

- **(220 – 40 – 55) x .60 + 55 = 130**

You can see that there is a large difference between these two figures. The Karvonen method is generally regarded as being the more accurate. Figure out which formula best suits your needs and use it consistently.

An aerobic session should last a minimum of 12 uninterrupted minutes. You should begin monitoring your pulse from the onset. With some exercises it may take you as long as five to ten minutes to reach the proper heart rate. In most cases, however, it shouldn't take you any more than three to five. You should train a minimum of three non-consecutive days per week and you can extend this to a maximum six days. If you have a problem gaining or maintaining muscle weight but desire to train aerobically, do the minimum amount of 12 minutes three times a week. If you're overweight, you should gradually (over the course of a few weeks) work up to the suggested maximums.

THE ONE-MINUTE HEALTH INDICATOR

Exercise scientists universally agree that monitoring your heart rate immediately following a workout will give you an excellent insight into the overall fitness level of your heart. Take your pulse immediately upon finishing an aerobic session and then take it once again exactly one minute later. Subtract the second reading from the first and divide it by 10. For example, suppose that your exercise heart rate is 137 and after you wait one minute your pulse has decreased to 85. Simply subtract 85 from 137. The number you're left with is 52. Then, divide 52 by 10 and you will come up with a figure of 5.2. The following list will clarify the meaning of this number.

HEART RATE INDICATOR	
Less than 2	Poor
2 – 3	Fair
3 – 4	Good
4 – 6	Excellent
6 or more	Super

CHAPTER 42

SEVENTEEN CARDIO EXERCISES

Try any and all of these cardiovascular activities to keep this part of your training fresh and to challenge your body in different ways.

Cardio exercises are an extremely important part of your training. We've compiled a comprehensive list of exercises that will best complement your muscle-building goals. Plan your aerobics around the following 17 exercises:

CROSS-COUNTRY SKIING

If you happen to live in an area where cross-country skiing is possible, then you should definitely hit the slopes. Cross-country skiing is one of the very best aerobic exercises – it works your heart hard but subjects your legs and back to little trauma.

NORDIC TRACK CROSS-COUNTRY SKIING EXERCISE

While this is not the same as skiing outside, it's a good replacement for days when the temperature is above 32 degrees Fahrenheit. The resistance you'll encounter while using it is directly proportional to your strength. The erect posture that you'll assume when using it also eliminates knee and high hip joint stress. Position the machine at greater degrees of incline for added intensity.

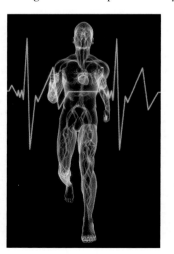

JOGGING

Jogging is one of the most popular forms of aerobic conditioning. The secret is to begin gradually and progress steadily. The primary goal of the graduated jogging plan for a beginner is to eventually jog one mile around a track. The most sensible approach to protecting previous muscle gains is to jog on two non-consecutive days per week (preferably on non-workout days) until you reach one mile.

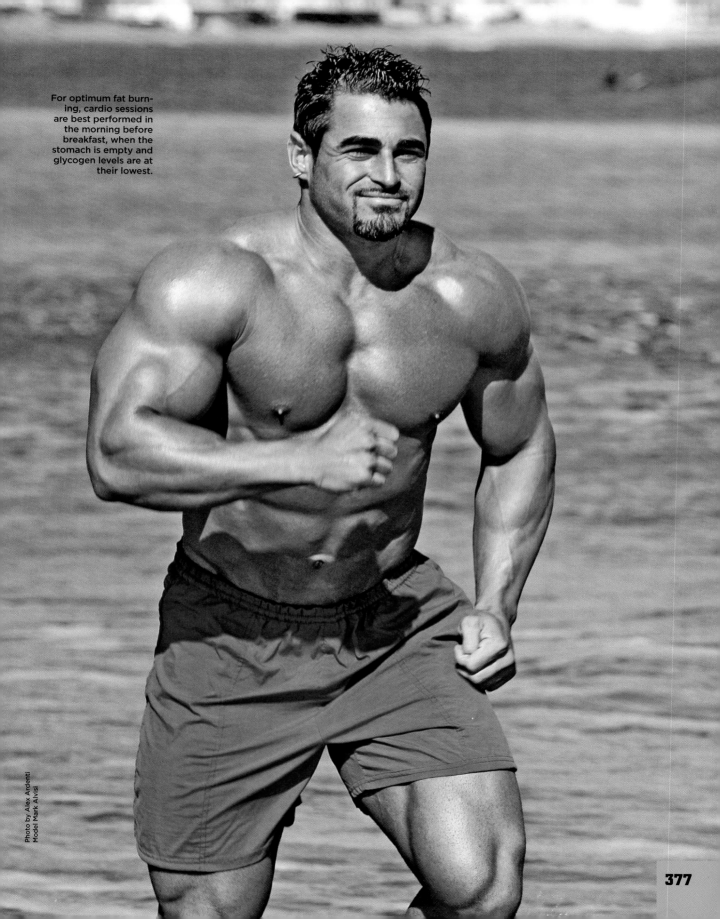

For optimum fat burning, cardio sessions are best performed in the morning before breakfast, when the stomach is empty and glycogen levels are at their lowest.

Photo by Alex Ardenti
Model Mark Alvisi

ONE-MILE GRADUATED JOGGING PLAN

JOGGING SESSION	YARDS JOGGED	YARDS WALKED
1	440	440
2	550	330
3	660	220
4	770	110
5	880 (or ½ mile)	440
6	990	330
7	1,100	220
8	1,210	110
9	1,320 (or ¾ mile)	440
10	1,430	330
11	1,540	220
12	1,650	110
13	1,760 (or 1 mile)	440

Depending on your stamina, recuperative ability and training priorities, you could continue with this jogging plan for an additional 13 sessions. If you do, you'll want to increase your jogging frequency to three non-consecutive days per week.

This jogging plan will, in most cases, eliminate the possibility of shin splints, however, this will be somewhat dependent upon the jogging surface. Ideally you should jog on a surface that has some give to it (grass, gym floors, beaches, etc.) as opposed to surfaces with no give, such as asphalt or concrete.

During a 1977 bodybuilding seminar, Frank Zane reinforced our conclusions regarding jogging. Frank said: "It gives you a superior hardness to your body and I think it adds a lot to your leg development." Frank added that "Another thing it does is increase your endurance, so it cuts down on your recuperation time between sets and this is helpful the last couple of months when you're training for a show."

JOGGING IN PLACE

Do this exercise on a soft carpeted area. Gradually work into using wrist and ankle weights as a means to increase your aerobic mechanism within the individual muscles of your upper and lower body. (Be sure to do this gradually or you could damage your tendons and/or liga-

ments.) If you want to add a little extra ab work during this workout, bring your knees high into your chest while forcefully tensing your abs. Jog in place for five minutes, take a two-minute rest and then jog in place for another five minutes.

WALKING

On the right you'll find a walking program that Eric Sternlicht, Ph.D. (founder and president of Simply Fit, as well as a regular magazine contributor) designed years ago.

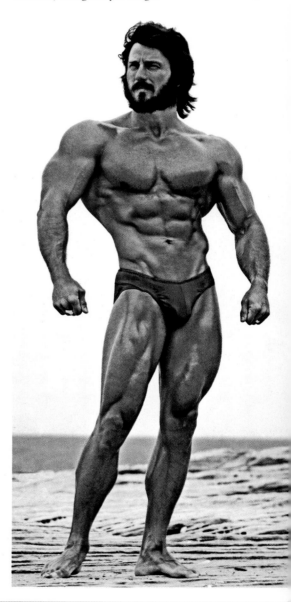

Model Frank Zane

Frank Zane was a strong supporter of jogging as part of bodybuilding workouts – it definitely worked for him.

GRADUATED WALKING PLAN

LEVEL	FREQUENCY (TIMES PER WEEK)	DISTANCE (MILES)	WALKING PACE (MILES PER HOUR)
Beginner	3	1–2	Moderate 3.0
Intermediate	4	2–4	Moderate 3.5
Advanced	5	3–5	Brisk 4.0–4.5

Another option to consider is power walking, which is simply walking as fast as you can (within your allowable aerobic training capacity of 60 to 80 percent of your targeted heart rate), taking the longest strides possible, rhythmically breathing in and out in sync with your strides. As you progress, you can go on more challenging terrain, go further or hold small hand weights.

CARDIO MACHINE INTERVAL TRAINING

Remember when we discussed the aerobic three minute system? That particular application was used as a warm up, but now we're going to change it up a bit so that you can get in some necessary aerobic conditioning. We suggest you do what's called the 30-30 System. Here's how it works: Using a stair stepper, stationary bike, treadmill or comparable machine, start at level 5. Go easy for 30 seconds (at about 60 to 65 percent of your target heart rate). Then work at a sprint pace for 30 seconds (80 to 90 percent of your target heart rate). At the end of this sprint and without resting, go back to an easy pace. Repeat this easy-hard 30-30 sequence without pausing for a total of 10 series on two non-consecutive (non-training) days a week. Every third workout, add one additional series of 30 seconds easy plus 30 seconds hard. Continue in this manner until you have reached your desired workout length.

10 SPEED CYCLING SPRINTS

This exercise expends approximately 300 calories per hour. The gear ratios on the bike give you the opportunity of selecting your own pedaling intensity. The higher gear ratios can stimulate extra muscle tissue growth in your thighs. If this isn't what you want, then you should select a lower gear and pedal faster. Some bodybuilders will do 10 sprints of 25 yards each and rest for one minute between each sprint. Upon completion of the 10 sprints, these bodybuilders rest for 10 minutes and begin another session of 10 sprints of 25 yards.

UPHILL WIND SPRINTS

Locate a hill that's fairly steep and at least 50 to 100 yards long. Perform consecutive uphill wind sprints on three non-consecutive non-training days per week using the Matt Furey (self-development and fitness author) way. In the first non-training day, do five consecutive uphill wind sprints of 50 to 100 yards. On the second non-training day, do seven uphill wind sprints and on the final non-training day do nine or ten uphill wind sprints.

GUERRILLA SPEED CARDIO SPRINTING

Some bodybuilders get fed up with their cardio program. They get on the cross walker and their cardio conditioning just seems to stay at the same level. They jog on the treadmill and never seem to get anywhere! We're going to let you in on a training secret that many amateur and pro bodybuilders as well as MMA fighters have been using for years to get into shape. It's called guerrilla speed cardio sprinting.

Find a field that's level. A soccer or football field would be a good choice, but you can also use a basketball court or an empty parking lot. Make sure you have decent shoes, and warm up with some high-knee jogging (to loosen up your glutes and hamstrings) and some jogging

Combine sprints with chin-ups and parallel bar dips for an intense 12-minute commando conditioning session.

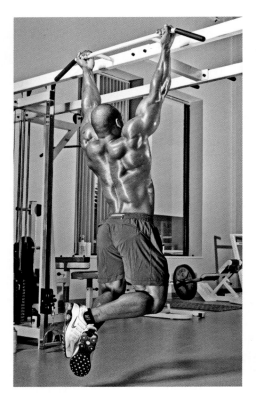
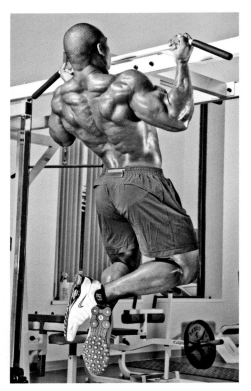

on your toes (to loosen up your calves) for intervals of 10 to 20 yards.

Start sprinting 20 to 25 yards. The only rest you should take is walking or jogging back the same distance that you just sprinted. When you get there, turn around and sprint again! At first, you'll only want to do five to seven of these sprints (resting one minute between each sprint). But after a couple of weeks, you should add two more sprints. Then, add two more sprints for every week thereafter until you're up to 15 to 20 sprints in a workout. One important thing to remember is that you should do these sprints only every three to four days because you have to recover. It's just like pumping the heavy iron.

Now obviously there are many variations – longer distances, shorter distances, sprinting up hills or stairs, mixing up distances in a workout – but you get the idea, right? If you do these regularly and with honest effort, your cardio fitness will go through the roof! On top of that, you could end up with a ripped Olympic sprinter-like lower torso.

You can even do sprints in sand. Jog for 30 seconds and then sprint for 30 seconds. Repeat the sequence until you've completed one five-minute cycle. In each workout thereafter, you should add an additional one-minute cycle until you are doing 12 one-minute cycles. At the conclusion of these sessions it's always important to cool down with a very slow jog of a quarter-mile and then do some stretching.

12-MINUTE COMMANDO CONDITIONING

The original concept of the 12-minute commando conditioning program was the brainchild of Ellington Darden, Ph.D. The objective is to get your heart rate up to between 160 and 180 beats per minute and to keep it there for at least 12 minutes. This can be accomplished by alternating bodyweight only chin-ups and parallel bar dips with 100 meter sprints. All of this should last around 12 minutes. The idea is to sprint 50 meters, turn around and sprint back. Then immediately do at least eight underhand chin-ups. If you can't do the eight underhand

Photos by Paul Buceta
Model Christopher White

chin-ups, perform as many as you can and then do the rest of them in negative style (where you step up on a bench and from the top position lower yourself down over the course of around eight seconds). Immediately upon completion of the chin-ups, sprint 50 meters and then turn around and sprint back. You should then immediately perform dips on the parallel bars using the same protocol as with the underhand chin-ups. A good guideline for these sprints is 16 seconds or less, which you most likely will be able to do three or four times.

You should try to do at least five or six chin-ups and parallel bar dips in negative fashion over the course of eight seconds. Remember that the alternating of the chin-ups and parallel bar dips with the 100-meter sprints should only

last around 12 minutes. Begin this program on two non-consecutive days per week (usually on a Monday and Thursday) separate from your regular weight training for about three to four weeks.

If you don't have access to chin-up and dip bars, then here's another quick fix substitute: Alternate the barbell clean and push press (12 to 20 reps) with an immediate sprint up a hill or several quick flights of stairs.

21-DAY GRADUATED SPRINT, WALK OR JOG PLAN

WEEK 1

On Monday, Tuesday and Thursday, sprint for 10 seconds and either walk or jog for two minutes. Repeat these instructions for a total of 10 cycles. On Wednesday, you should rest. On Friday, walk or jog for 90 seconds and sprint for 10 seconds. Repeat this for eight cycles. Saturday should see you sprinting for 15 seconds and walking or jogging for one minute. Do this for six cycles. Of course, as is usually the case, Sunday is reserved for rest.

WEEK 2

Pick a day and add five seconds to your sprints and also reduce your walk/jog by 10 seconds per interval.

WEEK 3

On the same day as Week 2, add another five seconds to your sprints and reduce your walk or jog by an additional 15 seconds. Tip: The 21-day graduated sprint outline is for flat terrain, but you could really up the ante by doing the sprints on a hellish hill.

ROPE SKIPPING

Rope skipping is a tremendous exercise. A couple of exercise equipment companies market weighted skipping ropes, which offer you the benefit of extra aerobic conditioning for your upper torso. Try to perform 70 to 80 jumps per minute (assuming that allows you to work at your active target heart rate) for a total of six to seven minutes. Consider this to be one set. Do two more sets, resting for one minute between each.

It may not look overly taxing, but skipping rope can give your cardiovascular system an incredible workout.

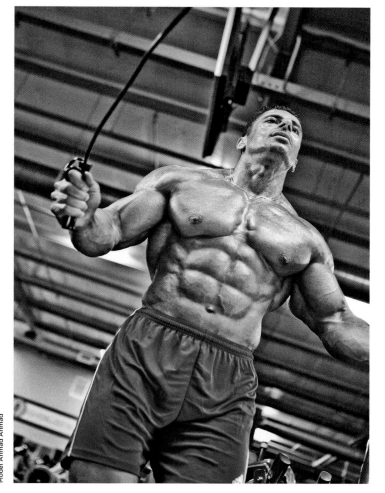

Photo by Alex Ardenti
Model Ahmad Ahmad

STAIR CLIMBING

Climbing eight to ten steps every five seconds is an excellent aerobic exercise, but descending those stairs may not keep your active exercise heart rate up to even its minimum requirements, so you should monitor this closely.

15-MINUTE RUNNING STAIRS CARDIO WORKOUT

Find a staircase that has at least 20 to 30 stairs. Walk up to the top of the staircase and then go down the stairs. Do this three to five times. After this warm-up, begin the workout.

Sequence 1: Sprint from the bottom of the stairs to the top as fast as possible

Sequence 2: Jog down to the bottom of the stairs

Repeat sequences 1 and 2 continuously for 15 minutes.

We realize this sounds way too simple, but you can make it more difficult by choosing longer flights of stairs. You also can jog a couple of miles before or after running stairs. The key to this exercise is that is you run up hard, thereby causing your body to release HGH.

Running stairs is great because you can do it almost anywhere: a local park, arena, community stadium, or even at your home or office.

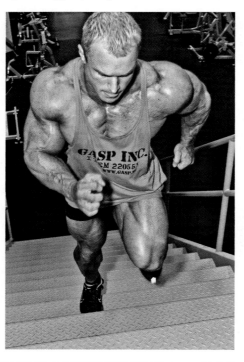

SWIMMING

Swimming is one of the priority exercises in physical therapy sessions. Swimming 50 yards per minute can result in 14 burned fat calories, and it's also stress free on your joints. In our opinion, a serious bodybuilder would never swim for fitness reasons because speed swimming challenges muscle density, causing you to lose size and pump.

AQUA JOGGING PROTOCOL

WORKOUT	TIME OF ALL-OUT EFFORT	TIME OF RECOVERY
No. 1	20 seconds	20 seconds
	25 seconds	25 seconds
	30 seconds	30 seconds
	35 seconds	35 seconds
	40 seconds	40 seconds
	45 seconds	45 seconds
	40 seconds	40 seconds
	35 seconds	35 seconds
	30 seconds	30 seconds
	25 seconds	25 seconds
	20 seconds	20 seconds
No. 2	60 seconds	30 seconds
	Perform cycle 4–6 times	

Alternate the above workouts from one session to the next.

Your heart rate can be used to ensure that you aren't going too easy. Remember, since you are running with resistance, your legs will not move as fast as they would on solid ground. Again, it is the effort you are gauging, not the speed. When aqua jogging, you should tilt your body forward slightly with your legs working in a piston-like fashion and your arms at your sides moving forward and back.

THE 40/20 AEROBIC SQUAT PROGRAM

Initially, this routine requires that you do a barbell back squat with a poundage that's 60 percent of your own bodyweight. You should do one full-squat rep every four seconds for a 40-second duration. Then rest for 20 seconds while utilizing the late Vince Gironda's oxygen

Photo by Rich Baker
Model Constantinos Demetriou

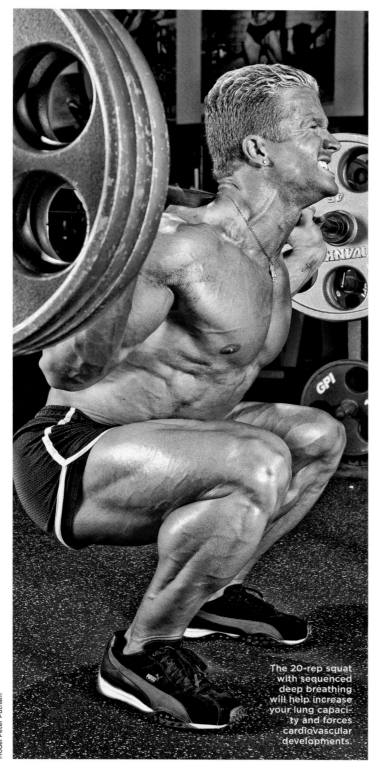

The 20-rep squat with sequenced deep breathing will help increase your lung capacity and forces cardiovascular developments.

Photo by Robert Reiff
Model Peter Putnam

saturation technique of taking five to ten deep breaths through pursed lips during your 20-second rest. The oxygen saturation technique offers some special benefits such as increased stamina, a lower heart rate and diminished acid levels in your body. Repeat the entire sequence another 19 times for a total of 20 minutes.

THE 20-REP SQUAT (DEEP-BREATHING STYLE)

Select a poundage in the barbell back squat that you know will seem quite heavy to you when you're performing your 10th rep. Begin your squats by filling your lungs with one deep breathe after each of the first five reps. On reps six through ten, breathe deeply twice. Remember that in order to keep your lungs full of air, you must always hold your very last breath as you begin your descent on any given repetition.

When you reach your 10th rep, you may begin to wonder if you'll be able to perform another one. As a result, between each of reps 11 through 15, you'll need to stop and take three deep breaths. This slight rest between reps is used primarily to refocus yourself for another rep. Rest will occur only in the quads, glutes and hamstrings. It will not occur in the anti-gravity muscles controlling balance, such as the abs, traps and spinae erectors. Thus, you may fail during a set as a result of fatigue in these particular muscles rather than your prime movers (quads, glutes, hamstrings). In the final five reps, you should breathe four times between reps.

You may need a couple of spotters to get you through the last few reps. You'll find that this method of squatting forces cardiovascular development and increases your lung capacity. Increased lung capacity suggests ribcage expansion and this can be accomplished by alternating lightweight breathing stiff-arm barbell pullovers (20 to 30 reps) with the 20-rep squats. For the purpose of ribcage expansion, you shouldn't use more than a 20-pound bar for the pullover. Anything heavier than this will restrict ribcage expansion. Do the barbell back squat for three sets of 20 reps superset with the breathing stiff-arm barbell pullovers for three sets of 20 to 30 reps each.

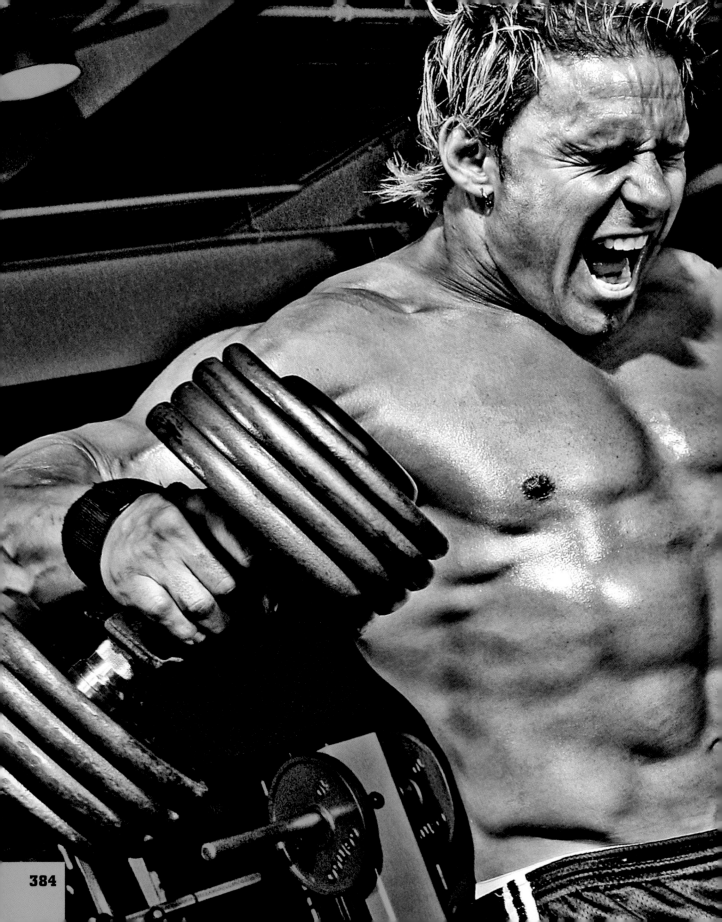

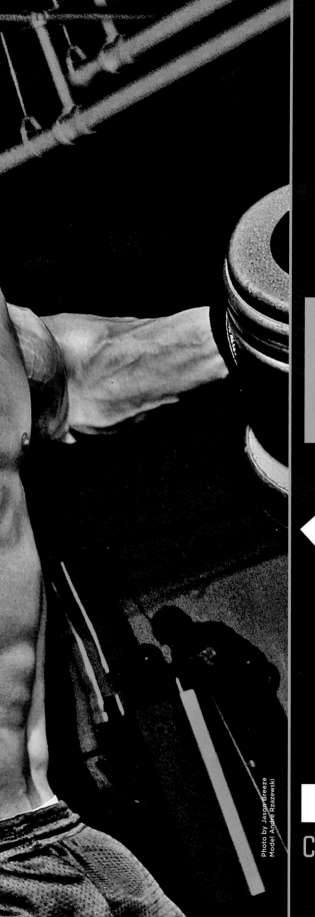

BOOK
13

Cherry Bomb Exercise Tips

CHAPTER 43

QUADS, HAMSTRINGS & CALVES

Tips, notes and exercises that will help you specifically target your leg muscles.

The next three chapters include an almost endless collection of the shortest, most explosive exercise tips and commentary ever published. These quick-start exercises have brought outstanding results to thousands of bodybuilders worldwide. Include these productive muscle-protection exercise tricks in your workouts and you'll see greater gains in no time.

QUADS
SQUATTING PROBLEMS

The barbell back squat and its variations should always be included in a weight-training program. There are, however, some problems you should be aware of when squatting.

Injuries to the Ligaments and Tendons Surrounding the Knee

The tendons and ligaments that surround your quads, hamstrings and calves are known for their lack of flexibility. Injuries are most prevalent when you're lifting more poundage than you're accustomed to using. Doing so may force you down in the bottom (low) position of the squat, which puts abnormal stress on your ligaments and tendons. As well, by squatting in an uncontrolled manner, you drop quickly through the descending phase of the movement and then literally rebound to the starting position.

Solutions

To overcome the lack of flexibility in your quads, hamstrings and calves, it's important that you do some stretching prior to squatting. Be sure to use a poundage that's within your present strength level and perform your squats properly, using strict form. Doing strict full-range squats with a weight you can control will subject your muscles to greater training intensity than if you use a weight that's too heavy.

Increased Glute or Buttocks Size from Squatting Movements

As with any other muscle, the gluteus maximus, or buttocks, may increase in size as a result of exercise. Generally, the area will grow in pro-

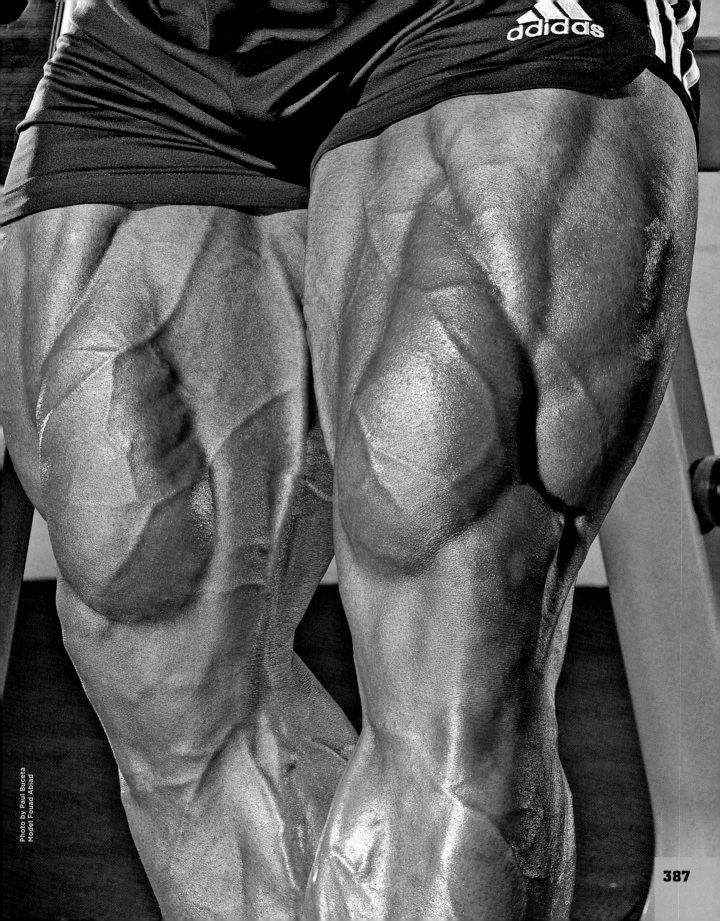

Photo by Paul Buceta
Model Fouad Abiad

387

portion to other muscles in the body, but there's a slight chance that you may have a predetermined genetic problem making this muscle larger in proportion to the other surrounding muscles. As a result, it's possible that you could add to your problems by going lower than parallel in your squats. What happens here is that your glutes, being stronger than your thighs, become greatly involved in the recovery part of the movement. Consequently, your glutes end up receiving more exercise stimulus than your quads and hamstrings.

Solutions

Squat to parallel and not below. This will help you overcome the potential problem of using your glutes to an excessive degree. It's also an acceptable way to prevent ligament and tendon injury in your knees. Another factor you must consider is that your glutes may appear to be larger than normal due to a lack of development in your hamstrings. If this is the case, do some priority training.

Sacroiliac Dislocation or Strain from Squatting

Sacroiliac dislocation or strain can be caused by carrying the barbell too high on the back of your neck. In turn, this puts massive pressure on your spine. Failure to maintain an upright posture during the squatting movement can also contribute to a serious back injury. What happens here is that you allow your back to form a hump-like structure. This, combined with the other squatting problems, causes the back of your spinal discs to open up while the front of the discs squeeze together. As a result, pressure on your discs is no longer distributed evenly, and in time one or more of these discs may rupture and squeeze out against a nerve. If steps aren't taken to correct these squatting problems, you may also suffer from spinal misalignment. The potential pain won't be pretty.

Solutions

Reposition the barbell. Instead of carrying the barbell high on your neck, position it low on your neck (powerlifter style) so it rests one inch below the top of the posterior deltoid. The problem of maintaining an upright position when squatting (this is very evident in

bodybuilders who have long thigh bones and a short upper torso) can be overcome in part by squatting with your heels on a two-by-four. Above all, make a concentrated effort to maintain an upright posture.

The potential for knee and spine injuries seem to be one of the more frequent excuses for not doing squats. If you follow the proper technique for squatting from beginning to end, you should have little risk of injury. As a matter of fact, we know of more people with deteriorated knees and spines resulting from a lack of use than from doing squats. Occasionally, a bodybuilder does suffer from a history of knee and lower back injuries associated with the squat or some other exercise. This could be caused by muscle insertions, a structural factor or from performing the exercise improperly. If squats really are impossible for you and you're not just using excuses because they're too tough, you'll have to find some other way to train your thighs.

Three Hyper Quad Workouts

Here are three hyper quad workouts that will not only add size, but also produce deep separations, striations and muscle hardness. All of these routines make use of the mother of all exercises – the barbell back squat. Use each of these workouts for a period of one month, once or twice per week. Rest assured, they've all been tested and they'll dramatically increase the size and strength of your quads.

THIG PROGRAM I
Powerlifter Style Barbell Squat – Add Poundage / Decrease Reps

Perform 10 sets in the following manner: Begin your first set with a poundage that will permit you 10 reps. Add 10 pounds to each succeeding set, decreasing the rep count by one. Perform as many reps as possible in the last set. You should rest for only one minute between sets.

Your basic foot positioning is important to your thigh development. For example, if you point your feet straight forward, you'll work the quadriceps; point them out, and your adductors or inner thigh will be stressed. If you point your feet inward (pigeon-toed), you'll achieve that outer sweep on the abductors.

THIGH PROGRAM II
Non-Lock Bodybuilder-Style Barbell Squat

Using strict form with tension, perform 10 sets of 20 reps. This program will produce that fibrous, thick, veiny look. It's important that you use a weight you can control and keep the weight moving. For example, if you're doing the non-lock barbell back squat, squat down slowly and with perfect control until your thighs are just below parallel to the floor. Begin to push yourself up, but just before you reach the knees-locked position, lower yourself back down. Ensure that the tension remains on the thigh muscles. Don't rest or pause at any point during any rep until the set is complete. The non-lock method of training can be used on many other bodyparts with equal success.

For lower-body development, nothing beats the squat.

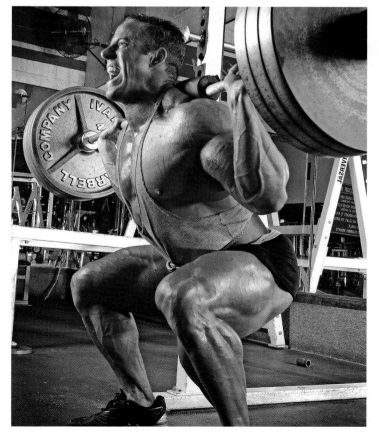

Photo by Irvin Gelb
Model Todd Jewell

THIGH PROGRAM III
Powerlifter-Style Barbell Squats – 5 sets x 8-10 reps
Non-Lock Bodybuilder Style Barbell Squats – 1 set x 10 reps (plus)

This program consists of doing powerlifter-style barbell squats followed by non-lock bodybuilder-style barbell squats. On the non-lock barbell back squat, you could try to add one rep in each workout session until you reach 30 reps. Here are some brief points to remember when doing the two styles of barbell squats:

POWERLIFTER-STYLE BARBELL BACK SQUAT

1. The bar rests low across your shoulders.
2. Your torso is bent forward.
3. Your feet are shoulder-width apart (or wider).
4. During the descent, your buttocks go back and your knees stay directly over your ankles. Lower your legs to remain perpendicular to floor.
5. Squat to parallel.

NON-LOCK BODYBUILDER STYLE BARBELL BACK SQUAT

1. The bar rests high on the trap muscles.
2. Your torso is erect.
3. Your feet are less than shoulder-width apart.
4. During the descent, your upper torso is upright (shoulders and hip joints are almost in line).
5. Your back is flat or arched in (lungs full and chest held high).
6. Squat below parallel. If you're not sure if you're squatting below parallel, imagine there is a marble positioned on the center of your quads. Continue squatting down until the marble would start rolling towards your hips. This mental trick should guarantee that the tops of your thighs will break parallel.

Notes on Squatting

Use a Smith machine when performing squats to eliminate stress on your glutes (buttocks) and hips. By using this apparatus, your hips will be in front of the bar and your torso will be leaning backward. If you don't have access to a Smith machine, bodyweight sissy squats will do fine. This particular method of squatting helps the hips to appear more slender.

DECLINE/INCLINE BARBELL BACK SQUAT

This exercise is done exactly the same way as the regular barbell back squat, but the difference is that your feet are positioned on an incline/decline anti-skid wooden platform, rather than flat on the floor. The wooden platform is made out of a piece of pre-cut ¾" x 2' x 14" structural plywood and three 3" x 12" support planks cut at a tapered angle to accommodate a variety of incline/decline (ranging from five to thirty degrees) foot placements.

There's no better feeling for your quads than when you step back from the squat rack and position your feet on the low end of the platform for some decline barbell back squats.

Proper body position on the sissy squat is with your upper torso and thighs in the same plane, with your knees moving forward.

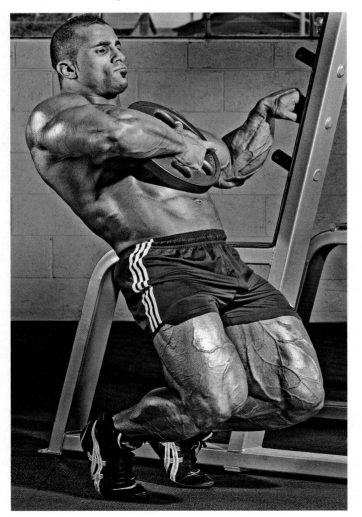

It's somewhat similar to doing squats with your heels on a 2x4, only better. If you want to target your hips and hamstrings, reverse the position and step forward midway onto the platform and then do some incline barbell back squats.

JUMPING SQUATS WITH DUMBBELLS

This exercise builds tremendous explosiveness for blasting out of the bottom position of the squat. Additionally, it will increase your vertical leap. Jumping squats are performed as follows: Hold a dumbbell in each hand (resting at your side) and then squat down to below parallel and jump up high. When you land, don't stop short. Immediately lower into a deep squat position and repeat for the remainder of your set.

SISSY SQUAT

Place your feet approximately 18 inches apart. Rise up on your toes (you can place a block of wood under your heels) and slowly lower yourself into a squat position. At the same time, you must lean back as far as possible, making sure your upper torso and thighs are in a straight line or in the same plane, with your knees moving forward. If your performance of this exercise is hampered by a loss of balance, lightly hold on to something stationary for support. Maintain continuous tension with absolutely no pause at all during the descent or ascent.

10 AND 2 O'CLOCK BARBELL SQUAT AND LEG PRESS

One of the best ways to develop inner thigh strength when doing any sort of squatting motion or leg press is to place your feet about shoulder width apart, but then rotate or turn your feet out to roughly 45 degrees. Rotate your hips correspondingly to save on the wear and tear on your knee. You should be imitating the foot stance of a penguin or Charlie Chaplin. Make sure you keep the 10 and 2 o'clock foot position through the whole exercise. Remember to push with your heels, not your toes. Here's a little-known trick that will help you to accomplish this. It's called the toe-curl squat trick. To acquire maximum power when

For the leg press, you can direct more focus on your quads and hamstrings by placing your feet high up on the platform.

ascending out of the bottom position of a barbell back squat, curl your toes up a fraction. This subtle move will give you a bit more drive through your heels. Using the 10 and 2 o'clock foot position as well as the toe-curl squat trick in your leg routine, you may not be able to move as much poundage as you're used to, but in time you'll exceed any poundage you were previously using and thereby make your inner thighs stronger.

Another thing you might want to try is to wrap a lifting belt around your mid thighs, buckle up and then force your thighs outward against the belt while squatting. Yet another method to strengthen your inner thighs is to simply place a basketball (let some air out so it has

some give) or medicine ball between your thighs and squeeze for 10 to 20 seconds. Relax and start the process all over again. Do a few sets.

QUAD-GLUTE-HAM LEG PRESS

Glutes and hamstrings receive stimulation when your feet are placed high on the foot platform, with your heels on the edge and your insteps extending off. When performing this exercise, push with your heels. The outer sweep of your quad (vastus lateralis) is stimulated by placing your feet wide and rotating out laterally from parallel to 45 degrees on the center of the platform. Push off on the balls of your feet during this exercise. The rectus femoris (frontal quad) is activated by taking a narrow, low

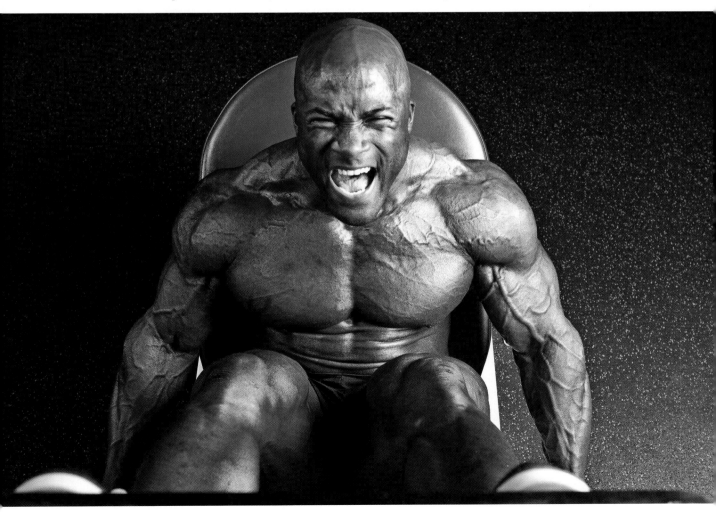

stance on the footplate with your feet facing straight ahead while you push off from the balls of your feet.

BOTTOM OUT LEG PRESS

Bottom out at the beginning of each rep and then press only to three-quarter lockouts. This will effectively stimulate your hamstrings and glutes. Another tip is to press to half lockouts, do a six second static contraction hold and bottom out. Don't do bottom outs if you have lower back issues.

HACK SQUAT FOOTPLATE SECRETS

A lot of bodybuilders don't take advantage of the foot plate. However, by simply adjusting it up or down you can dictate which aspect of your quad is targeted. For example, if the foot plate is adjusted upward approximately 45 degrees in relation to the floor, then you get more of a leg press action out of it. Your hips and outer quads will be stressed and there will be less emphasis on your vastus medalius.

If you want to develop steel-cord cuts, you should adjust the plate to a more horizontal plane (approximately 20 degrees in relation to the floor) thus turning the hack squat machine into a sissy squat medialis.

For the utmost in quad stretches, don't place your feet way out in front of you on the foot plate. Your feet should be as far down on the foot plate as possible (parallel to the hack guiding tracks). In this position, your heels will rise as you descend, but this is the exact angle you'll need for splitting the quad muscles. If you do this movement properly, you'll achieve steel cord cuts. But, if it's not done correctly, you may destroy your knees at the condyles (the bumpy part at the end of the bone) and where the tendons cross the knee joint. You may also cause micro tears in the ligaments along with excess bursa sac synovial flow.

THREE-WAY HACK SQUAT

Full squats don't always do the job when it comes to cutting and shaping your thighs. Three-way hack squats will provide the necessary added intensity to your upper-leg training sessions. Perform these on a hack squat machine.

Begin with your back flat, chin tucked into your neck and your feet parallel. Do seven full reps, keeping your knees very slightly bent at the completion of each. Follow that up with seven parallel reps with your heels touching and the front of your feet rotated out at a 10 and 2 o' clock positions. Your knees should be 20 inches apart. Complete the three-way hacks by doing seven full reps with your feet wide and off the foot plate of the hack slide machine. Do four sets of this 21-rep combination set. Tip: For that little extra in quad contraction, lift the front of your feet up toward your shins, rocking back or pushing through with your heels at the lockout of a hack squat or leg press. You should also squeeze your quads and glutes maximally for three seconds.

INNER-OUTER LEG EXTENSION

Work your inner quads by pulling your toes up toward your shins, leaning your upper torso forward and rotating your feet out to 45 degrees. Work your outer quads in the opposite manner. You have to extend your toes away from your shins, lean your upper torso back (you will have to slide a bit forward on the seat to accomplish this) and rotate your feet inward. Do a 20-second static contraction on the final rep of a set of leg extensions and then do a slow negative of five to eight seconds.

TENSILE CONTRACTION LEG EXTENSION

This exercise is divided into two parts. In the first part, lean your upper torso forward from vertical, at least 10 degrees or more, as a means to remove any assistance it might indirectly give to your quads. Slowly extend your lower legs upwards until your knees are totally locked and you can feel the frontal thigh muscles tightly contracted. The key is to keep your toes pointed up toward your shin all the way through the movement. Lower the weight slowly while maintaining tension on your quads.

The second part should begin in a similar fashion to the first part. Extend to within 30 degrees of complete extension. Instead of maintaining the forward posture of your upper

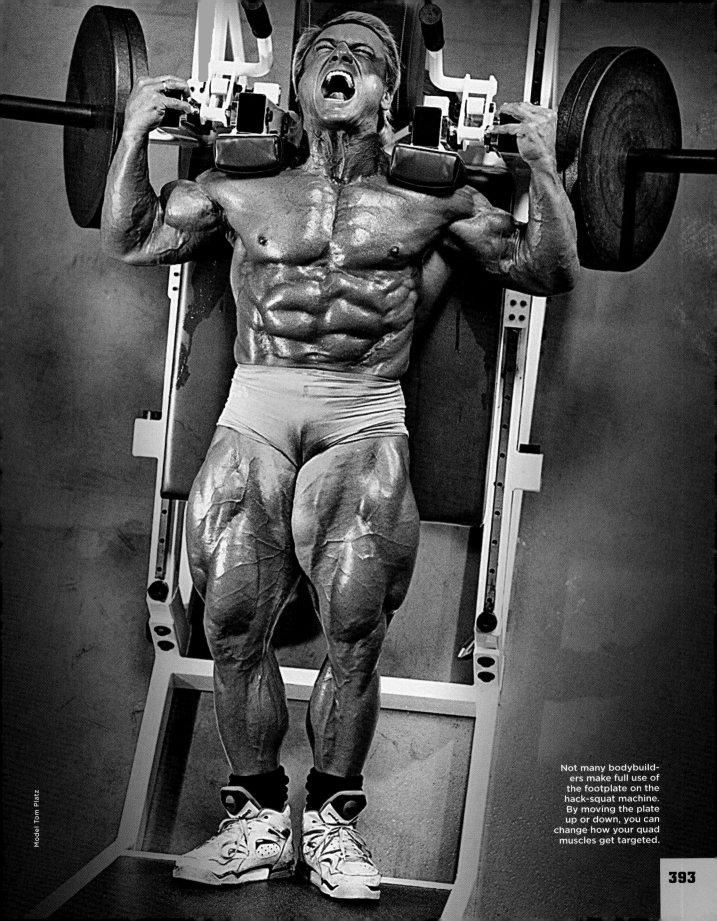

Model Tom Platz

Not many bodybuild-
ers make full use of
the footplate on the
hack-squat machine.
By moving the plate
up or down, you can
change how your quad
muscles get targeted.

torso, quickly lean back on the bench as a means to create dramatically more muscular force from your quads as your lower legs reach full extension. Hold the extension for five seconds, contracting your quads for all they're worth. Then, lower the weight slowly to the flexed-knee (starting) position.

Some bodybuilders may find that this exercise is painful on their knees, particularly where the patella tendon rubs against the two knobs at the bottom of the femur bone. There's one way to get around this problem. Perform machine leg curls first. Why? It seems that when leg curls are performed they appear to better lubricate your knees with synovial fluid than almost any other leg exercise.

INCLINE LEG EXTENSION

Raise your glutes six inches or more off the seat by grasping high on the seat back. Your legs will angle down at 45 degrees. Extend your lower legs and lockout at the top.

BARBELL LUNGE

Hold a barbell across your shoulders, just as you would for a barbell back squat. This can also be done in front-squat style, with the barbell placed high on your upper chest (clavicular area) so it's resting on the front deltoid. Stand as straight as possible with your feet about hip or shoulder-width apart. Keep the ball of your right foot stationary and lunge forward with your left leg, bending it at a 90 degrees or greater angle until your thigh is parallel to the floor. The step forward with your left leg should be a stride (for most bodybuilders this will be approximately three feet). This will allow your trailing right leg to be almost straight, but relaxed and slightly flexed. Push off hard, shifting your bodyweight backward with your left leg so you're standing in an erect position without having used your right leg. Maintaining an erect position is vital to obtaining maximum flexibility and flexion in your hip joints.

You can begin the next rep by placing the right foot forward, following the same procedure as described for the left leg, or you can do all your reps with one leg before starting with the other. As your flexibility improves, you can add some variety to this exercise by stepping up on an exercise bench with your leading leg.

LUNGE OPTIONS
Double-Rep Modified Barbell Lunge

Place one leg in front of you and the other about 35 to 40 inches behind you. Your feet should be six inches apart. Squat down until the kneecap of your trailing leg touches the floor and the thigh of your front leg is approximately parallel to the floor or slightly lower. Perform two reps in this manner and then switch legs for two more reps. Continue in this manner until you've completed all of your reps. To make the exercise go from ordinary to extraordinary, place an eight-inch-high wooden block in front of you on the floor and step up on it with your lead leg.

Power Barbell Lunge

To recruit some superhuman power, attach a 2' x 9" piece of six-inch-thick foam rubber to a wall (approximately six inches off the floor). Then secure a block of wood to the floor so when you're in the lunge position, your rear foot will be firmly supported with your heel snug against the thickest portion of the wooden wedge. The toe of your leading leg will be touching the wall, your kneecap and shin firmly in contact with the foam rubber. The wooden wedge and foam rubber are valuable training tools for successfully completing the double-rep modified lunge. The wedge prevents your rear foot from slipping, and your leading leg can't move forward because it's already secured against the piece of foam rubber. This rather unique method of performing the lunge will allow you to use 15 to 20 percent more poundage than the conventional method.

Rear Lunge

Cory Everson, the former six-time Ms. Olympia, loved doing lunges by stepping back with her rear leg rather than forward with her front leg. So to lead with your left foot, you would step back with your right, keeping it as straight as possible while still allowing the front left thigh to become parallel to the floor. Because of this unusual angle, use only mod-

Rotating your feet inward or outward on the lying leg curl will work different parts of the hamstrings.

Photo by Irvin Gelb
Model Chad Ray Martin

erate poundage. We do, however, know of some bodybuilding champions who do extremely high reps in this exercise with as much as 30 to 50 percent of their current full-squat one-rep maximum.

HAMSTRINGS
INNER-OUTER LYING LEG CURL

Your inner hamstrings are stimulated when your feet are rotated out at 45 degrees (heels close, toes wide). You can maintain this position throughout the set or you can change it up by allowing your toes to travel inward a few inches into the leg curl. At the top-contracted position, spread your toes as wide as possible and lower. Do the positive and negative phase of each rep slowly and deliberately.

You can work your outer hamstrings by rotating your feet to pigeon-toed position and extending your toes away from your shins. Another method of isolating the hamstrings when performing lying leg curls is to do them in the sphinx position. (Do not do the exercise this way if you have any lower back problems.) Rest your upper torso on the elbows or straight arms support. Maintain the sphinx position until your lower leg is nearing the vertical position, and then quickly drop your upper torso forward onto the bench while continuing the leg curl (remember to always tense your glutes) to the peak contraction position near your hamstrings. Hold the peak contraction for two seconds, making sure to maximally contract your hamstrings. Keeping your hamstrings tensed, slowly return your lower leg down to the start position. To avoid pain in your knees, don't let them hyperextend beyond straight (minus flexion).

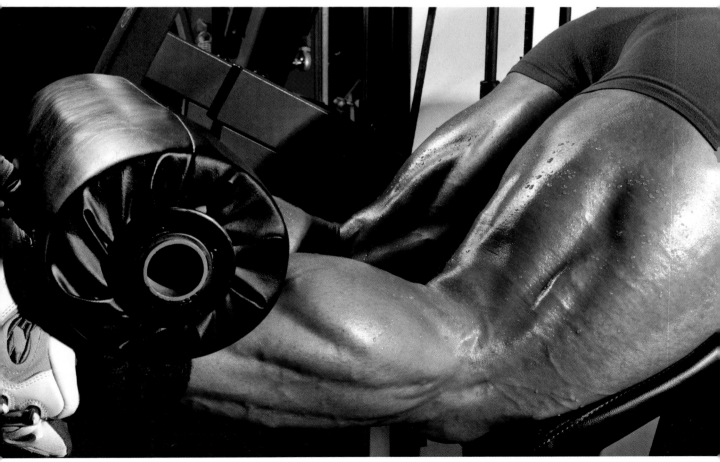

ONE-SIDE LEG CURL

Lie face down on the right side of the machine and do hamstring curls with your left leg under the foam normally used for your right leg. Then, reverse sides and do them with your right leg under the left-leg foam. This method offers a better muscular contraction in your hamstrings than when you lie in the machine the usual way and try to do one leg at a time.

HANGING LEG CURL

Place a flat exercise bench just in front of an overhead pull-up bar. Carefully step up on the bench and place the dumbbell between your ankles. Pinch the dumbbell tightly between your ankles, while at the same time flexing your feet toward your shins to further stabilize the dumbbell.

Reach overhead, tightly gripping the chinning bar with a shoulder-width, palms-forward (pronated) hand spacing. Next, ease yourself backward off the bench and let your entire body hang vertically, as if you were getting ready to do some pull-ups. Keep your thighs in line with your upper torso and, with a flexing action at your knee joint, curl your lower legs toward your buttocks as high as possible. Tense and squeeze your hamstrings for a second or two and then lower to a full extension. Remember not to use your hip flexors to pull your knees and thighs forward. Doing so will take away from the hamstring involvement (isolation). This movement doesn't lend itself to heavy poundage. You can also use ankle weights for this exercise, which allow for single-limb training – especially valuable for the hamstrings in your non-dominant leg, which could be as much as 20 percent weaker.

LEG EXTENSION STANDING HAMSTRING CURL

Stand between the roller pad and the seat, facing the seat. Stand on the right side of the machine for left leg hamstring curls. Move to the opposite side for your right leg. Doing this provides a continuous tension on your hamstring muscles. Be sure to have a training partner watch the roller pad as you perform the single leg hamstring curls. If you're aligned properly, there should be an almost undetectable movement of the roller pad. If you aren't aligned properly, adjust the movement arm accordingly so that it's positioned low on your Achilles' tendon, as it should be for all leg curl exercises.

If you're still not satisfied and want more leg curl variations, then position an incline sit-up bench lengthwise in a cable cross-over machine. Strap on some ankle cuffs, hook them to the end of the low pulley cable, twist around laying face down on the adjusted incline and

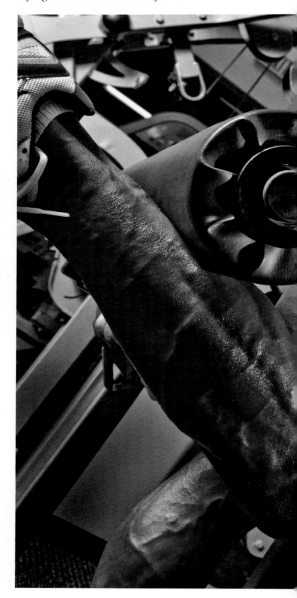

Photo by Paul Buceta
Model Hidetada Yamagishi

If you're going to use the leg extension to perform standing leg curls, make sure a spotter watches the roller pad to ensure your body stays properly aligned.

begin doing leg curls. You can also do leg curls on an incline sit-up or flat bench while holding a dumbbell between your feet.

Certain leg machines lend themselves to performing exercises for other bodyparts as well. Anterior/posterior neck flexion exercises and tibialis contractions (toe raises or pullbacks) are good examples. To perform anterior/posterior neck flexions, you should be lying in the opposite direction to when you're performing a leg curl (backwards). Simply re-

position either the back or front of the head on the roller pad of the movement arm. For tibialis calf contractions, you should sit upright on the leg curl machine facing the movement arm roller pad, with your legs straight and feet together extended off the end. Elevate your legs by centering a high-density pad or cushion behind your knee joints. Hook your toes underneath the roller pad and evenly flex the front of your feet toward your shins, lifting the movement arm.

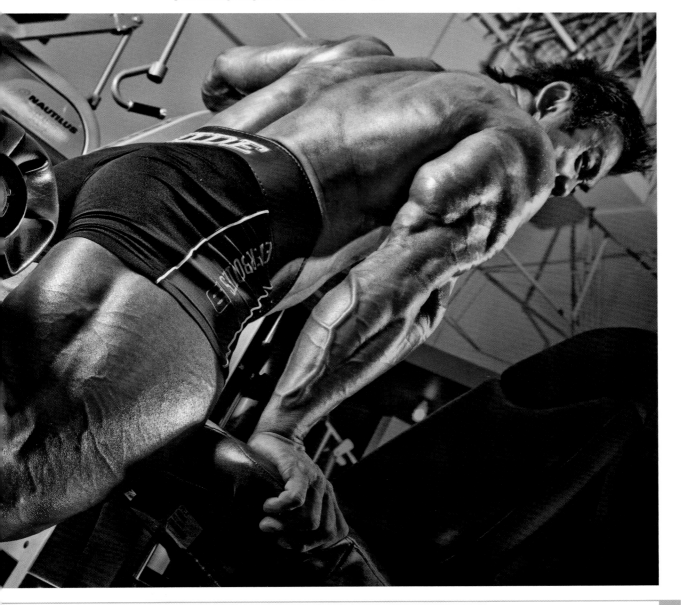

CALVES
CALF SYMMETRY

When it comes to calf improvement the biggest problems comes from neglect. Neglect mainly occurs because the calf muscle is nowhere near as responsive to training as such bodyparts as your biceps and chest. The lack of responsiveness is due to a number of factors. First, due to everyday activities of walking, running and just supporting your bodyweight, your calf muscles become very dense and tough. As a result, it's very difficult to break down these muscle fibers and spur them into new growth.

Another factor you must take into account is the intramuscular temperature of your calves. The temperature of your calves is about four degrees lower than that of many other muscles. The lower temperature is the result of gravity making blood circulation more difficult. With less circulation, growth in this particular muscle area is slower than it might be in other bodyparts.

Improper or inadequate contraction of the calf muscle when being exercised is yet another factor that contributes to slow growth. Using poundage in excess of what you're generally capable of on partial-range-of-motion movements (as opposed to strict full range of motion) is one of the main causes of inadequate contraction. It's very important that you use strict full range of motion in all of your calf exercises.

Some bodybuilding authorities suggest that your calf is like any other muscle in your body and can be worked with rep schemes of eight to twelve per set. We feel that your calves (and forearms) require more reps than many of the other muscle groups. Even using full range of motion, the movement is still short at best. As a result, more reps can be performed in the same amount of time as you spend on other exercises.

With so much focus on the quads and hamstrings, some bodybuilders miss out on any real development in their calves by not doing much specific work on the area.

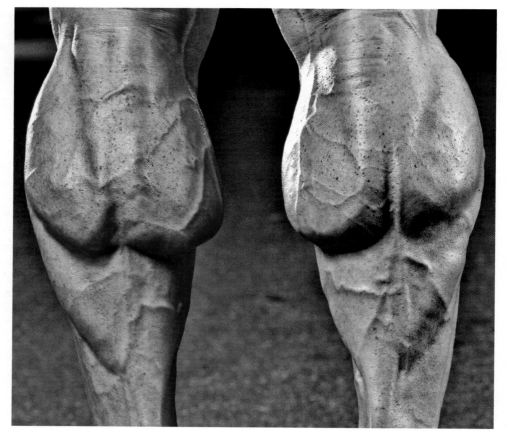

Photo by Robert Reiff
Model Ben Pukulski

Here's a simple but effective eight-point plan that will help you acquire calf growth and symmetry:

1. The most important apparatus you'll be using in your calf program is a block. The height of this block is very important. To allow for the proper stretching methods, it should measure at least half the length of your foot.

2. Your choice of shoes is important. Use shoes with flexible soles.

3. Always perform your calf raises on a block. Heel raises done from a flat-footed position (like the floor) tend to shorten the ankle tendon, which weakens the arch of your foot. There have even been some isolated cases of back problems with the flat-footed method of heel raises.

4. Place your feet close together (four to six inches apart measured from left to right big toes) when performing the various calf exercises. If they're far apart it makes the exercise more difficult because the ankle joint is moving through a shorter range of movement and can't be extended with as much force.

5. Don't do your heel raises with your feet pointed straight ahead. When you walk, your feet are normally pointed forward, and the idea here is to surprise the calf muscle with a new type of stress. Do the majority of your sets with your toes pointed outward (to work your inner calf) and inward at other times (to work your outer calf).

6. Do your set in a two-to-one ratio for the area of your calf needing the most development. For your inner calf, keep your bodyweight over the inside of your big toes. For your outer calf, keep the weight of your body on the outer edge of your foot.

7. Experiment with different calf routines and apparatuses until you find a program that works best for you.

8. Due to poor blood circulation in the calf region, it's a good idea to stimulate this bodypart constantly. There are two methods of providing this stimulation, as follows.

CALF STIMULATION METHOD I

Because the calf is a relatively small muscle and uses very little in the way of energy substrate, it can be worked very hard every day for up to three months. At the conclusion of this period, it would be a good idea to give your calves two weeks to allow them to soften up a bit before pursuing another three-month period of vigorous work.

The calf, like other muscle groups, must have periods of rest to spur growth. With this thought in mind, you should work your calves extremely hard every other day. This means using heavy poundage while maintaining strict form and a variety of exercises. On alternating days, just pump this muscle to increase the circulation capacity. Do this by performing three sets of bodyweight only one- or two-leg heel raises. Do your reps to absolute failure. On these pump days, you should always make a conscious effort to contract and stretch your calves to their absolute limit. When developing your calves, the stretching is as important as the contractions.

For best overall results, perform heel-raise and stretching movements keeping your knees in a slightly unlocked position. Slowly and with deliberation, rise as high as possible on your toes for each rep. It will help if you look straight up at the ceiling. Lower to the bottom position and then stretch even lower if possible. If there's a secret to calf development, it's the stretch at the bottom of the movement. After you've completed your calf routine, finish off with some bodyweight-only calf stretching. This should be done for at least 15 to 30 minutes on each foot. This movement should always be done on your calf block to benefit from a complete stretch.

Begin by putting all of your bodyweight on one leg. Keep your knees locked and your hips forward. Curl your toes up. Then, while standing on one leg, quickly bounce up and down to stretch your calf. Stretch at the bottom position until you cannot stand the pain. Then shift to your other leg. Alternate back and forth. Go easy when stretching because it can result in very painful and sore calves, particularly your first time.

Keep your rest periods short when performing calf exercises – only 30 to 45 seconds between sets.

After you've finished stretching your calves, place your calf block directly under your heels and rapidly raise and lower your toes (50 fast contractions) while keeping your heels on the board. This exercise will cause a cramping in your shin area (the tibialis anterior muscle). In the beginning, it will be enough to do this exercise without any added resistance. However, later you'll have to place added resistance on your toe area. In the end, you'll add to the appearance of your calf, especially when it's viewed from the front.

CALF STIMULATION METHOD II

You should rest for only 30 to 45 seconds between sets. These short rest periods will allow you to maintain a maximum pump in your calf. Many bodybuilders have found that applying an analgesic balm to their calf muscles between sets seems to help. On the days that you work your thighs, do your calf program immediately after your last set of thigh work. Heavy squats, leg presses and leg extensions are known for demanding huge amounts of blood and this is much needed for proper calf stimulation.

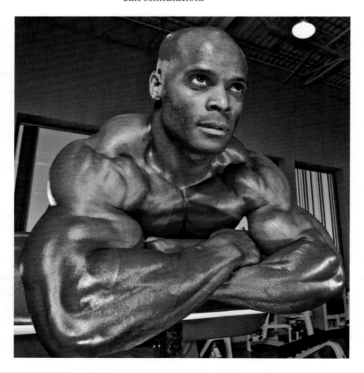

ALTERNATE HEEL RAISE

On a standing calf machine, lock your knees straight. Then, slowly and forcefully thrust your heels upward with the quick, powerful pull of your calves. Do this until the balls and heels of your feet are as close to vertical alignment as possible in the fully contracted position of the positive phase of the rep. Look up at the ceiling while doing this and try (if only mentally) to raise your heels even higher. You should feel the insteps shift forward at the apex of the movement (support pressure is over the balls of your feet and big toes).

Bend your right leg slightly (keeping your foot barely in contact with the calf block) so that your weight distribution shifts to the left side. Slowly lower your left heel until it's level with or below your toes (full stretch through the negative phase of rep). Do this until your foot feels as if it's going to be cut off at the metatarsal arch.

Change directions and, with your left leg straight, thrust your heel upward as high as possible into the top position of the positive phase of the rep. Straighten your right leg, shifting your weight fully to the right side calf support. Bend your left leg while slowly lowering the right heel down to the deep stretch position of the negative phase of the rep. Rise back up on your right leg to the top contracted position of the positive phase of the rep. Shift the weight fully to your left foot on the calf block. Bend your right leg and lower your left heel.

Once you get used to this exercise, you'll achieve a rhythm in your performance. It won't be jerky and there'll be no pauses during or between reps. Calf muscles actually re-engage themselves at every point of the rep. This exercise adapts quite efficiently to bodyweight-only standing heel raises.

FLEXED-KNEE SQUAT HEEL THRUST

This exercise (also known as calf squats or calf rock-ups) is a good one to use during the various phases of a calf workout. It helps keep muscle tension constant. But, more than that, it can create a continuous pump in your calves when you can't get to the gym or just don't have access to a standing or seated calf machine.

Photo by Paul Buceta
Model Morris Mendez

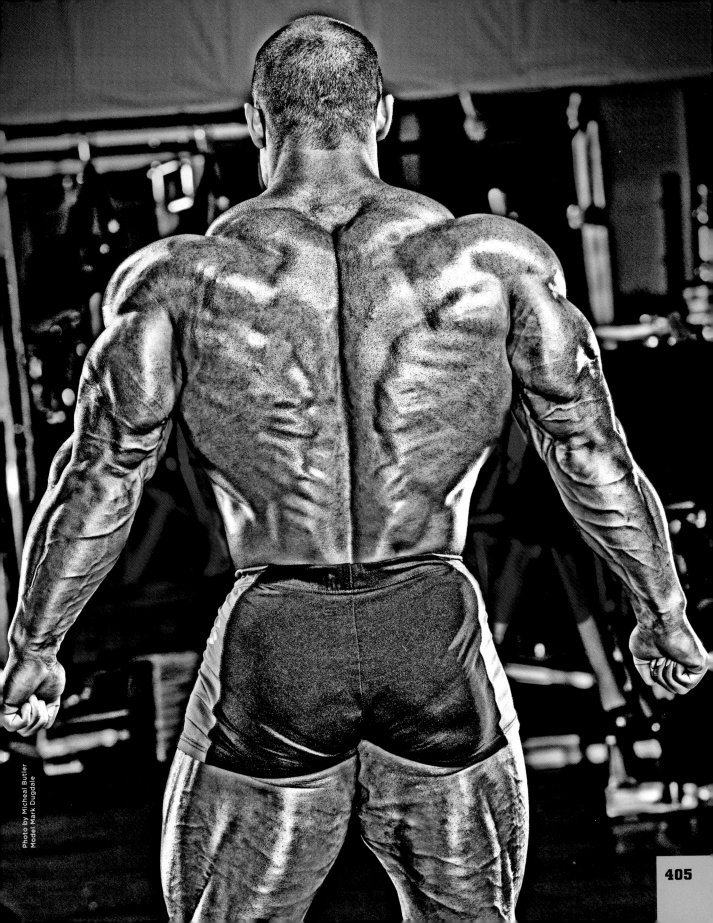

pulling the bar into your waist and squeezing the muscles of your mid-back. Remember to keep the poundage light and go for the stretch in your lats.

ALTERNATING DUMBBELL SHRUG

Hold a dumbbell in each hand, making sure your left and right sides are in contact with your upper thighs. As you shrug upward, rotate each of the dumbbells so they're at the sides of your body (neutral position) at the peak contraction (or top of the movement). If you want, you can also alternate shrugging one dumbbell at a time.

SEATED DUMBBELL SHRUG

Grasp a heavy dumbbell in each hand and position yourself on a flat bench with your legs outstretched. Your arms should be hanging straight down in line with your shoulders. Hold the dumbbells with a neutral hand position (palms facing and parallel to each other). This will give you the ability to perform the purest shrugging action possible. You should keep your arms perfectly straight during the movement, thereby ensuring that any biceps action is kept to an absolute minimum. With the dumbbells hanging as they are, the resistance is now in your center of gravity (middle of your upper torso).

The seated dumbbell shrug eliminates those little knee kicks that can occur toward the end of a grueling set of standing barbell shrugs. Always apply magnesium carbonate chalk to your hands prior to each set to make sure your vice-like grip on the bars never gives out before your traps become fully pumped. Sometimes using the chalk isn't enough, so you should consider using training straps for extra holding power.

CAMBERED OLYMPIC BAR SHRUG

Position a loaded cambered bar about 18 inches in front of the end of a secured flat exercise bench. Sit on the edge at the very end of the bench. With the cambered portion of the bar flipped in the down position and directly underneath your hamstrings, reach down with a knuckles-forward grip and firmly grasp the

bar an inch away from where the bends in the bar begin. With your upper torso in an upright position, take a deep breath and begin the shrugging motion. For an improved range of motion, use smaller diameter Olympic barbell plates (25 to 35 pounds as opposed to the 45 pounds). Similar to the seated shrug exercise, this exercise is one of the purest movements possible if you're looking to gain incredible trap muscle development.

LEE HANEY'S BARBELL SHRUG/ROW

Lee Haney, eight-time IFBB Mr. Olympia, popularized this hybrid exercise. Essentially, you hold a barbell behind your hips (just below your glutes) with a slightly greater than shoulder-width (palms-forward or palms-back) grip. Shrug your shoulders. Bend your arms and, leading with your elbows, pull the barbell to the mid-back region making sure that you squeeze your traps together. For a switch, instead of keeping your head in a neutral position (chin parallel to the floor), tuck your chin into the hollow of your neck (breastbone) or move your head (posterior flexion) to an extreme backward extension. Try to figure out which one of these head positions contributes to a better trap stimulus.

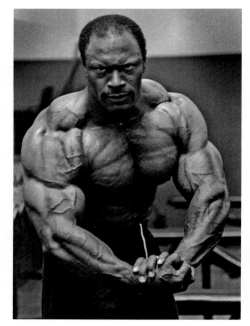

Lee Haney's own shrug-row mix did wonders for his traps development.

Photo by Jason Mathas
Model Lee Haney

LATS

If you're looking for optimum growth and shape in your lats, your best bet is to perform eight to twelve reps and keep your lats under continuous tension. Don't lock out your arms in your lat exercises – this will help you achieve this tension factor.

Go to the Exercise Selection Chart and take note of the lat exercises. Lat pulldowns and wide-grip pull-ups will add greater width to your lats, while heavy bent-over rowing will create the desired lat density or thickness. When you're performing barbell bent-over rows, it's a good idea to wear a lifting belt as it will help alleviate any abdominal pressure that might otherwise occur.

With each rep, concentrate on isolating and spreading your lats as much as possible. We mentioned the value of performing burns at the top contracted position of an exercise and it should be noted that these can also be done at the starting position. Try this in the lat pulldown and you'll find it works great for the separation of your back muscles.

The contracted position of the various lat exercises is equally important to your overall progress. On the final rep of a set, it's a good idea to hold the contracted position for six seconds. This practice is instrumental in recruiting neuromuscular nerve facilitation in your muscles. To shock your lats, try using the triangular approach. The idea here is to begin this program by using an overhead exercise such as the lat pulldown, which pulls your lats up and outward. After you've completed this exercise, perform another from-the-floor exercise such as heavy bent-over rowing, which will assist you in gaining upper-back thickness. Finish off the program with a horizontal pulley movement such as the seated row. This will add thickness and width from a different angle. Between sets, you might find it useful to perform 10 to 20 seconds of lat stretching.

Hanging lat stretches can help you develop your lats. Attach two pieces of heavy-stitched loops to your chin-up bar. Stand on a stool and loop your wrists through the webbing. Step off the stool and lower yourself to arms' length into a dead-hang position from the pull-up bar. Completely stretch your lats from this position. Work up to two minutes in this position per set. You could also use additional poundage around your waist for maximum intensity.

BEHIND-THE-NECK LAT PULLDOWN

Sit on the seat and tuck the tops of your thighs under the padded cross bar. Bend your lower legs backward so your feet (about shoulder-width apart with toes turned out slightly) are locked in behind you.

Reach up and grab a lat bar (either straight or angled), with your palms forward and almost double shoulder-width apart. This will ensure that your forearms are never parallel thus keeping maximum tension on your lats. Take a false grip (thumbs wrapped over the bar rather than under) and always make sure the bar is positioned high in the palm of your hands (near the base of the meaty part of the thumb). Lean back so your upper torso is in a straight line. Take a deep breath.

Use the path of most resistance by first pulling your shoulders down and back. Begin the actual pulling motion with your elbows (your hands only act as hooks in an extension of yourself to the bar), making sure your arms rotate out to your sides. Keep your elbows pointing down and to the rear. These actions will minimize biceps and forearm action. They'll also stimulate more lat involvement (as will visualizing yourself pulling the lat bar down through the center of your head).

As the bar touches the base of your neck, try to touch your elbows at an imaginary point behind your back. You must do this without hunching over. If you do it correctly, your shoulder blades will rotate inward. Imagine you're squeezing a tennis ball between your shoulder blades. Attaining this feeling means you're on the road to achieving maximum lat contraction.

Slowly, while exhaling, extend your arms back to the starting position. At this point you'll need to lean forward a bit, putting your shoulders into a semi-dislocated state (by moving your shoulder joint up) and stretch the scapulae attachments outward for maximum back width. Inhale and begin the next rep in the same manner as the first.

For the sake of variety, do front lat pull-downs as well, ensuring that the bar touches your chest below your sternal (low) pectorals. When performing these, arch your back and lean backward 30 degrees or so from vertical as the bar touches your chest. This exercise requires that your upper arms pull all the way in to the sides of your body. At times, you should take a narrow hand spacing of eight to twelve inches on the lat bar, using a supinated (palms up, curl) grip. This variation of the pulldown seems to work well and involves your lats in a unique way.

With any lat exercise, it's important to begin the pull exclusively with shoulder and lat action before bending your arms and involv-

ing your biceps. Always chalk your hands prior to gripping the bar and use power wrist straps to help minimize biceps involvement.

Recap

- Pull exclusively with your shoulders and lats.
- Be sure your feet are locked behind you.
- Keep your back arched.
- Point your elbows down and to the rear.
- Never extend your arms to the fully straight position.
- Concentrate on moving your shoulder joint up and down – if your shoulder joint stays in one place, most of the work shifts to your arms.

During the behind-the-neck lat pull-down, keep your elbows pointing downward and to the rear to minimize biceps and forearm involvement.

Photo by Dewie
Model Serge Nubret

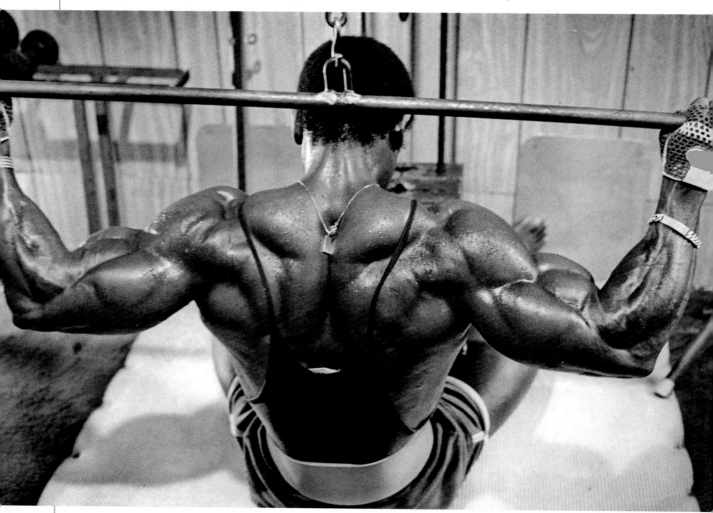

Maintain a very slight bend in your arms during the lat pulldown to eliminate torque and stress on your elbows.

Pro Tip #1

If you're trying to touch the back of your neck with the bar, don't drop your head or upper torso. Generally, if you're doing this, it indicates a couple of problems: Either the poundage is too heavy or there's an alignment issue.

Perform three- to five-second full contractions and extensions. It's a very good idea to occasionally do super-low reps at the rate of 10 seconds in the contraction phase and five seconds in the lowering phase.

When getting ready to do lat pulldowns, don't take a typical posture (facing the machine). Instead, face away from the machine and sit backwards on the seat with your lower back supported against the edge of the knee pad. You'll notice that the lat bar is hanging behind the plane of your upper torso and not in front of it. This alignment will virtually guarantee no protraction of your head (when pulling the bar to the base of your neck) or injury to your shoulder joint (glenohumeral joint). The glenohumeral joint is the most flexible joint in your body. Movement at this joint allows your arm to be raised and rotated. This joint connects the head of the humerus (your upper arm bone) to your shoulder blade.

Pro Tip #2

Lat bars with horizontal grip handles work well for developing sweeping lats.

Pro Tip #3

For a more complete scapulae attachment rotation, use a lat bar that allows you to position your little fingers higher than your thumbs. The upside-down lat pulldown bar will give this ability.

HIGH-PULLEY STRAIGHT-ARM LAT PULLDOWN

Using a light weight, grasp the bar (attached to an overhead cable pulley) with a shoulder-width, palms-down hand position. Step back (about four to five feet from the lat pulldown machine) until you feel a distinct stretch in your lats.

With your arms almost fully extended (a very slight bend in your arms will eliminate torque and stress on your elbows) and your

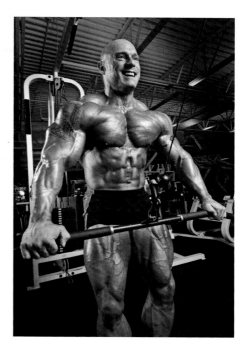

chest arched, bend your upper torso forward at the waist until it's parallel to the floor. Using a circular motion (keeping your arms straight and using your lats) bring the bar down toward your knees. Return your upper torso to an upright position. If you do this move correctly, you'll feel an incredible burn and pump in your lower lats.

PULLOVER MACHINE

Position yourself with your glutes, back and head against the seat back. Place your hands very close together, lightly grasping the bent yoke that attaches to each side of the movement arm. Don't place your elbows on the movement arm support pads, as is normally done. Take a deep breath and allow the movement arms to stretch your arms upward and back until they're near vertical.

Leading with your elbows, slowly squeeze out of the stretch position. Pull (with your lats) the movement arm forward and down in the positive phase of the rep, all the way to the most-extended position possible near your waist. Pause and force yourself to exhale. Breathe in again and very slowly allow the movement arm to return to the pre-stretch starting position.

Photo by Kevin Horton
Model Mark Antonek

LOWER BACK
CABLE PULL THRUST

Cable pull thrusts were popularized by Louie Simmons and the powerlifters at the Westside Barbell Club in Columbus, Ohio. They're an assist movement for garnering more strength in your lower back. Begin by attaching a triceps rope to the lowest pulley on the cable-crossover unit. Once you've selected your poundage, turn around and position your back toward the pulley cable.

Assume a shoulder-width stance and bend your upper torso forward from vertical (making sure to keep your lower back flat or slightly arched). Reach down between your legs (as if you were going to hike a football) and firmly grasp each end of the triceps rope. The palms of your hands should face each other and your arms should be slightly bent. Make sure the cable is tight (you'll have to adjust your distance from the floor pulley), as this will allow you to support the weight stack throughout the full range of the exercise motion.

Now it's just a matter of pulling on the rope and bringing your upper torso to an upright position. If you do this correctly, your hands will be positioned near your groin (it will mimic the lockout of a barbell sumo deadlift, where your arms are inside your thighs). Reverse the movement just described and allow your triceps rope to travel between your legs as far past your heels as possible. Repeat for the desired number of reps.

Keys to remember

1. Never lock out or straighten your arms. Bend your arms slightly at the elbow.
2. You can do this exercise with your knees locked (emphasizes the lower back involvement) or with a soft-knee bend (initiates gluteal involvement). Even though your goal is to develop your back, for the sake of variety, you may want to occasionally switch from a locked to soft-knee position. This will enable you to hit your muscle fibers from different angles.

The seated row is another effective back movement.

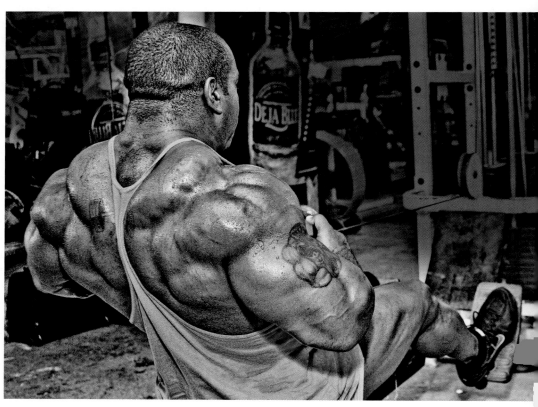

Photo by Jason Breeze
Model Johnnie Jackson

PRONE HYPEREXTENSION

We suggest you use prone hyperextensions for your lumbar region, but before you begin, keep the following ideas in mind: Stand within the confines of the bench unit, facing the padded platform. Lean forward onto it, allowing your lower legs (Achilles tendons) to rest against the restrainer pads or rollers. Be sure to have it adjusted so that when you're in the top position your legs are in alignment with the lumbar vertebrae. When your legs are improperly aligned downward, there's a potential for ruptured discs or pinched nerves. Adjust yourself so that the top edge of your pelvic girdle is in contact with the front edge of the platform and never beyond. Why? Because otherwise your hamstrings end up doing more work than your erectors.

Bend your upper torso (from your lumbar vertebrae to the top of your head) forward every five to ten seconds. Lightly rest your hands behind your head as if you're preparing to do ab crunches, or just cross your arms over your chest, touching your deltoids with your fingertips. Don't interlace your fingers, as doing so will limit your ability to arch backwards. Flex your hips while you arch your back in a swan-dive position. Never hump your back, and never bounce. Take a deep breath.

While holding your breath, raise your head as if you were trying to look up at the ceiling, and slowly contract and extend your thoracic and lumbar spine upward till your torso is at least level with your pelvic girdle. (Incidentally, some bodybuilders do barbell rows when in this position.) Hold this terminal point of contraction for five to ten seconds. If you wish, you can extend your spine 10 to 20 degrees beyond parallel to the floor. However, additional flexion of up to 30 to 45 degrees poses a potential danger to your vertebrae. Breathe out and begin the next reps. Perform up to 15 to 20 reps. As soon as you're able to perform this many reps, consider adding poundage in the form of a barbell plate held across your chest. Don't forget to work your abs because they can help absorb anywhere between 30 to 50 percent of the stress you place on your lower spine, especially when you're bending forward.

CHEST

Most bodybuilders rely too much on the supine bench press for chest development. In fact, it's actually better to do more incline barbell and dumbbell exercises, as both are known to work the upper chest area. The ideal degree of incline for this segment of your chest is approximately 35 to 45 degrees. Inclines beyond these figures stress the frontal or posterior deltoid excessively.

If you should decide to use dumbbells as a means of working your upper chest, be sure that all four parts of the dumbbell face each other (palms facing each other) when pressing. This will prevent your delts from kicking in. This same advice can be applied to flat supine and decline dumbbell presses. Dumbbells are excellent for obtaining a deeper, fuller stretch in your upper pecs.

FLAT DUMBBELL FLYE

Lie back on a flat bench. Hold a dumbbell in each hand with your palms facing at arms' length over your chest. To prevent injury to your elbows, keep your arms slightly bent. You might want to use an ace bandage or a neoprene elbow pad to add support to your elbow region.

Lock your wrists, (Fist in line with wrist)inhale and then slowly lower the dumbbells down and out to your sides in as wide an arc as possible in a parallel position to the floor. Next, extend (unlock) your wrists and continue to lower the dumbbells beyond parallel, only to where you feel a deep stretch in your pecs. With your wrists unlocked or extended back, you'll notice a stretch in your pecs' deepest-lying muscle fibers. To avoid injury to your biceps, rotator cuffs or pecs, reverse the direction slowly and then move the dumbbells back up following the same arc as before. As the dumbbells arrive at a position parallel to the floor, switch back to the locked-wrist position, continuing the arc toward the midline of your upper torso to the top-range contracted position. Exhale, and, as you bring the bells together at the top contracted position (like hugging a tree), flex your wrists again and force your pecs to squeeze and tense in a kind of static movement. Then, assume a locked-wrist position and begin the next rep.

ARNOLD'S FLAT DUMBBELL FLYE

To work the outer aspect of your pecs, stop the movement of the dumbbells about 12 to 15 inches apart at the top of the peak contraction. This concept can also be applied to the pec-deck and cable crossover exercises.

TRICK # 1
WRIST SUPINATION/PRONATION

This first precious little trick will help derail the overuse of same-motion dumbbell flyes and presses (incline, flat and decline). It'll also add some serious muscular development to your pecs. The trick is to experiment with supination and pronation of your wrists and foreams at the top of the movement. Alternate between supination and pronation from set to set.

Supinate your wrists/forearms: From palms facing each other at the top position of the dumbbell flye (or press), twist or turn your wrists so your pinky fingers turn inward and your palms are facing you. Mentally squeeze your elbows toward one another. Grip the dumbbell handles as tightly as possible and maximally squeeze and contract your pecs.

Pronate the wrists/forearms: From palms facing each other at the top of the dumbbell flye (or press), twist or turn your wrists so your hands flare outward (thumbs turn outward and palms face forward). Visualize the back of your hands facing each other. Obviously this can't happen, but it gives you an idea of how much effort you should put into the flaring of your hands.

Another way to grasp the concept of rotating your wrists when performing incline dumbbell flyes is to imagine doing the dual-end triceps rope extension lockout hand flare position.

TRICK # 2
DESCENDING INCLINE

Begin with the incline positioned at 55-degrees and do the dumbbell flyes for six to eight reps. Hold the dumbbells upright on top of your thighs and take a five- to ten-second rest while your training partner drops the incline down to 45 degrees. Do six to eight reps. Rest for five to ten seconds. Drop to 35 degrees and do six

When Arnold did flat dumbbell flyes, at the top position he'd stop the dumbbells when they were 12 to 15 inches apart.

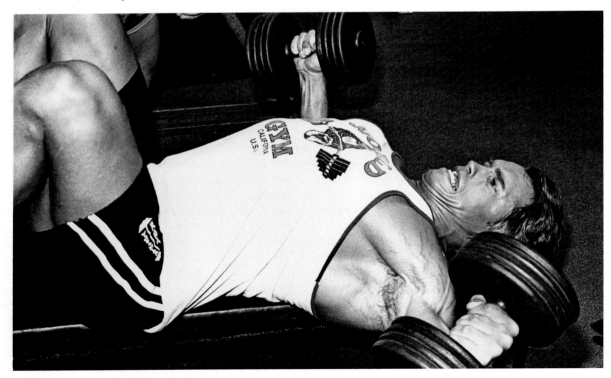

Model Arnold Schwarzenegger

to eight reps. Follow that up with five to ten seconds of rest before doing a final set of six to eight reps at 25 degrees. This completes one cycle. Do one or two more cycles in the manner described, resting for three minutes between each cycle.

The descending incline works great on dumbbell flyes and presses. It can also be applied to dumbbell curls. Don't be afraid to experiment with the descending degrees of incline. While we've suggested using 10-degree drops, you might find five degree drops more to your liking. Don't start higher than 55 degrees on the incline for flyes or presses because your deltoids will be receiving more of the stimulation than your pecs.

COSTA'S STRETCH-AND-GO TECHNIQUE

Choose poundage that will allow you to perform approximately 20 reps in the 30- to 40-degree incline dumbbell bench press. Begin by doing 10 full-range reps. In your 10th rep, lower the bells to your chest and hold them for 20 seconds. Do five more reps for another stretch of 15 seconds. Perform five more reps and on the fifth rep, just short of lockout, do a static hold for 20 seconds. Now do some lockout partial reps and finish off the set with five full reps. With a little imagination, this technique can be used with other exercises. It's just a matter of taking the time to find effective stopping points within the rep range.

A variation to the Leo Costa Jr. Stretch-and-Go Dumbbell Technique would be what Canadian amateur contest-winning bodybuilder Lee Hayward (www.leehayward.com) refers to as the 3 Minute Timed Flat Dumbbell Bench Press. Here is how it works: Take a pair of dumbbells 50 percent of the poundage you would use for 10 full-range-of-motion reps. For example if you use 100-pound dumbbells for 10 reps on the flat bench, use only 50 pounders. Begin by pressing the dumbbells to arms' length lockout above the chest. Do a static hold for 10 seconds, then lower the bells to the chest and again hold them for a 10-second static stretch. Now immediately press the dumbbells to arms' length. Repeat the described cycle eight more times for a total of three minutes. Take

no rest between the cycles. The time it takes to lower and lift the dumbbells does not count as part of the three-minute timing. This exercise is a tremendous finishing exercise for the chest.

LOW PULLEY UPPERCUT

1. Attach a D or stirrup handle to each end of the lower pulley cables on the cable crossover machine. Select a weight that will allow you to perform strict full-range-of-motion reps.
2. Grab hold of the D handles with your palms up and arms hanging fully and a bit out from the sides of your body (you'll almost look like you're trying to flare your lats out). Take a stance midway between and slightly to the front of the two low pulley stations with one foot about 2½ feet ahead of the other.
3. Bend your elbows 15 to 20 degrees. Arch your back and lean forward 10 degrees from the vertical position. Take a deep breath.
4. Simultaneously, in a scoop-like manner, bring your hands upward in a wide arc and inward toward the midline of your upper torso to a point where your pinkie fingers almost touch your upper chest, chin or slightly higher at your forehead. Focus on your inner and upper pecs, squeezing and contracting them fully for a second or two. Exhale and return to the start position. If you do the positive phase of the exercise correctly, it'll mimic a boxer throwing dual uppercuts. This exercise should never mimic a barbell curl motion.

HIGH-PULLEY CABLE CROSSOVER TRICKS

To work your outer pecs, stand in front of the machine. To stimulate the inner pecs, stand back slightly from the unit and make sure to cross your hands over at the finish position of each rep in an alternating fashion (right hand over left, left over right etc.) Your upper clavicular pecs are worked by holding your hands at chin level. To work your lower pecs, you must move your hands to waist level.

When doing standing cable crossovers, there should generally be a 10-degree bend at your elbows and your upper torso should be bent between 10 to 45 degrees forward from vertical. The cable crossover can also be done kneeling, which of course will minimize body swing and change the angle of the pull.

Here's another little trick: Instead of using the pulley cable D attachment or stirrup handles, substitute a single-grip triceps rope with rubber end, attaching one to each cable.

DUMBBELL DISLOCATES

Dislocates are a terrific exercise for opening up the deep breathing process in your lungs immediately after doing a set of high-rep barbell back squats. Put a pair of light dumbbells (10 or 15 pounders) on the floor at the front end of a flat exercise bench. Sit on the front end of the bench, bend over and, with a firm grip (palms facing inward), simultaneously pick up the dumbbells and lie back (supine) on the bench. Position the dumbbells in a stabilized upright position on your upper thighs, just below your groin area. With your arms straight and palms facing each other, take a deep breath and slowly (to avoid momentum) move your arms outward and back in a semi-circle (mimic a dumbbell lateral raise or snow angel movement). Instead of stopping the movement when your arms are in alignment with your shoulder joints, bring your arms all the way to an overhead position where both ends of the dumbbells touch.

Do not change your hand orientation during the movement. When the dumbbells touch overhead, the backs of your hands (knuckles) should face each other. However, if your shoulders are tight or jammed, turn your wrists halfway through the movement so the palms of your hands are facing upward at the top. Return to the starting position, slowly breathing out. Do 12 to 18 reps per set.

PRO TIP #1

Remember, the most important thing is that you're lying on your back on the bench. As your arms travel in an arc, they're parallel to the floor only slightly above your body. If you were to view your body sideways, your arms should barely rise or drop below the horizontal plane (sides) of your torso.

PRO TIP #2

Dumbbell dislocates can also be performed on an incline (deltoids bear the workload) and decline bench (lats are strongly activated). All of the bench angles mentioned (lying, incline and decline) will effect your ribcage development, but only if lighter dumbbell poundage is used (15 pounds or less). Anything heavier will cause the muscles around your ribcage to contract maximally and thus hinder ribcage expansion.

PEC DECK

Here are some pec deck variations and tips:

1. Adjust the seat six inches higher than normal. Instead of placing your forearms against the arm pads, make a karate-chop hand and place your palms directly on the pads. While holding your elbows high (perpendicular to the floor), squeeze the pads together with a crushing motion.

2. Another variation is to grip with each hand the bottom front corner of the movement arm pad and squeeze the pads together in a push/press fashion.

3. Stand in front of and facing the pec deck machine. Grasp the movement arms at shoulder level and do the crushing motion. Either one of these two ways of using the pec deck machine (seated or standing) will guarantee extra inner pec development. However, if it's the outer aspect of pec delineation you're seeking, then crush the pads to only 12 to 15 inches of closure.

4. To protect your shoulder ligaments, rotator cuffs and tendons, don't allow your elbows to hyperextend beyond the shoulder joint when you're in the starting position. Also, don't let your shoulder roll forward during the crushing phase of the movement.

5. Sit backwards in the pec deck machine with the front of your upper torso firmly pressed against the seat back. Hold your upper arms at shoulder level, pressing

Stick with lighter weights on the straight-arm dumbbell pullover – the main focus should be on achieving a deep stretch in your ribcage.

your elbows securely against the movement arm pads. Pull your arms backward as if you were pulling drapes apart. This reverse pec deck flye motion is a unique way to isolate and develop your rear deltoids.

STRAIGHT-ARM BARBELL PULLOVER

For complete chest development, always include some variation of the pullover to work your ribcage. In this case, the poundage you use isn't as important as really working for a deep stretch within your ribcage. The use of heavy poundage in the straight-arm barbell pullover tends to contract the lats. In turn, this con-

tracts against the rib cage. Likewise, your abs will contract against your ribcage if your feet remain on the floor. To counteract this, simply follow the foot isolation advice given for the flat dumbbell flyes. Another thing you can do to isolate the various muscles that might interfere with ribcage expansion is to relax your triceps muscles as much as possible when you begin to lower the bar over your head. The most advanced bodybuilder shouldn't have to use more than 50 pounds in this exercise. Beginners and intermediates should use much less. Remember, deep breathing and maximum ribcage expansion are the important considerations, not poundage lifted.

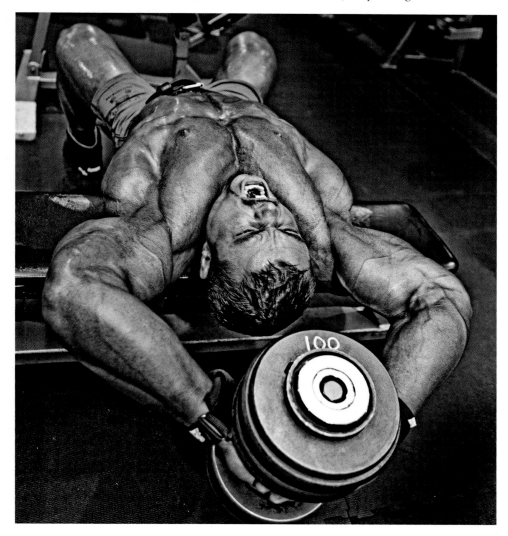

Photo by Paul Buceta
Model Dan Hill

RIBCAGE

Many of today's bodybuilders have some very glaring ribcage limitations. When we first started bodybuilding, Donne Hale, Chuck Sipes, John C. Grimek and the original publisher of *Iron Man* magazine, Peary Rader, used to say that to develop a complete fully-rounded chest, the ribcage bones must be stretched, pulled and expanded both by high-rep breathing barbell back squats and breathing pullovers. Bodybuilders from the '50s and '60s were obsessed with barbell back squats and barbell pullovers as a means to deepen and lift their ribcages,

which also helped them gain muscle mass. Of course, that's not to mention the role squats and pullovers played on internal hormonal factors like GH and testosterone release bathing the muscle fibers.

The bench press is often overlooked as a ribcage expander. Bodybuilders of the '50s and '60s were particularly bench press happy and they developed their ribcages because of a certain compensation and leverage factor. The heavy-duty bench-pressing bodybuilders always arched their spine during the lift, forcing their ribcage upward and thereby stretch-

During the '50s and '60s, bodybuilders spent a great deal of time stretching, deepening and lifting their ribcages as part of chest development.

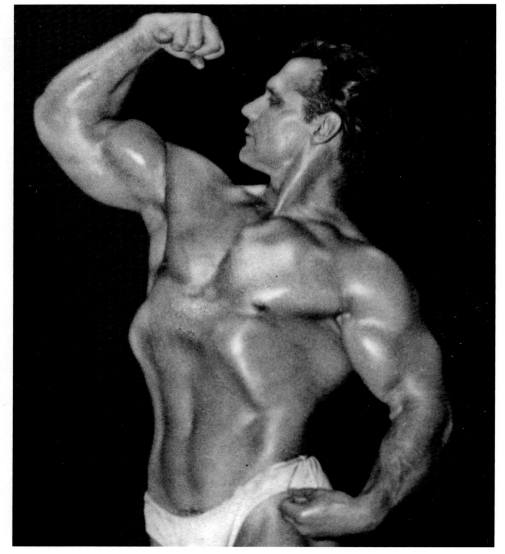

Model John Grimek

Chuck Sipes was one of the old-timers who favored breathing pullovers to expand and deepen his ribcage.

ing and lifting it to meet the bar. The visceral organs also vasodialated with an expanding force, pressuring the ribcage from within and thereby reshaping it. Of course with the advent of bench shirts, that type of ribcage involvement is non-existent. The use of steroids can also interfere with your ribcage lift because they can cause the ab walls to expand.

John C. Grimek believed you should put your feet up on the bench, causing the pelvic attachments of the rectus abdominis to release your ribcage and allow it to be lifted more easily when stretched in the pullover part of a compound torso stressor such as barbell pause squats and light deep breathing barbell pullovers. Dense abs can interfere with ribcage expansion and can camouflage the depth of your ribcage by adding girth to the waistline curve.

We're going to suggest an exercise that you might consider old, but if you're serious in your desire to increase the depth and breadth of your ribcage you should not ignore it. Probably the most effective chest stretching movement for ribcage expansion is the Rader chest pull. Created decades ago by the late Peary Rader, this exercise has generated tremendous results even when other methods failed. It's slightly difficult to properly describe, but once you learn it, it's easy to do and can be performed anywhere and at any time.

RADER CHEST PULL

Take a standing position in front of a pole, the edge of an open door or any other secure vertical object. Reach up about six inches above the top of your head and grasp the object. Your hands should be separated by about three inches or less and your arms should be straight (although some bodybuilders find that a stronger pull can be realized by bending their arms slightly). Now, pull down and inward (almost isometrically) with your hands while at the same time inhaling to your maximum capacity. Additionally, give a little jerk or yank while pulling, as this will increase the pull you feel in your chest.

Be sure to breathe into your upper chest cavity, never into your lower chest. Elevate your chest high and keep your head high and

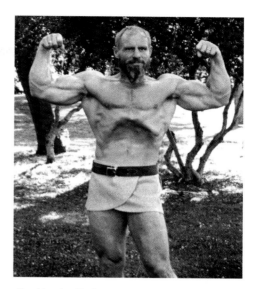

tilted back a little. Tense your front neck muscles – this helps to elevate your chest. You'll notice that your chest muscles are tensed and pulling hard. Your chest muscles (pectorals) do the lifting and pulling of your ribcage, thereby resulting in expansion. If you don't initially feel a little pain near your breast bone, you're not doing the movement correctly. You may be tensing your abs, which pulls the chest down and flattens it, thus preventing an effective pull from your chest muscles. You must keep your abs relaxed. When you can feel the pain around the breast bone, you'll know you're doing it correctly.

You will soon become very efficient at doing the exercise and getting the right effect. Your chest will feel high, arched and stretched after a session. Throughout the exercise, always remember to concentrate on spreading your ribcage as much as possible in all directions.

You should strive to do about 15 to 20 Rader chest pull reps immediately following each of the two sets of 20 to 30 barbell back squat reps. Remember, don't squat on empty lungs and don't crowd your squat poundage. Also, the weight isn't all that important. What's important is the way you breathe. Follow this plan of pairing breathing barbell squats with the Rader chest pull and in a very little time you'll achieve ribcage development that will surpass your wildest dreams.

DELTS

HOMEOSTATIC STANCE OVERHEAD BARBELL PRESS

This method was invented by a chiropractor named Dr. Sipple as a way to almost instantly increase your strength. Simply put, you take your regular stance in the overhead barbell press but with one slight adjustment: Position one foot (usually your shortest leg) approximately three inches ahead of the other, and with your feet adducted or slightly turned in. When you alter your stance in this way, the working muscles seem to harmonize with one another. There's also no knee pain or pre-existing stress on your lower back. If you elect to give the homeostatic stance a try, back off your normal exercise poundages for at least a month so that you can get accustomed to this new position. After a month of adapting, you can resume using your old poundages.

SPECIAL BARBELL PUSH-PRESS TECHNIQUE

Assuming you're doing a strict overhead barbell press with no serial distortion such as a knee thrust to get the weight moving, then we would suggest you do the old reliable barbell push-press (also called the heave or power press) as a basic assistance movement to derail the sticking point in the strict overhead press. There's a subtle difference in the performance of the push-press as compared to the more conventional pressing movement. To initiate movement in the push-press, bend your knees about six inches and then, with a dynamic thrust, extend your legs while simultaneously pushing or heaving the bar straight up to just short of lockout position overhead.

One special push-press technique that some advanced bodybuilders use to conquer an ascending sticking point is performed with a weight that's between five and twenty percent in excess of their best strict 1RM. They take this weight off an adjustable squat rack or power rack adjusted to standing chest height, and from their shoulders they push-press the weight up to just short of lockout. Then, they slowly lower the bar down to the sticking point and do an isometric hold for a six-second count. They return the bar to the squat rack and take a six-second rest before performing another. They perform six reps in this fashion. Try this technique one training day a week.

75-DEGREE INCLINE SEATED FRONT OR BEHIND-THE-NECK OVERHEAD BARBELL PRESS

In both of these exercises, use an adjustable bench and incline the seatback to 75 degrees. Using a 75-degree incline as opposed to a 90-degree incline will reduce AC joint pressure and potential for injury. You could also apply this change to the use of dumbbells. You can also help prevent injury by lowering the bar just to the tops of your ears and no lower when doing the behind-the-neck barbell press.

Use a bench height that will permit your legs to bend at a 90-degree angle. This will help you prevent cramping in your hip region, which occurs when your legs are at lesser angles than advised.

RUSSIAN SEATED ALTERNATING DUMBBELL OVERHEAD PRESS

Sit on the floor with your legs outstretched and slightly spread apart. Brace your lower back securely against the end of a stationary flat exercise bench. Bring dumbbells to the start position of the overhead press. Rotate and pull your shoulders back as if you were stand-

Slightly adjusting the incline on the seated front overhead barbell press from 90 to 75 degrees will reduce joint pressure and decrease the risk of shoulder injury.

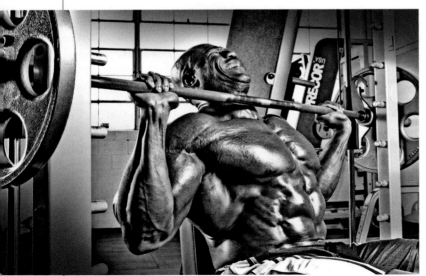

Photo by Paul Buceta
Model Joel Stubbs

ing at attention. This subtle move helps eliminate the shoulder pain often associated with this exercise. Also, contract your thigh and ab muscles. Take a couple of deep breaths and be sure to hold the last one. You're now ready to begin a six-step process.

1. Press the left dumbbell to an arm-extended overhead position. At two-thirds of the way to lockout, forcefully expel the air from your lungs.
2. Inhale and press the right dumbbell to an extended overhead position, expelling the air from your lungs.
3. Bring the left dumbbell down to the start position.
4. Inhale and, without pausing, press the left dumbbell to overhead arms length while breathing out.
5. Lower the right dumbbell to the start position.
6. Inhale and, without pausing, press the right dumbbell to overhead arm's length.

The Russian alternating dumbbell overhead press maintains maximum tension on the deltoid complex because one arm is always in an overhead top contracted static rest position while the other one lowers and presses up again. In the more common version of the exercise, when one dumbbell is being pressed overhead, the other dumbbell is at the shoulder in a rest position. As a result, there isn't as much tension on your deltoids. To make the Russian version even more effective for stimulating your middle delts, keep your palms facing forward and your elbows out to your sides. Most importantly, remember that the little finger side of the dumbbell should be higher than the thumb side of the dumbbell. This requires taking an off-center grip on the dumbbell handle, with your little finger snug against the inside plate. The off-center grip works very effectively on flat dumbbell bench presses, keeping maximum tension on your pecs as opposed to your triceps. Alternating reps as described (where one arm is always in the top contracted rest position) can also be used in dumbbell bench presses or flyes (incline, flat or decline position) for your chest, lateral raises for your delts and two-arm alternate dumbbell rows for your lats.

Once you get accustomed to the lower back/bench supported version of the Russian alternate dumbbell press, increase the difficulty of the exercise by eliminating the bench support altogether. Doing this will put demands on the body core and further round out your deltoid development.

AMERICAN SEATED BEHIND-THE-NECK BARBELL PRESS
The American seated behind-the-neck barbell press is an excellent alternative to the Russian seated alternating dumbbell press. Your posture should be the same as it is for the Russian exercise (sit on the floor, legs stretched and slightly spread apart and back supported), except instead of using dumbbells, you'll use a barbell. A training partner will have to correctly position a barbell in your hands. Your elbows should be directly under your hands (knuckles facing the ceiling) and pointing out to your sides and down. Take a deep breath and press the barbell overhead. At two-thirds of the way to lockout, forcefully expel the air from your lungs.

At the arms-overhead position, hold the barbell for a slow count of six. Take a deep breath and hold it. Then lower the bar back to the base of your neck while exhaling. Breathe in again. This is called double oxygen saturation. The bar barely touches the base of your neck before the next rep begins.

If you want, you can occasionally press the barbell only four to six inches above your head rather than going to complete lockout. Also, if you feel your shoulders are being compromised in any way, lower the barbell to the bottom of your ears rather than the base of your neck. As an added measure of security, you might want to forgo the seated behind-the-neck barbell press in favor of the more shoulder-friendly front barbell overhead press.

SEATED OVERHEAD PRESS MACHINE
Instead of facing out with overhead handles to the front of your torso, sit facing into the unit with the overhead handles behind your upper torso.

WIDE-GRIP BENT-OVER ROW

There are many good posterior deltoid exercises, but bodybuilding champions have found the wide-grip bent-over row works this area most effectively. This exercise has always been thought of as a lat developer. However, as long as it's done slowly, smoothly and in strict style it works the rear deltoid very well. Instead of pulling the barbell into your stomach region, try pulling it to your throat with your elbows out to your sides.

BARBELL UPRIGHT ROW/SHRUG

Begin with your feet shoulder-width apart and flat on the floor. Bend your knees slightly and keep your bodyweight over your heels. Your upper torso should be 10 to 20 degrees forward from vertical at your hips. Put your head in a neutral position with your eyes looking straight ahead. Use an overhand (knuckles forward) shoulder-width grip on the bar. Take a deep breath and contract your abs. From a dead hang (arms and wrists straight) start po-

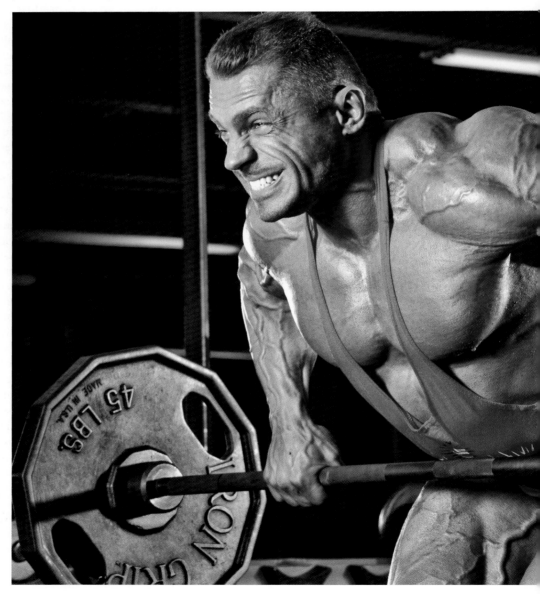

Photo by Paul Buceta
Model Evgeny Mishin

Taking a wide grip on the bent-over row will work your rear delts to the max.

sition, and with the bar close to your body throughout, begin the barbell upright row or pull by leading with your elbows, which travel upward, out to your sides and slightly back. Continue pulling the bar to your lower pec line. Shrug your traps and hold the contracted position for one or two seconds. Exhale and smoothly lower the bar to the start position. This completes one rep.

Some information suggests that exercises such as the overhead barbell press, behind-the-

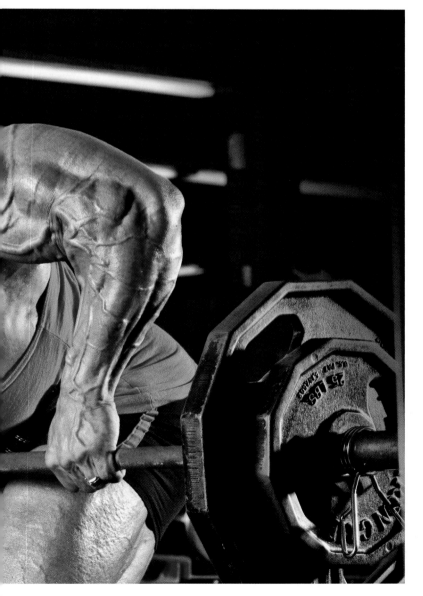

neck barbell press and the upright row aren't biomechanically pure and clinically safe exercises. These exercises are thought to be a common source of shoulder injuries, as well as acutely inflamed and impinged (trapped) tendons and bursa. Injuries occur because these exercises make the shoulder complex move into a position of external rotation, which goes against the way the shoulder actually functions. However many bodybuilders do the exercises mentioned with no apparent shoulder issues.

For a change of pace, instead of doing barbell upright rows, do low-pulley cable rows. Use a dual-grip rope with rubber ends.

REBOUND BARBELL UPRIGHT ROW

When you can't do any more reps in the upright barbell row, then it's time to use the shock/rebound technique (SRT) as a means of getting a few extra reps. For the sake of variety, instead of keeping the bar close to your body during the pull upward, pull it away from your body by about 10 inches.

First, get about six to eight pre-cut 1" by 12" by 24" high-density sponge rubber pads. Place a stack of three or four on the floor just outside the edge of each foot. To get the maximum rebound effect, be sure the rubber pads are positioned so the bottom edge of the barbell plates hit directly in the middle of them.

Do the barbell upright row as previously described but with one difference: As lactic acid paralysis sets in during the final reps, you'll desperately feel like you can't do another rep in the upright row from the dead hang start position. To combat this problem, quickly lower the barbell toward the floor, bouncing it very quickly off the stacks of high-density sponge rubber pads. The rebounding of the barbell plates off the pads allows your delt muscles to momentarily reset themselves for another effort on the upward row and thereby accelerate past the dead-hang position.

Continue pulling, leading with your elbows, until the bar again reaches the lower pec line. Pause for a second and then lower the barbell, initiating the shock/rebound technique (SRT) for another extra rep. You could also occasionally try kneeling rebound upright rows.

PRONE INCLINE DUMBBELL ROW

This movement is an excellent direct stimulant for the hard-to-hit posterior (rear) head of your deltoid. Lie face down on an adjustable incline bench set at a 60-degree angle. Keep your chin on the bench throughout the movement. Hold a pair of dumbbells in your hands at arms' length (hanging beneath the bench) with the two inside bells touching. Pull the dumbbells up as high as you can go. Return the dumbbells to the dead-hang position and then begin the next rep.

The facedown dumbbell row allows you to work your rear delt and lower trapezius from a new angle with heavier poundages.

Two-Step Delt Developer x 10

Are you having a problem gaining decent poundage on the standing dumbbell lateral raise? If so, then quit doing them and try this:

STEP #1

While standing with your arms hanging fully extended, have a training partner place an adjustable strap around your body just below the lower pec line. The strap should be cinched tight so it won't fall down, but not so tight that it restricts movement. Now in an isometric manner, contract your delts while trying desperately to force your arms out laterally against the belt. Hold the isometric contraction for six seconds and then relax. Repeat this twice more. Perform the isometric delt movement for three sets of six seconds and for a total of 10 training sessions. You may be surprised to find that whatever poundage you were previously using on the dumbbell lateral raises (prior to the isometric delt movement sessions) will now seem absurdly light.

STEP #2

Upon completion of the 10th and final training session, go back to doing the dumbbell lateral raise and its variations.

DUMBBELL LATERAL RAISE

To ensure that you're working the lateral or side deltoid, point the front of the bells slightly downward as you reach the crucifix position of the movement. This will isolate the lateral delt without letting the anterior or front delt kick in. It's important that you do this because dumbbell lateral raises are instrumental in giving the illusion of greater shoulder width. Since they're a leverage-type exercise, they don't allow you to handle much weight (as opposed to shoulder pressing movements). However, they've proven to be the best type of exercise for isolation of the lateral deltoid. On all lateral movements, your arms should be unlocked to relieve excess pressure and strain on the elbow insertions.

ONE-DUMBBELL LEAN-AWAY LATERAL RAISE

Stand with your feet together and the left side of your body a couple of feet away from a secured vertical upright support such as a doorframe or power rack. Hold a dumbbell in your right hand, letting your arm hang down fully at your side. With your left hand, grasp the vertical upright support at about shoulder height and lean out sideways to arm's length. The angle of your body in relation to the upright support should be approximately 30 to 35 degrees.

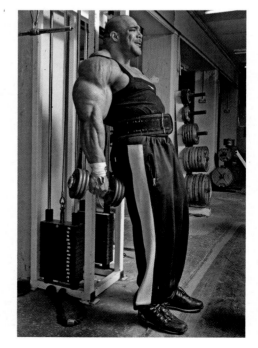

Photos by Kevin Horton
Model Zack Khan

PRO TIP #1

Do half of the reps with your palm down and then rotate your wrist to a palm forward/thumb up position. This subtle change will cause your shoulder girdle to tilt back and shift the tension from your lateral to your frontal delt complex.

PRO TIP #2

When doing the one-dumbbell lean-away lateral raise, imagine that you're desperately trying to reach out and touch the far wall in the gym. This little imaginary trick will do wonders for increasing muscle tension in your deltoid.

PRO TIP #3

For a change of pace, you could occasionally do the low-pulley cable lean-away lateral raise on a cable crossover machine. Or, you could do a one-dumbbell lateral raise while lying sideways on an incline bench or angled sit-up board.

When doing lateral raises, make sure your arms remain unlocked so you don't put any extra pressure or strain on your elbow insertions.

5 X 10 X 5 STANDING DUMBBELL LATERAL RAISE

Beginning with the dumbbells held behind your back (with dumbbells parallel and touching each other at both ends), do five sets of 20 reps. In each set you should do five full-range reps, 10 partial reps (constant tension with six- to eight-inch movements) and finish off with five full-range reps.

CHARLES GLASS' THREE PART FRONT/INWARD/ LATERAL DUMBBELL RAISE

Charles Glass, IFBB pro and superstar trainer, created and popularized this form of dumbbell raise. It combines two different movements in one fluid repetition. Sit upright on an exercise bench with your arms hanging, holding a dumbbell in each hand with a suitcase or neutral-hand grip.

Part 1: Simultaneously raise your arms upward in a semi-circular motion to shoulder level. Rotate your arms to a pronated hand position (knuckles up/palms down). Pause for two seconds.

Part 2: Move the dumbbells inward to the midline of your chest. The inner face of the dumbbell plates should touch. Pause for a sec-

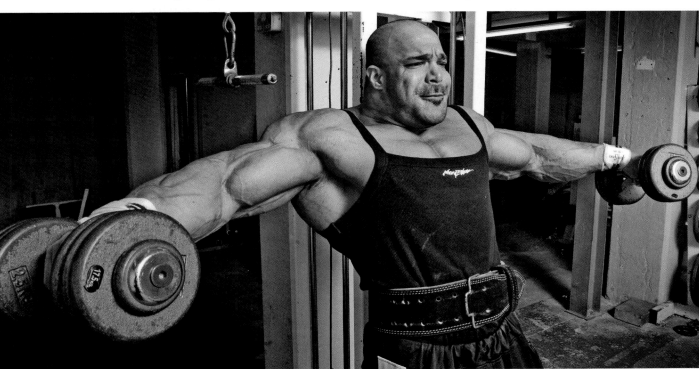

ond while contracting maximally your inner pecs. **Part 3:** Move the dumbbells outward to your sides at arms' length and lower (four-second negative) to the near starting position.

This exercise is terrific for the development of the anterior/lateral delt and inner pec tie-in. Do three sets of ten, eight and six reps.

PRO TIP #1

Lift your ribcage high and keep your shoulders down and back.

PRO TIP #2

Maintain a bend in your elbows to reduce joint stress and better target the lateral delts.

PRO TIP #3

Lower the dumbbells just short of arms' length. Doing this will keep adequate tension on your deltoid.

SUPINE BARBELL FRONT RAISE

This exercise is similar to a standing barbell front raise except you're lying on a bench. Hold a barbell over your chest as you would in a flat barbell bench press, using your normal bench press grip. Lower the barbell to your upper thighs (arms always remain straight) until it just barely touches. Lift the barbell back to the overhead position and repeat for the number of reps you plan to do. This movement is terrific for generating deltoid power in the various bench press exercises. You can also do this on an incline bench.

BARBELL PLATE FRONT RAISE

Pick up a barbell plate (whichever size plate suits your strength level) with one hand on each side. Stand in an upright position with your back and head firmly against an upright post or wall. Hold the plate at arms' length so its rounded edge is in contact with the front of your thighs. Take a deep breath and, with your arms straight, lift the plate forward and up (in a semi-circle) in a strict slow deliberate manner to arms' length over your head. Pause momentarily, exhale and then lower the plate in the reverse manner to the front of your thighs. Inhale and begin the next rep.

SUPERMAN DUMBBELL FRONT RAISE

This exercise can be divided into two parts: **Part 1:** Position a pair of dumbbells approximately two feet in front of the end of a flat exercise bench. Lie face down on the bench facing the dumbbells. Reach down and grasp the dumbbells with a pronated (palms-down) grip. With the dumbbells still on the floor, push your arms forward until they're completely outstretched in front of you. Take a deep breath and lift the dumbbells simultaneously until your arms are parallel to the floor. (This exercise looks like a Superman flying formation.) Forcefully contract and squeeze your delts for around two seconds, then breathe out and lower the dumbbells to the floor. Repeat the sequence for the desired number of reps. **Part 2:** Make them work harder for you: On the final rep of a set, instead of lowering the dumbbells back to the floor, sweep your outstretched arms out to your sides (laterally) and all the way back until the dumbbells are even with your torso. Lower the dumbbells to the floor and back up.

SUPERMAN DUMBBELL PARTIAL FRONT RAISE

Forgo the use of the flat exercise bench and do these raises while lying on the floor, arching your back simultaneously as your extended arms rise off the floor. Pause for a couple of seconds at peak contraction and lower the dumbbells to the floor. Depending on your flexibility, the range of motion will be approximately half of that of the previous exercise.

Here's an idea: Do Superman dumbbell front raises to positive failure while lying prone on the bench. Then finish off a set on the floor. Immediately continue doing some training-past-the-burn, short-range reps to positive failure.

LATERAL RAISE MACHINE

Stand in front of a lateral raise machine. Place the back of your forearms – from your elbow joints to your knuckles – firmly against the arm pads. Incline your upper body about 10 degrees forward from vertical and begin doing the reps, leading with your elbows and raising both arms until they're parallel to the

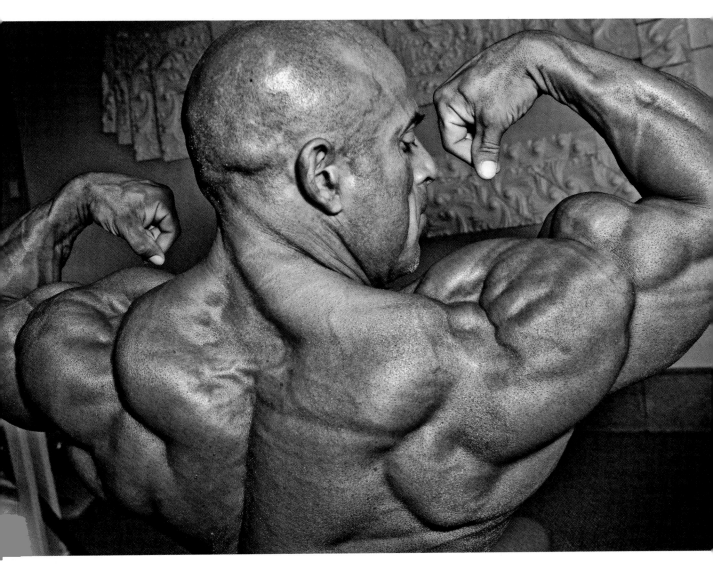

A key part of delt training is working all three heads – front, middle and rear – to ensure equal development and proportion.

floor. If you aren't sure if you're leading with your elbows, simply place an index card securely between the pads and your elbows. If your elbows are not absolutely tight against the support pads, the index cards will fall to the floor and you will not be leading with your elbows.

The standing version of this exercise works the posterior and lateral heads of your deltoids in a more vigorous manner than the more common seated version. The best part about using these machines is that the movement can be done one arm at a time in alternating fashion, resulting in maximum tension from all your muscles.

HIGH-PULLEY CABLE ROWS TO FOREHEAD

This little gem of an exercise will add some serious development to your rear deltoids. Attach a 20-inch exercise bar to the high pulley. Take an overhand grip on each end of the bar. Step back far enough so the cable is taut. With your arms straight and in alignment with your shoulder joints, rhythmically pull the bar until it almost touches your forehead (the arm orientation should mimic the L-lateral raise) and return to the start position. Make sure your arms don't drop below parallel to the floor.

CHAPTER 45

TRICEPS, BICEPS, FOREARMS, ABS & NECK

Recommendations, approaches and exercises to tackle your arms, midsection and neck.

TRICEPS

Triceps are an impressive muscle group, making up two-thirds of your upper arm mass. Biceps may get the attention, but real bodybuilders know triceps are where big arms come from. When training your triceps you need consistency and total concentration. To get massive, you must concentrate on the muscle group you're working. You must work all the muscle fibers in your triceps. Next time you enter a gym, take a moment to notice how many people are goofing off or talking. When you reach the gym it should feel like you're entering another world where nothing exists but muscle building.

Triceps exercises can be divided into three types. In each session, you should use at least one exercise from each of the following groups:

1. Palms facing away from your body – Triceps pressdowns on the lat pulldown bar or the standing barbell French press.
2. Palms facing your body – Reverse-grip cable extensions and kickbacks.
3. Palms parallel to your body (suitcase grip) – Parallel bar dips and triceps pulldowns with rope are ideal exercises.

You have countless grip variations to choose from, and for even more options you can work on a flat, incline, decline or standing bench. Still, the key is the use of exercises from each one of the groups. This will ensure you're working all the muscle fibers in your triceps and the end result will be bigger arms.

LYING BARBELL EXTENSION (SKULLCRUSHER)

When performing this exercise, also known as the skullcrusher, use an EZ-curl bar rather than a straight bar. The EZ-curl bar will help to eliminate elbow and triceps injuries because of its more favorable mechanical leverages.

Lying supine on an exercise bench, take a grip on the bar with your hands spaced three to five inches apart. Keep your fists in line with your wrists. Fully extend your arms above your chest and then move them to

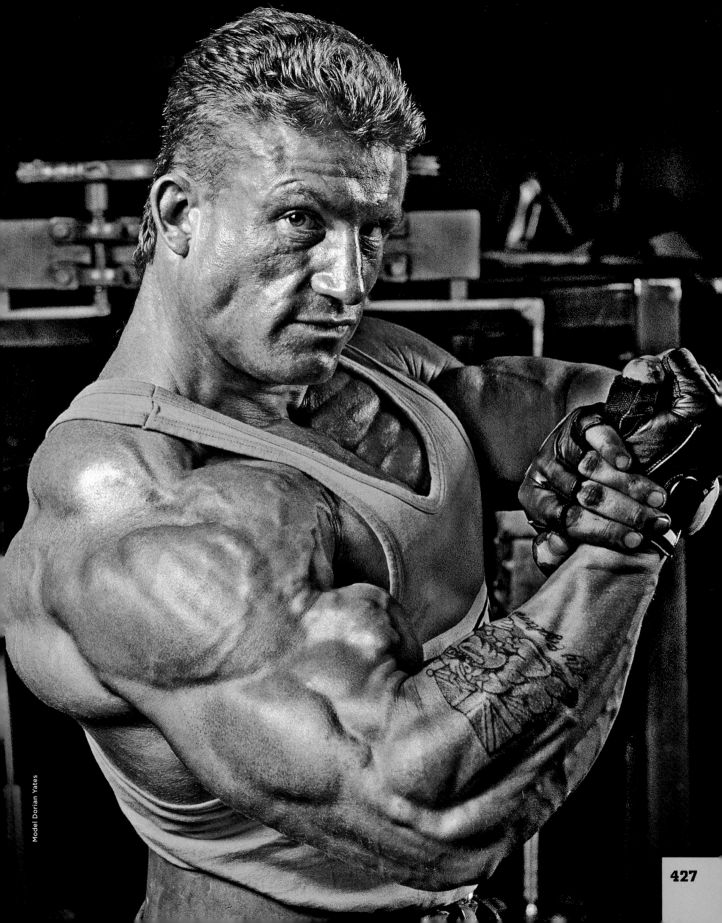

Model Dorian Yates

427

a 45-degree angle (in relation to your head). The reason for the 45-degree angle is to reduce the risk of injury and pain in your elbow. You'll feel a slight stretch in your triceps. Keep your elbows pointed toward the ceiling and your upper arms still. Take a deep breath and slowly lower the barbell until it touches the bench surface behind your head (or at the very least your arms should be at a 90-degree angle at the elbow joint). Don't bounce the barbell at this low position. Contract your triceps, fully extending your elbows to lockout and contraction. The barbell should be at a slight angle above and beyond your head. Exhale quickly and then take another deep breath before performing another rep. Finish your set by doing close-grip EZ-curl bar bench presses – do half the reps you did for skullcrushers. For example, if you did eight skullcrushers then do four close-grip bench presses to finish off the set.

On the barbell close-grip bench press, make sure to keep your elbows tucked into your sides while lowering the bar to your upper chest and then back up. While a hand spacing of three to five inches seems to work well when using the EZ-curl bar for close-grip bench presses, it doesn't work quite as well when using a straight exercise bar. Use a slightly less than shoulder-width hand spacing when performing your reps with a straight bar.

A regular exercise bench is fine as long as you have some way to rack the weight upon the completion of a set. If you don't, we suggest you use a bench that's roughly six inches off the floor. This low bench will allow you to lift the barbell off the floor without injuring yourself.

With this and all other triceps exercises, maintain a locked-wrist position. Don't allow your wrists to bend back into extension. If you make this mistake, you're sure to experience triceps tendonitis (inflammation and soreness), which will most certainly hamper your training efforts.

TWO-PART CABLE PULLEY EXTENSION

Do triceps pressdowns while facing the cable unit. When you reach positive failure – and without letting go of the bar or rope – turn your

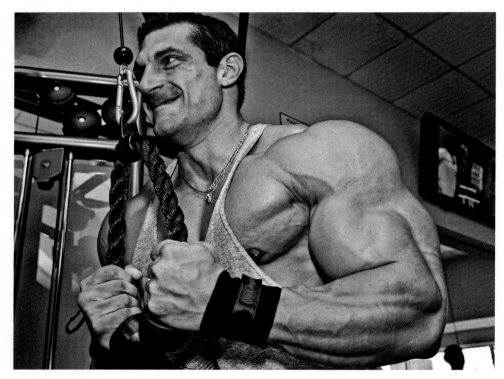

You can use various cable attachments as a way to target the three triceps heads in slightly different ways.

Photos by Rich Baker
Model Brian Yersky

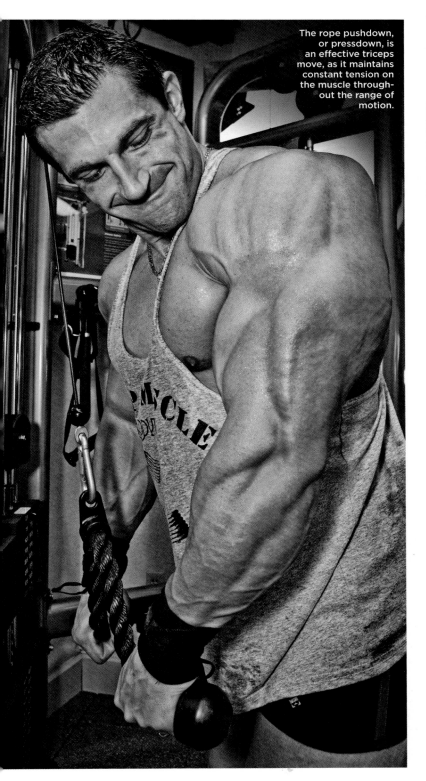

The rope pushdown, or pressdown, is an effective triceps move, as it maintains constant tension on the muscle throughout the range of motion.

back to the pulley unit. Take a soft-knee split stance and bend your upper torso forward from 45 to 90 degrees. Continue doing cable pulley extensions using a measured movement strategy to work all three heads of your triceps.

Long head: The first 30 to 45 degrees of a rep.

Lateral head: The first 60 degrees of a rep.

Medial head: The final 30 degrees of a rep.

Note: If you use the rope, begin the movement in the stretch position with your wrists rotated so the back of your hands face forward. As you extend your arms, rotate your wrists so your palms face forward at lockout.

CLOSE-GRIP BEHIND-THE-NECK BARBELL PRESS

This exercise will build your triceps while saving your elbow joints from unnecessary stress. It places a great deal of tension on the largest head of your triceps muscle – the medial or outer head. Use a false (thumbless) grip about four to six inches apart on a barbell. Keep your elbows wide throughout the exercise. Don't forget that this exercise can cause elbow injuries. Remember to press the weight upwards, lock out hard and tense your triceps forcibly at the top of each repetition. Lower the bar to behind your head.

PUSHDOWN WITH ROPE

Using the rope attachment, extend your arms from 30 degrees below parallel (to the floor) to lockout, ensuring that your medial triceps head will receive maximum stimulation. Working the triceps pushdown with the rope in a range from 30 degrees above parallel to 30 degrees below works the lateral head of your triceps. You can also do this movement using an underhand curl grip.

Try the following training procedure next time you work your triceps: Perform a set of 12 reps of strict triceps pressdowns using a medium amount of poundage. Next, add more poundage and perform three or four sets using just the lower (lockout) half of the movement. Use a movement of about six inches with heavy poundage. After the half-pressdowns, decrease the poundage and perform one set of 12 reps.

BICEPS
STRICT STANDING BARBELL CURL

This exercise is a favorite among many of today's top physique champions because it develops spellbinding biceps size and muscularity. Quite possibly the best test of true biceps strength or power is the standing barbell curl.

Potential in the strict standing barbell curl will vary from an average of 72 percent of your best strict press overhead to as much as 85 percent. Proper performance of this exercise and the two other biceps blasters (seated incline bench dumbbell curls and the standing one arm dumbbell concentration curl) will unlock yet another secret to rapid biceps growth.

It's just too simple to advise a bodybuilder to do a barbell curl in the prototypical way. You can't expect to work for the feel of the muscle and discover the muscular pathways when all you have is incomplete and superfluous stock technique instructions. Little things like a twist of your wrist, pulling down your shoulder, lifting the weight either a little forward or backward or holding the barbell mo-

Among bodybuilders, the standing barbell curl is a bread-and-butter move for biceps.

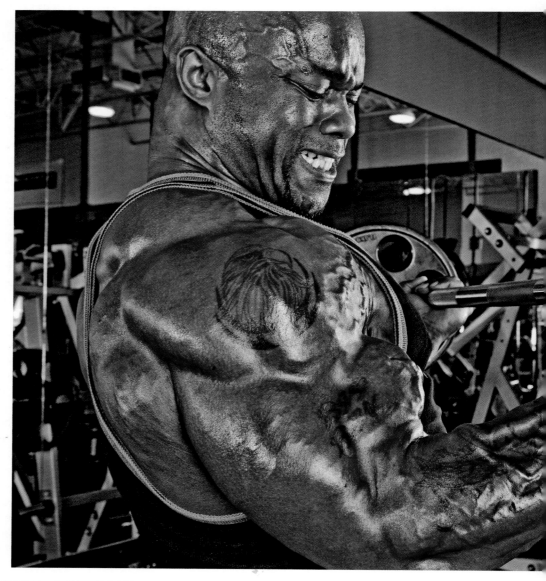

mentarily at the peak contraction of the movement can make all the difference between building mediocre biceps and gigantic ones.

We cannot emphasize enough how important it is to do this exercise with strict form. The regular standing barbell curl is probably the second most abused exercise next to the bench press. Many bodybuilders use exaggerated body movements, vigorously accelerating or moving their upper torso (shoulders and back) and thrusting their hips forward in an abrupt, jerking action while swinging (not

curling) the weight up in an attempt to gain some mechanical advantage in order to bypass the sticking point or resting inertia.

This snappy way of curling decreases maximum tension in your muscle because the weight isn't being lifted against gravity, but rather by momentum. When the movement is performed in the manner described, it's called cheat curls and it shouldn't be confused with the advanced training principle known as controlled cheating.

Begin the starting point of the strict standing barbell curl by loading up a standard barbell with the exact assortment of weights you'll be using, be it for the specific warm-up or actual growth zone sets. Many bodybuilders prefer to use an EZ-curl bar. This can lessen pain and make the exercise easier to perform if you have joint issues, but using this bar also takes some of the biceps action away because of the change in supination. Use a straight bar if biceps growth is your primary consideration.

While standing in front of the barbell with a shoulder-width or slightly wider foot placement, bend your knees very slightly while bending forward at the hip joint and grasp the barbell with a supinated (palms facing away from your body) shoulder-width grip. Now come up to an erect vertical and stabilized position. Keep your heels in contact with the floor and your knees very slightly unlocked throughout each set. Fully extend your arms and wrists, with the bar touching or resting against your upper thighs. Look straight ahead with your chin parallel to the floor.

Using shoulder-width hand spacing maximizes the resistance of gravity by putting your shoulders, arms and hands in a straight line of pull. When you keep your elbows in close and tight to your body, the short head of your biceps is maximally contracted, and when you develop this muscle to its fullest potential you can improve your biceps peak. Finally, muscles are uniquely structured with nerves throughout, so when the message is sent from your brain to your muscle, the whole muscle contracts. The nerves that control your biceps activate both long and short heads. Using too wide a hand spacing can stress elbow joints.

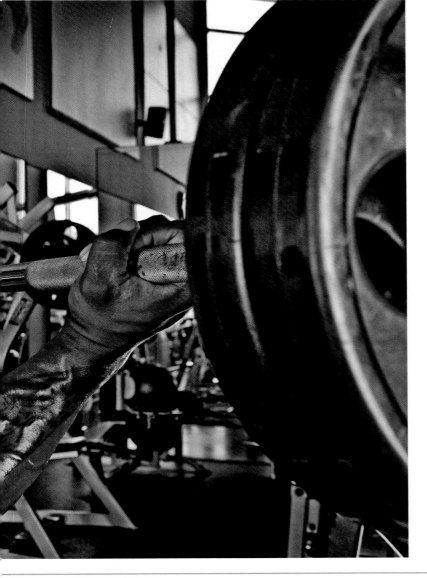

Photo by Greg James
Model Ben White

Begin the curling action by taking a deep breath, expelling the air slowly as the barbell begins to pass the horizontal during the positive contraction phase of the movement. Lift and thrust your chest forward during this movement. If you feel you must to take the tension off your forearms, then open your hands slightly. Tighten your grip on the bar, as if you were actually trying to crush it (this is a little-known secret for squeezing out a couple of extra reps at the end of a set). Extend your wrists upward, so your hands (palms up) precede your wrists. Now strongly flex at your elbow joint while tensing your biceps muscles, moving the barbell in a semi-circular motion forward and upward toward your chin rather than to the top of your collarbone or neck. This will help to keep intra-muscular tension on your biceps and not allow gravity to dictate the movement (where it could fall into your collarbone or neck region and shut off the continuous tension effect). Forcefully contract and squeeze your biceps (biceps and forearms touching) at the completion of the upward curling movement and hold for a count of one.

You have a couple of alternatives to choose from with regards to your elbow positioning and its corresponding movement. You can keep your upper arm vertical and aligned with your body or angled slightly back so they remain behind the bar throughout the entire movement. When your elbows are as vertical and motionless as possible throughout the movement, your deltoids tend to stay out of the action, which allows for more isolation on the belly of your biceps. You can substantially add to the isolation by dropping your shoulders and pulling them back.

On the other hand, you can raise your elbows to a position parallel to the floor near the completion of the upward curling movement to produce the greatest tension by increasing the resistance. An additional advantage to pushing your elbows up is that it helps in creating peak and separation between your biceps and deltoids, especially when you squeeze and contract your biceps for three to four seconds at the top of the movement.

Now that you've curled the barbell in an arc to your chin, lower it to arms' length in a semi-circle, pushing out and downward. Once the rep is over, your elbows should be straight and locked with zero degrees of flexion. At this point you are able to take maximum advantage of contraction and circulation of your biceps by pre-stretching. This kicks in a larger number of muscle fibers than normal, which can't help but enhance biceps growth stimulation. The full-range-of-motion stimulus offers a number of immediate benefits, includ-

Always keep the motion controlled on both the positive and negative phase of each rep.

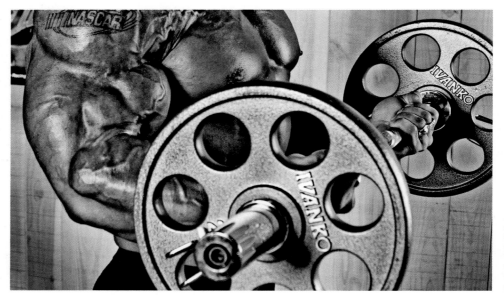

Photo by Irvin Gelb
Model Lee Preist

ing maximum muscle contraction, optimal rate of blood flow for a super pump and the ability of increased flexibility while adding additional muscle size. Be sure to stretch for half a second between each rep.

To add an element of ultra strictness to the standing barbell curl exercise, lean your body and head back against a wall or upright post and position your legs at an outward angle from your hips to the floor. This will keep your upper torso from moving forward or back. Another little technique you'll find beneficial is to curl the barbell upward and then lower it slowly in drag fashion as in the body-drag curl.

PREACHER BENCH BARBELL CURL

These curls are superior for developing the low biceps connection. The angle of the preacher bench should be anywhere between 45 and 90 degrees. Your body position and hand spacing are extremely important factors in your success with these curls. The top of the padded bench should be two to four inches below the lower pec muscle. This position will allow you to develop nice round biceps, as opposed to sinking the top of the preacher bench directly under your armpits near your upper pecs, which will encourage flat biceps. To some degree, the hand and elbow placement and spacing you choose when doing this exercise determines which segment of the muscle you'll be working. Here are three examples:

1. Biceps peak contraction – Use a 12- to 14-inch spacing between your elbows on the bench surface and between your pinkie fingers on the bar. Instead of curling to your collarbone, drop your head down into a chin-in-neck position. Continue curling the bar over your head and ending near the nape of your neck. If you've done this correctly, the belly of your forearms will be folded on top of your biceps. Forcefully squeeze your biceps for two seconds. Mentally squeeze your elbows inward as a means of creating an extra bit of tension or load on your biceps.
2. Inner biceps – Keep your elbows 20 inches apart and your hands three to four inches apart.

3. Outer biceps – Keep your elbows close together and your hands wide apart.

To further up the biceps muscle gain, try sitting down when performing the preacher bench curl. Maintain constant tension on your muscle, especially at the bottom position. If you relax at the bottom of the movement, it is very easy to hyperextend your elbows.

ONE ON ONE WITH WEIS

I have always enjoyed performing the preacher bench barbell curl (Scott curl). Back in the early '70s, I made a rookie bodybuilding mistake where I would anchor the preacher bench so the top of it was as far up under my armpits as possible.

My arms were anchored so deep that my elbows extended off the bottom edge of the preacher bench. At the time, I felt this was the best way to work the biceps through a strict and complete range of movement. After a period of time all I received for my efforts was hyperextended elbows and extremely flat biceps, instead of the round look that I was working so hard for.

I checked with Vince Gironda. He told me the proper way to use the preacher bench is to place it so the top is three inches lower than your low pectoral line. It worked great this way. I developed nice round biceps and eliminated elbow hyperextension because my elbows were in contact with the bench in this new position. My poundage even increased.

SEATED BARBELL CURL

Sit on a flat exercise bench with a barbell resting on top of your thighs, your upper arms and elbows at your side (never move your elbows from this position) and palms up. Now curl the barbell up toward your chest. Obviously, the bar can't be brought to touch your chest if your elbows don't move. As a result, your biceps will experience great cramping at the high contracted position of the curl. Lower the barbell to your thighs (just barely touching).

SEATED NEGATIVE BARBELL CURL

This exercise is an excellent negative-accentuated workout for really trashing your biceps. It also keeps exceptional tension on your biceps, which makes the exercise even more effective. Your biceps will get no rest with this one.

First, load a barbell with just enough poundage that you'll be able to perform five to seven curls. Set the bar on the floor in front of the end of a flat exercise bench and then sit on the bench. Lean forward and grab the bar with a shoulder-width, palms-up, curl grip. Position the bar on your lap while maintaining the curl grip. Take a large breath and hold it. Bend forward at your hip joints, bringing your torso forward and down to where the top of your biceps fold against your forearms and your hands are securely against your upper chest.

In an almost rocking motion, lift your upper torso to a vertical position, keeping your arms locked into place so the bar comes up like it's a part of your torso. This looks like the upward motion of the seated good morning exercise except for the position of the bar.

Exhale and begin doing a five- to eight-second negative rep, fighting gravity as you lower the bar to your lap. Inhale, bend forward and repeat. Continue doing reps until you can't manage to do a rep over five seconds. You'll feel your biceps work on each negative rep and by the time you've finished the final rep you'll have a huge pump in your biceps.

INCLINE BARBELL CURL

Adjust the seatback on a bench to a 45-degree incline. Lie back on the bench with a barbell in your hands positioned on the top of your thighs. Curl the barbell but only three-quarters of the way up and then lower it to the start position. Don't let the bar touch your thighs. Doing this partial curl exercise will have your biceps under maximum tension and it'll feel like they're trying to burst right out of your skin!

LAP BARBELL CURL

Bodybuilders occasionally become disappointed with the size of their biceps. They try many different exercises, but sometimes they just don't see results and feel like giving up. For the first time ever, we're going to reveal an unknown exercise that will cause a rage in your biceps.

This most unusual exercise was taught to us by Donne Hale of Miami, Florida. It's an excellent exercise for keeping maximum tension on your biceps throughout every rep of a set. The exercise is called the lap barbell curl.

Prep: Load a five-inch exercise bar with plenty of five or ten-pound plates on each side. Next, sit on the floor and form a 90-degree angle of your upper chest/lower torso (thighs), positioning your back against a wall with your feet together and your legs completely outstretched. Have a training partner hand the barbell to you. Take a shoulder-width curl grip on the bar. Hold the barbell with the backs of your forearms resting on top of your thighs. If you take a wider grip, the bar will be resting on your thighs. The set is performed in two parts:

Part 1

Using a moderately fast, controlled, non-pausing rep cadence, curl the barbell to the top curl shoulder position, squeeze and cramp your biceps for a second and then immediately reverse the procedure, lowering the barbell to the starting position and touching the top of your thighs. This completes one rep. Don't pause. With no body momentum, go right into the next rep, continuing till you've done about eight to failure.

Part 2

By now your biceps should be screaming for mercy as a result of the blood pump and massive lactic acid build up. You might not think you can do any more reps, but you can by decreasing the range of movement. Instead of starting the curl from the top of your thighs with your legs outstretched, bend your knees slightly, pulling them an inch or two toward your chest, thereby decreasing the distance between your chest and upper thighs. Do a few reps to momentary failure. Pull your knees a couple more inches towards your chest and do some more curls. Continue until the distance between your knees and chest is so short that you're curling the bar only an inch or two.

3 PRO TIPS

1. Lap barbell curls can be performed in a super-slow five seconds up and five seconds down rep cadence..

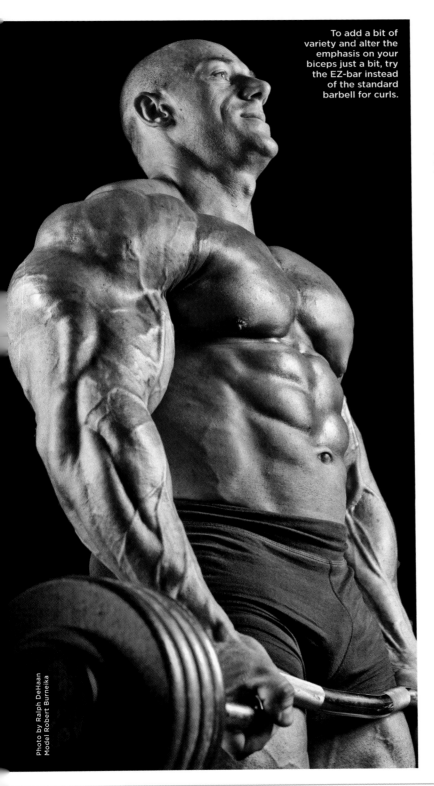

To add a bit of variety and alter the emphasis on your biceps just a bit, try the EZ-bar instead of the standard barbell for curls.

Photo by Ralph DeHaan
Model Robert Burneika

2. For some added tension on your biceps lower the bar to within one-quarter to one-half inch of your thighs. Rest the barbell on top of your thighs only at the beginning of the first rep and at the conclusion of the last rep.
3. You can also do lap barbell curls in reverse curl fashion.

REBOUND STANDING BARBELL CURL

When you can't do any more curls in the regular manner, forcefully lower the barbell to the floor applying concepts of the Shock/Rebound Technique (SRT) mentioned earlier for the rebound barbell upright row.

THE BODY DRAG CURL

This specialized movement helps bring out the cephalic vein, which is the thick, straight (comparably) vein that runs from the frontal deltoid down your biceps to your forearm. A prominent cephalic vein always makes your arm look thicker, more muscular and generally more impressive. Plus, this exercise develops the lateral head or "leaf" of your biceps. To execute a proper body drag curl, bend over and firmly grasp a five-foot barbell with a false (thumbless) grip wider than shoulder width (collar-to-collar in extreme cases).

Hold the bar at arms' length, your fists aligned with your wrists (wrists straight). Hold your arms tight against the sides of your body at all times (no forward and up movement). Your elbows can, however, travel back behind the plane of your torso. Hold your shoulder girdle down and back, your chest arched and your chin parallel to the floor. Keep the bar in contact with your torso, both on the drag/curl upward and the return downward to the start position. Contract your abs and glutes throughout the movement to generate more biceps strength.

Inhale slowly through your nose. Forcefully contract your biceps muscles. Slowly exhale through pursed or puckered lips (as if you are going to whistle). Lower the bar slowly, dragging down your body. Remember to maintain proper form throughout this movement. Being precise will target more muscle fibers.

SQUATTING LOW PULLEY CABLE CURL

Face the low-pulley machine. Attach a 20-inch revolving bar to the end of the cable. Choose a poundage on the weight stack that you'll be able to use for at least four reps. Next, stand three feet away from the machine and position your feet shoulder-width apart. Squat down and grasp the bar with a palms-up false (thumbless) grip, placing your elbows on your knees. Slowly begin doing cable curls in the top 3/5 range of the movement (don't fully extend your arms), tensing your biceps maximally at the top.

RUSSIAN LOW PULLEY CABLE CURL

Instead of facing the machine, turn your back to it. Assume a body position with your feet slightly wider than shoulder-width apart. Bend your legs slightly and move your upper torso forward from a vertical to horizontal position. Keep your lower back flat or slightly arched. Reach down between your legs (kind of like you're hiking a football) and firmly grasp the 20-inch revolving bar, with a palms-up, false grip. Brace your elbows against the inside of your thighs very near your knees. Make sure

the cable is taut (you'll have to adjust your distance to about two feet from the pulley), as this will allow you to support the weight stack throughout the curling motion. Maintain the body position previously described. Now it's just a matter of curling the weight.

DANTE TRUDEL LOW-PULLEY CABLE CURL WITH LAT BAR

This exercise is a creation of Dante Trudel, the innovator of Doggcrapp Training. Hook a 48-inch lat pulldown bar to a low-pulley cable. Reach down and take a curl grip (palms up), as near the cambered bends as possible. Stand up tall, making sure the cable is taut (you'll have to adjust your distance to about two feet from the pulley), as this will allow you to support the weight stack throughout the curling motion. Lean your upper torso forward about 20 to 30 degrees from vertical and arch your back. With the bar hanging at arms' length and your elbows positioned slightly in front of your body, curl it upwards till it touches your forehead, contract the biceps and lower the bar slowly to the starting position.

A D-handle is an ideal attachment to use for low-pulley cable curls.

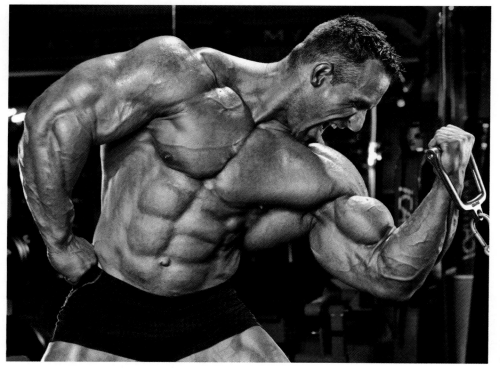

Photo by Robert Reiff
Model Armin Scholz

SQUATTING/BARBELL CURL

If you don't have access to a pulley apparatus, you can do the movement quite efficiently using a five-foot barbell and mimicking the curling procedure described for the cable version. Using this exercise here's a cool little triset biceps shocker routine you might want to try:

Squatting Barbell or Pulley Cable Curl	3 x 5
Straight-Bar Wide-grip Barbell Curl	3 x 5
Preacher Bench Barbell Curl	3 x 5

Perform these three exercises one set after another with absolutely no rest. Rest for 60 to 90 seconds after completing the fifth rep of the third exercise. Repeat the exercises in triset fashion, as described, two to five times depending on your energy, endurance and sanity. If you want another secret to a better biceps pump, simply do a set of barbell shrugs prior to doing a set of curls.

ROTATION DUMBBELL CURL

Lie back on a 45- to 50-degree incline bench and hold a dumbbell in each hand with a regular curl grip and your arms hanging straight. Your elbows should be tight against the sides of your ribcage. Rotate your arms until your forearms are in a lateral plane with your body, as if you were doing rotations. Curl the dumbbells upward (forearms move upward laterally) to your shoulders, lift your elbows slightly to increase the tension on the biceps, and lower.

SEATED INCLINE BENCH DUMBBELL CURL

Sit on an adjustable incline bench, reach down toward the floor and grasp a dumbbell with each hand. Use a thumbless grip with an off-center hand placement where the little finger of each hand is touching the inside plate of the dumbbell. Lie back on the incline bench so your head and the back of your upper torso are both in full contact with the bench back. Your glutes should remain in contact with the seat of the bench during every set. Your arms should be in a fully extended, elbows-locked position and motionless in a dead-hang pose. The palms of your hands should be facing one another (neutral grip) with the dumbbells parallel to each other.

This basic position will vary slightly depending on the angle of the incline. The incline range for this particular exercise can be from as little as 15 to 20 degrees to as much as 45 degrees. At the 15- to 20-degree angle, the spot where your upper biceps separates from the deltoid complex will be maximally stressed. As well, this lower incline adjustment creates a dynamic stretch reflex, which really activates the motor units in the muscle for huge biceps gains.

Inhale deeply. Curl the dumbbells in a semi-circular motion or wide arc toward the deltoids in a thumbs-up style until your forearms approach a 90-degree angle to your body. At this point, begin to slowly supinate (by twisting your wrist and rotating with your wrist) the little-finger side of both dumbbells until they touch the deltoids. Push your elbows up as described for the previous exercise. Exhale and lower the dumbbells in exactly the reverse manner described for the upward curling phase of the exercise.

The effect of the supination (rotation of the palms of your hands and twisting your wrists from facing the body to palms up) is very beneficial for developing the peak of your biceps, while the actual seated incline dumbbell curl lends itself to developing the belly of your biceps.

3 X 3 ALTERNATING DUMBBELL CURL

Do three sets of nine reps in the following manner: While holding a dumbbell in each hand, do three continuous curls with only your right arm (looking to your right wrist will make you have a better muscle contraction). Once these are completed, do three curls with your left arm. Go back and forth nonstop until you've done nine reps with each arm. This constitutes one set. Take a short rest and then do two more sets.

The most unusual part of this exercise sequence is that the forearm of your non-curling arm is supposed to be held at a parallel position to the floor, thus contracting your biceps in isometric fashion. For a change of pace, try doing 3 x 3 preacher bench alternating dumbbell curls. Or for even more of a challenge, do them on the vertical side of the preacher bench.

CHEST-SUPPORTED INCLINE DUMBBELL CURL

Sit backwards on an incline bench set to 45 degrees, supporting your chest against the seat back. With dumbbells in your hands and your arms hanging fully extended, slowly curl the weight, supinating your wrist at the top of the movement. Lower and repeat.

STANDING ONE-DUMBBELL CONCENTRATION CURL

Standing near a high flat exercise bench or dumbbell rack, position your feet at least shoulder-width apart. With your knees slightly bent (soft knee), lean forward at your hip joint and grasp a dumbbell in your right hand. Bring your upper torso to a position that's approximately 45 degrees to the floor. With your knees still slightly bent, place your non-exercising hand on a support device such as the flat exercise bench, using the top of a seat back or even your own knee for back support and to brace your upper torso.

Extend your curling arm with the dumbbell hanging between your legs, utilizing a regular palms facing away from the body grip. You can't cheat at all because your arm is hanging free in this modified version of the concentration curl. Inhale deeply and flex your elbow joint, moving the dumbbell with biceps contractile force in an arc across the midline of your upper body until the little finger side of the dumbbell touches the left deltoid. Squeeze and contract your biceps for a full two count at the completion of the upward curling movement.

Make a determined effort to keep your upper arm perfectly vertical during both the positive and negative curling sequence. Slowly expel the air from your lungs and lower the dumbbell to the beginning zero degree flexion starting position. Repeat for the desired number of reps with your right hand, then switch to your left hand and begin the entire starting point and movement performance over again.

BICEPS/TRICEPS DUMBBELL COMBO

This special exercise combination, best known for garnering a biceps peak and adding triceps stimulation, was taught to us by the late Ernest F. Cottrell in 1975. The exercise is a bit tricky because it requires considerable coordination, but once you master it, you'll be thrilled beyond description. Your arms will have new size, shape and appearance, including a pronounced biceps peak.

As the name of the exercise suggests, you'll be doing a combination of a biceps concentration curls and triceps kickbacks in one continuous movement using a single dumbbell. Here's a brief description of how the exercise is performed when using your right hand:

1. Start by standing beside a flat exercise bench and bend your upper torso forward to a 45-degree angle. With your knees just slightly bent, place your left foot ahead of your right and keep them about shoulder-width apart. Place your non-involved (left) open hand on top of the bench as a means to support your upper torso. Hold a dumbbell in your right hand, letting your arm hang down fully extended, palm facing forward.

2. Dumbbell concentration curl: Take a deep breath and, without moving your elbow to the front or rear (keep it as vertical and stationary as possible), curl the dumbbell. Use your biceps to force it up as high as possible. Squeeze and contract your biceps for a full two seconds at the completion of the upward curling movement.

3. Elbow transition: With your arm still in the top curl position, move or raise your elbow back so that your upper arm, from your elbow to your shoulder, is just above the horizontal plane.

4. Dumbbell kickback: With your upper arm (from your elbow to your shoulder) as stationary as possible, extend your forearm back until your entire arm is straight and in line with your upper back or just slightly higher. Turn your wrists ever so slightly, so the thumb side of the dumbbell is higher than the little finger side. This subtle twist of the wrist will transfer even more tension to your triceps. Squeeze and contract your triceps for a full one count.

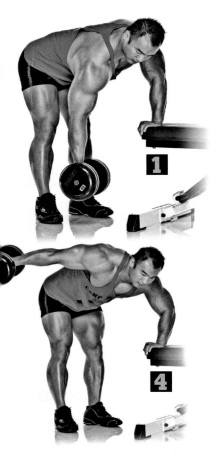

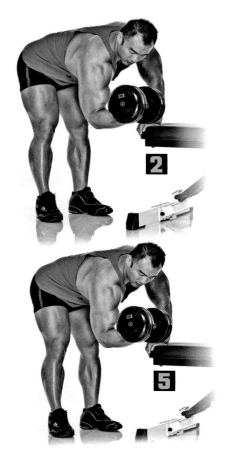

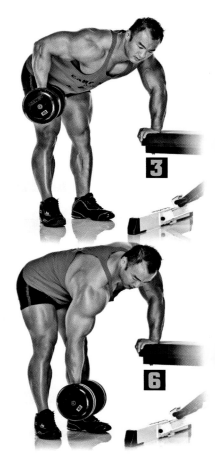

Your goal with biceps and triceps training is to add size and shape, but you also want to achieve balance between the two muscle groups and symmetry from left to right.

5. Top curl position: Exhale and lower your forearm to a vertical position (done correctly there will almost be a 90-degree angle between your upper and lower arm). Next, lower your upper arm from your elbow to your shoulder, to a vertical position (your forearm is now parallel or slightly above to the floor). Squeeze and cramp your biceps into the top curl position.

6. Lower and repeat: Now lower the dumbbell from the top curl position down to the fully extended arm-hang starting position. With no swing and a steady rhythm, immediately repeat the whole process for the desired number of reps with your right hand. Then switch the dumbbell to your left hand and reverse your position (so your right hand is supporting your upper torso). Begin the entire movement all over again.

The combination of one biceps concentration curl and one triceps extension constitutes one rep. With this exercise you'll find you can use more weight with your biceps than your triceps. For example, you might be able to do 10 reps in the dumbbell concentration curl phase of the movement using 50-pound weights, but you may only be able to perform one or two reps in the dumbbell triceps kickback or extension with that same weight. This dilemma is easy enough to solve by simply using the poundage of the weaker exercise for both the combined biceps and triceps movement. This will cause a different problem, as your biceps won't get enough stimulation with the lighter poundage. The solution is to simply do each dumbbell concentration curl rep more slowly and stricter than the dumbbell triceps kickbacks. Speeding through any move in virtually any program will only cheat you out of whatever gains you're striving to accomplish.

FOREARMS

Forearm power is very much a matter of intense mental concentration. Because less energy is used during your workout and the recovery time between workouts is minimal, you'll find it's easier to work frequently at gaining forearm size and power than with some other larger bodyparts such as thighs. If it's your goal to develop great gripping power, we suggest you try some of these proven exercises.

ONE-HAND BARBELL DEADLIFT

This exercise is performed in a straddle-lift style, where the loaded bar is positioned between your legs on the floor. Reach down, grasp the bar in the center and stand up. Use a hook grip, since this keeps your hand from slipping as much as it would with a standard grip. By hook grip, we mean taking a good grip with your fingers (index and middle) wrapped around the end of your thumbs. You may feel discouraged when you first do this exercise because the grip seems to be the limiting factor, but as you continue to train you'll find your grip getting progressively stronger.

SLIDING PINCH GRIP WITH OLYMPIC PLATES

Take two metal Olympic plates (begin light and work up to using two 45 pounders) and place them together so the smooth surfaces are on the outside. Now, without the aid of chalk on your hands, pinch-grip the plates and walk until your grip fails. Perform this exercise anywhere from one to three times with each hand. Measure your progress in this sliding pinch grip exercise by determining the distance you walk and by poundage increases. If you don't have access to Olympic plates, you can load up two heavy dumbbells, then lubricate the palms of your hands generously with petroleum jelly and walk around with the dumbbells until you just can't hold them any longer. Do this for at least three attempts. Make sure to wear protective footwear with these exercises, and hold the plates/dumbbells to the side so they will fall on the floor.

SUSTAINED POWER GRIPPING

Use a heavy-duty hand gripper. Squeeze the handles together and hold for two minutes. Place a piece of leather between the closed handles to provide full closure; leather will fall out if grip weakens. You can even tie a small weight (three to five ounces) to this leather and hang from a 12-inch length of twine. Alternate your hands when doing sustained power gripping. As your strength increases, do these exercises for progressively longer sessions. Never reduce your sustained power gripping.

Much like calves, forearms are often an overlooked and undertrained bodypart.

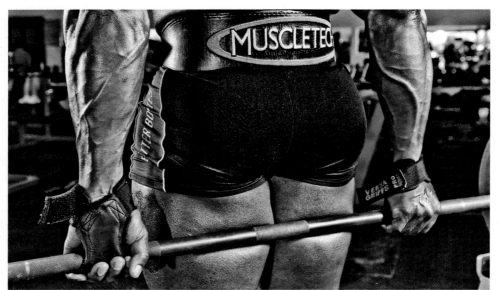

Photo by Michael Butler
Model Johnnie Jackson

WRIST ROLLER

The wrist roller is about 10 to 20 inches long and made of solid hardwood (called a dowel). It's a couple of inches in diameter and has a hole in its center where you tie a cord or knotted clothesline, which should be about 50 to 60 inches long. On the other end of this knotted cord, you'll find a barbell plate loading system consisting of a snap link and plate holder.

Before beginning your workout, set an exercise bar at shoulder height on a set of squat stands. Load an appropriate amount of poundage on the wrist roller. Using a palms-down grip, firmly grasp the wrist roller with both your hands. The weight should be on the floor with roughly a foot of slack in the cord. Be sure to support your wrists over the middle of the exercise bar. Once in that position, extend your arms forward at shoulder height. This will help keep your deltoids from becoming overly fatigued before your forearms have had a chance to be properly worked. If you can't picture this position, just imagine what you look like when you complete a barbell front raise.

Now that you're all set, wind the cord by turning the dowel, using your forearm muscles. Continuously roll your hands forward until the weight touches the dowel. At this point, clench your forearms. Hold that clenched position for just a brief second and then steadily roll your hands back in the opposite direction until the weight returns to the floor. You have now completed one cycle. Repeat the cycle two more times.

STANDING EZ-BAR REVERSE CURL

Load a comfortable weight on the EZ-bar. Using a palms-down, shoulder-width false grip, firmly grasp the bar. Get into an erect and stabilized vertical position with your chin parallel to the floor and your feet shoulder-width apart. Make sure your elbows are locked inward above your hips throughout the exercise. The bar should be resting against your upper thighs with your arms hanging and your wrists straight. Inhale. Tense your forearms and flex at your elbow joint, curling the weight in an upward semi-circle motion toward your shoulder or chest area until your forearms are parallel to the floor. During this action, slowly expel the air in your lungs. Lower the bar to the starting position and inhale. This completes one rep.

Never curl the bar past the point where you're feeling maximum tension. If maximum tension occurs at the upper chest level, don't push through to shoulder level. Remember to bend your knees so that you decrease the potential of suffering a lower back strain. You also shouldn't be making any additional unnecessary movements such as thrusting your hips, moving your upper torso or swinging the weight to gain a mechanical advantage. If you're using momentum to assist you, you'll only be cheating yourself. Your goal should be to ensure that your forearms are feeling maximum tension throughout the exercise.

RECTANGULAR FIX

This specific type of reverse barbell curl was used by legendary strongman George F. Jowett to dramatically improve his grip. The improvement was so incredible that he was amazingly able to grip and overhead press a 160-pound anvil by the horn using only one hand.

To begin, warm up with two sets of eight to ten light-heavy reverse curl reps using regular style. Don't forget to rest for one minute between sets. Now, start with the barbell at the top position of the reverse curl exercise and lower it until your forearms are parallel to the floor. Hold it there for three to five seconds. Then, without the assistance of momentum, return the barbell to the starting position. This concludes one rep. Try doing three or four sets of five reps in this manner. To eliminate any unnecessary elbow movement, use a belt to strap your arms to your sides.

BARBELL REVERSE-WRIST CURL

The barbell reverse-wrist curl is a specialized movement that not only produces a fantastic pump in your forearms, but also stimulates the hard-to-hit brachialis anticus that lies between your biceps and triceps.

Stand with your feet less than shoulder-width apart and using a slightly wider than shoulder-width palms-down grip (not thumbless). Rest the bar against your thighs at arms' length. Bend your wrists down and toward your body as hard as you can, and tense your forearm flexor muscles to their absolute maximum. Straighten your wrists and go back to the dead-hang position for a very slight pause, and then do a regular, strict reverse curl. Remember to keep your elbows close to your body. Do four sets of 12 repetitions.

DECLINE BARBELL (PALMS UP) WRIST CURL

If you're interested in an exercise that will primarily develop size in the belly of your forearm, then you'll want to try the decline barbell wrist curl. Place a wooden or concrete beam block under the end legs of one side of a padded flat exercise bench. If possible, you might want to place the block against a wall so you'll experience the least amount of movement possible from either the block or the bench. Once you've accomplished this, rest a bar with the appropriate poundage at the foot of the bench. Remember to use a bench low enough that it will allow you to perform a wrist curling action, but high enough so the plates don't touch the floor when your wrists hyperextend. Your best bet to ensure this is using a forearm bench.

Sit, facing the barbell, at the declined end of the bench. Grasp the bar using a fairly loose grip, thumbs under the bar and hands roughly six inches apart. Rest your elbows and the back of your forearms on the padded bench. Also remember to keep your elbows against the inside of your thighs and lean your upper torso forward until you've established an angle of less than 90 degrees between your upper and lower arms. If you feel pain in this position, then you should place your forearms on the top of your thighs.

Flex your wrists and forearm muscles while curling the barbell as high as possible (roughly 60 degrees to horizontal). Pause in this peak contraction position for two seconds before slowly lowering the bar back to the starting position or just below the edge of the bench. This concludes one rep. Repeat this for the desired amount of reps and sets.

When performing this exercise you should always remember to inhale and hold that breath while you lift the barbell and then exhale while you are returning the barbell to the starting position. How you hold the bar and your hand positioning is crucial to your success. Don't let the bar roll down to your fingers at the end of the rep. If you allow this to happen, you'll be working your fingers as opposed to your forearms and it'll also be placing tremendous stress on your wrists, leaving you highly susceptible to tendonitis. It's also important not to squeeze the bar. Doing so could cause your tendons to tighten too much and thereby not allow your wrists to flex up or fully return to the starting position. Keep a loose grip and you'll reap the rewards of full contraction and the complete range of motion required to properly perform this exercise. Remember to lift and lower your arms in as close to an even rhythm as possible and rest for 45 seconds to a minute between sets.

Tip: If you're planning on doing any barbell or dumbbell bench presses, overhead presses, bent-over rows, power cleans, deadlifts or any other movement requiring gripping strength or stability, then don't perform any forearm exercises as it will comprise your gripping strength.

ONE-DUMBBELL WRIST CURL (PALM UP, UPPER ARM PARALLEL)

Find a decline (20 to 30 degrees) bench and load a dumbbell with a manageable poundage. Once you've accomplished this, rest the dumbbell at the foot of the bench. Place the back of your forearm along the top of your thigh while performing this exercise. Your hand and wrist should extend past your knee. Your upper arm should be as close to parallel with the floor as possible. If you're having problems getting into this position, simply twist or lean your torso forward. By doing this, you should experience a much stronger muscle contraction than you would have if you performed the exercise the standard way.

Now that you know how, it's time to spring into action. Reach down with one hand and, with your thumb firmly against the inside of the

Forearm exercises are best scheduled last in your workout. Pre-exhausting your forearms before moving on to other bodypart training will only decrease your grip strength on subsequent movements.

plate (or off-center), take a palm-up grip on the bar. By lifting it in this off-center manner you are able to target a specific point of your forearms. If you don't want to use an off-center grip but still want the benefits, simply add a quarter-pound weight (or washers) on one side of the bar and you will create the same type of imbalance. With the exception of this off-center grip, everything else about performing this exercise will mirror a regular palms-up wrist curl.

While performing this exercise you should flex your wrist and contract your forearm muscles as you curl the dumbbell as high as you possibly can. The typical range of wrist action should allow you to get about 60 degrees to horizontal. When you get to this position, pause for two seconds. Slowly lower your hand so it goes back down below the edge of your knee and be sure to use this part of the exercise to exhale.

FOREARM TRAINING SECRETS

If there's a secret to any wrist-curling movement, it's to keep your hips higher than your knees and your elbows higher than your wrists. Lean forward until the angle between your biceps and forearms is less than 90 degrees. Assuming the wrist curl is done in a palms-up position, the flexor muscles in your forearms will effectively be isolated. Perform the exercise with your palms down and you'll isolate the extensor muscles.

You can develop greater gripping strength by increasing the diameter of your barbell and dumbbell bars. You can do this by purchasing a material called Armaflex (be sure to ask for the 1 1/8- or 1 1/4-inch inside diameter size) from your local plumbing or heating store. Generally, you'll want to cut two pieces of this material slightly longer than the width of your hand. Increasing the diameter of your exercise bars with Armaflex will make you grip the bar extra tight. As a result, it will help build a tenacious grip. Another way you can use Armaflex is on your squat bar. It will add some comfort to the bar as it sits on your shoulders for a set of 20-rep squats.

Above all, remember that your grip is important when performing many barbell and dumb-

bell exercises, so don't work your forearms first. Round out your workout program with forearm and grip exercises as the last group of exercises performed in your daily workout.

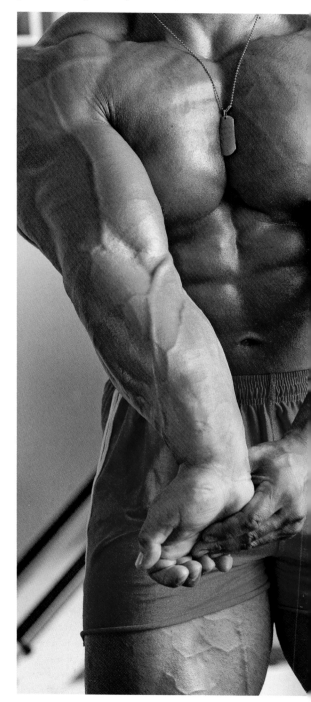

Photo by Ralph DeHaan
Model Ray Arde

ABDOMINALS

Abs are often the last muscle group to be given quality training time. Yet no other bodypart can give your physique that finished and mature look like a ripped, cut-up six pack. Anyone can have a trim waist by following the proper techniques. The basic functions of the abdominals are to pull your ribcage and pelvis together and keep your torso stable. Properly toned abs assist in keeping your pelvis at the proper angle (up and back) and this keeps your spinal column straight.

SIX FACTS ON ABS

1. Many exercises classified as abdominal exercises don't contribute much to the abdominal stimulation, but instead work your hip flexor muscles.

2. An exercise will qualify as an abdominal exercise if your feet aren't secured to the floor. When your feet are anchored, there's a gravitational pull on your legs which means your hip flexors receive the majority of the work. Any movement beyond 30 degrees from the start position of the exercise will increase hip flexor activity. This can be a very serious issue if you have back problems.

3. If you have back issues, structure your abdominal program around crunch variations and the lying six-inch leg raise. The crunch is one of the purest frontal abdominal exercises in existence.

4. Your abdominals are slow-twitch muscles. They're known for endurance-type training, so you should perform high reps. You generally will want to do 15 to 25 reps per set, though this does vary somewhat from the abdominal programs listed in this book.

5. Many bodybuilders feel that because abdominal muscles are slow-twitch they should do their reps slowly, but repetition speed has nothing to do with whether muscles are fast or slow twitch. We recommend that you do your ab exercises slowly for behavioral reasons. It turns out that if we tell bodybuilders to do their exercises at a medium cadence, most will tend to do them (especially the crunch) ballistically, using momentum rather than muscle power. Experimentation has revealed that most of the bodybuilders who do abdominal exercises correctly, and actually realize maximum benefits from them, have been instructed to do the movement slowly. Of course, there's the other school of thought that suggests you use the speed you like. More important than the speed of the rep is that you do the exercises deliberately, consciously using your abdominal muscles.

6. The best abdominal reducer is a proper diet. If you don't follow a proper clean diet, all your exercises will be for nothing.

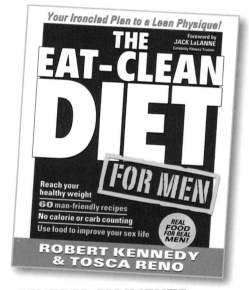

GENERAL COMMENTS

For developing density, thickness and hardness in your abs, perform more sets and fewer reps (five to ten sets of eight to ten reps) using weight. Vary the angles you hit your abs from. On an abdominal apparatus such as the roman chair, you can intensify the movement by putting a six-inch block of wood under the front of the unit. Your back should never break parallel to the floor on the roman chair movement because too much stress is then placed on your lower back.

Don't do abdominal work before a heavy squatting or deadlift session. You need your

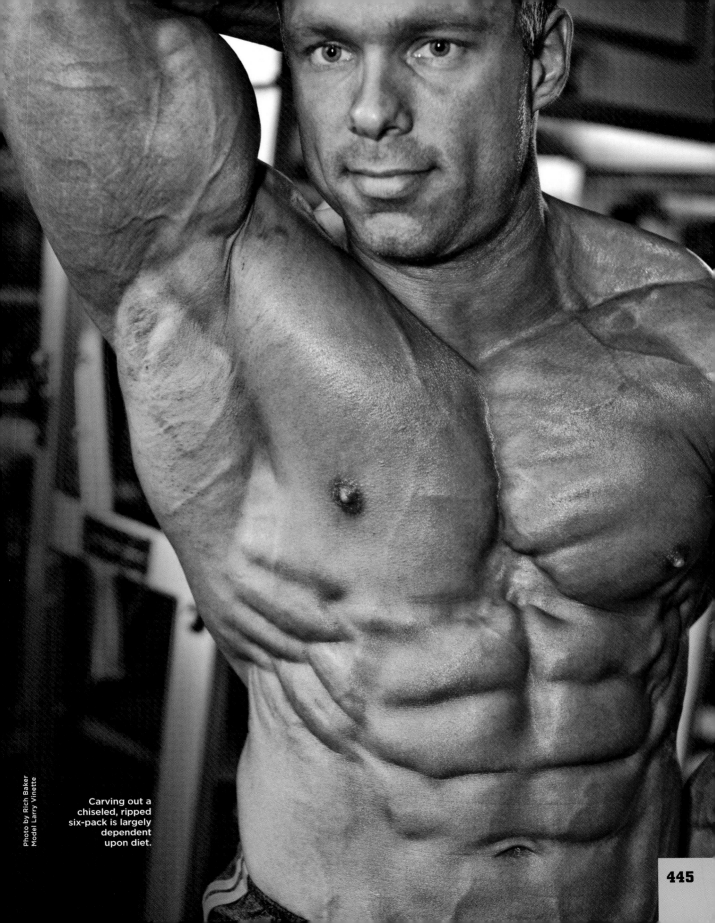

Carving out a chiseled, ripped six-pack is largely dependent upon diet.

abs and lower back (your core) for stability during these workouts. Your core is also used in many overhead pressing movements, and helps support your torso in exercises such as the barbell curl.

LYING SIDE CRUNCH

Lie flat on the floor and turn both of your knees slightly to the left side with your right thigh bent at a 90-degree angle and your calf propped up on top of a flat exercise bench. Your left leg should also be similarly bent with your calf hugging the underside of the bench. Place your right hand behind your head with your elbow forward. Put your left hand on the upper abs/intercostals you're working (establishing a mind-to-muscle connection).

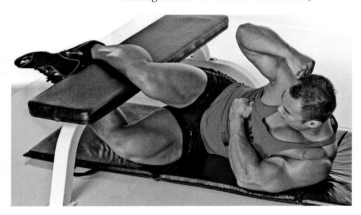

Take a deep breath and then exhale as you curl and rotate your upper torso (shoulders and upper back) to the left, till your right elbow touches the outside of your right knee. Hold this position for two seconds while maximally tensing your abs. Inhale and allow your upper torso to return back to the floor. Repeat the sequence for as many reps as possible. Reverse your leg positioning on the bench and repeat the sequence, only this time you'll be curling and rotating your torso to the right. Maintain abdominal tension throughout the exercise set. Never let your abdominal muscles relax.

STANDING JUMPS OVER A BROOMSTICK

An unusual choice, this is one of the finest and simplest ab exercises we've ever come across.

Place two sturdy chairs almost the length of a broomstick apart. Lay a broomstick securely across the seats of these chairs. Be sure to inhale before each jump and exhale forcefully when your knees are in the tucked position.

BROOMSTICK FORWARD AND BACK JUMPS

Stand in front of the broom handle and jump over it explosively. Simultaneously pull your upper thighs up as close to your chest as possible, then split-second cramp or squeeze your abdominal muscles hard as if you were doing a hanging reverse crunch. Upon landing with bent knees do a quick turn around and jump back over the handle in the same fashion. Be sure to inhale prior to beginning the movement and exhale forcefully at the contracted position.

BROOMSTICK LATERAL JUMPS

Stand beside the broomstick and jump sideways to the opposite side of the stick. Upon landing, immediately jump to other side. The idea is to jump at a height that will allow you to forcibly crunch your ab complex. Gradually raise the broomstick height to accomplish the desired crunch contraction. Determine the sets and reps for this exercise by how your ab muscles respond to the movement.

MINI-TRAMPOLINE AB CRUNCH

For this super ab exercise, sit in the middle of a trampoline with your palms next to your hips. Drop your head down to a chin-in-neck position. Through pursed lips, exhale. At the same time, raise your legs (knees locked and toes pointed forward) and bring them back until your knees are in front of your face. From this position, forcefully suck in your abs, thereby contracting them. Return to the starting position. Be sure to keep the small of the back in contact with the surface of the trampoline at all times. Eventually try to work up to 10 sets of 20 reps, resting for only five seconds between sets. If you don't have a mini-trampoline available, then your next option would be to do crunches or reverse crunches on an exercise ball.

Photo by Gregory James
Model Carl Cheung

SQUAT AB CRUNCH

Take a slightly wider than shoulder-width stance and squat as low as you can go with your knees spread wide apart. Place your arms inside your legs with your palms flat on the floor. While looking straight ahead and keeping your shoulders relaxed, exhale. Then, thrust your hips forward. This movement will be very short, but you'll feel a strong contraction in your abs. Hold this contraction for a count of 10. Relax and take a deep breath. Repeat the sequence until there's a deep muscle ache in your abs.

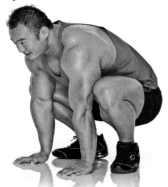

ABDOMINAL VACUUMS

This exercise can be performed seated or standing, as long as you're doing it on an empty stomach. Bend your knees slightly and lean forward at your waist (hump the upper back). Place your chin on your chest and your hands on top of your thighs and then press downward and outward. Avoid lifting your ribcage or expanding your chest. Relax your abdominal muscles. Sharply expel as much air as possible from your lungs. Suck your abdominals (stomach) in and out several times (a minimum of 10 times or until your abs ache), mentally trying to pull it into and behind your ribcage. Inhale and then begin the procedure all over again. Repeat the described series five to ten times, twice per day. As you begin becoming more adept at performing abdominal vacuums, with both hands on the tops of your thighs, gradually press downward. Then press outward with only one hand on your thigh. This results in a single isolation effect on one side of your abs. An even more advanced version is to alternately press your hand on one

The abdominal vacuum was a technique used to train the ab muscles to suck inward.

thigh, then the other. This will cause your abdominals to move from one side to the other.

AB ASSAULT WORKOUT

This ab assault training routine will help you maintain your existing level of development and push it beyond.

Exercise #1	
Reverse Crunch	3 sets x 15 reps – Hold 5, then 10

Exercise #2	
Cross Bar Crunch	1 set x 25 reps, 20, 15 – Hold each for five seconds.

Exercise #3	
Twisting Crunch (elbow to opposite knee)	2 sets x 40 reps on each side

REVERSE CRUNCH

Lie back on a flat exercise bench, your butt just peeking off the bottom. Reach overhead and grip the end of the bench. Cross your legs and lift until your thighs are perpendicular to your body.

Without swinging, use your abs to lift your butt off the bench (in a contracted position) by approximately eight inches. Breathe out.

In a controlled manner, lower your legs until your heels barely touch the floor, then lift again.

Upon completion of the fifth rep (in the top position), hold for five seconds. Do 10 more reps and hold in the top position for a 10-second count. This completes one set. Do two more sets.

CROSS-BAR CRUNCH

Lie on your back on the floor. You can position your lower torso in one of two ways: Either rest your calves on a bench or bed in such a way that your thighs are virtually vertical or simply cross your legs in the air while lying on the floor. Either of these positions will keep your hip flexors from participating in the actual movement.

Hold a broomstick behind your neck and clasp your hands (interlocked) behind your head. This will keep your arms well back and in line with your upper torso, which will keep your ab muscles under a greater tension than when your elbows are allowed to come forward. Exhale all the air out of your chest. This will help create tension in the abdominals. Now crunch. While you're doing this (and remember that your back must never go beyond 30 degrees off the floor, which will be only a few inches at most), mentally try to curl your pelvis and lower ribs until they touch for maximal contraction of your frontal abdominals. You won't actually be able to do this, but the mental focus will certainly help you acquire a tight crunch. Hold this position and repeat. It's important for you to realize that your hands behind your head should be relaxed at all times through the movement and they shouldn't assist in any way.

1. After performing 25 reps, hold the up position for five seconds.
2. Do 20 more reps and hold for five seconds.
3. Do 15 more reps and hold for five seconds. At this point, you should rest.

NECK

The neck is composed of soft muscle tissue. This tissue is very responsive to training and not much work is needed to increase its size and strength. One to two months of specialization will usually be enough. After a properly initiated program, your gains can be maintained with as few as one or two workouts per week. Neck work will increase the blood supply to your brain and also aid in the reduction of a double chin.

NECK STRAP HARNESS

Commercial Gym: Using a neck-strap harness and the low cable on a crossover unit, seated cable rowing or preacher cable machine, you can do the following exercises:

1. Put the neck-strap harness on your head. Next, sit on a bench while facing the machine and attach the cable to the neck strap. Now it's just a matter of moving your head (posterior flexion) from the

FAT BUSTER DIET PLAN FOR SIX-PACK ABS

FIVE MEALS ABOUT THREE HOURS APART

MEAL	UNDER 195 POUNDS	OVER 195 POUNDS
1	Oatmeal w/milk or Cream of Wheat (70 gm) 4 egg whites 1 banana Coffee or tea	Oatmeal w/milk or Cream of Wheat (100 gm) 6 egg whites 1 banana Coffee or tea
2	1 can white tuna (rinsed 3 times) 2/3 cup rice (cooked) 2 tbsp. low-cal Italian dressing	1-1/2 cans white tuna (rinsed 3 times) 1 cup rice (cooked) 2 tbsp. low-cal Italian dressing
3	1 plain baked potato 1 piece fruit (apple, orange, banana, or 16 grapes) 1/2 cup low-fat cottage cheese	1 plain baked potato 1 piece fruit (apple, orange, banana, or 16 grapes) 1/2 cup low-fat cottage cheese
4	1½ chicken breasts or 5-6 oz. lean meat 1 potato (Idaho or sweet) large salad 3/4 to 1 cup vegetables (broccoli, cauliflower, carrots, spinach, asparagus)	2 chicken breasts or 8 oz. lean meat 1 potato (Idaho or sweet) large salad 3/4 to 1 cup vegetable (broccoli, cauliflower, carrots, spinach, asparagus)
5	When you reach a bodyfat level that you're happy with, you may add an extra meal (similar to meal 4). Add this extra meal for only two days and then delete it for one. Repeat this sequence.	When you reach a bodyfat level that you're happy with, you may add an extra meal (similar to meal 4). Add this extra meal for only two days and then delete it for one. Repeat this sequence.
Snacks	You may have any one of the following snacks, once per day: An eight-ounce yogurt, one piece of fruit, a four-ounce low-fat frozen yogurt, plain popcorn or a half-cup of cottage cheese.	

chin-in-neck position to an extreme backward extension and then forward. Reverse your position (and neck strap) so you're sitting with your back to the machine. Move your head (anterior flexion) from the extreme backward extension forward to the chin-in-neck position and back.

2. Readjust the neck-strap harness on your head and, while sitting sideways (right side of body facing the machine), pull your head (lateral flexion) from one shoulder (right) to the other (left) and back. Then reverse the position so the left side of your body faces the machine. Pull your head (lateral flexion) from one shoulder (left) to the other (right) and back.

Home Gym: The most obvious use of the neck strap harness is to begin in a seated position in a sturdy chair. Position the harness over your head with the weight in front of you. Lean your upper torso forward and brace your hands on your upper thighs. Begin with your head down (chin in neck), move it to an extreme backward extension and then forward again.

The next exercise is to stand up and reverse the neck strap harness so that the weight is behind you. Hold the harness so that it doesn't slip off your head, but don't assist the actual movement with your hands. With your head as far backward as possible, move it forward to the chin in the hollow of your neck and then back.

NECK BRIDGES
One of the most effective ways to build up the back of your neck is by doing the static and rocking neck bridges as follows:

STATIC NECK BRIDGE
Lie on your back with your head on the floor. You may use a pillow for comfort. Now, using the strength of the neck muscles alone, bridge or raise your body off the floor. Your back will be completely off the floor and arched, and your feet should be directly under your knees. If you haven't been doing neck exercises on a regular basis, the most you'll want to do is to hold this position without any further movement. Your goal over the next few weeks should be to work up to holding the bridge posture for three or four minutes.

ROCKING NECK BRIDGE
Now you're ready for some neck bridge movements, which consist of getting into the position described and rocking back and forth from the top of your head as far toward the forehead as possible. Lower yourself back to the floor until your back is touching again. This concludes one rep. Work up to 25 reps for a couple of sets. When you accomplish this goal, it's time to begin slowly using progressive weight resistance in which you hold a barbell plate or light barbell over your chest while performing the neck bridge. Some of

Just one to two months of training the neck area, with exercises such as neck bridges, will increase its size and strength in the soft muscle tissue.

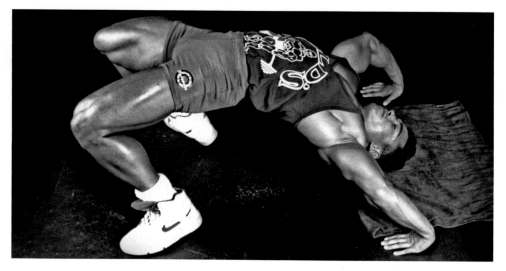

Photo by Irvin Gelb
Model Danny Hester

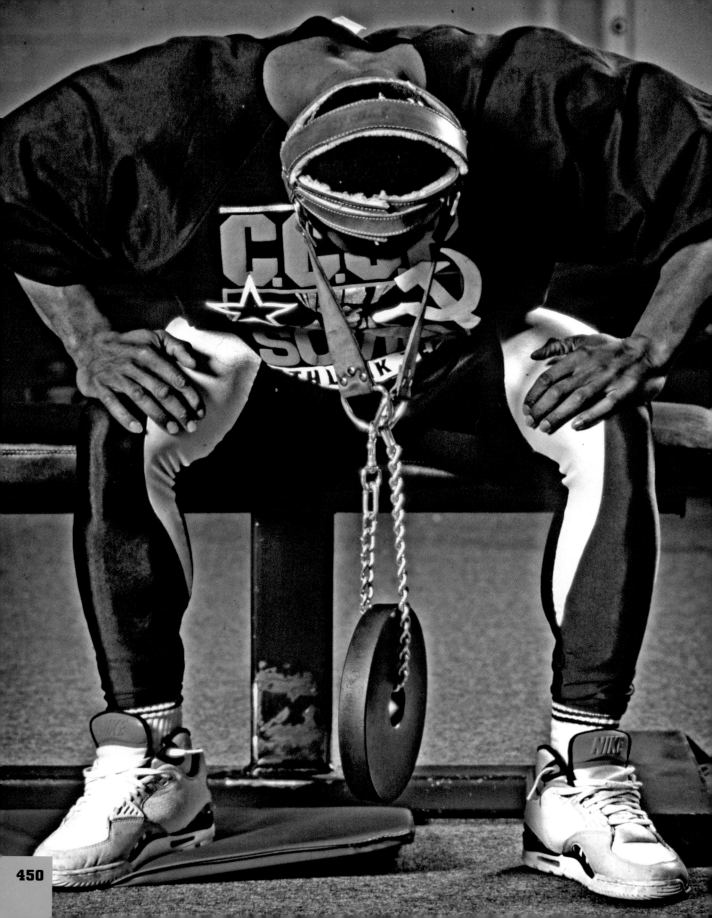

the old-time strongmen used to position themselves in the neck bridge position and perform a modified barbell bench press.

One of the best ways to work the front of your neck is to lie flat on your back on a bench, with your head extended over the end of it. Then, rest a folded towel on your forehead for padding and place a barbell plate on top of it. Holding the plate with your hands, and using neck action alone, lower and extend (posterior extension) your head as far back as possible. Then, smoothly lift your head upward and toward your chest to achieve anterior flexion, thereby working the front of your neck.

MANUAL RESISTANCE NECK WORK

There are numerous ways to work your neck with partner-assisted resistance movements. Many bodybuilders forgo the weighted neck exercises in favor of partner-assisted movements.

The most common fault we find with this approach, or other similar dynamic tension methods, is that you may have the capacity to endure 100 pounds of neck resistance for a one-rep maximum in the posterior extension of the movement. Unfortunately, your training partner may only apply 80 pounds of resistance (which is appropriate for eight to twelve reps). Other times, your training partner may apply the appropriate weight. Of course, a muscle will only begin an adaptive response at a minimum of 35 percent of your one-rep maximum. In this case, that would be 35 pounds. If your training partner doesn't provide that amount of resistance, you wouldn't be meeting the demands of your muscles.

Now, the next potential set is dramatically different. Your training partner's mind just isn't into the workout, and during this set he begins to apply 125 pounds of resistance. Naturally, this exceeds your strength capabilities in the back-of-the-neck movement (posterior extension) and because of that, an injury could occur. Remember, your limit was 100 pounds for a one-rep max and if your partner provided 125 pounds, that's a 25 percent increase. Of course this is all hypothetical, but as you can see, there's no real consistency or method to accurately measure the resistance applied by

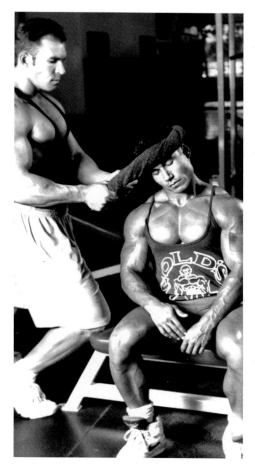

a training partner. Even the various dynamic tension methods in which you apply resistance to yourself have the same type of problems.

Progressive resistance weight training, body-weight-only exercises or any other method in which you can measure resistance or force applied is the better approach to training.

CLOSING THOUGHTS ON NECK WORK

There are other more advanced exercises such as headstands with your feet against a wall, prone (face down) and supine (face up) neck and body supports between two chairs, but the ones we've listed will do nicely for now. Don't try and include all of these exercises into one workout. Instead, select one or two different ones (three sets of 12 to 15 reps of each) for each neck training session. You'll enjoy the variety and your neck will respond better.

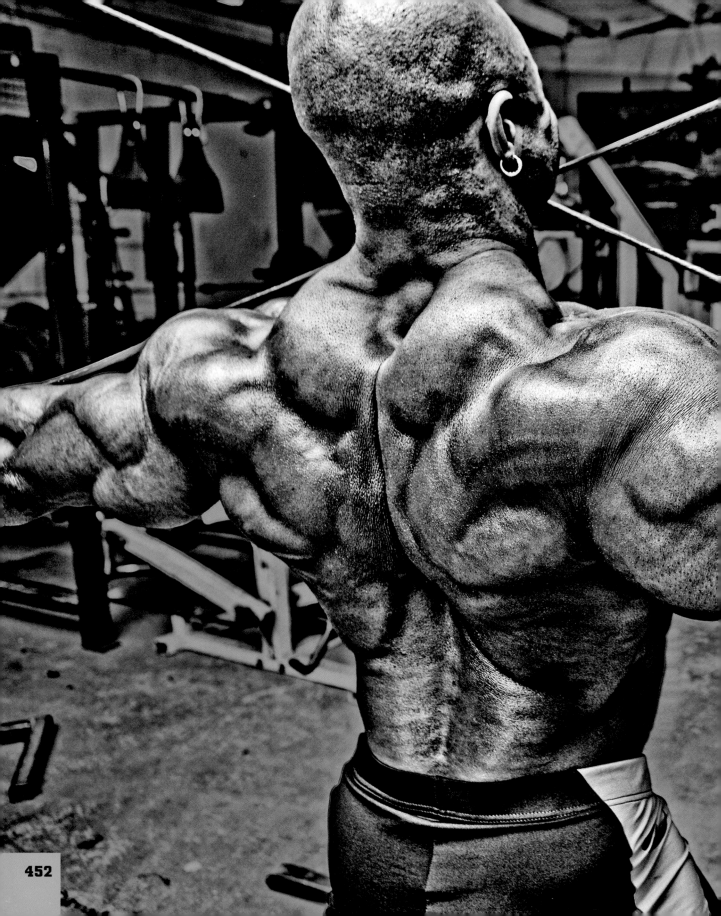

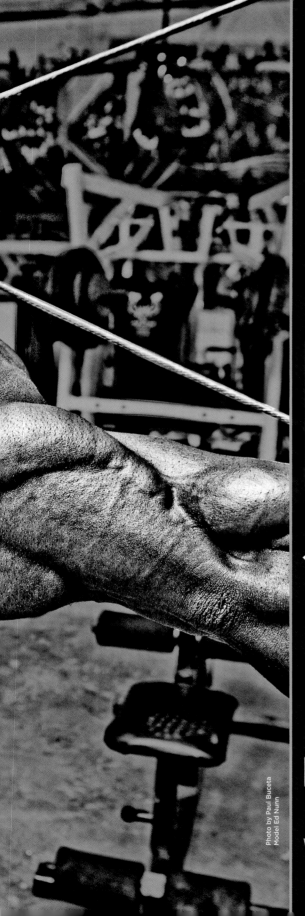

BOOK
14

Questions and Answers
with Robert and Dennis

CHAPTER 46

QUESTIONS & ANSWERS WITH ROBERT AND DENNIS

Two pros in their own right offer advice, information and guidance to help you advance with your bodybuilding.

As an added bonus, here are some of the most thought-provoking e-mails, letters and phone calls that we've received, along with our most insightful answers.

BRUTALLY HUGE MUSCLE MASS IN 30 DAYS.

Q) *Hi. I've been pumping iron for a little over a year. I read all the bodybuilding magazines but it's confusing. It seems like there are dozens of companies selling supplements. The magazines have loads of training articles, but there doesn't seem to be any consistency to them. One guy says don't do more than one set per exercise while another talks about doing mega sets. Some of them suggest doing exercises on machines usually found in larger gyms.*

I don't have a large cash flow, so I don't want to experiment with all kinds of different supplements to figure out what's going to help me put on muscle. And I sure don't have the time to try out all the bodybuilding routines. I live far from a major town so I don't have access to lots of equipment.

The bottom line is that I want a food supplement and a training program that will help me pack on freaky huge muscle and with power to spare, without using steroids and without any fancy equipment. Can you give me a helping hand?

A) It seems there are as many training programs and different types of supplements as there are bodybuilders. The following is an exercise program and supplement that has proven to work for the majority of amateur bodybuilders. You didn't include your bodyweight, measurements or strength levels, so we can't tailor a specific program to your actual wants and needs, but the 3-8-12 Method For Gaining Muscle Mass In 30 Days and the Get-Big Drink will produce some very shocking muscle gains for you.

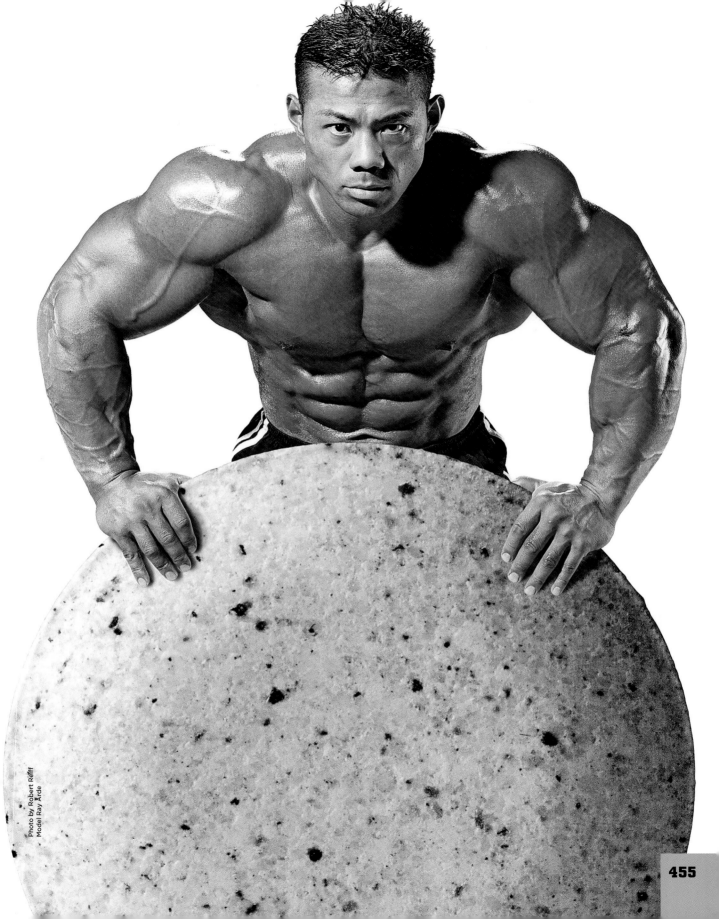

455

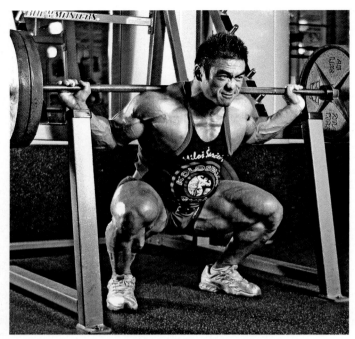

The wide-stance barbell back squat is one of eight core growth moves in the 3-8-12 methods.

3-8-12 METHOD FOR GAINING MUSCLE MASS IN 30 DAYS

Training Frequency: Three non-consecutive days per week

Number of Exercises: Eight anabolic core growth

Total Training Sessions: 12

WEEK 1, DAY 1

General Warm-Up: Five minutes on an exercise bike or other cardio machine, walking fast or active stretching.

1. Barbell Back Squat – Wide Stance
Specific Warm-Up

> **Set 1:** 12 Reps x 30% 1RM
> (Rest for 90 seconds)
> **Set 2:** 6 Reps x 60% 1RM
> (Rest for 90 seconds)

Gain Factor Sets

> **Set 1:** 6 Reps x 85% 1RM
> (Rest for 60 seconds)
> **Set 2:** 8 Reps x 80% 1RM
> (Rest for 60 seconds)
> **Set 3:** 10 Reps x 75% 1RM
> (Rest for five minutes)

Use the barbell plate front raise to perform gain factor sets.

2. Flat Bench Barbell Press
Specific Warm-Up

> **Set 1:** 12 Reps x 30% 1RM
> (Rest for 90 seconds)
> **Set 2:** 6 Reps x 60% 1RM
> (Rest for 90 seconds)

Gain Factor Sets

> **Set 1:** 6 Reps x 85% 1RM
> (Rest for 60 seconds)
> **Set 2:** 8 Reps x 80% 1RM
> (Rest for 60 seconds)
> **Set 3:** 10 Reps x 75% 1RM
> (Rest for five minutes)

3. Barbell Plate Front Raise
Gain Factor Sets

> **Set 1:** 10 Reps (Rest for 60 seconds)
> **Set 2:** 10 Reps (Rest for 60 seconds)
> **Set 3:** 10 Reps

WEEK 1, DAY 2

General Warm-Up: Five minutes on an exercise bike or other cardio machine, walking fast or active stretching.

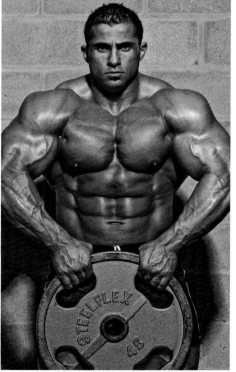

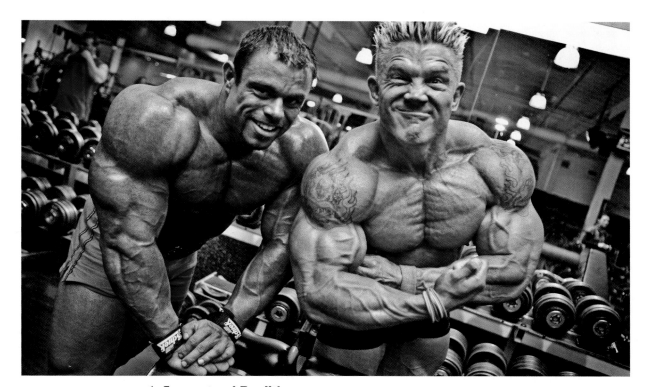

Photo by Paul Buceta
Models Dan Hill and Andy Haman

1. Conventional Deadlift
Specific Warm-Up
Set 1: 12 Reps x 30% 1RM
　　(Rest for 90 seconds)
Set 2: 6 Reps x 60% 1RM
　　(Rest for 90 seconds)
Gain Factor Sets
Set 1: 6 Reps x 85% 1RM
　　(Rest for 60 seconds)
Set 2: 8 Reps x 80% 1RM
　　(Rest for 60 seconds)
Set 3: 10 Reps x 75% 1RM
　　(Rest for five minutes)

2. Standing Barbell Overhead Press
Specific Warm-Up
Set 1: 12 Reps x 30% 1RM
　　(Rest for 90 seconds)
Set 2: 6 Reps x 60% 1RM
　　(Rest for 90 seconds)
Gain Factor Sets
Set 1: 6 Reps x 85% 1RM
　　(Rest for 60 seconds)
Set 2: 8 Reps x 80% 1RM
　　(Rest for 60 seconds)

Set 3: 10 Reps x 75% 1RM
　　(Rest for five minutes)

3. Barbell Shrug
Specific Warm-Up
Set 1: 10 Reps x 50% 1RM
　　(Rest for 90 seconds)
Gain Factor Sets
Set 1: 6 Reps x 85% 1RM
　　(Rest for 60 seconds)
Set 2: 8 Reps x 80% 1RM
　　(Rest for 60 seconds)
Set 3: 10 Reps x 75% 1RM

WEEK 1, DAY 3
General Warm-Up: Five minutes on an exercise bike or other cardio machine, walking fast or active stretching.

1. Barbell Back Squat – Narrow Stance
Specific Warm-Up
Set 1: 12 Reps x 30% 1RM
　　(Rest for 90 seconds)
Set 2: 6 Reps x 60% 1RM
　　(Rest for 90 seconds)

Gain Factor Sets
> **Set 1:** 6 Reps x 85% 1RM
> (Rest for 60 seconds)
> **Set 2:** 8 Reps x 80% 1RM
> (Rest for 60 seconds)
> **Set 3:** 10 Reps x 75% 1RM
> (Rest for five minutes)

2. Parallel Bar Dip With Added Weight
Specific Warm-Up
> **Set 1:** 12 Reps x 30% 1RM
> (Rest for 90 seconds)
> **Set 2:** 6 Reps x 60% 1RM
> (Rest for 90 seconds)

Gain Factor Sets
> **Set 1:** 6 Reps x 85% 1RM
> (Rest for 60 seconds)
> **Set 2:** 8 Reps x 80% 1RM
> (Rest for 60 seconds)
> **Set 3:** 10 Reps x 75% 1RM
> (Rest for three minutes)

IFBB pro Kai Greene knows all about gaining max muscle.

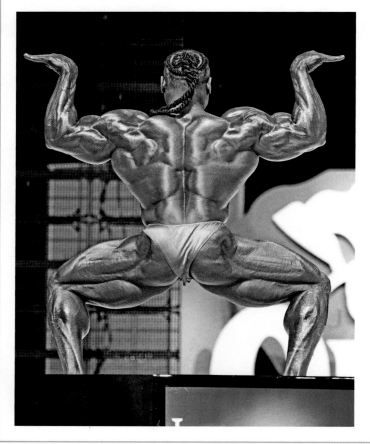

3. Bent-Over Row
Specific Warm-Up
> **Set 1:** 10 Reps x 50% 1RM
> (Rest for 90 seconds)

Gain Factor Sets
> **Set 1:** 6 Reps x 85% 1RM
> (Rest for 60 seconds)
> **Set 2:** 8 Reps x 80% 1RM
> (Rest for 60 seconds)
> **Set 3:** 10 Reps x 75% 1RM

WEEK 2, DAY 1
General Warm-Up: Five minutes on an exercise bike or other cardio machine, walking fast or active stretching.

1. Barbell Back Squat – Wide Stance
Specific Warm-Up
> **Set 1:** 12 Reps x 30% 1RM
> (Rest for 90 seconds)
> **Set 2:** 6 Reps x 60% 1RM
> (Rest for 90 seconds)

Gain Factor Sets
> **Set 1:** 6 Reps x 85% 1RM + 10 pounds.
> (Rest for 60 seconds)
> **Set 2:** 8 Reps x 80% 1RM + 10 pounds.
> (Rest for 60 seconds)
> **Set 3:** 10 Reps x 75% 1RM + 10 pounds.
> (Rest for five minutes)

2. Incline Bench Barbell Press
Specific Warm-Up
> **Set 1:** 12 Reps x 30% 1RM
> (Rest for 90 seconds)
> **Set 2:** 6 Reps x 60% 1RM
> (Rest for 90 seconds)

Gain Factor Sets
> **Set 1:** 6 Reps x 85% 1RM
> (Rest for 60 seconds)
> **Set 2:** 8 Reps x 80% 1RM
> (Rest for 60 seconds)
> **Set 3:** 10 Reps x 75% 1RM
> (Rest for three minutes)

3. Bent-Over Row
Specific Warm-Up
> **Set 1:** 10 Reps x 50% 1RM
> (Rest for 90 seconds)

Gain Factor Sets

Photo by Jason Breeze
Model Kai Greene

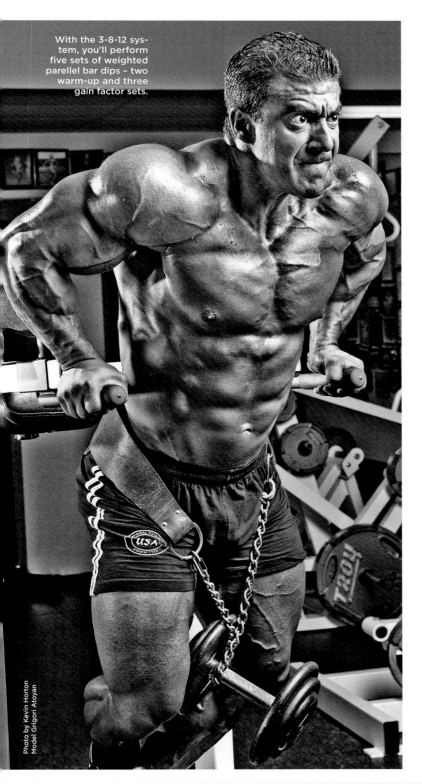

With the 3-8-12 system, you'll perform five sets of weighted parellel bar dips – two warm-up and three gain factor sets.

Photo by Kevin Horton
Model Grigori Atoyan

Set 1: 6 Reps x 85% 1RM + 5 pounds.
    (Rest for 60 seconds)
Set 2: 8 Reps x 80% 1RM + 5 pounds.
    (Rest for 60 seconds)
Set 3: 10 Reps x 75% 1RM + 5 pounds.

WEEK 2, DAY 2

General Warm-Up: Five minutes on an exercise bike or other cardio machine, walking fast or active stretching.

1. Conventional Deadlift

Specific Warm-Up
    Set 1: 12 Reps x 30% 1RM
        (Rest for 90 seconds)
    Set 2: 6 Reps x 60% 1RM
        (Rest for 90 seconds)

Gain Factor Sets
    Set 1: 6 Reps x 85% 1RM + 10 pounds.
        (Rest for 60 seconds)
    Set 2: 8 Reps x 80% 1RM + 10 pounds.
        (Rest for 60 seconds)
    Set 3: 10 Reps x 75% 1RM + 10 pounds.
        (Rest for five minutes)

2. Standing Barbell Overhead Press

Specific Warm-Up
    Set 1: 12 Reps x 30% 1RM
        (Rest for 90 seconds)
    Set 2: 6 Reps x 60% 1RM
        (Rest for 90 seconds)

Gain Factor Sets
    Set 1: 6 Reps x 85% 1RM + 5 pounds.
        (Rest for 60 seconds)
    Set 2: 8 Reps x 80% 1RM + 5 pounds.
        (Rest for 60 seconds)
    Set 3: 10 Reps x 75% 1RM + 5 pounds.
        (Rest for three minutes)

3. Barbell Shrug

Warm-Up
    Set 1: 10 Reps x 50% 1RM
        (Rest for 90 seconds)

Gain Factor Sets
    Set 1: 6 Reps x 85% 1RM + 10 pounds.
        (Rest for 60 seconds)
    Set 2: 8 Reps x 80% 1RM + 10 pounds.
        (Rest for 90 seconds)
    Set 3: 10 Reps x 75% 1RM + 10 pounds.

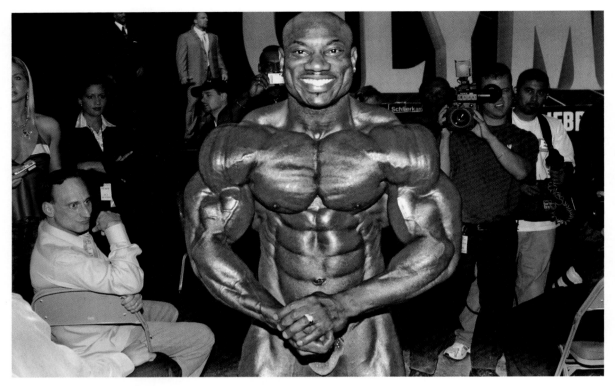

IFBB pro Dexter Jackson shows off his impressive mass and proportionate physique.

WEEK 2, DAY 3

General Warm-Up: Five minutes on an exercise bike or other cardio machine, walking fast or active stretching.

1. Barbell Back Squat – Narrow Stance
Specific Warm-Up
 Set 1: 12 Reps x 30% 1RM
  (Rest for 90 seconds)
 Set 2: 6 Reps x 60% 1RM
  (Rest for 90 seconds)
Gain Factor Sets
 Set 1: 6 Reps x 85% 1RM + pounds.
  (Rest for 60 seconds)
 Set 2: 8 Reps x 80% 1RM + 10 pounds.
  (Rest for 60 seconds)
 Set 3: 10 Reps x 75% 1RM + 10 pounds.
  (Rest for five minutes)

2. Parallel Bar Dip With Added Weight
Specific Warm-Up
 Set 1: 12 Reps x 30% 1RM
  (Rest for 90 seconds)
 Set 2: 6 Reps x 60% 1RM
  (Rest for 90 seconds)

Gain Factor Sets
 Set 1: 6 Reps x 85% 1RM + 5 pounds.
  (Rest for 60 seconds)
 Set 2: 8 Reps x 80% 1RM + 5 pounds.
  (Rest for 60 seconds)
 Set 3: 10 Reps x 75% 1RM + 5 pounds.
  (Rest for three minutes)

3. Barbell Plate Front Raise
Gain Factor Sets
 Set 1: 12 Reps (Rest for 60 seconds)
 Set 2: 12 Reps (Rest for 60 seconds)
 Set 3: 12 Reps

WEEK 3, DAY 1

General Warm-Up: Five minutes on an exercise bike or other cardio machine, walking fast or active stretching.

1. Barbell Back Squat – Wide Stance
Specific Warm-Up
 Set 1: 12 Reps x 30% 1RM
  (Rest for 90 seconds)
 Set 2: 6 Reps x 60% 1RM
  (Rest for 90 seconds)

Photo by Raymond Cassar
Model Dexter Jackson

Gain Factor Sets

> **Set 1:** 6 Reps x 85% 1RM + 20 pounds.
> (Rest for 60 seconds)
> **Set 2:** 8 Reps x 80% 1RM + 20 pounds.
> (Rest for 60 seconds)
> **Set 3:** 10 Reps x 75% 1RM + 20 pounds.
> (Rest for five minutes)

2. Standing Barbell Overhead Press

Specific Warm-Up

> **Set 1:** 12 Reps x 30% 1RM
> (Rest for 90 seconds)
> **Set 2:** 6 Reps x 60% 1RM
> (Rest for 90 seconds)

Gain Factor Sets

> **Set 1:** 6 Reps x 85% 1RM + 10 pounds.
> (Rest for 60 seconds)
> **Set 2:** 8 Reps x 80% 1RM + 10 pounds.
> (Rest for 60 seconds)
> **Set 3:** 10 Reps x 75% 1RM + 10 pounds.
> (Rest for three minutes)

3. Bent-Over Row

Specific Warm-Up

> **Set 1:** 10 Reps x 50% 1RM
> (Rest for 90 seconds)

Gain Factor Sets

> **Set 1:** 6 Reps x 85% 1RM + 10 pounds.
> (Rest for 60 seconds)
> **Set 2:** 8 Reps x 80% 1RM + 10 pounds.
> (Rest for 60 seconds)
> **Set 3:** 10 Reps x 75% 1RM + 10 pounds.

WEEK 3, DAY 2

General Warm-Up: Five minutes on an exercise bike or other cardio machine, walking fast or active stretching.

1. Conventional Deadlift

Specific Warm-Up

> **Set 1:** 12 Reps x 30% 1RM
> (Rest for 90 seconds)
> **Set 2:** 6 Reps x 60% 1RM
> (Rest for 90 seconds)

Gain Factor Sets

> **Set 1:** 6 Reps x 85% 1RM + 20 pounds.
> (Rest for 60 seconds)
> **Set 2:** 8 Reps x 80% 1RM + 20 pounds.
> (Rest for 60 seconds)

> **Set 3:** 10 Reps x 75% 1RM + 20 pounds.
> (Rest for five minutes)

2. Parallel Dips With Added Weight

Specific Warm-Up

> **Set 1:** 12 Reps x 30% 1RM
> (Rest for 90 seconds)
> **Set 2:** 6 Reps x 60% 1RM
> (Rest for 90 seconds)

Gain Factor Sets

> **Set 1:** 6 Reps x 85% 1RM + 10 pounds.
> (Rest for 60 seconds)
> **Set 2:** 8 Reps x 80% 1RM + 10 pounds.
> (Rest for 60 seconds)
> **Set 3:** 10 Reps x 75% 1RM + 10 pounds.
> (Rest for three minutes)

3. Barbell Plate Front Raise

Gain Factor Sets

> **Set 1:** 14 Reps (Rest for 60 seconds)
> **Set 2:** 14 Reps (Rest for 60 seconds)
> **Set 3:** 14 Reps

WEEK 3, DAY 3

General Warm-Up: Five minutes on an exercise bike or other cardio machine, walking fast or active stretching.

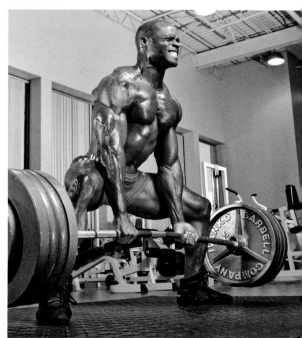

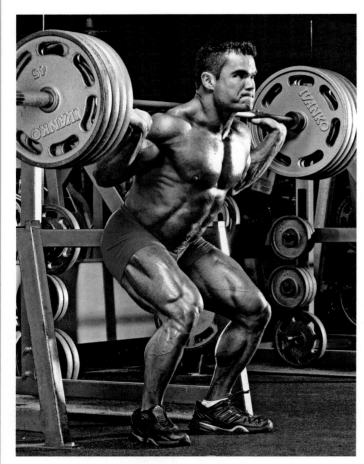

This program includes another version of the barbell back squats – with a narrow foot stance.

1. Barbell Back Squat – Narrow Stance
Specific Warm-Up
    Set 1: 12 Reps x 30% 1RM
        (Rest for 90 seconds)
    Set 2: 6 Reps x 60% 1RM
        (Rest for 90 seconds)
Gain Factor Sets
    Set 1: 6 Reps x 85% 1RM + 20 pounds.
        (Rest for 60 seconds)
    Set 2: 8 Reps x 80% 1RM + 20 pounds.
        (Rest for 60 seconds)
    Set 3: 10 Reps x 75% 1RM + 20 pounds.
        (Rest for five minutes)

2. Flat Bench Barbell Press
Specific Warm-Up
    Set 1: 12 Reps x 30% 1RM
        (Rest for 90 seconds)
    Set 2: 6 Reps x 60% 1RM
        (Rest for 90 seconds)

Gain Factor Sets
    Set 1: 6 Reps x 85% 1RM + 10 pounds.
        (Rest for 60 seconds)
    Set 2: 8 Reps x 80% 1RM + 10 pounds.
        (Rest for 60 seconds)
    Set 3: 10 Reps x 75% 1RM + 10 pounds.
        (Rest for three minutes)

3. Barbell Shrug
Specific Warm-Up
    Set 1: 12 Reps x 50% 1RM
        (Rest for 90 seconds)
Gain Factor Sets
    Set 1: 6 Reps x 85% 1RM + 20 pounds.
        (Rest for 60 seconds)
    Set 2: 8 Reps x 80% 1RM + 20 pounds.
        (Rest for 60 seconds)
    Set 3: 10 Reps x 75% 1RM + 20 pounds.

WEEK 4, DAY 1
General Warm-Up: Five minutes on an exercise bike or other cardio machine, walking fast or active stretching.

1. Barbell Squat – Wide Stance
Specific Warm-Up
    Set 1: 12 Reps x 30% 1RM
        (Rest for 90 seconds)
    Set 2: 6 Reps x 60%
        (Rest for 90 seconds)
Gain Factor Sets
    Set 1: 6 Reps x 85% 1RM + 30 pounds.
        (Rest for 60 seconds)
    Set 2: 8 Reps x 80% 1RM + 30 pounds.
        (Rest for 60 seconds)
    Set 3: 10 Reps x 75% 1RM + 30 pounds.
        (Rest for five minutes)

2. Parallel Bar Dip With Added Weight
Specific Warm-Up
    Set 1: 12 Reps x 30% 1RM
        (Rest for 90 seconds)
    Set 2: 6 Reps x 60% 1RM
        (Rest for 90 seconds)
Gain Factor Sets
    Set 1: 6 Reps x 85% 1RM + 15 pounds.
        (Rest for 60 seconds)
    Set 2: 8 Reps x 80% 1RM + 15 pounds.
        (Rest for 60 seconds)

Set 3: 10 Reps x 75% 1RM + 15 pounds.
(Rest for three minutes)

3. Bent-Over Row
Specific Warm-Up
Set 1: 10 Reps x 50% 1RM
(Rest for 90 seconds)
Gain Factor Sets
Set 1: 6 Reps x 85% 1RM + 15 pounds.
(Rest for 60 seconds)
Set 2: 8 Reps x 80% 1RM + 15 pounds.
(Rest for 60 seconds)
Set 3: 10 Reps x 75% 1RM + 15 pounds.

WEEK 4, DAY 2
General Warm-Up: Five minutes on an exercise bike or other cardio machine, walking fast or active stretching.

1. Conventional Deadlift
Specific Warm-Up
Set 1: 12 Reps x 30% 1RM
(Rest for 90 seconds)

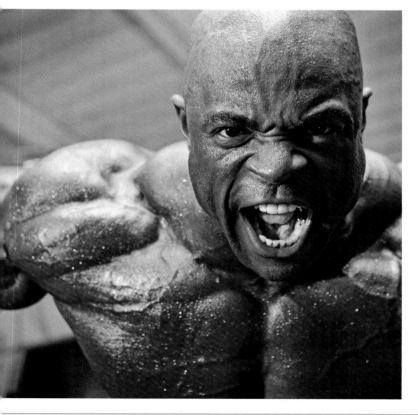

Photo by Paul Buceta
Model Ed Nunn

No one said adding substantial mass was easy!

Set 2: 6 Reps x 60% 1RM
(Rest for 90 seconds)
Gain Factor Sets
Set 1: 6 Reps x 85% 1RM + 30 pounds.
(Rest for 60 seconds)
Set 2: 8 Reps x 80% 1RM + 30 pounds.
(Rest for 60 seconds)
Set 3: 10 Reps x 75% 1RM + 30 pounds.
(Rest for five minutes)

2. Incline Bench Barbell Press
Specific Warm-Up
Set 1: 12 Reps x 30% 1RM
(Rest for 90 seconds)
Set 2: 6 Reps x 60% 1RM
(Rest for 90 seconds)
Gain Factor Sets
Set 1: 6 Reps x 85% 1RM + 10 pounds.
(Rest for 60 seconds)
Set 2: 8 Reps x 80% 1RM + 10 pounds.
(Rest for 60 seconds)
Set 3: 10 Reps x 75% 1RM + 10 pounds.
(Rest for three minutes)

3. Barbell Shrug
Specific Warm-Up
Set 1: 10 Reps x 50% 1RM
(Rest for 90 seconds)
Gain Factor Sets
Set 1: 6 Reps x 85% 1RM + 30 pounds.
(Rest for 60 seconds)
Set 2: 8 Reps x 80% 1RM + 30 pounds.
(Rest for 60 seconds)
Set 3: 10 Reps x 75% 1RM + 30 pounds.

WEEK 4, DAY 3
General Warm-Up: Five minutes on an exercise bike or other cardio machine, walking fast or active stretching.

1. Barbell Back Squat – Narrow Stance
Specific Warm-Up
Set 1: 12 Reps x 30% 1RM
(Rest for 90 seconds)
Set 2: 6 Reps x 60% 1RM
(Rest for 90 seconds)
Gain Factor Sets
Set 1: 6 Reps x 85% 1RM + 30 pounds.
(Rest for 60 seconds)

Set 2: 8 Reps x 80% 1RM + 30 pounds.
(Rest for 60 seconds)

Set 3: 10 Reps x 75% 1RM + 30 pounds.
(Rest for three minutes)

2. Standing Overhead Barbell Press
Specific Warm-Up

Set 1: 12 Reps x 30% 1RM
(Rest for 90 seconds)

Set 2: 6 Reps x 60% 1RM
(Rest for 90 seconds)

Gain Factor Sets

Set 1: 6 Reps x 85% 1RM + 15 pounds.
(Rest for 60 seconds)

Set 2: 8 Reps x 80% 1RM + 15 pounds.
(Rest for 60 seconds)

Set 3: 10 Reps x 75% 1RM + 15 pounds.
(Rest for three minutes)

3. Barbell Plate Front Raise
Gain Factor Sets

Set 1: 16 Reps (Rest for 60 seconds)
Set 2: 16 Reps (Rest for 60 seconds)
Set 3: 16 Reps (Rest for 60 seconds)

TRAINING NOTES

1. Don't do any exercises for the full week before beginning this 30-day program.
2. Train for three non-consecutive days per week.
3. All poundage percentages are based on an unfatigued one-rep maximum.
4. If you can't perform the barbell back squat, replace it with the leg press.

THE GET-BIG DRINK

This drink contains approximately 3,000 calories and 200 grams of protein that's sure to assist you in your goal of getting massive. Mix one to two cups of weight gain protein powder with two quarts of whole milk and two cups of skim milk powder. Then, add two whole eggs and four tablespoons of natural peanut butter and half a brick of natural ice cream (choose your own flavor). Also add one medium banana, four tablespoons of melted milk powder and six tablespoons of corn syrup. Pour the mixture into pitchers and drink 10 glasses per day. It may sound like a lot, but it's what you need.

POWER BODYBUILDING TECHNIQUES

Q) *In the '90s, I attended a shape-training seminar that Robert Kennedy conducted at the Solid Sweat Gym in Berkeley, California. It remains one of the most information-packed seminars I've ever had the privilege of attending. The comment with regard to thinking in terms of shaping muscles rather than seeing how much weight you can handle was indeed most insightful.*

Shape training has helped me to become a contest-winning bodybuilder, but after the competitive season is over I'd like to train for an upcoming powerlifting meet. I understand that the three big lifts are the squat, bench press and deadlift. What would be the best way to switch gears from shape training to a power-training program?

A) To begin with, you'll want to make your training conditions the least complicated as possible. Wear a lifting belt and supportive lifting shoes. For the time being, stay away from wearing any power gear such as lifting suits and knee wraps. Make use of a conventional exercise bar as opposed to an Olympic bar. Here are comparisons of the two types of training for each of the big lifts.

SHAPE-TRAINING BARBELL SQUAT

Place the bar high on your trapezius. Your foot placement should be slightly less than shoulder-width apart. Your upper torso should remain erect or as near a vertical plane as possible during the descent to just below parallel. Keep your glutes in alignment with your body. Your knees should travel over the instep of your foot.

POWER-STYLE BARBELL SQUAT

Place the bar low on your trapezius – an inch or so lower than the top of your deltoid. Your feet should be at least shoulder-width apart or in some cases, even wider. Your upper torso should be arched, but you can allow it to bend forward from vertical during the descent phase of the squatting movement. Have your glutes drift back, and keep your lower leg perpendicular to the floor from the knee down. The power squat obtains maximum leverages and strength output from your hip, quad and lower back.

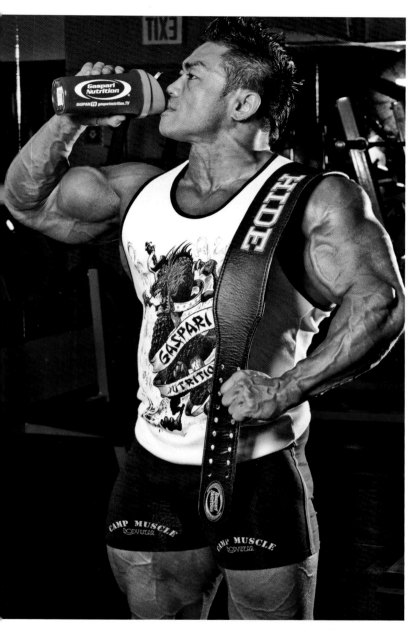

Photo by Paul Buceta
Model Hidetada Yamagishi

Pre- and post-workout protein shakes are crucial to fuel your body and muscle tissue.

SHAPE-TRAINING BENCH PRESS

Lying on a flat bench, cross your lower legs and draw them up so your thighs form a 90-degree angle to your upper body. Take a wide hand spacing (36 inches between your index fingers). Take a deep breath, unrack the barbell and, with your elbows and upper arms directly in line under the bar (or in line with your shoulder joint), lower the bar slowly to the lower neck or cla-vicular area. Pause for two seconds. Press the bar back up, directly in alignment with your sternum-clavicle area.

POWER-STYLE BENCH PRESS

On the power style bench press, plant your feet firmly on the floor rather than having them off the floor. Arch your back as much as possible while lifting, keeping your head, shoulders and glutes in contact with the bench surface. Inhale and lower the bar to your chest, about a half an inch below your nipples. This shouldn't take any more than two seconds. Your upper arms should be flared out. Press to lockout. On your last set of benches, and in the final three reps, pause with the weight on your chest for 10 sec-onds on the first rep. In the second set, pause for five seconds, and pause for three seconds in the third rep.

MODIFIED (STIFF-LEG) DEADLIFT

Perform this exercise while standing on a se-cure platform that's high enough that the bar touches the instep of your foot. With just a very slight bend of your knee joint, and while keep-ing your back arched (never rounded), pivot at your hip joint as you pull the bar upward to lock-out. Lower and repeat.

POWER-STYLE DEADLIFT

In this variation of the deadlift you will not use a platform. Use as much knee bend as neces-sary to allow you to perform your lift. On the final rep of your last set, hold the lockout posi-tion for five seconds. Gradually work up to 20 seconds. In other sessions, rather than holding the barbell and locking out, simply lower the bar to within four inches of the floor and hold this static position for a five-second count.

During the power bodybuilding phase of your training, make use of a lifting suit, belt and wraps. The pause methods in the bench press and squat should never be used for more than one workout per week and for no more than four to six weeks. The shape training exercise reps should be done at a slow (even super-slow) to moderate speed in order to produce strength and cosmetic development of the muscle. On the other hand, reps should be done explosively to recruit as many white fast-twitch muscle fibers as possible. Unless you're doing pauses, use the touch-and-go method (absolutely no pauses) to recruit a stretch reflex for explosiveness. How soon you switch from one type of training to another is strictly up to you.

DEADLIFTING DOWNHILL

Q) *A few weeks ago I found an old book in the library entitled* Hepburn's Law. *The deadlift program it offered looked interesting so I thought I'd give it a shot.*

This program is really tough! The first workout I warmed up with four sets of eight reps in the deadlift and then did three big ones. With the same weight, I then did seven sets of two reps. After these, I dropped the pounds to something I can perform for six mind-blowing reps. I did the first set for six reps, the second set for five reps and then a third, fourth and fifth set for four reps each and a sixth set for three reps. Finally I do a pump-out set with a weight I can handle for 10 reps. That's my first workout. The workouts stay pretty similar but I increase weight. I'm into my eighth workout today. I'm only doing this deadlift program twice a week.

I end up with my head hitting the pillow for nine to ten hours every night. This program really takes a lot out of me. Don't get me wrong – I like to work hard. I want to keep up with the program but do you have any advice to make it seem a little easier, especially when I get to my eighth workout and I am doing eight sets of three reps?

A) We're well aware of the strength programs that Doug Hepburn, the former world's strongest man, once used. They're brutally hard. Let's see if we can help you solve your problem. Would you agree that it's much easier to move an object downhill than to move it uphill?

To lift an object, in your case a very heavy barbell, you must defy gravity. It's easier to lift a heavy weight if you're in the center of gravity. In a squatting movement, where the bar is on the back of your neck and head, you can put yourself into the center of gravity quite simply by wearing squatting shoes with a minimum heel height of three-quarter inches or as much

as one-and-a-half inches. You must do the exact opposite with the deadlift – your toes should be higher than your heels. Place a two-foot-long two-by-four under the front of your feet. This puts you in a position to pull backwards, with the end result being that it gives you the feeling of deadlifting downhill.

MICRO-BURST CHEST WORKOUT

Q) *I'm going to be working on an oil rig for the next three months and the only workout equipment is a lousy 100-pound barbell and a pathetic flat exercise bench. I like doing big bench presses (225 pounds for eight reps), but that's going to go to hell with nothing more than a stupid 100-pound barbell. What would you do if you were me?*

A) What would we do if we were you? We'd go stick our head in a bucket of water and take 10 deep breaths. Like Martin Burney said in the movie, *Sleeping with the Enemy,* "Think!" Since you're obviously not thinking, here's what you can do with that so-called worthless 100-pound barbell. In the next three

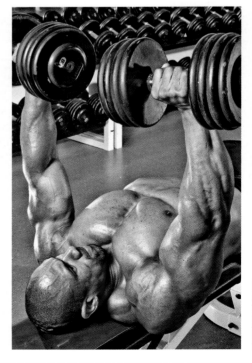

Photo by Paul Buceta
Model Marlon John

Even with limited equipment, you can still piece together a challenging and effective workout.

months (and twice per week on non-consecutive days) do flat barbell bench presses with the 100 pounds for no more than two sets. Do as many reps as possible. Always try to do more than you did in your last workout! In other words, don't settle for less than at least one additional rep in each set per workout. You should then rest for two to three minutes between the first and second set. Upon completion of the second set, strip the bar completely of all poundage and position it securely on the floor. Use some type of wedge on either side of the collars to keep the bar from moving.

Get into a regular push-up position and grasp the bar with your regular bench press hand spacing. Then do one or two sets of the bodyweight-only exercise for as many reps as possible. Follow the instructions given for the barbell bench press. Do as many reps as possible on each set and try to add one additional rep to each set in each workout. Put your feet up on the bench for even more resistance.

You'll experience a tremendous pump from this micro-burst chest workout. Even better, at the end of the three months you'll retain most of the previous gain factor of your 225 pounds for eight reps and you may even see an increase in poundage or reps.

BUILDING BARNDOOR LATS

Q) *Recently, my workout partner and I decided we wanted to develop more width to our lats, so we started a high-intensity lat cycle. The lat program consists of four lat exercises performed one after another without any rest whatsoever. We began with behind-the-neck pull-ups using an overhand grip on the bar. Our hand spacing was about 12 inches wider than our shoulders. Our goal was to perform 12 reps.*

Next we did bent-over rows with a curl grip. Our hands were spaced four inches apart at the center of the bar. We did 12 reps. After that, we did barbell bent-arm pullovers with our hands spaced 12 inches apart. Once again our goal was 12 reps. Our final exercise was a negative-only chin-up with a normal underhand shoulder-width grip. We tried to do 12 very slow reps and when we were able to do more than 12, we'd hook a 25-pound dumbbell on our chin/dip belt.

The program worked pretty well for my partner, but I had a problem with getting any type of a pumped feeling or muscle contraction in the behind-the-neck pull-up. Do you think it's a leverage problem or is it neuromuscular efficiency? I would appreciate any advice you can send my way.

A) The main problem with the behind-the-neck pull-ups (or most chinning type movements) is that they're only half movements. In your case, you are getting only a 60-degree range of movement out of the behind-the-neck pull-ups and even less if you take a wider grip. The last exercise you mentioned is probably a little better because you can get approximately 120 degrees range of movement. Half pull-ups or chins don't produce maximum results.

Drop the program you're doing and begin performing pull-ups to your chest or sternum area. Don't take much more than a shoulder-width grip. Arch your back while pulling yourself up – an absolute must because it forces your lats to pull down and back.

If your chest is concave and your back is rounded (as they are when doing behind-the-neck pull-ups) you'll end up working your pecs and teres major – not your lats. Your upper arms (triceps) should be touching the sides of your outer lats and your elbows should be pulled back to your sides. Now you should be touching your high arched chest below the low pec line to the bar. Lower yourself very slowly and touch your feet to the floor after each rep.

Actually strive to take the entire weight of your body on your feet. Spring up and touch your chest to the bar again and again. Having your feet on the floor and springing up will help you in the beginning when you can't pull high enough. Later on as you become more efficient at this exercise, stop allowing your feet to touch the floor. This exercise is the best for getting a full muscle contraction in your lats.

ARM-A-GETTIN'

Q) *Hello Mr. Weis and Mr. Kennedy. Are the arms the easiest or hardest part of the physique to develop? Does a person's bodyweight determine arm growth? Do you think small wrists* *interfere with building large arms? Finally, does arm size and strength have a bearing on how successfully you're able to train the other muscle groups in your body? Thanks for your help.*

Packing on size, increasing strength and carving shape into your biceps in quite attainable with the right strategies.

A) Building muscle, especially arm size and strength, isn't as complex or mysterious as one might think. Arms are second only to chest in responsiveness. Furthermore in over 90 years in the iron game it's been our obser-

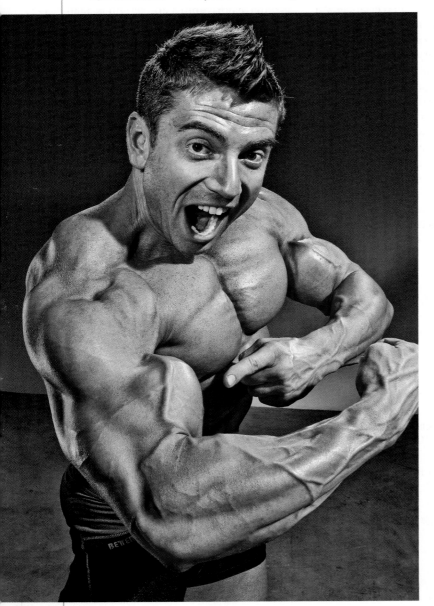

vation that most bodybuilders, from rookies to advanced levels, devote approximately 75 percent of their training efforts to pecs, arms and lats, while their delts, quads and abs receive only 20 percent and their forearms and calves receive a paltry 3.5 percent. Even more sadly, the lower back and neck come up dead last, receiving only 1.5 percent of a bodybuilder's training effort.

Your bodyweight does help determine arm growth. If you're in good shape and have low bodyfat, you must add more overall bodyweight in order to elicit a spurt in arm growth. There's no doubt that you can gain a bit of size through direct arm training, but the most meaningful gains in arm development will come from a gain in overall bodyweight, something that's accomplished most efficiently by including a compound exercise for each of the major and minor muscle groups of your body. Just a 10-pound gain in overall bodyweight can ignite a one-inch gain in arm size.

Small wrists don't interfere with molding massive arms! We've known of many natural bodybuilders who've had average to small wrists and made insane arm-size gains.

Finally, there's a definite relationship between arm development and strength to total body development. If your arms are lacking in strength (which is related to size), you simply won't be able to perform heavy barbell rowing, deadlifts or shrugging movements using maximal poundage.

HERCULEAN ARMS IN 10 MINUTES

Q) *I just found out that I'll be doing some 14-hour shifts for the next couple of weeks. Not only that, but I'll have to commute to work an hour each way. What this means is that I'm not going to have time to get in a decent workout and I'm worried!*

I know you guys are going to think I'm just training a favorite muscle group when I tell you this, but my biceps and triceps are sadly lacking behind the rest of my development. What I desperately need is an extra-quick arm routine. Anything you guys might have up your sleeves would be greatly appreciated.

Photo by Robert Reiff
Model Binais Begovic

A) Origins and insertions of the tendon muscle attachments can dictate the relative efficiency of the muscle group and its ultimate growth potential. A more common reason for muscle unresponsiveness is that many bodybuilders don't train the lagging muscle with the same intensity (as a result of the lack of response), all while upping the intensity on other muscles that are showing more distinct improvement almost daily.

It's always a good idea to reevaluate your current and past training programs. Analyze the number of sets, reps and variety of exercises you've done. The training frequency is also important. As well, it's a good idea to reflect on the type of daily activities you were doing in addition to your arm training both when there was growth and when there wasn't. You may have been overtraining your arms through your daily practices. A good muscle-building diet is also important, as is sleep. Getting eight to ten hours each day is important to muscle growth, but for the time being that's out of the question given your 14-hour shifts and daily commute.

Because time is your primary concern we suggest that you superset one-arm dumbbell leaning curls and dips on the parallel bars for 10 quick sets. Use the routine below three times per week and do it for at least one month.

We'll assume that this program will be the only training you'll have the time or energy to do during your two weeks of 14-hour shifts. However, when you go back to your regular workout programs after this two-week stint, you should do the 10 supersets at the conclusion of your workout. Do this arm routine only, with no other arm work thrown in. Be sure to up your intake of first-class proteins at a rate of one gram per pound of lean muscle mass. The program goes like this:

1. Three sets of eight to ten reps.
2. Increase poundages.
3. Two sets of five to seven reps.
4. Increase poundages.
5. Five sets of three to five reps.

There you have it. A few points worth remembering: Do the rep scheme stated for both the curls and the dips as a superset. Do each exercise with absolutely no rest other than the time it takes to change the poundage requirements. Due to the intensity of the program, you may need to decrease the poundage at some point within the final five supersets. On the tenth superset, decrease the poundage and do 15 to 20 reps on each exercise for the ultimate maximum pump. In the parallel bar dips, this may mean just doing them with your bodyweight only.

You may have other exercises in mind that are far more effective than the two suggested. If that's the case, use them. The choice is yours. Just be sure all your equipment is set up and ready to go before your workout. Then experience the ultimate journey into Herculean arm development in only 10 minutes!

THE HARDGAINER

Q) *Can you guys help me with my weight. I'm 5 feet 8 inches and have a small bone structure. I've been taking some of the weight-gain formulas that are on the market, but none of them seem to do me much good, even though they seem to help other members of the gym where I train. I weigh 140 pounds and I'm unable to gain any more weight. What should I do?*

A) Have you given some of the muscle-gaining programs featured in issues of *MuscleMag* a fair shake? In other words, have you tried one of the programs for at least six weeks to see whether it can help you? Most weight-gaining programs will make some bodybuilders gain fast, but there are some who find it very difficult to gain weight. They have to be more patient and continue on the program somewhat longer. Although small bones will prevent you from becoming a superheavyweight, it shouldn't prevent you from gradually gaining 10, 20 or 30 pounds of solid muscle.

To gain muscular bodyweight you have to train hard, rest hard and eat hard. In other words, you have to work hard in the gym but not overtrain, do as little physical activity as possible when you're not training, get lots of sleep and lots of food. Eat a well-balanced diet that contains plenty of protein, and be sure to supplement your diet with one or two protein shake meals. A fine weight-gain shake can be made with one cup of milk, a half cup of cream, one tablespoon of wheat germ, one banana, a couple of tablespoons of natural peanut butter and a scoop of whey protein. Throw in a scoop of ice cream if you like.

CONTINUOUS GAINS

Q) *I think I've found the perfect solution for bodybuilders looking to making continuous gains in size and strength. What if I combine the components of Leo Costa Jr.'s Titan Training System, Larry Scott's Bio Phase Feedback system, Iron Man's Positions of Flexion and Mike Mentzer's Heavy Duty approach to training?*

It's really exciting to think about the unlimited possibilities of making continued gains in bodybuilding literally nonstop. What do you think about this sensational new brainstorm in training? I can't wait for your comments.

A) Most of the training systems, techniques, principles and exercises in use today are well over 50 years old and in some cases hundreds of years old. Of course, there are many new pieces of training equipment giving bodybuilders the opportunity to work muscles with greater variety. However, if you read a book on kinesiology, you'll learn the function of how muscles work and realize that the training systems you mentioned in your letter approximates that function. We've always been of the opinion that recommending a certain number of exercises, sets and reps for most bodybuilders is generalizing.

Once past the beginner's stage, each bodybuilder presents an entirely different challenge. What suits you might not suit another. All of the training systems you mentioned are terrific contributions to the ongoing evolution of bodybuilding and it will be up to you to find out what suits you best and which exercises, sets and rep combinations bring you the best gains. No bodybuilder experiences continuous gains, although you can figure out ways to make gains come as steadily as possible. Every bodybuilder could form a graph of gains, with a quick start, slow rises, a leveling off, a slight drop, a small gain, another leveling off and so on.

SECRETS OF CHAMPIONS

Q) *I read all the bodybuilding magazines and try many of the super-intense training techniques that are published hoping that they'll quickly add mass. I've tried everything for the past two years and my gains have literally been nothing. You want to know what I think? I think the muscle magazines are keeping the secrets the champion bodybuilders really use to build muscle mass. What's the real secret of building muscle?*

A) If you're merely associating muscles with champion bodybuilders, you've overlooked, ignored or missed something else that these champions all have in abundance. It's called mind power. Their tremendous energy, willpower, concentration and determined mind directs their every physical effort when in the gym. The might of the mind is their secret training tool to achieving behemoth bulk, power, size and strength. The champions don't sap their energy or demoralize their being with the thought of failure. Rather they have sublime self confidence and calm poise. They know they'll complete the set of curls if it kills them, and the end result will be awesome rock-hard biceps. They have the will to succeed and you can see it. They give it everything they've got, and then some.

You can't overlook the power of the mind when it comes to your training. It seems invincible and it is. When a champion releases this giant power it seems to accomplish results in only a few minutes that would ordinarily take weeks of hard training for the rest of us to achieve. Concentrate intensively as you work out and avoid having your mind wander. Force yourself into every set and it can't help but shorten your path to attaining your goal.

That's the secret. But you also have to stick with a program for a while before you can see whether or not it works. If you've tried every program you've read about in the last two years then what did you do, spend one workout on each program? Give a program at least four weeks and up to six weeks before switching to another. You can bet these pro bodybuilders you're looking at didn't switch their programs around every time they went to the gym.

THE PROS AND CONS OF MACHINES

Q) *I've read most of your articles and books and I notice that the routines you guys write about have pretty much always stressed the use of compound, multi-joint exercises and free weights. Why did all these machines spring up if free weights are so much more versatile and effective? What are the pros and cons of the strength-training machines that you see in today's health clubs?*

A) We've been acquainted with bodybuilders who have used machines exclusively for three months, doing heavy negatives and the associated training principles. Some mighty impressive poundages were hoisted using these machines, but upon a return to using free weights only, these bodybuilders found strength losses of between 10 and 20 percent. The reality is that free weights involve the little nuances of timing, balance and coordination – something machines don't offer.

Most machines are primarily mono-planar devices, meaning there's only one path a given movement can take. If you had a dollar for every time a person brags that he can bench press 325 pounds (on a machine) and when challenged can barely lift 225 with a free barbell, you'd be rich.

Machines are excellent for select rehab situations and for some specific exercises difficult to do with free weights, such as leg curls and leg extensions. Cables, too, are very useful in a

No matter what your school of thought, there are upsides and downsides to machines.

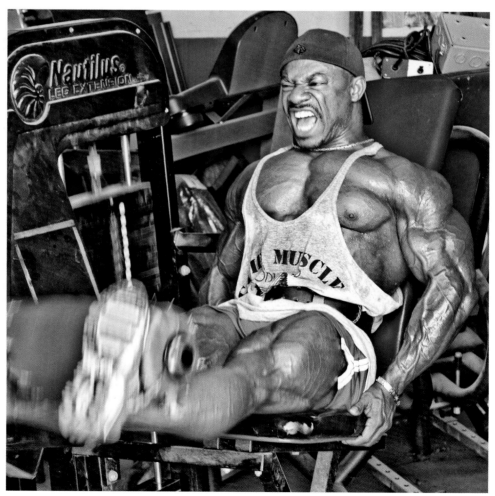

Photo by Paul Buceta
Model Richard "Tricky" Jackson

weight-training program. Machines are a valuable addition, but cannot be the core of a person's weight training in a multi-dimensional world. Use free weights about 80 percent of the time and machines for the remaining 20 percent.

PSYCHO WORKOUTS

Q) *What's the most unthinkable psycho workout you've ever personally experienced?*

A) The answer is Dennis B. Weis' Psycho Workout. I had to think about what you just asked me for about a half of a micro-second. The most psycho workout I've ever done was in the late 1980s at Monster Maker Gym in Inglewood, California. Under the direction of owner "Big" Jack O'Bleness, this gym had a reputation for creating a stable of natural drug-free contest-winning bodybuilders. An inner-circle joke about the Monster Maker Gym was that if you could survive one of Jack's sinister workouts, he would give you a body bag as a souvenir.

Welcome to my nightmare as I recall my adventure in that foreboding dungeon of a gym. Prior to the workout I remember saying to myself that there was nothing Jack could do to me that my bodybuilding mentor Donne Hale hadn't already done to me in the late '60s. Heck, I could still easily do 400 pounds in the barbell back squat rock bottom for 20 reps and the conventional barbell deadlift with 500 pounds for 10 reps.

I'm going to go into a bit of detail describing the workout, but it's been over 20 years since that adventure and my memory fails me as to the poundages and reps I used on most of the exercises with one exception. That exercise is the barbell clean and push-press. Before the workout "Big" Jack loaded an Olympic bar with a quarter on each side for a total of 105 pounds (including collars) and told me that's what I would be using for the barbell clean and push-press. I remember asking if that was some kind of joke weight? "I am the Yukon Hercules from Alaska for crying out loud," I said, and the only response I heard was diabolical laughter.

He told me not to worry, as the workout would last only 45 to 60 minutes. "Big" Jack then surprised me a little when he told me I would be doing the barbell clean and push-press between each cycle of a muscle group, as a means to stimulate my cardiovascular system. He added that I would be doing between 12 and 20 reps of this exercise. The mechanics suggest cleaning the barbell to the shoulders with as much leg action as necessary, starting the push with a drive of the legs by bending and then straightening them quickly, before finishing by pressing the barbell to straight arms' length overhead. In his sadistic way, he told me to be careful and not hyperventilate. That was so nice of him to tell me that. It's time to begin the workout, Monster Maker style.

First up, I had to do the barbell clean and push-press for 20 reps, then immediately without a rest it was on to some leg extensions before moving straight to the hack squats. That completed one cycle and it really was no big deal until Jack shouted for me to immediately begin a second and then third cycle.

"Big" Jack said there would be absolutely no rest between exercises because I was a famous bodybuilding writer and had better be in top-notch condition to complete a challenging workout. After this series of exercises was completed, Jack had me do the barbell clean and push-press for another 20 reps before moving on to some leg curls and standing calf raises for three cycles. I should mention that the rep ranges for the quad and hamstring exercises were somewhere between 5 and 25 reps while the calf exercise had a rep range of 15 to 40.

Next up was the barbell clean and push-press for 15 reps, and then on to barbell curls and triceps pressdowns for three cycles, rep ranges between five and twelve. That concluded the day of training Monster Maker style. Sure I had to fight through a brutal pain barrier as I pushed my body to the limit, but I have to say this had to be the most effective deep-muscle training I've ever endured.

I was breathing like a racehorse, taking three to six breaths between each rep of the barbell clean and push press. Believe me, that Olympic barbell I was using felt like it was loaded up with three big wheels (45 pounders) on each side instead of 25 pounders. The sweat poured off me in buckets as I struggled mightily with what I'd thought was a joke weight of 105 pounds for 15- to 20-rep sets. Four hundred pound dirt squats for 20 reps never felt that heavy!

You won't believe what Jack said after the workout. He invited me to come back in a couple of days for another Monster Maker workout, this time for my chest, back and shoulders using, of course, the barbell clean and push-press for 20 reps at the beginning of each cycle. I politely declined, explaining I had a return ticket to fly out of LAX to my hometown of Ketchikan, Alaska the next day. Thank God! Actually Jack O'Bleness is a dear friend of mine whom I wouldn't hesitate to go to every time my primary goal is to get into top-notch condition fast.

ROBERT KENNEDY'S PSYCHO SUPER-STRENGTH PROGRAM

Here is the honest but brutal six days per week psycho super-strength program developed by a Canadian, the late Doug Ivan Hepburn. Doug was the world's strongest man and the World Olympic Weightlifting Champion in 1953 without the use of any kind of anabolic steroids. Between 1950 and 1956, at a height of 5'9" and a bodyweight that fluctuated between 260 and 305 pounds (arms, 20 ¼"; chest, 55"; thighs, 30"), Doug did some incredible lifts that 99 percent of today's top lifters would be hard pressed to do. His top lifts during the 1950s looked like this:

DOUG HEPBURN'S TOP LIFTS

Squat: 760 lbs.

Bench Press: 580 lbs.

Deadlift: 700 lbs.

Barbell Curl: 260 lbs.

Dumbbell One-Hand Holdout: 120 lbs.

Right-Arm Press (37 reps): 120 lbs.

Two-Handed Dumbbell Press: 157 lbs. each

Barbell Press (10 reps): 300 lbs.

Kneeling Press: 320 lbs.

Press Behind Neck: 330 lbs.

Jerk Press: 460 lbs.

Two-Handed Dumbbell Crucifix: 110 lbs. each

The following is Doug Hepburn's super strength program. It has produced eye-opening second-to-none results for those who have dared to follow it:

MONDAY

Exercise 1 – Barbell Back Squat

Warm up with a weight that allows you five consecutive reps. After that, perform four single reps, increasing the poundage with each single repetition so on the fourth rep you are lifting a near-1RM poundage. Continue with the final poundage and strive to increase the number of repetitions by one rep only in each succeeding training session until a maximum of three single repetitions can be performed. Note: Don't attempt to perform more repetitions than advised, as this practice could cause staleness.

Exercise 2 – Conventional Barbell Deadlift

For the following exercises, you should do the same sets and repetitions as in the barbell back squat routine, but for the upper body your weight increases should be only five pounds.

Once you can manage the required number of reps, increase the warm-up and the four single repetitions by five to ten pounds and again strive for the required three single reps. After you've accomplished this, do it again.

When you've completed the above portion of the exercise routine, decrease the poundage to do five sets of three consecutive repetitions in the barbell back squat and conventional deadlift. Strive to increase the number of repetitions by one in each exercise and in each training session.

For example, assuming that you do the five sets of three consecutive reps, then in the following training period you should perform four consecutive repetitions in the first set and three in the remaining four sets. Then follow that up by performing five consecutive reps in the first set, four in the second set and three in each of the remaining three sets. The succeeding training session would require you to perform five consecutive repetitions in the first set, five in the second set and three in the remaining three sets. Continue in this manner until you can perform the required five sets of five consecutive repetitions and then increase the poundage and repeat from the process from the beginning. Note: The instructions regarding the number of sets and poundage increases should be applied to all exercises in each daily training routine. In the majority of cases, the poundage used in the heavy single repetitions and the sets of consecutive repetitions will increase proportionally.

As training progresses you'll encounter occasions when you fail to succeed with the required addition of single repetitions. It's normal and may not be staleness (overtraining). Proceed with the sets of consecutive repetitions. If you are still not improving, discontinue training until the following training period. If the stale condition persists in the following exercise sessions, take a week off. If even this fails to correct the stale condition, reduce all training poundages and perform the minimum number of repetitions. Note: When striving for a repetition gain you may take a second attempt. This is recommended when the failure was almost successful.

TUESDAY
Upper-Body Routine
Exercise 1 – Flat Bench Barbell Press
Exercise 2 – Barbell Curl

WEDNESDAY
Lower-Body Routine
Exercise 1 – Barbell Back Squat
Exercise 2 – Conventional Deadlift

THURSDAY
Upper-Body Routine
Exercise 1 – Press Overhead From
*   Squat Stands*
Exercise 2 –Barbell Curl

FRIDAY
Lower-Body Routine
Exercise 1 – Barbell Back Squat
Exercise 2 – Deadlift

SATURDAY
Upper-Body
Exercise 1 – Flat Bench Barbell Press
Exercise 2 – Barbell Curl

SUNDAY
Press Overhead From Squat Stands

This program is designed expressly for those in above-average physical condition and familiar with weight training. If you experience difficulty following this training routine, follow the preparatory exercise routine outlined for a period of six weeks before concentrating on the super-strength course. Use the same principle of poundage increment in the preparatory training routine, but perform five sets of five consecutive repetitions, increasing from a minimum of three to a maximum of five reps in the final set.

Use the following procedure when you have temporarily discontinued the heavy single repetitions because of staleness. Warm up with five consecutive reps in the normal manner then perform five sets of three consecutive repetitions, increasing the poundage each set so you are performing a maximum of two consecutive reps in the sixth set. Strive to increase the number of repetitions in the final set by one. When you can get three repetitions in the sixth or final set, increase the poundage in the warm-up and subsequent sets proportionally so again you can get no more than two reps in the last set. Then, repeat as outlined on Monday, Wednesday and Friday.

MONDAY
Exercise 1 – Flat Bench Barbell Press
Exercise 2 – Conventional Deadlift
Exercise 3 – Barbell Back Squat
Exercise 4 – Barbell Curl

WEDNESDAY
Exercise 1 – Overhead Barbell Press
*   From Stands*
Exercise 2 – Conventional Deadlift
Exercise 3 – Barbell Back Squat
Exercise 4 – Barbell Curl

FRIDAY
Exercise 1 – Flat Bench Barbell Press
Exercise 2 – Conventional Deadlift
Exercise 3 – Barbell Back Squat
Exercise 4 – Barbell Curl

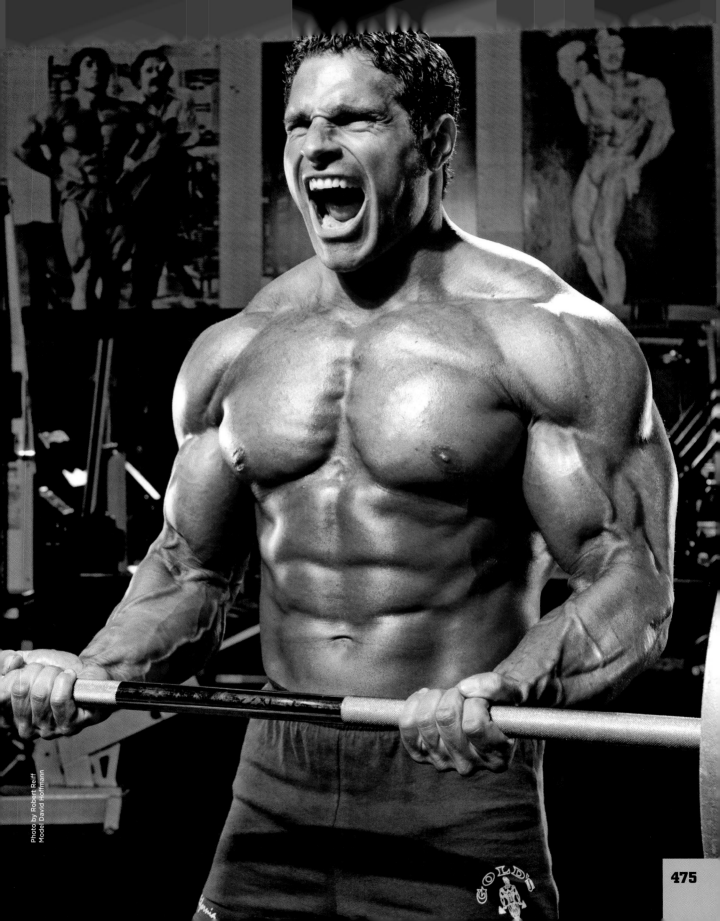

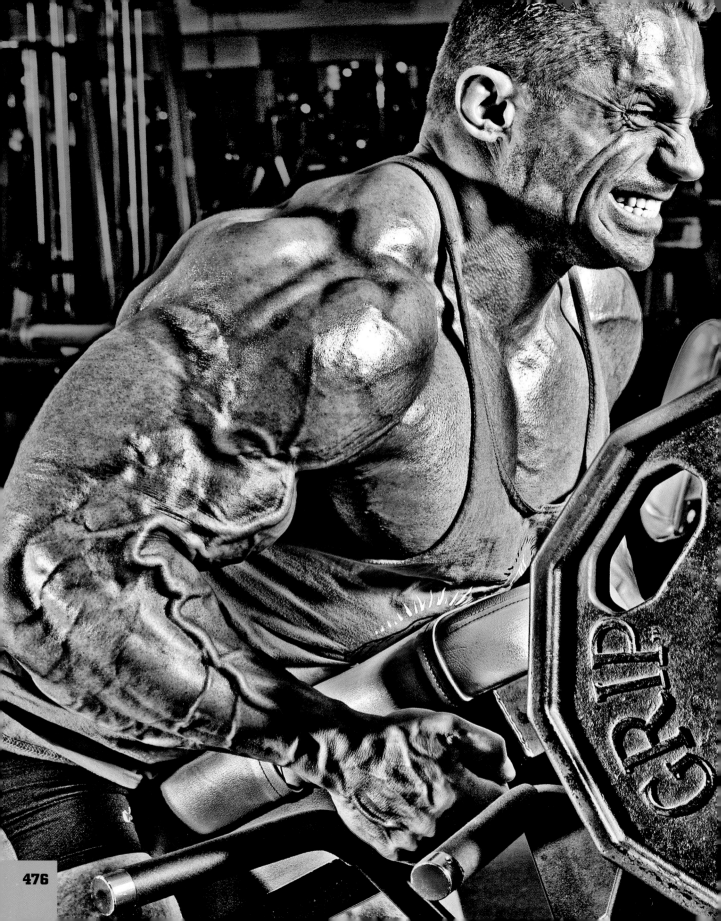

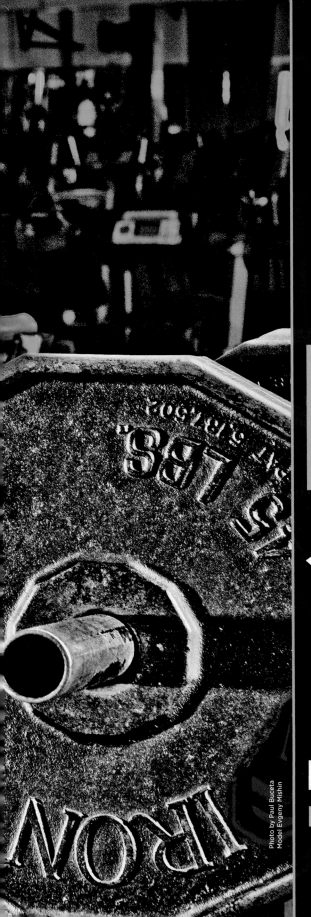

BOOK
15

Holistic Training Guide

CHAPTER 47

CHARTS AND FINAL COMMENTS

Huge & Freaky Muscle Mass and Strength *can* be *yours*.

The following is a collection of exercises and training guidelines that's sure to come in handy on your road to building huge and freaky muscle mass and strength in record time.

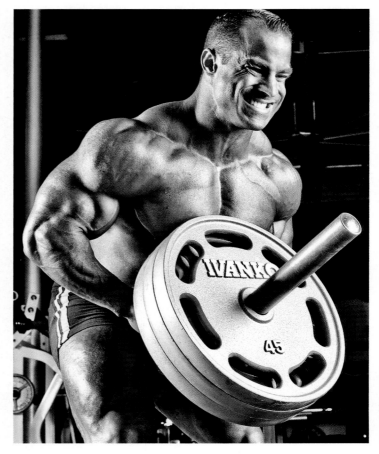

Photo by Ralph DeHaan
Model Mark Dugdale

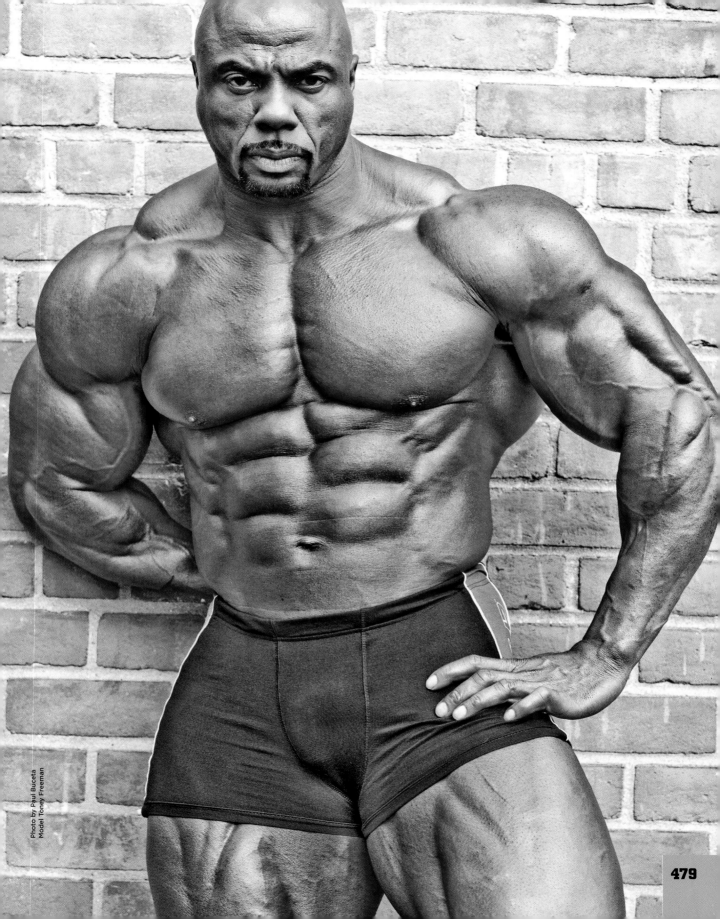

HOLISTIC EXERCISE SELECTION CHART

This chart will be helpful in determining which muscles you are working within a particular exercise, especially when your focus is on a lagging muscle group.

BODYPART(S)	GROUP 1 CORE GROWTH (COMPOUND) EXERCISES	GROUP 2 MUSCLE SPECIFIC (ISOLATION) EXERCISES	GROUP 3 TENDON STRENGTH EXERCISES

THIGHS General	• Power-Style Squat
	• Leg Press
	• Half Box Squat
	• Olympic-Style (High Bar) Squat
		• One-Leg Squat
		• Roman Chair Squat
		• Sissy Squats:
		  1. Bodyweight only
		  2. Add poundage
			• Power Rack:
			Barbell Back Squat
			  1. 1/8, 1/4, 1/2
			  2. Negatives
			  3. Isometric/Barbell-
			    timed holds.
			  4. Heavy supports

Quads	• Barbell Front Squat	• Leg Extension Two Legs/Single Leg Note: The above exercises can be performed in full range of motion with a timed static hold on the final rep. The reps can also be performed in non-lock style.	

Hams		• Leg Curl
		  Lying/Seated/
		  Standing
		• Dumbbell Leg Curl
		  Lying/Incline
		• Stiff-Leg Deadlift
		  3/5 mid-range	

Adductors (Inner Thighs)		• Ballet or Plie Squat
		  Wide stance with feet
		  rotated outward 45°
		• Cable Leg Squeeze
		  Inner thigh pull with
		  low-pulley cable
		• Isometric Inner-Thigh
		  Squeeze basketball
		  between knees
		• Adduction Machine
		  Inner thigh pull	

Adductors (Outer Thighs)		• Abduction Machine
		• Cable Abduction
		  Side leg lift
		• Abductor Machine
		  Outer-hip pull	

Sartorius		• Squats
		  Any variety of squats
		  make this muscle thick.	

Glutes		• One-Leg Kickback
		  1. Low-pulley cable
		  2. Ankle weights
		• Lunges
		  1. Barbell/Dumbbell
		  2. Smith Machine
		• Bench Step-Up
		  1. Barbell/Dumbbell	

HOLISTIC EXERCISE SELECTION CHART

This chart will be helpful in determining which muscles you are working within a particular exercise, especially when your focus is on a lagging muscle group.

BODYPART(S)	GROUP 1 CORE GROWTH (COMPOUND) EXERCISES	GROUP 2 MUSCLE SPECIFIC (ISOLATION) EXERCISES	GROUP 3 TENDON STRENGTH EXERCISES

BACK	• Bent-Over Row
	• Deadlift
	  1. Conventional Style
	  2. Sumo Style
	• Barbell Power Clean
	  Hang clean
		• Bent-Arm Pullover
		  EZ or straight bar
		• Straight-Arm
		  Cable Pulldown
			• Power Rack Pull

Traps	• Dead Hang
	• Clean
	• Snatch
	• High Pull
	• Wide-Grip Upright Row
		• Shrug
		  Barbell/Dumbbell
			• 1/4 Barbell Shrug
			  Works rhomboids

Lower Traps		• 45-Degree Bent-Over Barbell Shrug	

Upper Lats		• 45-Degree Lat Pulldown
		• Wide-Grip Lat Pulldown
		  Works long strand
		  of lat
		• Wide-Grip Pull-up
		  Palms forward
		  or parallel
		• Long T-Bar
		  Leverage Row
		• Alternating
		  Dumbbell Row
		• One-Arm
		  Dumbbell Row	

Middle Lat		• Cable Row
		• Prone Dumbbell Row
		  On a 20-inch
		  high bench
		• Racing Dive Lat Pull	

Lower Lat	• Close-Grip
	  Pull-Up to Chest
	  (Sternum Pull-Up)
	• Close-Grip
	  Bent-Over Row
	  (Palms up and down)
		• Lat Pulldown
		  With a parallel grip	

Spinal Erectors	• Stiff-Leg Deadlift	• Hyperextension
		  30-inch high bench
		• Barbell Good Morning
		  Standing/Seated	

HOLISTIC EXERCISE SELECTION CHART

This chart will be helpful in determining which muscles you are working within a particular exercise, especially when your focus is on a lagging muscle group.

BODYPART(S)	GROUP 1 CORE GROWTH (COMPOUND) EXERCISES	GROUP 2 MUSCLE SPECIFIC (ISOLATION) EXERCISES	GROUP 3 TENDON STRENGTH EXERCISES
CHEST	• Flat Bench Press Barbell/Dumbbell	• Power-Twister • Pec-Deck • Expander Chest Pull	• 1/4 Benches • Negatives
Upper Pecs	• 40-Degree Incline Barbell Press to Neck	• Incline Dumbbell Flye • High-Pulley Cable Crossover	
Middle Pecs	• 20-Degree Barbell Press to Neck • Barbell or Dumbbell Bench Press	• Flat Bench Dumbbell Flye	
Lower Pecs	• Decline Barbell Press	• Decline Dumbbell Flye • Pec Dip • Low-Pulley Cable Crossover	
Ribcage		• Straight-Arm Pullover Barbell/Dumbbell with light weight. • Dumbbell Dislocates • Decline Pullover Barbell/one dumbbell only	
Serratus	• Overhead Barbell Press • Pullover	• Serratus Pull on Lat Machine	
Deltoids	• Overhead Press Barbell/Dumbbells • Seated or Standing Behind-the-Neck Press • Forward and Back Barbell Press Standing or seated		• Power Rack Work
Anterior (Front)	Influenced greatly by the above exercises and all pressing movements for the chest	• Standing Front Raise Barbell/Dumbbell • Supine Flat-Bench Front Raise Barbell/Dumbbell	
Lateral (Medial or Side)		• Dumbbell Lateral Raise Standing/Seated • Dumbbell L-Lateral Raise • Cable Lateral Raise Standing/Kneeling One or two-arm style • Cable Upright Row Shoulder-width grip	

Posterior (Rear)		• Bent-Over Lateral Raise
		  1. Bent over 90 degrees
		  2. Try expander cables
		 • Cable Lateral Raise Bent over 90 degrees
		 • Prone Lateral Raise Dumbbells on a 45-degree incline bench
		 • Prone Bench Dumbbell Raise to Rear	

HOLISTIC EXERCISE SELECTION CHART

This chart will be helpful in determining which muscles you are working within a particular exercise, especially when your focus is on a lagging muscle group.

BODYPART(S)	GROUP 1 CORE GROWTH (COMPOUND) EXERCISES	GROUP 2 MUSCLE SPECIFIC (ISOLATION) EXERCISES	GROUP 3 TENDON STRENGTH EXERCISES
BICEPS	• Heavy Barbell or Dumbbell Curl • Chin-Up Palms-facing grip	• Expander Cable Curl	• Cheat Barbell or Dumbbell Curl

High Biceps	• Chin-Up Palms facing 4″ grip	• Barbell or Dumbbell Spider Curl
		  1. On a vertical 90-degree side of a preacher bench
		  2. Seated Close-Grip (4-inch)
		• Bent-Over Barbell Curl
		• Concentration Curl	

Middle Biceps	• Kneeling Bench Curl • Seated Barbell Curl • Body Drag Curl	• Dumbbell Bench Curl • 45-Degree Incline Dumbbell Curl • Seated Dumbbell Curl	
Lower Biceps		• Preacher Bench Curl Barbell/Dumbbell • 25-degree Incline Dumbbell Curl • Dumbbell Hammer Curl Thumbs up	
TRICEPS		• Expander Cable Archer Movement	
Outer Triceps (Lateral)	• Barbell French Press Lying/Seated/Standing • Narrow-Grip (12-inch) Press to Neck	• One-Arm Extension Lying/Seated/Standing • Dumbbell Kickback One or two arms	
Inner Triceps (Long Head)	• Parallel Bar Dip • Bench Dip	• Triceps Pressdown	
Medial Head (Near Elbow)	• High-Pulley Cable Triceps Extension		
FOREARMS	• One-Hand Deadlift • Zottman Dumbbell Curl Pinch Grip	• Wrist Roller Movement • Squeeze Rubber Ball • Forearm Gripper Machine • Hand Grippers	
Flexors	• Barbell or Dumbbell Wrist Curl Palms up	• Decline Barbell Wrist Curl Palms up	
Extensors	• Barbell Reverse Curl	• Barbell Wrist Curl Palms down • Decline Barbell Wrist Curl Palms down • Expander Cable Reverse Curl • Barbell Preacher Reverse Curl	

HOLISTIC EXERCISE SELECTION CHART

This chart will be helpful in determining which muscles you are working within a particular exercise, especially when your focus is on a lagging muscle group.

BODYPART(S)	GROUP 1 CORE GROWTH (COMPOUND) EXERCISES	GROUP 2 MUSCLE SPECIFIC (ISOLATION) EXERCISES	GROUP 3 TENDON STRENGTH EXERCISES
ABDOMINALS Upper Abs		• 45-Degree Incline Sit-Up Weight behind head • Rope Crunch	
Middle Abs		• Crunch • Roman Chair Sit-Up To parallel only • Knee Pull-In	
Lower Abs		• Hanging Leg Raise • Lying Leg Raise • Reverse Crunch	
Obliques		• Twisting Leg Raise • Twisting Crunch • Side Jackknife	
CALVES	• Standing Calf Raise • Leg Press Toe Press	• One-Leg Heel Raise	
Upper Calves		• Donkey Calf Raise • Hack Machine Calf Raise	
Front Calves		• Tibialis Contraction	
Lower Calves	• Seated Calf Raise	• Calf Stretching	

NECK		• Various Neck Bridges
		   Initially bodyweight
		   exercises and advance
		   to barbell resistance
		• Neck Strap	

The rope crunch specifically targets the upper-ab region.

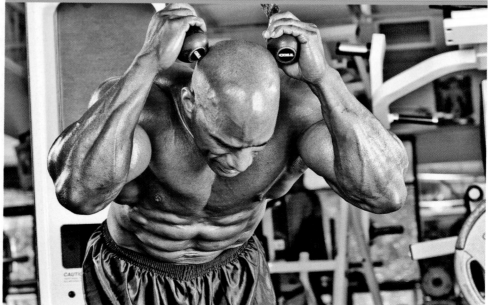

Photo by Jason Breeze
Model Darrem Charles

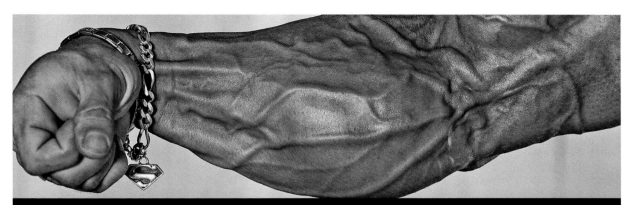

THE HOLISTIC TRAINING GUIDE

REQUIREMENTS	PHASE A: ENDURANCE	PHASE B: STRENGTH/ ENDURANCE	PHASE C: SIZE/STRENGTH	PHASE D: POWER
Workloads	60–78% of 1-rep max	80% of 1-rep max	84–88% of 1-rep max	88–92% of 1-rep max
Repetitions	15–30	8–12	6–8	3–5
Sets	2–6	3–4	3–5	3–4
SPEED OF EACH REP				
1. Positive (Up)	2 or 10 seconds	2 seconds	2 seconds	Explosive
2. Negative (Down)	4 seconds	4 seconds	4 seconds	2–4 seconds
Pause Between Reps	5–10 seconds or option: 1–2 seconds	1–2 seconds	1–2 seconds	1–2 seconds
REST BETWEEN SETS				
1. Core Growth (Compound) Exercise	1½–2 minutes	2–3 minutes	3–6 minutes	3–8 minutes
2. Muscle-Specific (Isolation) Exercise	1–1½ minutes	1–2 minutes		
3. Tendon Exercise			3–8 minutes	3–8 minutes
Rest Between Body-Part Workouts	Minimal	Minimal	Minimal	Minimal
REST DAYS BETWEEN MUSCLE GROUPS				
1. Thighs	Minimal	2–3 days	2–3 days	5 days
2. Lower Back	Minimal	2–3 days	2–3 days	5 days
3. Chest	Minimal	2–3 days	2–3 days	3–4 days
4. Latissimus	Minimal	2–3 days	2–3 days	
5. Trapezius	Minimal	2–3 days	2–3 days	
6. Deltoids	Minimal	2–3 days	2–3 days	
7. Biceps	Minimal	2–3 days	2–3 days	
8. Triceps	Minimal	2–3 days	2–3 days	
9. Forearms	Minimal	2 days or less	2 days or less	
10. Abdominals	Minimal	2 days or less	2 days or less	
11. Calves	Minimal	2 days or less	2 days or less	
12. Neck	Minimal	2 days or less	2 days or less	
EXERCISE PER MUSCLE GROUP				
1. Beginner	Optional	1 Compound exercise	Optional	None
2. Intermediate	Optional	1 Isolation exercise	1 Compound exercise	Optional
3. Advanced	Optional	2 Isolation exercises	1 Compound exercise	Optional

Photo by Irvin Gelb
Model Lee Priest

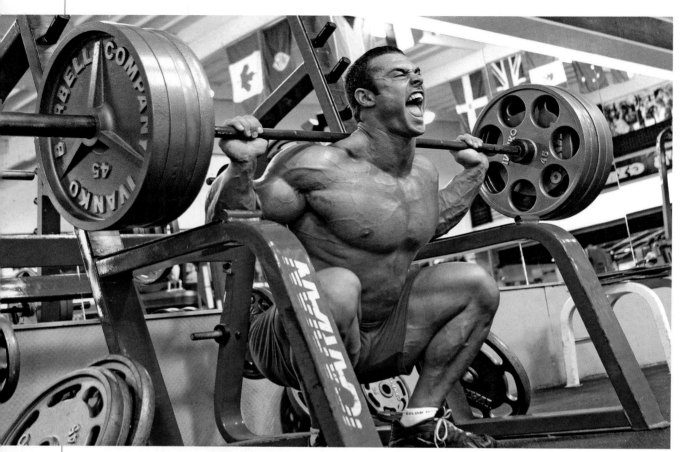

Regardless of your level of training experience, squats rank as the No. 1 single exercise.

FINAL COMMENTS

If you want to gain massive muscle mass, strength and overall better health, you'll only be able to accomplish this with an insatiable passion and will to learn everything there is to know about your body. You must gain knowledge and use it wisely. With that in mind, we conclude this book with 10 fundamental principles that will help you in your future bodybuilding training.

1. Strive to obtain a symmetrical and proportionate physique.
2. Squats are the most important single exercise for a beginner, intermediate or advanced bodybuilder.
3. Learn all you possibly can from the various bodybuilding magazines and journals, as well as the numerous books and courses pertaining to the subject.
4. Study and learn everything there is to know about nutrition and clean eating.
5. Talk to others who are devoted to the sport of bodybuilding.
6. Always stay informed on the new ideas and developments in the field.
7. Believe in yourself and your ability to succeed in bodybuilding.
8. Never rate yourself in comparison to others. Be the very best that you can be.
9. Strive to better your past performances and goals.
10. Don't make an excuse to miss a workout. Excuses are at the root of most bodybuilding (and other) failures.

Hopefully, the information we have provided you with in this book will aid you in the pursuit of muscular magnificence. And remember, to achieve such muscularity it must be a holistic effort – mind, body and spirit. Now go for it! We're behind you all the way.

Photo by Irvin Gelb
Model Frank McGrath

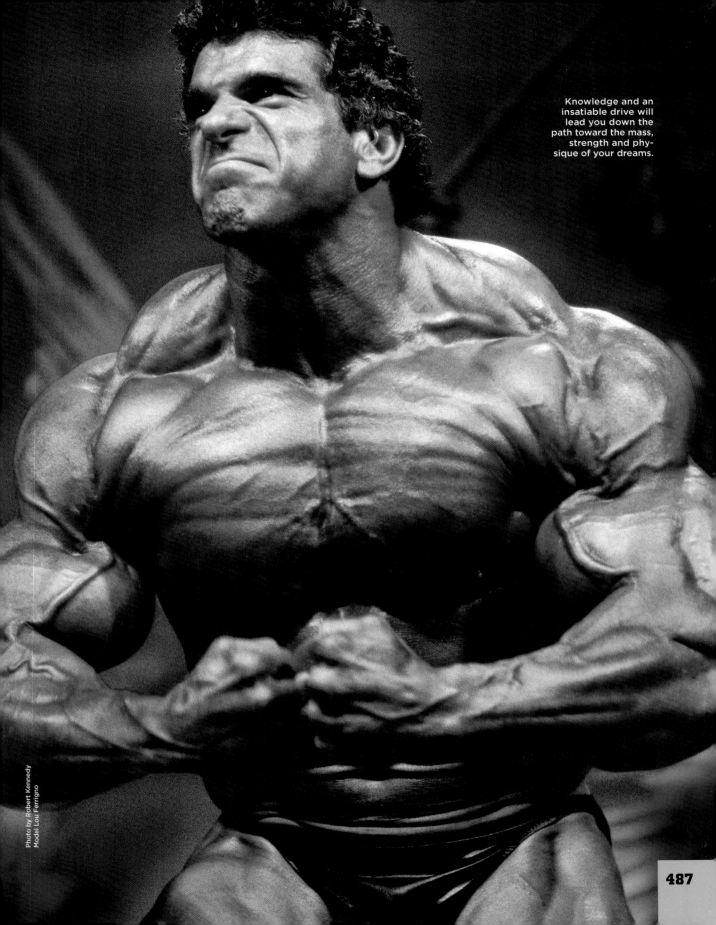

Knowledge and an insatiable drive will lead you down the path toward the mass, strength and physique of your dreams.

INDEX

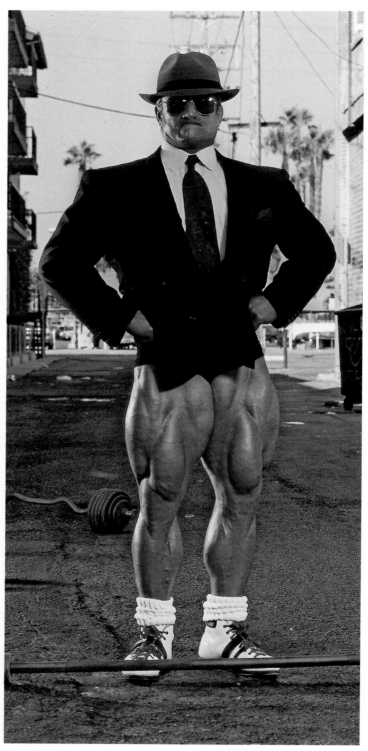

Model Tom Platz

A

B

C

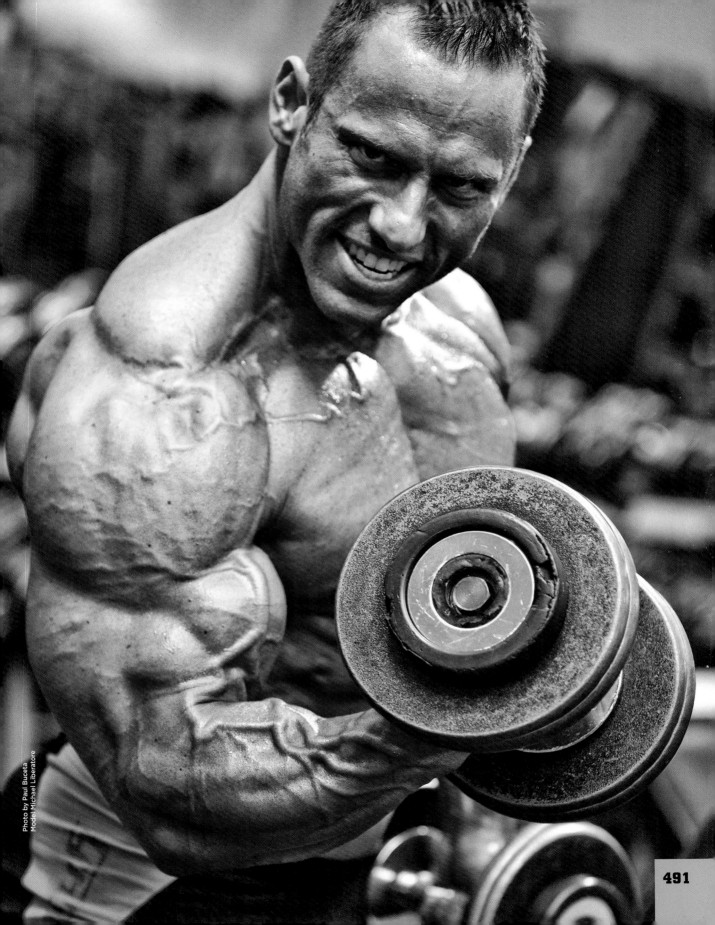

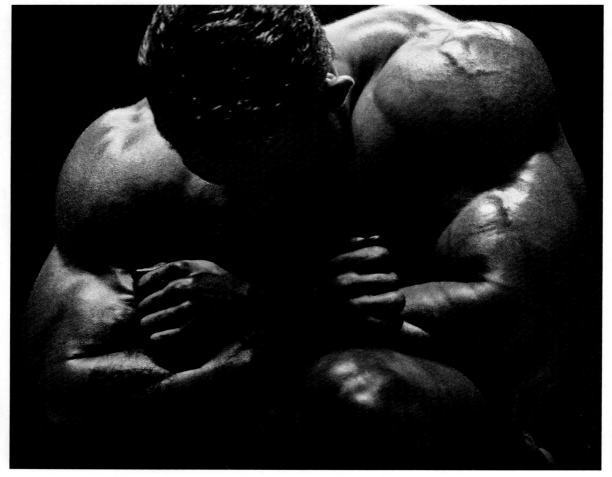

Model Dorian Yates

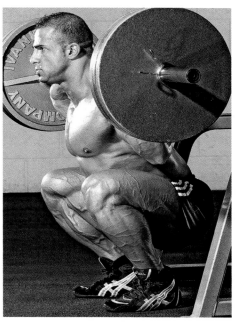